Innovative Therapies for Pancreatic Cancer

Pallavi Singh
Graphic Era University, India

Shiva Prasad Kollur
Amrita Vishwa Vidyapeetham, India

Raghavendra G. Amachawadi
Kansas State University, USA

IGI Global
Scientific Publishing
Publishing Tomorrow's Research Today

Vice President of Editorial	Melissa Wagner
Director of Acquisitions	Mikaela Felty
Director of Book Development	Jocelynn Hessler
Production Manager	Mike Brehm
Cover Design	Jose Rosado

Published in the United States of America by
IGI Global Scientific Publishing
701 East Chocolate Avenue
Hershey, PA, 17033, USA
Tel: 717-533-8845 | Fax: 717-533-7115
Website: https://www.igi-global.com E-mail: cust@igi-global.com

Library of Congress Cataloging-in-Publication Data

LCCN: 2025021838 (CIP Data Pending)
ISBN13: 9798337314693
Isbn13Softcover: 9798337314709
EISBN13: 9798337314716

British Cataloguing in Publication Data
A Cataloguing in Publication record for this book is available from the British Library.

Table of Contents

Detailed Table of Contents

Pancreatic cancer remains one of the deadliest malignancies due to late diagnosis, aggressive progression, and limited treatment efficacy. This chapter explores key molecular pathways—KRAS, Hedgehog, Notch, Wnt/β-catenin, TGF-β, JAK/STAT and their roles in tumorigenesis, progression, and resistance. It highlights recent pharmacological advances, including KRAS G12C inhibitors, SMO antagonists, gamma-secretase inhibitors, β-catenin and TGF-β receptor inhibitors. Multi-pathway targeting agents and synergistic strategies with chemotherapy, immunotherapy, and radiotherapy are discussed. Clinical trials and case studies illustrate improved outcomes and resistance management. Challenges such as tumor heterogeneity, toxicity, and lack of biomarkers are critically examined. Innovative solutions like advanced drug delivery, multi-omics, and AI-driven discovery are proposed. The chapter reviews the translational journey of pathway-targeting therapies and discusses emerging tools like liquid biopsies and ctDNA for treatment monitoring.

Pancreatic cancer is among the deadliest of all cancers in the world, for other contributors in addition to its late-stage diagnosis and poor prognosis and limited therapeutic efficacy are the high mortality rate concerning this type of cancer.

Recently, new findings from microbiome investigations point toward the mighty role of microorganisms in the initiation of pancreatic carcinogenesis and pancreatic tumors progression while also posing chronic challenges in treatment responsiveness. Traditionally believed to be free of all microbial life, the pancreas is now revealed to host an aberrant microbiome predominantly sourced from the gut and oral cavity, which inflicts large-scale modifications in its microenvironment. Current dysbiosis promotes chronic inflammation, immune evasion, and carcinogenesis. Several pathogenic species such as Helicobacter pylori, Porphyromonas gingivalis, and some members of Proteobacteria are rightly considered causative of increased pancreatic cancer risk through mechanisms that relate mainly to inflammation, immune suppression, and genotoxic metabolites. Together with that, the emergence of intratumoral bacteria is implicated in chemoresistance chiefly due to the bacterial cytosine deaminase-mediated degradation of gemcitabine. In addition, microbial effluents like Lipopolysaccharides (LPSs) and secondary bile acids would induce tumor-promoting NF-κB and TLR4 signaling. The emerging concept of the tumor microbiome also presents an avenue for novel therapeutic approaches.

Pancreatic cancer is one of the most fatal tumours, with few therapeutic choices and a low survival rate. This emerging dataset considers the microbiome an essential contributor to the genesis and pathogenesis of pancreatic cancer. The gut and tumor-associated microbiomes can influence pancreatic tumorigenesis primarily through immune regulation, inflammation, and metabolic pathways. Most importantly, dysbiosis, defined as microbial imbalance, has been associated with pancreatic cancer, opening up a potential avenue for prevention and treatment. Probiotic and prebiotic supplementation, faecal microbiota transplantation, and auditory species targeting are some intervention possibilities that can achieve modification of microbiomes for improving immune surveillance, constraining inflammation, and enhancing chemotherapeutics and immunotherapy responses. Furthermore, microbial profiling could be a diagnostic tool in identifying high-risk patients and predicting treatment outcomes. This chapter covers the following aspects: complex interaction between the microbiome and pancreatic cancer, and its application in possible preventive and therapeutic maneuvers against the disease being engineered in the future. New approaches to understanding pancreatic cancer therapy harness microbiota, but the final clinical promise will require further proof. Constraining certain bacteria may enhance the efficacy of traditional chemotherapies and modern immunotherapies such as immune checkpoint inhibitors. Microbial profiling might serve as a new and up-and-coming reliable non-invasive diagnostic tool to screen individuals at high risk for pancreatic cancer and predict therapy outcomes.

B. Lokeshwari, Department of Microbiology, Sacred Heart College, Tirupattur, India
M. Divya, Department of Microbiology, Sacred Heart College, Tirupattur, India
U. Subhalakshmi, Department of Microbiology, Sacred Heart College, Tirupattur, India
P. Prakathi, Department of Microbiology, Sacred Heart College, Tirupattur, India

Pancreatic Cancer (PC) has a five-year survival rate of fewer than 5% due to its late-stage diagnosis, poor prognosis, and significant resistance to traditional therapy. Nanotechnology has become a game-changer, providing novel medicinal and diagnostic approaches to address these issues. Since pancreatic tumours have extensive stromal barriers, this allows for precision targeting of cancer cells, reduces off-target effects, and improves drug delivery systems. In order to increase the effectiveness of treatment, nanoparticles, including metallic, lipid, and polymeric varieties, are essential. Gold, quantum dots, and superparamagnetic iron oxide are examples of nanoparticles that improve the sensitivity and specificity of early tumour detection in diagnostics. Advanced nanocarriers, like liposomes and polymeric nanoparticles, are used therapeutically to encapsulate RNA interference inhibitors and chemotherapeutic drugs (like gemcitabine and paclitaxel), enhancing their pharmacokinetics, stability, and bioavailability. When coupled to nanoparticles, targeting ligands like peptides and antibodies improve selectivity for cancer cells, and stimuli-responsive systems enable regulated drug release that is triggered by the tumour microenvironment (e.g., pH, enzymes). Key resistance mechanisms like as hypoimmunogenicity, stromal desmoplasia, altered drug transport, and cancer stem cell survival are also addressed by nanotechnology. Artificial intelligence also speeds up the design of nanoparticles, improves delivery, and makes customised treatment plans possible. Despite its potential, issues with stability, large-scale manufacturing, and possible toxicity need to be resolved in order to speed up clinical translation. With early diagnosis, focused therapy, and better treatment results, nanotechnology has the potential to completely transform PC management.

The neoplasm that develops in the pancreas is called pancreatic tissue cancer. According to recent research, the gut microbiota affects both the immune response and the effectiveness of treatment for PDAC. One tumor microenvironment that is extremely immunosuppressive is Pancreatic ductal adenocarcinoma (PDAC). By controlling both systemic and local immune responses, the microorganisms have a significant impact on oncogenesis, which in turn affects tumor growth and the effectiveness of treatment. The effectiveness of immunotherapy and chemotherapy may be impacted by the way some bacteria alter the activity of cytotoxic T cells and other immune components. Research indicates that the immune response can be shifted in favor of tumor suppression by modifying the microbiome through procedures like fecal microbiota transplantation. Modified immunological profiles have been connected to dysbiosis or imbalance in microbial populations, which could improve treatment results. The significance of microbial communities in cancer control is further highlighted by the fact that medications that deplete the microbiome can trigger anti-cancer immune responses. These discoveries open the door to novel treatments that target the microbiota to improve the effectiveness of pancreatic cancer treatment.

Pancreatic cancer is significant global issue due to high death rates, aggressive progression, and poor prognosis. The current treatments include surgical resection, chemotherapy, radiotherapy, and targeted therapies. Surgical resection offers the only potential for cure but is feasible in less than 20% of patients due to late-stage diagnosis. Chemotherapy regimens have improved survival modestly but are often limited by toxicity and chemoresistance. Radiotherapy is primarily used for local control in unresectable disease but has limited impact on overall survival. Targeted

Pancreatic cancer is one of the most aggressive and lethal malignancies, characterized by poor prognosis and limited therapeutic options. Despite advancements in surgical techniques and systemic therapies, the five-year survival rate remains dismal. Adjuvant has emerged as crucial components in the multidisciplinary treatment approach for pancreatic cancer, offering the potential to enhance therapeutic efficacy and improve patient outcomes. Adjuvants, substances that enhance the effects of primary therapies, play a pivotal role in the management of pancreatic cancer. These include Chemotherapy, Radiotherapy, Immunotherapy, and Targeted agents, Radiotherapy, often used as an Adjuvant to Systemic treatments, provides local control by targeting Residual cancer cells in the tumor bed. Additionally, advancements in Immunotherapy including Immune inhibitors and Cancer vaccines overcoming the Immune-suppressive tumor Microenvironment of Pancreatic Cancer. Targeted therapies, focusing on Mutations and DNA damage repair. Moreover, the integration of precision medicine and biomarker-driven approaches is refining the use of Adjuvants, enabling personalized treatment strategies. Challenges remain, including resistance to therapy, toxicity, and the heterogeneity of pancreatic tumors. In conclusion, adjuvants are integral to the contemporary management of pancreatic cancer, providing a pathway to improved survival and quality of life transforming the therapeutic application of this disease.

Pancreatic cancer remains one of the deadliest malignancies due to aggressive progression, early metastasis, and lack of reliable early detection. Advances in chemotherapy, targeted therapy, immunotherapy, nanomedicine, and organoid-based precision medicine offer hope. Neoadjuvant therapies have improved outcomes in

Preface

Pancreatic cancer is an extremely aggressive and challenging type of cancer, with a five-year survival rate of less than 10%. Effective therapy is difficult to achieve because this serious condition is often diagnosed at an advanced stage. Its biology is complex, and the tumors show resistance to standard radiation and chemotherapy. For a long time, the prognosis for pancreatic cancer has been poor due to the lack of effective treatments. However, recent advancements in therapies have brought new hope, and ongoing research is fostering a sense of optimism.

The book "Innovative Therapies for Pancreatic Cancer: Integrating Science, Treatment, and Hope" examines the novel approaches to treating this grave illness. This book will provide a understandable overview of the latest advances in treating pancreatic cancer, covering topics like immunotherapy, targeted therapies, gene editing, nanotechnology, and precision medicine. It also addresses the clinical, ethical, and personal dimensions of these innovative approaches, providing a well-rounded perspective on the progress and challenges in the field.

Central to this talk is the biology of pancreatic cancer. Different from numerous other cancers, pancreatic tumors usually possess a thick, fibrous stroma that restricts how well chemotherapy drugs can get and treat the cancer cells well. Also, the illness is fueled by changes in important genes like KRAS, TP53, and CDKN2A, which are hard to target and also cause the tumor to be very hard to treat. Since the tumor microenvironment is extremely immunosuppressive and actively prevents the cancer from being detected by the immune system, the immune system also has a difficult time fighting pancreatic cancer. Pancreatic cancer is very hard to treat due to these particular difficulties, but new scientific discoveries are to pass off these obstacles, giving patients new treatments and hope.

One of the most fascinating areas of pancreatic cancer research is immunotherapy, which aims to find and eradicate cancer cells by stimulating the body's immune system. Immunotherapies, such as immune checkpoint inhibitors, which have shown promise in treating other cancers like lung cancer and melanoma, are increasingly being considered for pancreatic cancer. However, because of their immunosuppressive milieu, pancreatic tumours have resisted these treatments. However, current studies are looking into how to boost the efficacy of checkpoint inhibitors by combining them with other therapies such radiation, chemotherapy, or targeted treatments. vaccinations for early-stage cancer that aim to improve the immune system's ability to target tumor-specific antigens show promise in their potential to overcome the immunological problems that typically prohibit immunotherapy from being a success in treating cancer.

Progress is also being made in the area of targeted therapy. These treatments function by obstructing particular chemicals or pathways that are essential for the growth and survival of cancer cells. Targeting the KRAS mutation, which is present in over 90% of instances of pancreatic cancer, has been a primary area of study. KRAS was thought to be "undruggable" until recently, however the discovery of KRAS G12C inhibitors has opened up new therapeutic options. These drugs work to prevent the mutated KRAS protein from encouraging the development of tumours. Treatments aimed at altering the tumor's vascular supply, preventing angiogenesis—the process by which tumours form new blood vessels—or obstructing. Examples of these targeted therapies include additional metabolic processes that support the development of cancer cells. As more of these medications go into clinical trials, customised therapy regimens are becoming a reality. Oncologists will be able to choose the optimum drugs as a result. According to the unique genetic profile of each patient. Also nanotechnology is showing great result in the treatment of pancreatic cancer.

The thick structure of the tumour makes it difficult for medications to reach cancer cells, but nanoparticles can be designed to do so more efficiently. More targeted drug delivery is made possible by nanomedicine, which reduces side effects and more therapeutic efficacy.

To increase the accuracy and effectiveness of these treatments, researchers are now looking into the possibility of mixing nanoparticles with radiation or chemotherapy. Furthermore, applying nanotechnology could enhance the ability to track the progress of real time monitoring of tumor response and progression.

Perhaps the most cutting-edge methods of treating pancreatic cancer are gene therapy and gene editing, and CRISPR-Cas9 and other technologies are leading the way in this revolution. These technologies make it possible to precisely alter genetic material, providing the potential to increase tumour cells' susceptibility to other treatments or to fix the mutations that cause pancreatic cancer. Theoretically, gene editing could change the genetic composition of a patient's cancer cells, increasing their receptivity to targeted medicines or perhaps stopping the cancer's resistance to existing therapies. Even though these technologies are currently in the experimental stage, they have the potential to transform pancreatic cancer treatment in the future and make the disease easier to control.

Precision healthcare, which involves tailoring treatment to an individual's genetic and molecular profile, is an essential part of the future of pancreatic cancer therapy. By sequencing tumor genomes and identifying specific mutations, clinicians can select the most appropriate treatments for each patient, offering a more personalized approach to care. This approach has already proven effective in other cancers, and ongoing research is showing that precision medicine may hold the key to overcoming the challenges of pancreatic cancer.

While these innovative therapies offer hope, there are significant hurdles to overcome. Access to these treatments is often limited by cost, geographic availability, and the availability of clinical trials. Moreover, the emotional and psychological toll of a pancreatic cancer diagnosis can add additional challenges, both for patients and their families. Despite these obstacles, the progress made in pancreatic cancer research in recent years has been remarkable, and the combination of immunotherapy, targeted therapies, gene therapy, and precision medicine offers unprecedented hope for the future.

Innovative Therapies for Pancreatic Cancer: Integrating Science, Treatment, and Hope willprovide readers with a comprehensive look at the cutting-edge therapies changing the landscape of pancreatic cancer treatment. Through a mix of scientific explanations, clinical trial data, patient stories, and expert insights, this book will educate and inspire patients, healthcare professionals, and anyone interested in the future of cancer care. By combining rigorous scientific research with the human experience of living with and treating pancreatic cancer, this book aims to offer both knowledge and hope, showing that with each new breakthrough, a cure may one day be within reach.

1. Educate patients and carers as the first target audience.

Give clear explanations of the newest therapies, including their working mechanisms. efficacy as well as possible side effects. Provide helpful advice for negotiating the complicated therapeutic environment, including alternatives for clinical trials and routine care.

2. Encourage Medical Professionals:

act as a resource to keep medical teams, nurses, and oncologists informed on the most recent developments in pancreatic cancer treatments. Provide case examples that illustrate the advantages and difficulties of using novel therapeutic strategies.

3. Encourage Scholars:

Describe the state of pancreatic cancer research today, considering advancements in gene editing, immunotherapy, CAR-T cell therapy, and precision medicine. Examine potential future paths with an emphasis on improving early pancreatic cancer detection and overcoming treatment resistance.

Chapters covered in this book signify many important points which are being provided below:

OVERVIEW OF CHAPTERS

Chapter 1: Molecular pathways and drugs involved in treatment of pancreatic cancer

The management of pancreatic cancer has long been one of oncology's most formidable challenges. The standard of care, while rigorously applied, is a multimodal strategy fraught with significant limitations. Surgical resection offers the only chance for a cure, yet it's an option for fewer than 20% of patients who present with localized disease. For the vast majority, systemic chemotherapy is the cornerstone of management, with aggressive regimens like FOLFIRINOX improving survival in both the adjuvant therapy and neoadjuvant therapy settings. Radiotherapy is also employed, often in combination with chemotherapy, for patients with locally advanced, unresectable disease. The efficacy of these treatments, however, is severely hampered by intrinsic and acquired chemoresistance. While targeted therapies have been developed, their benefit is confined to very small patient subsets defined by specific molecular alterations. This reality underscores a critical unmet need: the lack of robust biomarkers to predict treatment response, which complicates therapeutic decisions and contributes to the uniformly poor prognosis associated with this malignancy.

Chapter 2: Microorganisms involved in pancreatic cancer

This stark reality has forced a fundamental shift in research, moving from generalized treatments toward a granular understanding of the disease's root causes. The advancement in treatment is now increasingly reliant on a detailed understanding of its molecular underpinnings. Investigation into dysregulated molecular signaling pathways, such as those involving KRAS, PI3K/Akt, and MAPK, has paved the way for the development of targeted therapy. Unlike conventional chemotherapy, this approach utilizes drugs designed to specifically inhibit key proteins driving tumor growth. However, the complexity and heterogeneity of pancreatic tumors often lead to the rapid development of drug resistance, limiting the efficacy of single-agent treatments. Consequently, current research and active clinical trials are focused on evaluating novel strategies, including the use of multi-pathway inhibitors, to simultaneously block several oncogenic signals and overcome these adaptive resistance mechanisms.

Chapter 3: Utilizing the microbiome as a preventative or therapeutic for pancreatic cancer

While targeting the cancer cell's internal machinery is crucial, emerging evidence highlights that the tumour does not exist in a vacuum. A significant role is now attributed to the microorganisms involved in the pathogenesis of pancreatic cancer. The composition of the host microbiome, particularly in the gut and within the pancreas itself, is increasingly recognized as a critical factor influencing tumorigenesis. A state of dysbiosis, or a pathological imbalance in these microbial communities, has been strongly associated with disease development and progression. This link is substantiated by the discovery of distinct populations of intratumoral bacteria residing within the tumor microenvironment, suggesting a direct interaction with cancer cells. Mechanistically, these microorganisms are believed to contribute to carcinogenesis by promoting chronic inflammation and by producing bioactive microbial metabolites that can modulate host immune responses.

Chapter 4: Role of nanotechnology in pancreatic cancer

This growing understanding has naturally created promising new avenues for intervention. A primary therapeutic objective is to counteract the pro-tumorigenic state of dysbiosis by modulating the composition and function of the host's microbial communities. This has led to the exploration of microbiome-based therapy, which encompasses a range of strategies aimed at restoring a healthy gut ecosystem. Interventions currently under investigation include the administration of defined probiotics to introduce beneficial bacterial species, as well as the more comprehensive approach of faecal microbiota transplantation (FMT) from healthy donors. The overarching goal of these strategies is to leverage the microbiome not only as a preventative tool but also as an adjuvant therapy to enhance the efficacy of existing treatments.

Chapter 5: Microbiome immunomodulatory responses offer therapeutic potential against pancreatic cancer

Among the most exciting of these therapeutic avenues is the potential to modulate the host's immune system. Pancreatic ductal adenocarcinoma (PDAC) is notoriously resistant to treatment, partly due to a highly immunosuppressive tumor microenvironment that blunts the efficacy of immunotherapy. The host microbiome has been established as a critical regulator of the immune system's ability to recognize and combat malignancies, and the state of dysbiosis common in PDAC contributes to this immune evasion. Consequently, rationally modulating the microbiome represents a novel therapeutic strategy. The goal is to reverse this immunosuppressive state, aiming to restore anti-tumor immunity and potentially synergize with existing immunotherapy and chemotherapy regimens to improve patient outcomes.

Chapter 6: Standard treatment of pancreatic cancer and their limitations

This biomarker-driven, systems-level approach is the core principle of a broader strategy transforming oncology: precision oncology. The treatment paradigm for Pancreatic Cancer is shifting to match specific treatments to a tumour's molecular profile, moving beyond broad-spectrum chemotherapy to leverage Targeted Therapy. Progress has been difficult, largely because the vast majority of tumours are driven by historically "undruggable" KRAS Mutations. While early efforts targeting pathways like EGFR yielded disappointing results, the success of PARP Inhibitors in patients with BRCA mutations proves the concept's potential. That's why the hunt for predictive Biomarkers is now central to the field; they're essential for identifying the right patient for the right drug.

However, designing a precise drug is only half the battle; ensuring it reaches its target through the dense, hostile tumour microenvironment is another major hurdle. This is where nanotechnology is emerging as a transformative platform. Its application in nanomedicine offers novel solutions for early diagnosis through highly sensitive nanobiosensors and, in the therapeutic realm, a primary advantage in targeted drug delivery. Engineered nanoparticles serve as carriers to transport potent chemotherapy agents directly to the tumor, significantly enhancing drug efficacy while reducing the systemic toxicity that plagues conventional treatments.

Chapter 7: Combination therapies against pancreatic cancer for enhancing treatment effectiveness

The true potential of these innovations may lie not in isolation, but in combination. To enhance treatment effectiveness, innovative strategies that can overcome profound therapeutic resistance are required. One promising avenue involves pairing novel physical ablation techniques, such as Photo Thermal Therapy (PTT), with biological treatments. PTT induces potent localized cytotoxicity by using light-activated agents to generate lethal heat within the tumor. Crucially, this method of cell destruction can trigger an immunogenic response, sensitizing the cancer to Immune Therapy.

This approach can be further strengthened by incorporating Gene Therapy or employing Macrophage Targeted Therapy to reprogram the tumor's immunosuppressive microenvironment, creating a multi-pronged attack that simultaneously debulks the tumor and dismantles its defenses.

Chapter 8: adjuvants and their role in the treatment of pancreatic cancer

Supporting these primary treatments are adjuvants—agents designed to overcome the barriers created by the dense tumour microenvironment. They aren't standalone treatments but rather "helpers" that can, for instance, improve drug delivery systems or act as radiosensitizers, making the tumour more susceptible to damage from radiotherapy. In the context of immunotherapy, they can help remodel the immunosuppressive landscape, allowing immune cells to mount an effective attack. Ultimately, the strategic use of adjuvants aims to dismantle the defenses of the pancreatic cancer tumour, making it vulnerable.

Chapter 9: Emerging therapies - the future of pancreatic cancer treatment

Looking forward, the future of treatment hinges on dismantling this very Tumour Microenvironment (TME). Future strategies are moving beyond conventional chemotherapy, focusing instead on precision approaches where Nanomedicine offers the delivery systems to get Targeted Therapy and Immunotherapy past the TME's barriers. A key application for this powerful combination is in the Neoadjuvant Therapy setting, where these emerging treatments can be used to shrink tumors before surgery, potentially increasing the number of patients eligible for a curative resection.

Chapter 10: Precision treatment: the promise of targeted therapies against pancreatic cancer

Powering this entire evolution is the rise of Artificial Intelligence (AI), which is set to revolutionize management by tackling challenges from diagnosis to treatment. A primary focus is on early screening, where AI-powered algorithms can enable the tumour detection of subtle, early-stage lesions. Beyond detection, AI's strength lies in its capacity for prediction and determining prognosis by integrating complex data from genomics, pathology, and clinical records. Ultimately, this leads to the core promise of AI: creating truly personalized treatment plans, where algorithms help clinicians select the optimal therapeutic strategy for each unique patient.

Chapter 11: Role of artificial intelligence in the future of pancreatic cancer

While much of this represents the frontier of research, real-world case studies offer a hopeful glimpse into this future. These examples highlight the effectiveness of novel therapies, but they all share a common, critical starting point: early detection. The success of any therapeutic intervention is intrinsically linked to the stage at which it's diagnosed. The cases that follow demonstrate how combining timely diagnosis with advanced treatment protocols can lead to significantly improved outcomes, underscoring a fundamental truth: a breakthrough in treatment effectiveness isn't just about new drugs, it's about finding the disease early enough for those drugs to work.

While pancreatic cancer has long been one of oncology's greatest challenges, a new era of innovation is finally bringing hope to the horizon. This optimism starts with a foundational shift towards early detection, where AI and liquid biopsies are poised to find the disease at its most treatable stage. For those diagnosed, the future is moving away from brute-force chemotherapy and towards an intelligent, multi-pronged approach. It is this powerful convergence of precision medicine, nanotechnology, and immunotherapy that signals a true turning point in this difficult fight.

Chapter 12: Case Studies highlighting Promising Therapies and Their effectiveness in Pancreatic Cancer

Pancreatic cancer (PC) will soon become a leading cause of cancer death. Combined strategies for patients with unresectable, non-metastatic disease, which include chemotherapy and radiation, show promise. Proper application of these treatments can also increase the rate of radical resections in resectable. Alternative treatment have been shown to enhance survival and quality of life in fit patients suffering from metastatic disease. New locoregional treatment approaches are emerging as vital options in the multimodal strategy for patients. As of now, when compared to other cancer, targeted therapies have not demonstrated significant efficacy, either alone or in combination with chemotherapy and are therefore not incorporated into current clinical practice. Despite the promising outcomes of such studies in various tumors, immunotherapy is not yet included in the current therapeutic options for PC. We provide a review on (i) early detection, (ii) treatments, (iii) various biomarkers, (iv) focused treatments, and (v) future developments in PC to guide clinicians in managing PC.

Chapter 13: Hope on the horizon: the future of pancreatic cancer treatment

This chapter will focus on the future of pancreatic cancer research and the ongoing search for a cure. It will highlight the breakthroughs of the therapies and early-phase clinical trials to the development of more effective early detection methods. In order to highlight how grassroots initiatives, collaborations with healthcare institutions, and greater investment are influencing the next generation of therapies, the chapter will also look at the crucial roles that advocacy, funding, and patient involvement play in advancing research. Motivating stories of survivors who have overcome the odds will act as a powerful reminder of the strength and hope that drive the fight against pancreatic cancer. This chapter will provide a positive vision for the future by sharing these inspirational tales of tenacity and fortitude, highlighting the possibility that a cure for pancreatic cancer could one day be achievable with sustained research, teamwork, and willpower.

CONCLUSION

This book illustrates how ground-breaking treatments are transforming pancreatic cancer care by weaving together real-world experiences of patients and healthcare providers. It explores significant advances in immunotherapy, targeted therapies, precision medicine, and combination treatments, highlighting options that bring hope to patients who previously faced limited paths forward. Through these developments, readers gain insight into how science is reshaping outcomes for one of the most challenging cancers. This book serves a dual purpose: to inform readers about the cutting-edge scientific advancements in pancreatic cancer treatment and to offer hope through the personal stories of patients who are benefiting from these new therapies. It provides an in-depth exploration of the challenges and complexities involved in treating this aggressive disease, while also showcasing the real-life experiences of those navigating their journey with pancreatic cancer. By incorporating patient narratives, the book humanizes the scientific discourse, shedding light on the emotional and psychological toll of the disease, and illustrating how these innovations are not only changing lives but also restoring hope to those who once had few options.

Acknowledgement

We, the editors of this volume, wish to express our deepest gratitude to all those who have contributed to the successful completion of this book, *Innovative Therapies for Pancreatic Cancer*.

First and foremost, we extend our sincere thanks to all the contributing authors for their dedication, expertise, and commitment. Their scholarly contributions form the foundation of this work and have been a comprehensive resource on the subject. We also gratefully acknowledge the efforts of the reviewers, whose valuable feedback and constructive suggestions have helped us maintain the scientific rigor and quality of the chapters.

We take this opportunity to thank our respective institutions — **Graphic Era (Deemed to be University), Dehradun, Uttarakhand, India; Amrita Vishwa Vidyapeetham, Mysuru, Karnataka, India; and Kansas State University, Manhattan, USA** — for their constant encouragement, resources, and support that made this endeavour possible.

We also wish to acknowledge the assistance of **Ms. Bhawana Yadav**, Ph.D. scholar, and **Ms. Shreya Joshi**, B.Tech. A biotechnology student, whose sincere efforts in formatting and organizing the documents greatly facilitated the editorial process.

Finally, we are indebted to our families, colleagues, and well-wishers for their encouragement and support throughout this journey. We hope that this book serves as a meaningful contribution to the field and inspires further advancements in the treatment of pancreatic cancer.

Editors

Prof. (Dr.) Pallavi Singh

Dr. Shiva Prasad Kollur

Dr. Raghavendra G. Amachawadi

Chapter 1
Molecular Pathways and Drugs Involved in the Treatment of Pancreatic Cancer

Bhawana Yadav
Graphic Era University, India

Dhawani Maltonia
https://orcid.org/0009-0004-9112-6668
Graphic Era University, India

Ananya Singh
Graphic Era University, India

Shiva Prasad Kollur
https://orcid.org/0000-0003-3914-3933
Amrita Vishwa Vidyapeetham, India

Pallavi Singh
https://orcid.org/0000-0003-4537-4607
Graphic Era University, India

ABSTRACT

Pancreatic cancer remains one of the deadliest malignancies due to late diagnosis, aggressive progression, and limited treatment efficacy. This chapter explores key molecular pathways—KRAS, Hedgehog, Notch, Wnt/β-catenin, TGF-β, JAK/STAT and their roles in tumorigenesis, progression, and resistance. It highlights recent pharmacological advances, including KRAS G12C inhibitors, SMO antagonists,

DOI: 10.4018/979-8-3373-1469-3.ch001

gamma-secretase inhibitors, β-catenin and TGF-β receptor inhibitors. Multi-pathway targeting agents and synergistic strategies with chemotherapy, immunotherapy, and radiotherapy are discussed. Clinical trials and case studies illustrate improved outcomes and resistance management. Challenges such as tumor heterogeneity, toxicity, and lack of biomarkers are critically examined. Innovative solutions like advanced drug delivery, multi-omics, and AI-driven discovery are proposed. The chapter reviews the translational journey of pathway-targeting therapies and discusses emerging tools like liquid biopsies and ctDNA for treatment monitoring.

INTRODUCTION MODULE

Introduction to Pancreatic Ductal Adenocarcinoma (PDAC):

Over 90% of pancreatic tumors are pancreatic ductal adenocarcinomas (PDAC), an extremely deadly cancer with a pitiful 18% 1-year survival rate. The primary cause of dismal prognosis is the aggressive and asymptomatic character of the disease, which leads to most patients being discovered at an advanced stage. So, to detect pre-invasive neoplasm, enable early diagnosis, and creating an affordable screening technique is still a significant clinical problem, accurate biomarkers are therefore desperately needed. Genetic intricacy of PDAC impedes therapeutic advancements, and while palliative chemotherapy has made some strides, there are still few treatment choices available. A major advancement has been made by introducing regimens like FOLFIRINOX and gemcitabine/nab-paclitaxel. Some of the improvements have been seen from these therapies, but due to association with high toxicity, these are only suitable for younger, fitter patients (Xu et al., 2025).

In cases of PDAC that are locally progressed or borderline resectable, neoadjuvant therapy treatment administered before surgery has shown promise. More recent chemotherapy regimens may allow tumour downstaging, improving the chance of full (R0) resection, even though early studies did not demonstrate any survival advantage over adjuvant therapy (treatment following surgery). Strong data from randomized controlled studies is still required, though. Treatment choices for locally advanced, incurable PDAC include gemcitabine-based regimens, chemotherapy with FOLFIRINOX, or chemoradiotherapy. Although it does not perform better than systemic chemotherapy and frequently increases toxicity, chemotherapy-radiotherapy does provide a slight survival benefit over radiation alone (Hammel et al., 2016). Adding chemoradiotherapy after initial chemotherapy did not significantly improve outcomes, according to the LAP 07 trial, highlighting the need for more careful treatment selection.

For metastatic PDAC, palliation and survival prolongation have become new therapeutic objectives. The standard has long been gemcitabine, which is appreciated more for its controllable toxicity and symptom alleviation than for its effectiveness. When combined with other treatments, some minor increases are produced, like capecitabine or oxaliplatin, while regimens like FOLFIRINOX and gemcitabine with nab-paclitaxel have shown notable improvements in median survival (11.1 vs. 6.8 months and 8.5 vs. 6.7 months, respectively). These are only practical for patients who are performing better, though. An EGFR inhibitor called erlotinib was licensed in conjunction with gemcitabine after a phase III trial showed just a slight increase in survival. People who experienced a distinctive skin rash, its benefits are primarily limited to them, indicating that it may be a predictive biomarker (Catenacci et al., 2015). However, its routine use is limited due to increased toxicity and low efficiency.

Figure 1. Human Pancreas

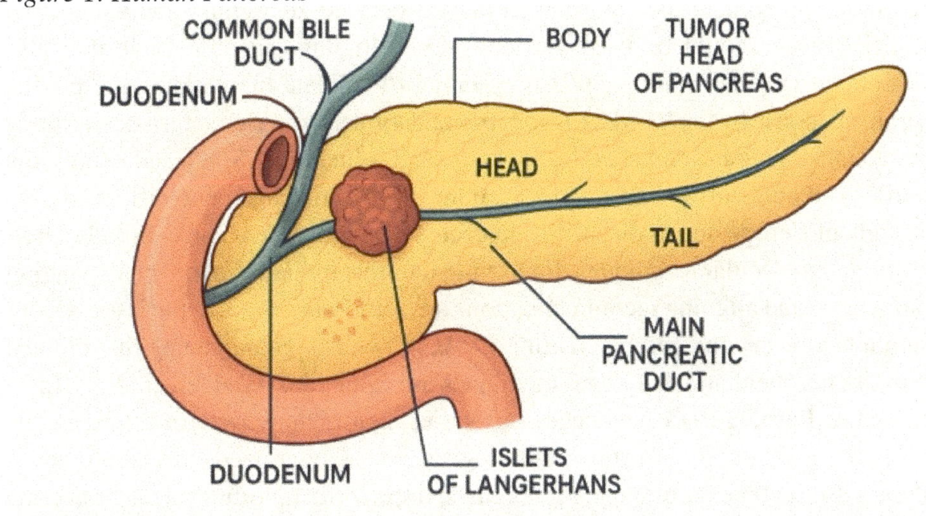

Patients who are usually performing well, about 40 - 50% of metastatic PDAC cases, are evaluated for second-line therapies. Certain regimens, like 5-FU with oxaliplatin or FOLFIRI, are effective, and gemcitabine might be used as a second-line treatment after FOLFIRINOX. It is essential to customize treatment based on the patient's age, condition, treatment, and nutritional status, since combinational therapies don't help those who perform poorly (EGOC >2). Nutritional support is essential to improve patients' outcomes, including the provision of enzymes in situations of pancreatic insufficiency. High genetic heterogeneity is seen in PDAC at the molecular level, with KRAS, p16, TP53, and SMAD4 mutations being common. No effective targeted medicines have been developed to target these genes, despite their ubiquity (Ryan et al., 2020). Chromatin remodelling, DNA damage repair (e.g., BRCA1/2), and axon guidance (e.g., ROBO1/2) are among the novel targets being studied. Additionally, EGFR, PI3K, and cancer stem cells (CSCs) are being investigated. Gemcitabine and tigatuzumab, two combinations that target CSCs, have demonstrated preclinical promise.

Tumour microenvironment, which is characterized by inadequate vascularization and thick stroma, can give rise to many treatment challenges. TGF-β inhibitors, Notch/Hedgehog pathway blockers, and pegylated hyaluronidase are some of the treatments that potentially target it, as it may act as a barrier to drug delivery. However, the latter has seen toxicity-related setbacks in clinical trials. The "stromal barrier" theory is still up for debate, although overexpression of SPARC in stromal fibroblasts offers another possible path (McGuigan et al., 2018).

To expedite medication development, clinical trial design needs to address the difficulties faced by PDAC. To evaluate and analyse medications for uncommon mutations, preclinical models such as patient-derived xenografts and genetically modified mice should be used and considered in stage-specific trials that also incorporate molecular imaging. It is essential to validate biomarkers that predict therapy response by the REMARK recommendations. Drug characteristics, stromal interactions, tumour uptake, and genetic context—including SNPs and expression profiles—should all be taken into account. PDAC management differs greatly throughout Europe due to disparities in access to standardized care, skilled radiologists, and molecular techniques. Improving interdisciplinary treatment, expanding trial access, and aligning recommendations are some ways to solve the issue. Cooperation can be encouraged by creating PDAC networks, guaranteeing that clinical trials are pertinent and that novel medicines are available. (Waddell et al., 2015).

Across Europe, PDAC management varies significantly due to differences in access to molecular tools, trained radiologists, and standardized care. Strategies to address this include harmonizing guidelines, improving multidisciplinary care, and enhancing trial access. Establishing a PDAC network can promote collaboration, ensuring clinical trials are relevant and new treatments are accessible (Saung et al., 2020).

PATHOPHYSIOLOGY & MOLECULAR FEATURES MODULE

Most patients have a bad quality of life since they are detected at a late stage by near the end of their lives. To improve the quality of life and treatment compliance, one should combine palliative care with chemotherapy early on. To improve the bleak prognosis for PDAC patients, ongoing efforts must concentrate on finding reliable biomarkers, investigating new targets, and standardising care.

1. Molecular Signal pathways in pancreatic Cancer:

Log2 FC: Fold change in normal vs. malignant (log base 2).
adj. p-val: FDR-corrected p-value (statistical significance).
TPM: Expression level normalized.
Mutation%: Propagation of patients with gene changes (TCGA or comparable).
Stage (Max): It is the highest clinical stage where expression or mutation is noted.
Role: Canonical biological role in the development of tumours.
Pathway: The gene participates in the major signalling route.
Prognosis: Clinical cohort correlation for overall survival.
Targetable: Is there a medication that targets this gene or any associated pathway?

Table 1. Key Differentially Expressed and Mutated Genes in Pancreatic

Gene	Log2 FC	adj. p-val	Expression (TPM)	Mutation %	Stage (Max)	Role	Pathway	Prognosis	Targetable?
KRAS	+2.5	0.0005	120.4	45%	III	Oncogene	RAS/MAPK	Poor	No (indirect)
TP53	-1.8	0.0056	98.7	60%	II	Tumor suppressor	p53 signaling	Poor	No
SMAD4	-2.2	0.0033	45.3	35%	IV	TGF-β modulator	TGF-β	Poor	No
CDKN2A	+1.4	0.015	67.2	25%	I	Cell cycle inhibitor	Cell cycle	Variable	Yes (CDK4/6 inhibitors)

KEY SIGNALLING PATHWAYS MODULE

1. KRAS Pathway:

Pancreatic ductal adenocarcinoma (PDAC) is considered one of the deadliest cancers with five survival rate of less than 10%. The high frequency of activating mutations in the KRAS oncogene is a characteristic of PDAC, which is essential for the development and spread of the tumour. It is essential to comprehend the molecular mechanisms behind KRAS mutations and their downstream effectors, especially the RAF-MEK-ERK and PI3K-AKT-mTOR pathways, for the development of targeted therapeutics (Ryan et al., 2020). KRAS mutations play an important role in the pathophysiology of PDAC because these mutations activate important signalling pathways that support the tumor development and survival.

Acting as a molecular switch, KRAS is a tiny GTPase that alternates between active (GTP-bound) and inactive (GDP-bound) states. Being the most prevalent, about 90-95% PDAC tumors include activating mutations in KRAS with G12D,

G12V, and G12R. Constitutive activation and sustained downstream signalling result from these alterations, which also affect KRAS's intrinsic GTPase function. Being influenced by oncogenic KRAS mutations, Apoptosis resistance, metabolic reprogramming, unchecked cell proliferation, and tumor microenvironment modification are some of the characteristics of PDAC pathogenesis (Sun et al., 2020). Several signalling pathways, including RAF/MEK/ERK and PI3K/AKT/mTOR, in addition to (Ishikawa et al., 2017). Additional pathways, including CDK5 and YAP/JAK/STAT3, are being controlled by the development of malignant cells from acinar or ductal cells promoted by KRAS mutations. (Caldas & Kern, 1995).

Figure 2. KRAS Signalling Pathway in PDAC

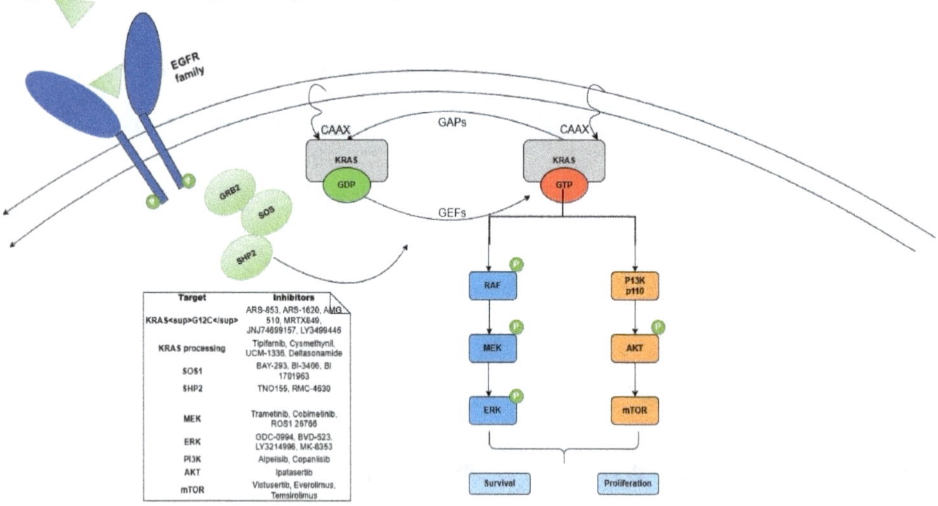

The RAF-MEK-ERK signalling cascade is the key downstream effector of KRAS. The plasma membrane is activated by KRAS, attracting RAF kinases, which start a chain reaction of phosphorylation in which RAF phosphorylates MEK1/2, which phosphorylates ERK1/2. The translocation and control of the expression of genes related to survival, differentiation, and cell cycle progression is performed by activated ERK in the nucleus. KRAS mutations in PDAC often result in an upregulation of the RAF-MEK-ERK pathway. It significantly influences the initiation and development of tumors by this route. Preclinical models of targeted therapy that use small-molecule inhibitors against elements of this system, such as MEK inhibitors (e.g., selumetinib, trametinib), have demonstrated promise. However, feedback loops and compensatory mechanisms that restart the route or activate alternate survival pathways have little clinical efficacy (Luo et al., 2023).

2. Hedgehog Signalling Pathway:

The hedgehog signalling pathway is an essential developmental regulator that preserves tissue patterning and stem cell fate throughout embryogenesis. The pathway is mainly dormant in adults but reactivates in a variety of malignancies, influencing the tumour microenvironment (TME) and aiding in carcinogenesis. The GLI transcription factors are activated by the interaction of the transmembrane protein Smoothened (SMO), the receptor Patched1 (PTCH1), and Hh ligands Sonic, Indian, and Desert Hedgehog in the canonical Hh pathway. Aberrant Hh activation has been associated with autocrine and paracrine processes in tumour biology.

The survival and growth of cancerous cells in several malignancies, such as glioblastoma, lung, pancreatic, and breast cancers, have been linked to hedgehog signalling. Paracrine signalling from stromal cells or by ligand-dependent autocrine loops in tumour cells is the cause of triggering of this pathway. (Yang et al., 2010).

Some ongoing research on breast cancer shows that epithelial-to-mesenchymal transition (EMT), which makes drug resistance and metastasis easier, is being encouraged by hedgehog signalling. Increased tumour aggressiveness and a poor prognosis are associated with high expression of SHH and GLI1. Invasion and migration of cells are promoted by the route in glioblastoma. SHH activation promotes the production of matrix metalloproteinase (MMP)-2 and MMP-9 via the PI3K/AKT pathway, which in turn promotes tumour invasion into neighbouring brain regions. In case of pancreatic cancer, paracrine hedgehog signalling from tumour cells actively surrounds stromal cells, indirectly supporting tumor proliferation. (Lee et al., 2014).

From the additional data, it has been indicated that Hh signalling has a role in the maintenance of cancer stem cells (CSCs). CSCs cause tumour initiation, treatment resistance, and recurrence. GLI1 and GLI2 transcription factors are increased in CSCs in colorectal and liver malignancies, which improves self-renewal and survival under treatment stress.

Hh signalling plays a significant role in the modification of the tumour microenvironment, in addition to its direct impact on tumour cells. Numerous non-malignant cells, including fibroblasts, immunological cells, endothelial cells, and extracellular matrix (ECM) constituents, are seen and observed in the TME. Hh signalling influences these components, which promote tumour growth. Cancer-associated fibroblasts (CAFs) that have GLI1 activated produce more growth factors and extracellular matrix proteins, which promote tumour cell migration and proliferation in breast cancer. Inflammatory cytokines like IL-6, in response to the SHH ligand from tumour cells, CAFs establish a tumour-supportive environment is released when the downstream signalling is triggered that stiffens the extracellular matrix (Linehan et al., 2024).

3. Notch Signalling Pathway:

The Notch signalling pathway, considered a highly conserved cell communication system, is essential for controlling cell fate decisions, proliferation, differentiation, and apoptosis during tissue homeostasis and embryonic development. Several abnormalities in this pathway have been linked to several malignancies, including pancreatic ductal adenocarcinoma (PDAC), which aid in the development, spread, and resistance to treatment of the tumour (Gao et al., 2017).

Notch signalling starts when the Notch receptors (Notch1–4) connect with their ligands (Jagged1, Jagged2, DLL1, DLL3, DLL4) on neighbouring and surrounding cells (Buchler et al., 2005). In response to ligand binding, the Notch receptor is cleaved twice by proteases: at first by a disintegrated and metalloproteinase (ADAM) family protease and then again by the γ-secretase complex. These cleavages release the Notch intracellular domain (NICD), which moves towards the nucleus and interacts with co-activators and the DNA-binding protein CSL (CBF1/Suppressor of Hairless/LAG-1), to control the transcription of target genes involved in cell proliferation, survival, and differentiation.

Dysregulation in PDAC, which is typically exhibited by Notch signalling, aids in the development of the tumour. In conjunction with oncogenic KRAS mutations, Acinar-to-ductal metaplasia (ADM), a precursor to PDAC, is promoted. (Buscail et al., 2020).

Pancreatic intraepithelial neoplasia (PanIN) lesions arise and proceed to invasive carcinoma because of this collaboration, making it easier for acinar cells to be reprogrammed into ductal-like cells(Sano et al., 2016). Tumor development and metastasis by modifying angiogenesis, immune cell infiltration, and stromal interactions are all supported by Notch signalling in the tumor microenvironment (Yabuuchi et al., 2013).

The Notch pathway has gained attention due to its significant involvement in PDAC pathogenesis as a possible therapeutic target. The two methods used for blocking Notch signalling are Monoclonal antibodies that target Notch receptors or ligands and γ-secretase inhibitors (GSIs). GSIs, including RO4929097 and MK-0752, have been assessed in preclinical and clinical trials. (Avila & Kissil, 2013).

Both the preclinical and clinical trials showed different results. Preclinical models showed that RO4929097 could stop tumor growth; however, clinical trials showed significant toxicity and poor efficacy, causing a delay in the ongoing research (Palagani et al., 2014). Similarly, in combination with chemotherapy,

MK-0752 had a moderate level of activity but was linked to negative side effects (Ma et al., 2013).

4. Wnt/β-Catenin Pathway:

The Wnt/β-catenin signalling system, a highly conserved cellular communication network, is crucial for stem cell maintenance, tissue regeneration, cell fate determination, and embryonic development. Cytoplasmic β-catenin is stabilized by Wnt ligand binding in its canonical form, which enables it to go into the nucleus and initiate target gene transcription (Murtaugh, 2008). Several cancers, which are strictly regulated under physiological settings, including colorectal, hepatic, pancreatic, and breast cancers, have been linked to dysregulation of this system occurs frequently because of mutations or aberrant signalling (S.P. et al., 2006).

Cross-talk with other pathways: -

The Wnt/β-catenin pathway interacts dynamically with various other signalling pathways, as it is not isolated.

NF-κB Pathway: This pathway can either activate or inhibit NF-κB, which affects inflammation and the development of cancer as it is reciprocally modulated with Wnt signalling and β-catenin (Ma & et al., 2013).

Notch, RTKs, and TGF-β Pathways: Results of these pathways are increased proliferation and resistance to apoptosis, improving β-catenin stability and activity (Ma et al., 2013).

Hippo pathway: It shows an interplay of actions to control carcinogenesis and organ growth, and co-modulation affects the course of cancer. (Ram Makena et al., 2019). Drug development efforts are Wnt signalling is suppressed by small molecule inhibitors such as WNT974 (LGK974), which block porcupine (PORCN), an enzyme necessary for Wnt ligand production. (Cui et al., 2012). Specifically limiting Wnt-driven gene expression without compromising normal tissue homeostasis, PRI724 interferes with the β-catenin/CBP connection. (Wang et al., 2009

). Using Antibodies: Vantictumab (OMP-18R5) inhibits Wnt ligand binding and pathway activation by targeting Frizzled receptors. Clinical trials have advanced for several diseases, including pancreatic and breast tumors. Novel Methods: Since β-catenin lacks a well-defined small-molecule binding site, proteolysis-targeting chimeras (PROTACs) and allosteric inhibitors have been developed to target it (Arensman et al., 2014). By facilitating the breakdown of β-catenin, PROTACs provide a novel way to prevent Wnt-driven oncogenesis (Javadinia et al., 2019).

5. TGF-β Signalling Pathway:

Tumor suppression role: -

TARGETED THERAPY STRATEGIES MODULE

TGF-β acts as a tumour suppressor in early-stage malignancies through apoptosis induction and cell growth inhibition. By activation of SMAD-dependent pathways, downregulation of oncogenes like c-MYC and transcriptionally activates cell cycle inhibitors like p15^INK4B and p21^CIP1. On this inhibitory action, the preservation of cellular homeostasis and the avoidance of unchecked cell proliferation are heavily dependent. (Villanueva et al., 1998). The tumour promotion role is that Cancer cells frequently become resistant to the suppressive actions of TGF-β as the tumour grows. (Shen et al., 2017).-β

Stimulates the epithelial-mesenchymal transition (EMT), increasing cell invasion, motility, and metastasis when the tumour reaches an advanced stage (Javle et al., 2014). Moreover, according to (Luo et al., 2023), .-TGF-β contributes to the immunosuppressive tumour microenvironment, stimulated by the development of regulatory T cells and preventing the proliferation and activity of cytotoxic T lymphocytes. This dual function of TGF-β in cancer is commonly known as the "TGF-β paradox" (Waters et al., 2018).

Figure 3. TGF-β Signalling Pathway in PDAC

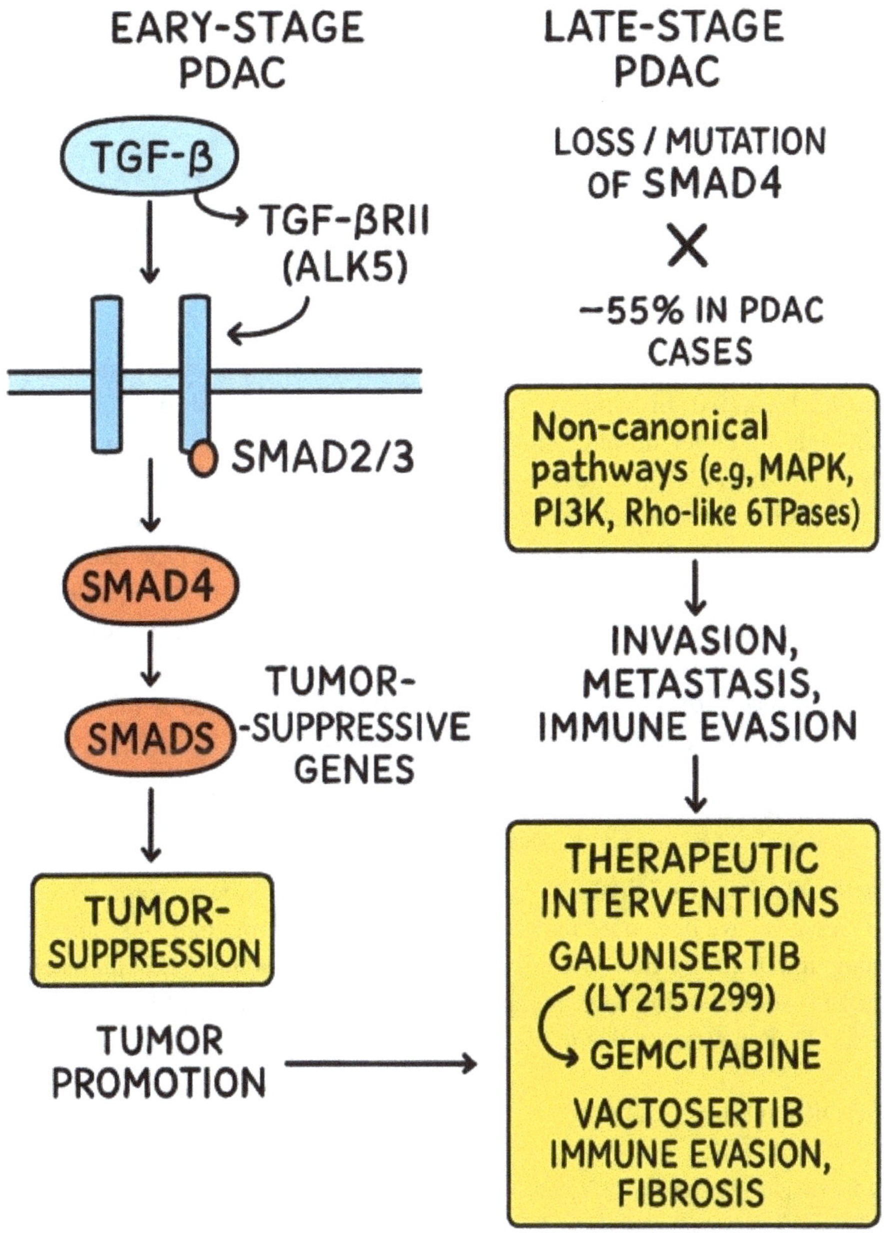

2. Drug Targeting key molecular pathways in PDAC:

Pancreatic ductal adenocarcinoma (PDAC) is a lethal malignancy with poor prognosis and limited treatment options. Owing to its complex molecular landscape, therapeutic efforts have increasingly focused on targeting dysregulated signalling pathways. Below is a comprehensive overview of key molecular targets and therapeutic strategies in PDAC, aligned with current research.

Inhibition of KRAS and Its Downstream Pathways:

A) KRAS G12C Inhibitors:

For more than 90% of PDAC cases, KRAS mutations are present, especially at codons 12, 13, and 61. In a limited percentage of PDAC patients, the G12C mutation remains a useful target, despite being more prevalent in non-small cell lung cancer. Covalent KRAS G12C inhibitors sotorasib (AMG 510) and adagrasib (MRTX849) have demonstrated therapeutic efficacy in malignancies with G12C mutations. To stop downstream signalling, their technique traps KRAS in its GDP-bound, inactive state. Although these inhibitors' limited application in PDAC is attributable to the number of mutations, their effectiveness has spurred efforts to create medications that target additional KRAS variations, like G12D, which is far more common in pancreatic cancer. Renowned KRAS G12D inhibitor RMC-9805 is presently undergoing preclinical development (Zhou et al., 2019).

B) MEK inhibitors:

In the RAS-RAF-MEK-ERK cascade, MEK1/2 are downstream effectors. PDAC models have been used to assess inhibitors like selumetinib and trametinib. Combination therapy with PI3K/mTOR inhibitors or immune checkpoint blockers is being researched to improve therapeutic response, even though MEK inhibition alone has limited efficacy due to route redundancy.

C) mTOR inhibitors:

A further downstream effector of KRAS signalling is the PI3K-AKT-mTOR axis. Tumour resistance and proliferation are facilitated by abnormal activation of this system. Clinical trials have assessed mTOR inhibitors such as everolimus; nonetheless, monotherapy outcomes have been underwhelming. To get around resistance mechanisms, combination approaches using autophagy or MEK inhibitors are being investigated.

Hedgehog Pathway Inhibitors

In PDAC, the Hedgehog (Hh) pathway, which is mostly engaged in embryogenesis, is reactivated. Signalling through the SMO (Smoothened) receptor is started by ligand binding (SHH, IHH), which eventually activates GLI transcription factors. Desmoplasia and immunological evasion are encouraged by this (Onishi & Katano, 2014).

Sonidegib and vismodegib are FDA-approved SMO antagonists that were first created to treat basal cell carcinoma. Preclinical models demonstrated that Hh inhibition improves medication distribution by reducing stromal density. However, the vismodegib and gemcitabine combination in the phase II clinical study did not show any improvement in PDAC survival (Catenacci et al., 2015). Complex interactions between the tumour and the stroma may be the cause of this, as they may encourage tumour growth when the stroma collapses. As a result, techniques for selective or temporary inhibition are being researched.

Notch Signalling Pathway

The Notch signalling pathway controls stem cell maintenance, proliferation, and cell destiny. Tumour development and treatment resistance are associated with abnormal Notch activation in PDAC. Inhibitors of gamma-secretase (GSIs). The cleavage of Notch receptors by the enzyme complex gamma-secretase enables the intracellular domains of these receptors to enter the nucleus and control gene expression. GSIs such as RO4929097 have undergone PDAC testing. Clinical trials were unsuccessful because of gastrointestinal damage and poor efficacy, despite preclinical results showing decreased tumor development. To improve results, current initiatives use GSIs in conjunction with immune checkpoint inhibitors or chemotherapy (Ristorcelli & Lombardo, 2010).

Wnt/β-catenin Pathway

In PDAC, another embryonic signalling axis is reactivated: the Wnt/β-catenin pathway. It contributes to invasion, chemoresistance, and stem cell maintenance. The transcription of carcinogenic targets is caused by aberrant nuclear accumulation of β-catenin. β-Catenin Small Molecule Inhibitors Certain agents, such as PRI-724 and ICG-001, prevent β-catenin from interacting with the transcriptional co-activator CBP (CREB-binding protein (Zeng et al., 2006). These compounds have demonstrated preclinical effectiveness in inhibiting the growth of tumours and downregulating Wnt target genes. There has been some success in early-phase clinical trials with PRI-724. The use of these inhibitors in combination with other medications is the topic of continuing research due to toxicity concerns and the complexity of the pathway.

Figure 4. Wnt/β-catenin Pathway in PDAC

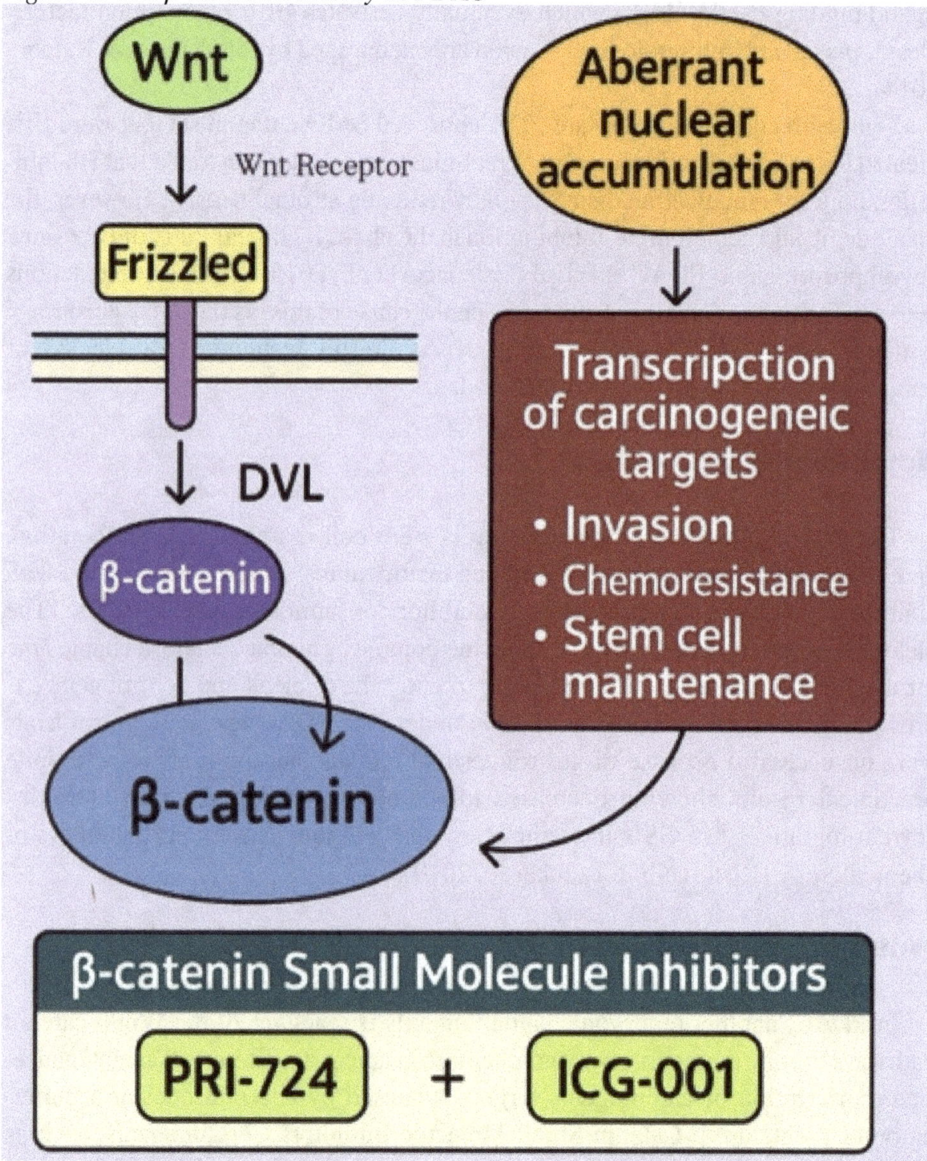

TGF-β Pathways

Signalling plays a dual role in PDAC, promoting tumour growth in advanced stages and suppressing tumours in early stages. SMAD4 mutations interfere with canonical TGF-β signalling and are found in around 55% of PDAC cases. Receptor Kinase Inhibitors of TGF-β A specific inhibitor of TGF-β type I receptor kinase (ALK5) is galunisertib (LY2157299). Gemcitabine alone did not enhance overall survival as much as galunisertib with gemcitabine did in phase II research (Melisi et al., 2018). According to this, TGF-β inhibition and chemotherapy might work in concert. Other inhibitors in clinical development target TGF-β-mediated immune evasion and fibrosis, such as vactosertib.

6. Immunotherapy and Combination Approaches Module

Emerging Multi-Way Pathway Targeting Agents

Because PDAC pathways are redundant and interact with one another, single-agent treatments frequently do not work. As a result, multi-pathway inhibitors and sensible medication combinations are becoming more popular. Two Inhibitors of PI3K/mTOR. When compared to single-pathway blockade, agents such as BEZ235 have greater efficacy by inhibiting both PI3K and mTOR concurrently. In xenograft models, these inhibitors reduce angiogenesis and tumour growth. Toxicology and feedback activation are still problems, though. Inhibitors of BET and Histone Deacetylase (HDAC). The potential of epigenetic modifiers, such as BET inhibitors (like JQ1) and HDAC inhibitors (like vorinostat), to alter several oncogenic pathways, including MYC, Notch, and NF-κB, has been investigated. These substances improve chemotherapy sensitivity, decrease fibrosis, and rewire the tumour microenvironment.

Combinations of Targeted Therapy and Immunotherapy. Immune checkpoint inhibitors by themselves are ineffective in PDAC because of its immunosuppressive milieu, although preclinical research has indicated that they may be effective when combined with drugs that target TGF-β, MEK, or CD40. Both anti-tumour immunity and tumour-promoting inflammation reduction are the goals of these combinations.

COMBINATION THERAPIES AND SYNERGISTIC APPROACHES

With its aggressive progression, late detection, and its ability for resistance to standard treatments, pancreatic ductal adenocarcinoma (PDAC) continues to rank among the deadliest cancers. Its treatment resistance is influenced by the thick stroma, genetic heterogeneity, and complicated tumor microenvironment (TME). To improve treatment effectiveness and get past resistance mechanisms, combination treatments that target several pathways at once have become viable tactics as a result.

Rationale for Combinational Therapies

Due to compensatory mechanisms and system redundancy, monotherapies that target only one pathway have had little success in PDAC. As an example, the effectiveness of the treatment is reduced when focusing just on the KRAS pathway frequently results in activation of other survival pathways. Consequently, combining drugs that target different pathways or processes may have synergistic effects that improve tumor suppression and go past resistance. In addition, the immunosuppressive TME in PDAC reduces the efficiency of immunotherapies. By modifying the TME, immunotherapeutic drugs can be used in conjunction with chemotherapy or targeted therapies to promote immune cell infiltration and activity. For instance, Immunogenic cell death can be caused by chemotherapy, resulting in the tumor antigens and increasing the effectiveness of immune checkpoint inhibitors.

Targeting Multiple Pathways Simultaneously

A) KRAS and the downstream pathway:

Downstream pathways like PI3K/AKT/mTOR and MAPK are activated because KRAS mutations are common in PDAC. Although going after KRAS directly has been difficult, combining inhibitors of downstream effectors has shown promise. For example, it has been shown from the preclinical models that simultaneous inhibition of PI3K and MEK (a part of the MAPK system) produces synergistic effects that improve tumor suppression.

B) Hedgehog and notch pathways:

Cancer stem cell maintenance and the desmoplastic response in PDAC are facilitated and maintained by the Hedgehog and Notch signalling pathways. Two examples of inhibitors that target these pathways and have demonstrated minimal effectiveness when used alone are SMO antagonists for hedgehog and gamma-secretase inhibitors for notch. However, to improve drug distribution and disturb the supportive TME, their combination with chemotherapy has been investigated. (Kelleher, 2011).

Combining Targeted Therapies with Chemotherapy

To increase the cytotoxic effects on tumor cells and maybe lessen systemic toxicity, targeted treatments are combined with chemotherapy. For example, erlotinib, an EGFR inhibitor, and gemcitabine, a nucleoside analog, together showed a slight increase in survival when compared to gemcitabine alone. Underscoring the need for more potent pairings, the advantage was modest, though.

Another strategy is to combine the chemotherapy with drugs that target the DNA damage response.

In BRCA-mutated PDAC, for example, PARP inhibitors have been used in conjunction with platinum-based chemotherapy to promote tumor cell death by utilising the idea of synthetic lethality.

Immunotherapy and Pathway Modulation

Although treatment of cancer has been transformed by immunotherapy, the immunosuppressive TME has hampered its effectiveness in PDAC. The following are some methods to improve immunotherapy's effectiveness in PDAC:

Checkpoint inhibitors to boost the immune responses. Although the effectiveness of PD-1/PD-L1 inhibitors as monotherapies has been limited, their combination with radiation therapy or chemotherapy is being investigated (Cao et al., 2021).

To elicit an immune response antigen unique to the tumor, cancer vaccines are designed. The effectiveness of these treatments can be increased by chemotherapy or checkpoint inhibitors.

Adoptive cell therapy to enhance the infiltration and permanence of modified T cells, research is being done on PDAC using techniques such as CAR-T cell therapy in conjunction with substances that alter the TME.

Targeting immunosuppressive cells to alleviate immunosuppression, agents targeting regulatory T cells, myeloid-derived suppressor cells, and tumor-associated macrophages are being combined with immunotherapies.

CHALLENGES & LIMITATIONS MODULE

Emerging multi-pathway targeting Agents

The creation and development of substances that can target several different pathways at once offers a space for possible therapy options for PDAC. Dual PI3K/mTOR inhibitors, for example, can disrupt two important survival pathways at the same time to overcome the dual resistance mechanism (Ryan et al., 2020). To improve specificity and efficacy, fusion proteins and bispecific antibodies are also being developed to target a variety of different pathways and antigens.

Challenges and Limitations in Targeting Pathways

Targeting specific molecular pathways in pancreatic cancer is one of the most explored areas in research today, but it comes with a long list of challenges. One of the major challenges is how different these tumors can be, and not just varying from patient to patient, but even within a single tumor. Some types of cancer cells can be responsive to a certain drug, while others do not, which ultimately makes it hard for one treatment to be effective across the board.

Another obstacle must be how quickly resistance develops. For instance, in pancreatic cancer, the KRAS mutations are widespread, but many different forms of this mutation do not have effective drugs yet. And even when we do find something that works initially, the tumor often finds a way to adapt, either by switching on backup pathways or changing how it behaves at the molecular level. The surrounding of the tumor's environment makes things even harder. Pancreatic tumors are often wrapped in thick, fibrous tissue that acts like a shield, which not only blocks drugs from reaching the tumor but also helps the cancer to hide from the immune system and resist treatment.

And then there comes the issue of the side effects. Normal and healthy cells are also affected by the drugs that are used to target the cancer pathway, which means that the patients can ultimately experience harmful side effects and especially if they are already in a fragile state due to late-stage cancer or any other health issues. This limits how much of a drug can be given safely.

Nowadays, we also face a serious gap when it comes to biomarkers, which are the biological clues that help doctors choose the right treatment for each patient. While a few exist, like BRCA mutations for certain targeted therapies, most patients do not have any clear markers that tell us what will or will not work for them.

Clinical Trials and Drug Development Module

Also, cancer cells are smart as they rely on complex networks of signalling pathways. If you block one, they often just activate another route to survive, which means that using only one drug is usually not enough, and combination treatments are likely to be more effective but more complicated to develop and test. Science has made progress in understanding pancreatic cancer at the molecular level, but turning that knowledge into effective, long-lasting treatments remains a major challenge.

On top of all these challenges, one major difficulty researchers face is the lack of precision in current treatment approaches. Even when treatments are developed to specifically target known mutations in pancreatic cancer, the way these tumors behave can be incredibly unpredictable. What works well in one patient may do very little in another, and that unpredictability makes clinical trials difficult to design. It is not easy to determine in advance which patients are most likely to benefit, and this uncertainty adds a layer of complexity to developing effective therapies (M.B. et al., 2020).

Timing is another major challenge in the diagnosis. Pancreatic cancer is usually diagnosed at an advanced stage, often after it has already spread. This delay severely limits treatment options. Targeted therapies that might have had more impact earlier in the disease often do not work as well once the cancer has progressed. The disease is typically aggressive, less responsive, and hard to manage by the time treatment starts.

On top of everything, collecting the right kind of tissues for research is not easy. Pancreatic tumors are tucked away deep in the body, making them difficult to access. As a result, researchers often must work with very limited or poor-quality samples. This makes it tough to study the cancer properly, slowing down efforts to determine where targets are most effective for treatment.

Progress is still being made. Researchers are gaining a better understanding of how these tumors grow and adapt, and they are testing new drug combinations and looking for better and more efficient ways to get treatments directly into the tumor. Every step is bringing us closer to more personalised and effective therapies in this long and complex journey. There is no universal fix, but there is hope, and science is moving in the right direction because pancreatic cancer is diagnosed late when it has already spread, and options and time are limited.

UNDERSTANDING PRECLINICAL AND CLINICAL RESEARCH IN PANCREATIC CANCER

Pancreatic cancer, especially the common and aggressive type known as Pancreatic Ductal Adenocarcinoma (PDCA), is extremely hard to treat. Scientists have been working hard to find better ways to fight it, and one area they have been focusing on is the process of angiogenesis, which is how tumors create new blood vessels to feed themselves and grow, and blocking this process seems like a smart way to starve the tumor. Researchers have been testing in the lab a range of ideas and then in real patients. Many different drugs have been tested to see if they can slow or stop the growth of blood vessels in pancreatic tumors in early research that has been done in labs or with animals. For example, one drug, Sunitinib, stood out because it targets multiple cancer-related pathways all at once. In mouse models, it did not just slow tumor growth, but it also changed the way the tumor interacted with its environment.

Another drug, Verteporfin, usually used for eye problems, turned out to have surprising anti-cancer effects. It was able to disrupt a sneaky trick that some tumors use to mimic blood vessels, helping them survive even when the blood supply is cut off. Verteporfin helped shrink tumors and make them more vulnerable to treatment by targeting this process.

Researchers have also been tackling the low-oxygen (hypoxic) environment inside tumors, and this environment activates certain survival signals in cancer cells. Drugs that block HIF-1α, a major player in hypoxia, have been tested and have shown promising tumor-slowing effects. (Zhang et al., 2017). Another research is focused not just on the tumor itself, but the surrounding tissue and supportive cells, known as the tumor microenvironment. In pancreatic cancer, dense fibrous tissue surrounds the tumor, making it hard for drugs to reach their target. Scientists have been experimenting with ways to weaken this protective barrier. For example, using bisphosphonates, drugs originally used for bone disease, combined with chemotherapy has helped slow down these support cells and reduce blood vessel growth.

After success in the lab, many of these treatments moved into clinical trials. One example is Sorafenib, a drug that blocks blood vessel growth. When the drug Gemcitabine is combined with chemotherapy, some patients respond better, especially those with lower levels of a blood marker called LDH. This suggests that certain markers in the blood might help predict who will benefit from these drugs (Bloomston et al., 2002).

Another treatment, Elpamotide, aimed to boost the immune system to attack tumor blood vessels. Some patients who had strong reactions at the injection site lived longer, hinting that the body's immune response might play a bigger role than expected.

Drugs like Everolimus, which target a pathway that helps cancer cells grow and divide, which on tested with chemotherapy and showed manageable side effects. Bevacizumab, which is one of the drugs that target blood vessel growth, had mixed results, but interestingly, patients who developed high blood pressure while on the drug seemed to do better (Craven et al., 2016). This unusual reaction might serve as a clue to which patients are responding well.

In case of neuroendocrine tumors (a less common type of pancreatic cancer that tends to grow more slowly but has more blood vessels), drugs like Sunitinib, Pazopanib, and Bevacizumab showed better results. These treatments helped slow the cancer and improve survival in some patients (Annese et al., 2019).

Overview of Preclinical Models for Pathway-Targeting Drugs

Any new cancer drug must be thoroughly tested in the lab before it reaches patients. For pancreatic cancer, especially the aggressive type like Pancreatic Ductal Adenocarcinoma (PDCA), researchers rely on preclinical models to explore how well a drug works and whether it is safe. In vitro cell line studies and genetically engineered mouse models (GEMMs) are the two commonly used models, and these tools are essential for studying drugs that target specific pathways, such as those involved in tumor angiogenesis (blood vessel formation) (Bloomston et al., 2002).

In vitro studies are often the first step. Scientists grow pancreatic cancer cells in dishes and test how they respond to different drugs, and these experiments are fast and cost-effective, allowing researchers to focus on specific cancer pathways. For example, drugs like Sunitinib and Verteporfin have been tested this way. Researchers can observe changes in cell growth, survival, and the expression of genes related to angiogenesis, such as VEGF and HIF-1α, with the help of these studies. One of the benefits of using the cell lines in the experiment is that we can use the ability to control the environment completely. Scientists can modify drug doses, quickly spot patterns, and study different pathways. However, the behaviour of cancer is observed differently in a human body and a petri dish. Immune cells, blood vessels, and the surrounding tissue are all absent in these models with which the tumor interacts. This is the reason why in vitro studies are often performed on animal models (Nisar et al., 2022).

To study cancer in a setting that more closely mimics the human body, Genetically Engineered Mouse Models (GEMMs) are often used by researchers. Genetic mutations like those seen in human pancreatic cancer, like KRAS AND TP53 mutations, are carried by these mice. And as a result, this causes the tumors to behave and develop just like those in humans. Drugs that target angiogenesis are studied by GEMMs because it is especially used for that. A great example is the RIP-Tag2 mouse model, which is used to study pancreatic neuroendocrine tumors. Researchers tested drugs like nintedanib and clodronate in these mice and found that they could block blood vessel formation and reduce tumor size. These models also allow researchers to observe how tumors adapt over time. Some pancreatic tumors escape anti-angiogenic treatment by forming vessel-like structures without actual blood vessels, a process called vasculogenic mimicry, or by using nearby normal vessels, known as vessel co-option. The ability to test drug combinations, such as pairing anti-angiogenic agents with chemotherapy, makes GEMMs especially valuable, which helps researchers predict not just how effective the treatment is, but also how the tumor environment might influence the outcome.

Both in vitro and mouse models are critical in the journey of developing new treatments. While in vitro studies offer just fast insights into how a drug affects cancer cells, mouse models show how those effects play out in living organisms. Together, they give scientists the evidence they need to move forward into clinical trials and one step closer to better therapies for pancreatic cancer.

Key Completed Clinical Trials in Pancreatic Cancer: Wins, Losses, and Lessons Learned

Over several years, numerous clinical trials have aimed to improve outcomes for pancreatic cancer patients, and many by targeted key biological pathways like angiogenesis. Although there have been some encouraging results, many have also exposed how tough and unrelenting this disease truly is (Nisar et al., 2022).

One of the most notable breakthroughs came with Sunitinib, which is a multitargeted tyrosine kinase inhibitor. Sunitinib was first introduced as a cancer treatment and later found its way into trials for patients with pancreatic neuroendocrine tumors (PNETs), a rarer type of pancreatic cancer that is often easier to manage. The results were promising; patients saw a meaningful improvement in how long their disease stayed under control, which ultimately led to the drug being approved for use in this specific group. While it was not a cure-all, it offered a much-needed sense of hope for those who previously had very few options.

Everolimus is another example, a drug designed to target the mTOR pathway, which plays a key role in how cancer cells grow and develop blood vessels. When tested in patients with pancreatic neuroendocrine tumors (PNETs), it showed real promise by slowing down how quickly the tumor progresses. What made it especially significant was the way it highlighted how targeted treatments can truly make a difference when the therapy is tailored to the tumor's specific biology.

Pazopanib has also shown some encouraging results in this area. Although it has not been officially approved for pancreatic cancer, studies in patients with neuroendocrine tumors revealed noticeable improvements. It works by targeting several pathways involved in blood vessel growth, and some patients, especially those who did not respond to earlier treatments, benefited from it. These kinds of outcomes remind us how crucial it is to match the right treatment with the right patient, particularly when dealing with targeted therapies. In these cases, success was not just about the drug itself. But about matching the drug to the biology of the tumor (Robatel & Schenk, 2022).

On the other side, many trials aimed at pancreatic ductal adenocarcinoma (PDCA) did not meet expectations. One example is the widely studied drug Bevacizumab, an antibody that targets VEGF (a key molecule in angiogenesis). While it worked well in other cancers, large phase III trials combining Bevacizumab with gemcitabine in PDCA patients failed to show any significant survival benefit.

Another disappointment came with Axitinib, another VEGF pathway blocker. Despite encouraging results in earlier trials, the larger studies did not replicate the same benefits in overall survival. Similarly, attempts to combine Sorafenib, a multi-kinase inhibitor, with chemotherapy did not produce the hoped-for results, though interestingly, some subgroups with specific biomarkers like low LDH levels seemed to fare better.

These setbacks did not mean the science was flawed, but rather highlighted the complexity of pancreatic tumors, especially how they interact with their surrounding environment. And the lesson is simply that blocking one pathway often is not enough. Tumors find ways around the roadblocks. That is why researchers now focus more on combination therapies, better biomarkers, and personalized approaches (Aslan et al., 2018).

Ongoing Clinical Trials: A Forward-Looking Perspective

Pancreatic Ductal Adenocarcinoma (PDCA) continues to be one of the most difficult cancers to treat, but there is hope on the horizon as a wave of clinical trials is currently underway, aiming to bring in next-generation therapies. These trials are exploring not just one approach but a spectrum of options, ranging from gene-targeting drugs to novel immunotherapies and personalised vaccines (Wenzel et al., 2024).

A key area of current focus is targeting KRAS mutations, which are present in over 90% of PDAC cases. While Kras G12C accounts for a small fraction of these mutations, early studies using drugs like *sotorasib* and *adagrasib* have shown promise in small patient groups. The *CodeBreaK 101* and *KRYSTAL-1* trials are now looking at combining these agents with other treatments to boost efficiency. Meanwhile, new drugs like MRTX1133 and RMC-9805, which target the more common KRAS G12D mutations, are under evaluation in early-phase trials (NCT05737706, NCT06040541), marking an important step in addressing a previously "undruggable" target.

There is an increasing interest in comprehensive RAS pathway inhibition beyond single mutations. This includes attempts to target pan-RAS mechanisms and associated downstream signalling elements such as MEK and RAF. Drugs are being tested either as standalone agents or in combination, trying to shut down the redundant backup systems that cancer cells often activate when one pathway is blocked.

On the immune front, adoptive cell transfer therapies like *CAR-T* and *TCR-T* are being developed to recognize and attack pancreatic cancer cells. These treatments are personalized by targeting specific tumor markers, such as KRAS G12D/G12V, TP53, and mesothelin. While still early, some trials have already shown partial responses and stable disease in patients who previously failed conventional therapies. Trials like NCT04146298 and NCT03745326 are currently assessing safety and response rates in these settings.

Vaccine strategies are also gaining traction. A good example is *auto gene cevumeran*, a custom-made mRNA vaccine designed to target specific tumor markers. It is currently being tested alongside chemotherapy and immune checkpoint drugs in patients with either resected or advanced pancreatic cancer. Other vaccines like GVAX and dendritic cell-based therapies are also getting renewed attention, especially in combination approaches aimed at boosting the body's immune response.

Some ongoing trials are focusing on patients whose tumors have trouble repairing DNA, particularly those with changes in the *BRCA* or *PALB2* genes. These studies are looking at using PARP inhibitors to help control the disease. In some cases, they are testing these drugs alongside immunotherapies, hoping the combination might work better by overcoming resistance, like in the POLAR trial NCT04666740).

Another important focus is ongoing research is the area around the tumor itself, often called the tumor microenvironment. Scientists are exploring new treatments that can block signals or structures that help the tumor hide from the immune system and resist therapy. For example, drugs like *CD40 agonists* and *CCR/CCR5 inhibitors* are being tested to help make the tumor more visible and vulnerable to treatment.

FUTURE TRENDS AND TECHNOLOGIES MODULE

These ongoing trials show a clear move toward more personalised treatment approaches in pancreatic cancer, based on the unique biology of each patient's tumor. By combining tools like genetic testing, immune system analysis, and targeted drugs, researchers are working to overcome the long-standing challenges in treating PDCA disease. While many of these treatments are still in early stages, the range and depth of today's trials give real hope that better options could be on the way soon.

Why have many treatments failed in Clinical Trials for Pancreatic Cancer?

Many treatments for Pancreatic Cancer that looked promising in early research have unfortunately failed to succeed in clinical trials. This is mainly because pancreatic cancer is extremely complex and aggressive, with multiple genetic changes driving its growth. Targeting just one pathway is often not enough, as cancer cells find ways to survive by activating other pathways (Neoptolemos et al., 2018).

The design of clinical trials themselves has also contributed to disappointing results. Trials often include patients with highly advanced disease and poor overall health, making it difficult to demonstrate clear benefits from new therapies. Additionally, a lack of reliable biomarkers for patient selection has led to trials that enroll diverse patient groups without matching treatments to the specific molecular profile of their tumors.

Another big reason is the tumor's ability to develop resistance. Even when the drug initially works, the cancer can change or adapt, making the treatment ineffective over time. The presence of a defense and protective tumor environment also blocks drugs from reaching the cancer cells and weakens the immune system's ability to fight the disease (Waddell et al., 2015).

Additionally, most pancreatic cancers are diagnosed very late, when the disease is already too advanced for targeted treatments to work well. Clinical trials also often include patients with different genetic profiles without matching the right drug to the right patient, reducing the chances of success. Finally, many experimental treatments come with serious side effects that limit how much of the drug can be safely given. All these factors together explain why progress has been slow, and highlight the need for better patient selection, combination therapies, and early detection to improve future outcomes.

Novel Therapeutic Targets in Pancreatic Cancer

One of the most critical areas of progress in pancreatic cancer research is the identification of new molecular targets. Traditional chemotherapy has limited effectiveness, so newer, more precise treatments are being explored. A prime target is the KRAS gene, mutated in over 90% of PDAC cases. While KRAS mutations have long been considered "undruggable," recent breakthroughs in targeted inhibitors, particularly those aimed at KRAS G12C, have shown promise in preclinical and early clinical trials. Beyond KRAS, other genetic alterations are also under investigation. For example, CDKN2A deletions and SMAD4 inactivation are common in pancreatic tumors and have been linked to poor prognosis. These mutations affect cell cycle regulation and the TGF-β signalling pathway, making them attractive targets for therapeutic intervention. Additionally, PRMT5 inhibitors show potential in patients with MTAP-deleted tumors, a subset of PDAC characterized by loss of tumor suppressor function (Neoptolemos et al., 2018; Xu et al., 2022).

Other emerging targets include Claudin 18.2, NGR1 fusions. And the DNA damage repair pathways, such as those associated with BRCA1/2 mutations. In BRCA-mutated patients, PARP inhibitors like Olaparib have demonstrated benefit by exploiting synthetic lethality mechanisms, especially when used as maintenance therapy after initial chemotherapy (Kleeff et al., 2016).

Efforts are also being made to reactivate the immune system within the hostile tumor microenvironment. Pancreatic cancer is notoriously resistant to immunotherapies due to its desmoplastic stroma and low immunogenicity. However, newer strategies, such as combining immune checkpoint inhibitors with vaccines, CD40 agonists, or oncolytic viruses, are being evaluated to improve immune infiltration and effectiveness.

Advances in Drug Delivery Systems

Another challenge in pancreatic cancer therapy is the dense stromal barrier surrounding the tumour. This fibrotic tissue hinders drug penetration, reducing treatment efficacy. Innovative drug delivery systems are being designed to overcome this barrier and improve therapeutic outcomes (Nishimoto, 2022).

One such advancement is the use of nanoparticle-based drug carriers. These systems allow for targeted delivery of chemotherapeutic agents directly to the tumor, minimizing toxicity to healthy tissues and increasing the concentration. Gemcitabine is a good example already in clinical use. Other approaches involve liposomes, dendrimers, and biodegradable polymers designed to slowly release drugs in the tumour microenvironment (Conte & Caude, 2022).

Enzyme-based therapies also aim to dismantle the fibrotic barrier. PEGylated hyaluronidase, for instance, has been tested to break down hyaluronic acid in the extracellular matrix, improving drug perfusion and access to cancer cells (Cui et al., 2015). Although some trials have faced setbacks, the concept continues to hold potential when combined with cytotoxic and targeted therapies.

In addition to physical drug carriers, researchers are exploring stimulus-responsive systems that release their content in response to specific tumour characteristics such as pH, enzymes, or heat, providing another layer of specificity and control.

Integration of Artificial Intelligence in Drug Discovery

In recent years, artificial intelligence (AI) has begun to reshape the landscape of medical research, particularly in how we approach the discovery and development of new treatments for diseases like pancreatic cancer. By analysing enormous amounts of data that range from genetic profiles and protein expression to medical imaging and clinical outcomes, AI tools can identify connections that would be nearly impossible for humans to detect manually, and they can do so with remarkable speed (Kenner et al., 2021).

Drug repurposing is one of the most exciting applications of AI in this field, which involves finding new uses for medications that are already approved for other conditions. Using machine learning techniques, researchers can scan through large datasets to spot drugs that may also be effective against pancreatic tumours, dramatically cutting down the time and cost typically required to bring new treatments to trial. In addition, AI can assist scientists in designing entirely new drug compounds by predicting how these molecules might interact with specific genetic mutations found in pancreatic cancer (Pourmousa et al., 2025).

AI is also making strides in diagnosis. For instance, advanced computer models can now interpret CT and MRI scans with exceptional precision. These systems are trained to recognize even the smallest irregularities in pancreatic tissue, abnormalities that may be too subtle for the human eye to catch. As a result, this technology has the potential to help detect cancer at an earlier stage, which is critical, given that many patients are diagnosed only after the disease has progressed (Kenner et al., 2021).

CONCLUSION MODULE

Moreover, AI-powered models are being developed to help predict how a patient is likely to respond to certain treatments or how their disease may progress. By collecting information from pathology reports, laboratory tests, genetic markers, and previous treatment outcomes, these systems can offer insights that support more personalized treatment decisions, ultimately leading to better care and fewer unnecessary harmful side effects.

Role of Liquid Biopsies and Circulating Tumour DNA

In pancreatic cancer, traditional tissue biopsies often pose a challenge due to the deep and inaccessible location of the pancreas. As a result, obtaining samples safely and effectively can be difficult. In response, a new method known as liquid biopsy has emerged, offering a less invasive and more practical solution. This technique involves analysing a simple blood sample for markers such as circulating tumour DNA (ctDNA) or circulating tumour cells (CTSs), providing valuable information about the cancer without needing surgery (Hussain et al., 2025).

One of the major advantages of ctDNA testing is its ability to detect specific genetic mutations related to the tumour. This not only aids in diagnosis but also helps monitor how the disease responds to treatment. By tracking mutation over time, particularly those in genes like KRAS, which is frequently mutated in pancreatic cancer, doctors can determine whether a treatment is working or if the tumour is developing resistance. This ongoing monitoring allows for quicker adjustments in therapy, often before changes would appear on scans or traditional lab tests.

Liquid biopsies are also gaining attention for their potential to identify tiny traces of cancer that may remain after surgery or chemotherapy, a condition known as minimal residual disease (MRD). If ctDNA is found after what was thought to be the curative procedure, it could signal the need for additional treatment or closer observation, offering a chance to act before the cancer grows back (Chen et al., 2021).

As this technology continues to evolve, it is becoming more accurate, more affordable, and more integrated into regular cancer care. The hope soon, liquid biopsies will become a standard part of managing pancreatic cancer, allowing for more precise and timely treatment decisions.

Looking ahead, the outlook for pancreatic cancer treatment is gradually improving. With innovations like liquid biopsies, targeted therapies (Strimpakos et al., 2008), advanced drug delivery methods, and personalized treatment strategies, the approach to this disease is becoming more patient-focused and effective. While serious challenges still exist, such as resistance to treatment, tumour complexity, and late diagnosis, these advances represent a move toward turning pancreatic cancer into a more manageable condition. Continued research and collaboration are key to realizing that goal.

Figure 5. Role of Liquid Biopsy and Circulating Tumor DNA in Pancreatic Cancer

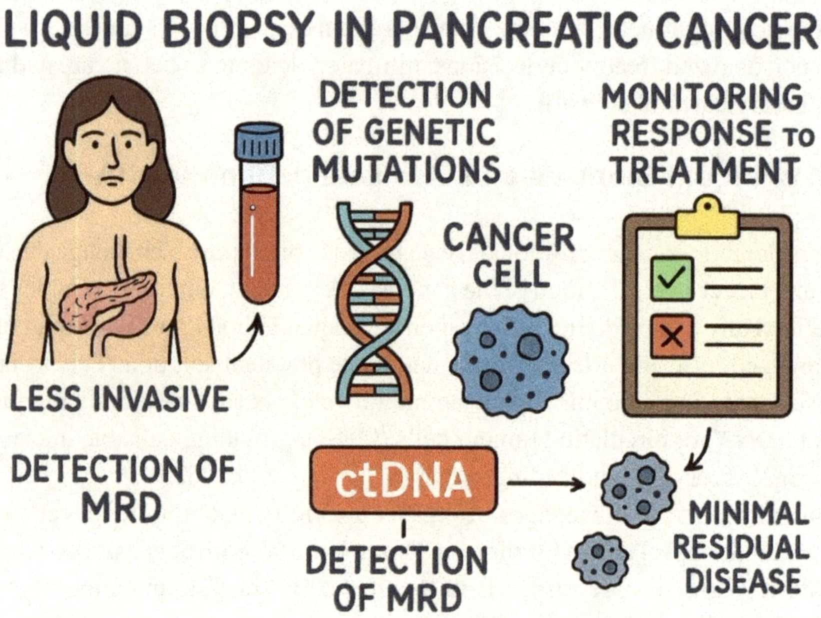

FUTURE DIRECTIONS, EMERGING TRENDS, AND RECENT ADVANCES IN BIOMARKERS

Pancreatic cancer, especially the common type known as pancreatic ductal adenocarcinoma. Pathway redundancy, drug resistance, need for combination therapies

(PDCA) (O'Reilly & Buckley, 2024) are still among the deadliest cancers worldwide. Even though research is ongoing and treatments have come a long way, survival rates remain very low. That is mainly because the disease is usually found late, spreads quickly, and often does not respond well to standard treatments (Haller, 2002). As science advances, several promising avenues are emerging, aimed at overcoming the limitations approaches. These include novel therapeutic targets, cutting-edge drug delivery systems, the application of artificial intelligence in drug discovery, and the use of liquid biopsies for non-invasive cancer monitoring (Wenzel et al., 2024).

One of the most precise challenges in pancreatic cancer remains the difficulty of detecting the disease at an early, treatable stage. Recent years have seen significant progress in the search for diagnostic biomarkers that could allow for earlier identification and better monitoring of pancreatic cancer, particularly pancreatic ductal adenocarcinoma (PDAC). Several recent studies (Lee et al., 2014), including those by, have highlighted the potential of KRAS mutation detection in plasma as a minimally invasive method to help guide clinical decisions.

In addition to the genetic mutations, there is growing interest in examining DNA methylation patterns in circulating cell-free DNA (cfDNA). Abnormal methylation-chemical changes to DNA that can switch genes on or off- may serve as another early signal of pancreatic cancer. Studies have shown that measuring these changes through blood samples could improve early detection when combined with other biomarkers (Cao et al., 2023).

Beyond ctDNA, researchers are also exploring the role of microRNAs, exosomes, and metabolomic signatures as possible diagnostic tools. These biomarkers, detected in blood or other body fluids, may complement existing markers like CA 19-9 (Kim et al., 2023), which, while commonly used, lack sensitivity and specificity for early diagnosis. Parallel to advances in blood-based diagnostics, developments in imaging technology are also helping to improve early detection. Tools like computed tomography (CT), magnetic resonance imaging (MRI), and endoscopic ultrasound (EUS) remain central to diagnosing pancreatic cancer. However, artificial intelligence is now being used to analyse imaging data in new ways. By applying AI-driven radiomics (Vétil et al., 2023), researchers can extract subtle patterns from scans that may not be visible to the human eye, potentially identifying cancer earlier or predicting how aggressive it might be.

REFERENCES MODULE

Conclusion

Pancreatic Cancer is, without a doubt, one of the most difficult battles a person can face. Especially the most common form, pancreatic ductal adenocarcinoma (PDAC), patients are often met with a diagnosis that comes late, at a point when treatment options are limited and the disease has already progressed. It is a cancer that tends to move quietly, without obvious symptoms, until it is too far along. That is one of the reasons survival rates have stayed low for so long, despite decades of research and effort (Gopinathan et al., 2015).

Science has made meaningful progress in understanding what makes this cancer so stubborn, from its complex genetic makeup to the protective tissue that surrounds tumors and makes drug delivery so hard. Researchers now know that no single treatment is likely to work on its own. Instead, the focus is moving toward combination approaches, mixing traditional chemotherapy with newer options like targeted drugs, and even experimental cancer vaccines (Adiseshaiah et al., 2016).

We are also learning that the biology of each patient's tumour matters. Treatments like PRAP inhibitors for patients with BRAC mutation, or KRAS inhibitors for specific subtypes, show that when we match the right therapy with the right patient, real results can follow. It is no longer about just treating cancer; it is about understanding it at a deeper level and personalizing the fight (Zhou et al., 2019; Zhang et al., 2017; Luo et al., 2023).

Immunotherapy, a treatment that has shown incredible results in other cancers, has not had the same success in pancreatic cancer, yet. But researchers are not giving up. They are trying new combinations: pairing immune-based treatments with chemotherapy or agents that alter the tumour's environment to make it more vulnerable. There is also growing excitement around therapies like CAR-T, which use a patient's immune cells to attack the cancer directly (Cao et al., 2021).

One of the most encouraging developments is the rise of liquid biopsies, a simple blood test that can give doctors a real-time picture of how the tumor is behaving. These tests can catch important changes early, even before a scan would show something, allowing treatment to be adjusted faster. They are also being used to check if any cancer is left after surgery, helping guide follow-up care and possibly preventing recurrence (Linehan et al., 2024).

And let us not forget how far drug delivery has come. In the past, getting medicine into the actual tumour was a major hurdle. Now, with innovations like nanoparticles and special enzymes that break down the tumor's dense shield of tissue, drugs can reach their target more effectively, and with fewer side effects for the patient.

Even artificial intelligence is stepping into the picture. It is helping researchers comb through massive amounts of data, find patterns that humans might miss, and even predict which treatments could work best for a specific individual (Pourmousa et al., 2025). It is not science fiction anymore; it is becoming part of how we approach real-world cancer care. Still, it is important to be honest that we are not there yet. Pancreatic cancer is incredibly complex. It adapts, it resists, and it often does not play by the rules. Many patients are still diagnosed too late, and some tumours do not respond the way we hope. But even with these setbacks, what we have now that we did not before is direction and a growing sense of possibility.

The future is not guaranteed, but it is looking brighter. With every trial, every experiment, every patient who participates in research, we move a little closer to better answers. Maybe one day, not too far off, pancreatic cancer will not be a certain end, but another fight that patients can win (Wenzel et al., 2024).

REFERENCES

Adiseshaiah, P. P., Crist, R. M., Hook, S. S., & McNeil, S. E. (2016). Nanomedicine strategies to overcome the pathophysiological barriers of pancreatic cancer. *Nature Reviews. Clinical Oncology, 13*(12), 750–765. DOI: 10.1038/nrclinonc.2016.119

Annese, T., Tamma, R., Ruggieri, S., & Ribatti, D. (2019). Angiogenesis in pancreatic cancer: Pre-clinical and clinical studies. *Cancers (Basel), 11*(3), 381. DOI: 10.3390/cancers11030381

Arensman, M. D., Kovochich, A. N., Kulikauskas, R. M., Lay, A. R., Yang, P. T., Li, X., Donahue, T., Major, M. B., Moon, R. T., Chien, A. J., & Dawson, D. W. (2014). WNT7B mediates autocrine Wnt/β-catenin signaling and anchorage-independent growth in pancreatic adenocarcinoma. *Oncogene, 33*(7), 899–908. DOI: 10.1038/onc.2013.23

Aslan, M., Shahbazi, R., Ulubayram, K., & Ozpolat, B. (2018). Targeted therapies for pancreatic cancer and hurdles ahead. *Anticancer Research, 38*(12), 6591–6606. DOI: 10.21873/anticanres.13026

Bloomston, M., Zervos, E. E., & Rosemurgy, A. S.II. (2002). Matrix metalloproteinases and their role in pancreatic cancer: A review of preclinical studies and clinical trials. *Annals of Surgical Oncology, 9*(7), 668–674. DOI: 10.1007/BF02574483

Büchler, P., Gazdhar, A., Schubert, M., Giese, N., Reber, H. A., Hines, O. J., & Friess, H. (2005). The Notch signaling pathway is related to neurovascular progression of pancreatic cancer. *Annals of Surgery, 242*(6), 791–801. DOI: 10.1097/01.sla.0000189115.94847.f1

Buscail, L., Bournet, B., & Cordelier, P. (2020). Role of oncogenic KRAS in the diagnosis, prognosis, and treatment of pancreatic cancer. *Nature Reviews. Gastroenterology & Hepatology, 17*(3), 153–168. DOI: 10.1038/s41575-019-0245-4

Caldas, C., & Kern, S. E. (1995). K-ras mutation and pancreatic adenocarcinoma. *International Journal of Pancreatology, 18*(1), 1–6. DOI: 10.1007/BF02825415

Cao, D., Song, Q., Li, J., Jiang, Y., Wang, Z., & Lu, S. (2021). Opportunities and challenges in targeted therapy and immunotherapy for pancreatic cancer. *Expert Reviews in Molecular Medicine, 23*, e21. DOI: 10.1017/erm.2021.26

Cao, L., Huang, X., Yu, J., Liao, Z., & Zhang, J. (2023). Cell-free DNA methylation markers in plasma for early detection of pancreatic cancer. *Biomarker Research, 11*(1), 88. DOI: 10.1186/s40364-023-00528-y

Catenacci, D. V.. (2015). Randomized phase IB/II study of gemcitabine plus placebo or vismodegib in patients with metastatic pancreatic cancer. *PLoS One*, *10*(4), e0127770. DOI: 10.1371/journal.pone.0127770

Chen, L., Xu, Z., Li, Q., Feng, Q., Zheng, C., Du, Y., Yuan, R., & Peng, X. (2021). USP28 facilitates pancreatic cancer progression through activation of the Wnt/β-catenin pathway via stabilising FOXM1. *Cell Death & Disease*, *12*(10), 887. DOI: 10.1038/s41419-021-04163-z

Chen, X., Zeh, H. J., Kang, R., Kroemer, G., & Tang, D. (2021). Cell death in pancreatic cancer: From pathogenesis to therapy. *Nature Reviews. Gastroenterology & Hepatology*, *18*(11), 804–823. DOI: 10.1038/s41575-021-00486-6

Conte, M., & Cauda, V. (2022). Multimodal therapies against pancreatic ductal adenocarcinoma: A review on synergistic approaches toward ultimate nanomedicine treatments. *Advanced Therapeutics*, *5*(11), 2200079. DOI: 10.1002/adtp.202200079

Craven, K. E., Gore, J., & Korc, M. (2016). Overview of pre-clinical and clinical studies targeting angiogenesis in pancreatic ductal adenocarcinoma. *Cancer Letters*, *381*(1), 201–210. DOI: 10.1016/j.canlet.2015.11.047

Cui, J., Jiang, W., Wang, S., Wang, L., & Xie, K. (2012). Role of Wnt/β-catenin signaling in drug resistance of pancreatic cancer. *Current Pharmaceutical Design*, *18*(17), 2464–2471. DOI: 10.2174/13816128112092464

Gao, J., Long, B., & Wang, Z. (2017). Role of Notch signaling pathway in pancreatic cancer. *American Journal of Cancer Research*, *7*(2), 173.

Gopinathan, A., Morton, J. P., Jodrell, D. I., & Sansom, O. J. (2015). GEMMs as preclinical models for testing pancreatic cancer therapies. *Disease Models & Mechanisms*, *8*(10), 1185–1200. DOI: 10.1242/dmm.021055

Haller, D. G. (2002, December). Future directions in the treatment of pancreatic cancer. [). WB Saunders.]. *Seminars in Oncology*, *29*(6), 31–39. DOI: 10.1016/S0093-7754(02)70024-9

Hammel, P., Huguet, F., Van Laethem, J. L., Goldstein, D., Glimelius, B., Artru, P., Borbath, I., Bouché, O., Shannon, J., André, T., Mineur, L., Chibaudel, B., Bonnetain, F., & Louvet, C. (2016). Effect of chemoradiotherapy vs chemotherapy on survival in patients with locally advanced pancreatic cancer controlled after 4 months of gemcitabine with or without erlotinib: The LAP07 randomized clinical trial. *Journal of the American Medical Association*, *315*(17), 1844–1853. DOI: 10.1001/jama.2016.4324

Hussain, M. S., Prajapati, B. G., Gandhi, S. M., Sharma, M., Kapoor, D. U., Elossaily, G. M., & Garg, S. (2025). Overcoming obstacles: The role of lipid nanocarriers in therapeutic approaches for pancreatic cancer. *BioNanoScience*, *15*(2), 262. DOI: 10.1007/s12668-025-01873-y

Ishikawa, T., Okayama, T., Oka, K., Mizushima, K., Yasuda, T., Sakamoto, N., & Itoh, Y. (2017). The JAK/STAT pathway is involved in the upregulation of PD-L1 expression in pancreatic cancer cell lines. *Oncology Reports*, *37*(3), 1545–1554. DOI: 10.3892/or.2017.5399

Javadinia, S. A., Shahidsales, S., Fanipakdel, A., Joudi-Mashhad, M., Mehramiz, M., Talebian, S., Maftouh, M., Mardani, R., Hassanian, S. M., Khazaei, M., Ferns, G. A., & Avan, A. (2019). Therapeutic potential of targeting the Wnt/β-catenin pathway in the treatment of pancreatic cancer. *Journal of Cellular Biochemistry*, *120*(5), 6833–6840. DOI: 10.1002/jcb.27835

Javle, M., Li, Y., Tan, D., Dong, X., Chang, P., Kar, S., & Li, D. (2014). Biomarkers of TGF-β signaling pathway and prognosis of pancreatic cancer. *PLoS One*, *9*(1), e85942. DOI: 10.1371/journal.pone.0085942

Kelleher, F. C. (2011). Hedgehog signaling and therapeutics in pancreatic cancer. *Carcinogenesis*, *32*(4), 445–451. DOI: 10.1093/carcin/bgq280

Kenner, B., Chari, S. T., Kelsen, D., Klimstra, D. S., Pandol, S. J., Rosenthal, M., Rustgi, A. K., Taylor, J. A., Yala, A., Abul-Husn, N., Andersen, D. K., Bernstein, D., Brunak, S., Canto, M. I., Eldar, Y. C., Fishman, E. K., Fleshman, J., Go, V. L. W., Holt, J. M., & Wolpin, B. (2021). Artificial intelligence and early detection of pancreatic cancer: 2020 summative review. *Pancreas*, *50*(3), 251–279. DOI: 10.1097/MPA.0000000000001762

Kim, J., Bamlet, W. R., Oberg, A. L., Chaffee, K. G., & Petersen, G. M. (2023). CA 19-9 and emerging biomarkers for the early detection of pancreatic cancer. *World Journal of Gastroenterology*, *29*(10), 1387–1400.

Kleeff, J., Korc, M., Apte, M., La Vecchia, C., Johnson, C. D., Biankin, A. V., Neale, R. E., Tempero, M., Tuveson, D. A., Hruban, R. H., & Neoptolemos, J. P. (2016). Pancreatic cancer. *Nature Reviews. Disease Primers*, *2*(1), 16022. DOI: 10.1038/nrdp.2016.22

Lee, J. J., Perera, R. M., Wang, H., Wu, D. C., Liu, X. S., Han, S., Fitamant, J., Jones, P. D., Ghanta, K. S., Kawano, S., Nagle, J. M., Deshpande, V., Boucher, Y., Kato, T., Chen, J. K., Willmann, J. K., Bardeesy, N., & Beachy, P. A. (2014). Stromal response to Hedgehog signaling restrains pancreatic cancer progression. *Proceedings of the National Academy of Sciences of the United States of America, 111*(30), E3091–E3100. DOI: 10.1073/pnas.1411679111

Linehan, A., O'Reilly, M., McDermott, R., & O'Kane, G. M. (2024). Targeting KRAS mutations in pancreatic cancer: Opportunities for future strategies. *Frontiers in Medicine, 11*, 1369136. DOI: 10.3389/fmed.2024.1369136

Liu, L., Huang, X., Shi, F., Song, J., Guo, C., Yang, J., Liang, T., & Bai, X. (2022). Combination therapy for pancreatic cancer: anti-PD-(L) 1-based strategy. *Journal of Experimental & Clinical Cancer Research : CR, 41*(1), 56. DOI: 10.1186/s13046-022-02273-w

Luo, Q., Hu, Z., Zhao, H., Fan, Y., Tu, X., Wang, Y., & Liu, X. (2023). The role of TGF-β in the tumor microenvironment of pancreatic cancer. *Genes & Diseases, 10*(4), 1513–1524. DOI: 10.1016/j.gendis.2022.10.019

Ma, J., Xia, J., Miele, L., Sarkar, F. H., & Wang, Z. (2013). Notch signaling pathway in pancreatic cancer progression. *Pancreatic Disorders & Therapy, 3*(114), 1000114. DOI: 10.4172/2165-7092.1000114

McGuigan, A., Kelly, P., Turkington, R. C., Jones, C., Coleman, H. G., & McCain, R. S. (2018). Pancreatic cancer: A review of clinical diagnosis, epidemiology, treatment, and outcomes. *World Journal of Gastroenterology, 24*(43), 4846–4861. DOI: 10.3748/wjg.v24.i43.4846

Melisi, D.. (2018). Galunisertib plus gemcitabine vs. gemcitabine for first-line treatment of unresectable pancreatic cancer: A randomized phase II study. *British Journal of Cancer, 119*(10), 1208–1214. DOI: 10.1038/s41416-018-0246-z

Murtaugh, L. C. (2008). The what, where, when, and how of Wnt/β-catenin signaling in pancreas development. *Organogenesis, 4*(2), 81–86. DOI: 10.4161/org.4.2.5853

Neoptolemos, J. P., Kleeff, J., Michl, P., Costello, E., Greenhalf, W., & Palmer, D. H. (2018). Therapeutic developments in pancreatic cancer: Current and future perspectives. *Nature Reviews. Gastroenterology & Hepatology, 15*(6), 333–348. DOI: 10.1038/s41575-018-0005-x

Nisar, M., Paracha, R. Z., Adil, S., Qureshi, S. N., & Janjua, H. A. (2022). An extensive review of preclinical and clinical trials of oncolytic virus therapy for pancreatic cancer. *Frontiers in Oncology, 12*, 875188. DOI: 10.3389/fonc.2022.875188

Nishimoto, A. (2022). Effective combinations of anti-cancer and targeted drugs for pancreatic cancer treatment. *World Journal of Gastroenterology, 28*(28), 3637–3643. DOI: 10.3748/wjg.v28.i28.3637

O'Reilly, E. M., & Buckley, C. W. (2024). Next-generation therapies for pancreatic cancer. *Expert Review of Gastroenterology & Hepatology, 18*(1–3), 55–72.

Onishi, H., & Katano, M. (2014). Hedgehog signaling pathway as a new therapeutic target in pancreatic cancer. World journal of gastroenterology. *World Journal of Gastroenterology, 20*(9), 2335. DOI: 10.3748/wjg.v20.i9.2335

Palagani, V., Bozko, P., El Khatib, M., Belahmer, H., Giese, N., Sipos, B., Malek, N. P., & Plentz, R. R. (2014). Combined inhibition of Notch and JAK/STAT is superior to monotherapies and impairs pancreatic cancer progression. *Carcinogenesis, 35*(4), 859–866. DOI: 10.1093/carcin/bgt394

Pourmousa, M., Jain, S., Barnaeva, E., Jin, W., Hochuli, J., Itkin, Z., Maxfield, T., Melo-Filho, C., Thieme, A., Wilson, K., Klumpp-Thomas, C., Michael, S., Southall, N., Jaakkola, T., Muratov, E. N., Barzilay, R., Tropsha, A., Ferrer, M., & Zakharov, A. V. (2025). AI-driven discovery of synergistic drug combinations against pancreatic cancer. *Nature Communications, 16*(1), 4020. DOI: 10.1038/s41467-025-56818-6

Ram Makena, M., Gatla, H., Verlekar, D., Sukhavasi, S., & Pandey, K., M., & C. Pramanik, K. (. (2019). Wnt/β-catenin signaling: The culprit in pancreatic carcinogenesis and therapeutic resistance. *International Journal of Molecular Sciences, 20*(17), 4242. DOI: 10.3390/ijms20174242

Ristorcelli, E., & Lombardo, D. (2010). Targeting Notch signaling in pancreatic cancer. *Expert Opinion on Therapeutic Targets, 14*(5), 541–552. DOI: 10.1517/14728221003769895

Robatel, S., & Schenk, M. (2022). Current limitations and novel perspectives in pancreatic cancer treatment. *Cancers (Basel), 14*(4), 985. DOI: 10.3390/cancers14040985

Ryan, M. B., Fece de la Cruz, F., Phat, S., Myers, D. T., Wong, E., Shahzade, H. A., Hong, C. B., & Corcoran, R. B. (2020). Vertical pathway inhibition overcomes adaptive feedback resistance to KRASG12C inhibition. *Clinical Cancer Research, 26*(7), 1633–1643. DOI: 10.1158/1078-0432.CCR-19-3523

Sano, M., Driscoll, D. R., DeJesus-Monge, W. E., Quattrochi, B., Appleman, V. A., Ou, J., Zhu, L. J., Yoshida, N., Yamazaki, S., Takayama, T., Sugitani, M., Nemoto, N., Klimstra, D. S., & Lewis, B. C. (2016). Activation of WNT/β-catenin signaling enhances pancreatic cancer development and the malignant potential via up-regulation of Cyr61. *Neoplasia : an International Journal for Oncology Research*, *18*(12), 785–794. DOI: 10.1016/j.neo.2016.11.004

Saung, M. T., Muth, S., Ding, D., & Armstrong, T. D. (2020). Targeting the tumour microenvironment in pancreatic ductal adenocarcinoma: Rationale and current status. *Cancers (Basel)*, *12*(5), 1156. DOI: 10.3390/cancers12051156

Shen, W., Tao, G. Q., Zhang, Y., Cai, B., Sun, J., & Tian, Z. Q. (2017). TGF-β in pancreatic cancer initiation and progression: Two sides of the same coin. *Cell & Bioscience*, *7*(1), 1–7. DOI: 10.1186/s13578-017-0168-0

Strimpakos, A., Saif, M. W., & Syrigos, K. N. (2008). Pancreatic cancer: From molecular pathogenesis to targeted therapy. *Cancer and Metastasis Reviews*, *27*(3), 495–522. DOI: 10.1007/s10555-008-9134-y

Sun, C.. (2020). Targeting Wnt signaling in cancer stem cells for cancer therapy. *Pharmaceuticals*, *13*(6), 137. DOI: 10.3390/ph13060137

Vétil, R.. (2023). Non-redundant combination of hand-crafted and deep learning radiomics: Application to early detection of pancreatic cancer. *Scientific Reports*, *13*(1), 2175.

Villanueva, A., García, C., Paules, A. B., Vicente, M., Megías, M., Reyes, G., de Villalonga, P., Agell, N., Lluís, F., Bachs, O., & Capellá, G. (1998). Disruption of the antiproliferative TGF-β signaling pathways in human pancreatic cancer cells. *Oncogene*, *17*(15), 1969–1978. DOI: 10.1038/sj.onc.1202118

Waddell, N., Pajic, M., Patch, A. M., Chang, D. K., Kassahn, K. S., Bailey, P., Johns, A. L., Miller, D., Nones, K., Quek, K., Quinn, M. C. J., Robertson, A. J., Fadlullah, M. Z. H., Bruxner, T. J. C., Christ, A. N., Harliwong, I., Idrisoglu, S., Manning, S., Nourse, C., & Grimmond, S. M. (2015). Whole genomes redefine the mutational landscape of pancreatic cancer. *Nature*, *518*(7540), 495–501. DOI: 10.1038/nature14169

Waddell, N., Pajic, M., Patch, A. M., Chang, D. K., Kassahn, K. S., Bailey, P., Johns, A. L., Miller, D., Nones, K., Quek, K., Quinn, M. C. J., Robertson, A. J., Fadlullah, M. Z. H., Bruxner, T. J. C., Christ, A. N., Harliwong, I., Idrisoglu, S., Manning, S., Nourse, C., & Grimmond, S. M. (2015). Whole genomes redefine the mutational landscape of pancreatic cancer. *Nature*, *518*(7540), 495–501. DOI: 10.1038/nature14169

Wang, Z., Li, Y., Kong, D., Banerjee, S., Ahmad, A., Azmi, A. S., Ali, S., Abbruzzese, J. L., Gallick, G. E., & Sarkar, F. H. (2009). Acquisition of epithelial-mesenchymal transition phenotype of gemcitabine-resistant pancreatic cancer cells is linked with activation of the notch signaling pathway. *Cancer Research*, *69*(6), 2400–2407. DOI: 10.1158/0008-5472.CAN-08-4312

Waters, A. M., & Der, C. J. (2018). KRAS: The critical driver and therapeutic target for pancreatic cancer. *Cold Spring Harbor Perspectives in Medicine*, *8*(9), a031435. DOI: 10.1101/cshperspect.a031435

Wenzel, P., Mogler, C., Görgülü, K., & Algül, H. (2024). Pancreatic Cancer: Current Concepts, Trends, and Future Directions. *The Turkish Journal of Gastroenterology : the Official Journal of Turkish Society of Gastroenterology*, *36*(2), 69–81. DOI: 10.5152/tjg.2024.24544

Xu, H., Banerjee, P., Khan, S. A., Ahsan, F., Yadav, D., & Das, S. (2025). Unveiling circulating targets in pancreatic cancer: Insights from proteogenomic evidence and clinical cohorts. *iScience*, *102304*. Advance online publication. DOI: 10.1016/j.isci.2025.102304

Xu, Z. H., Wang, W. Q., Lou, W. H., & Liu, L. (2022). Insight of pancreatic cancer: Recommendations for improving its therapeutic efficacy in the next decade. *Journal of Pancreatology*, *5*(02), 58–68. DOI: 10.1097/JP9.0000000000000093

Xu, Z. H., Wang, W. Q., Lou, W. H., & Liu, L. (2022). Insight of pancreatic cancer: Recommendations for improving its therapeutic efficacy in the next decade. *Journal of Pancreatology*, *5*(02), 58–68. DOI: 10.1097/JP9.0000000000000093

Yabuuchi, S., Pai, S. G., Campbell, N. R., De Wilde, R. F., De Oliveira, E., Korangath, P., Streppel, M. M., Rasheed, Z. A., Hidalgo, M., Maitra, A., & Rajeshkumar, N. V. (2013). Notch signaling pathway targeted therapy suppresses tumor progression and metastatic spread in pancreatic cancer. *Cancer Letters*, *335*(1), 41–51. DOI: 10.1016/j.canlet.2013.01.054

Yang, Y., Tian, X., Xie, X., Zhuang, Y., Wu, W., & Wang, W. (2010). Expression and regulation of the hedgehog signaling pathway in pancreatic cancer. *Langenbeck's Archives of Surgery*, *395*(5), 515–525. DOI: 10.1007/s00423-009-0493-9

Zeng, G., Germinaro, M., Micsenyi, A., Monga, N. K., Bell, A., Sood, A., Malhotra, V., Sood, N., Midda, V., Monga, D. K., Kokkinakis, D. M., & Monga, S. P. (2006). Aberrant Wnt/β-catenin signaling in pancreatic adenocarcinoma. *Neoplasia : an International Journal for Oncology Research*, *8*(4), 279–289. DOI: 10.1593/neo.05607

Zhang, Q., Lou, Y., Zhang, J., Fu, Q., Wei, T., Sun, X., Chen, Q., Yang, J., Bai, X., & Liang, T. (2017). Hypoxia-inducible factor-2α promotes tumor progression and has crosstalk with Wnt/β-catenin signaling in pancreatic cancer. *Molecular Cancer*, *16*(1), 1–14. DOI: 10.1186/s12943-017-0689-5

Zhang, Y., Zhou, M., Wei, H., Zhou, H., He, J., Lu, Y., Wang, D., Chen, B., Zeng, J., Peng, W., Du, F., Gong, A., & Xu, M. (2017). Furin promotes epithelial-mesenchymal transition in pancreatic cancer cells via Hippo-YAP pathway. *International Journal of Oncology*, *50*(4), 1352–1362. DOI: 10.3892/ijo.2017.3896

Zhou, P., Li, Y., Li, B., Zhang, M., Liu, Y., Yao, Y., & Li, D. (2019). NMIIA promotes tumor growth and metastasis by activating the Wnt/β-catenin signaling pathway and EMT in pancreatic cancer. *Oncogene*, *38*(27), 5500–5515. DOI: 10.1038/s41388-019-0806-6

Zhou, Y., Shan, T., Ding, W., Hua, Z., Shen, Y., Lu, Z., Chen, B., & Dai, T. (2018). Study on mechanism about long noncoding RNA MALAT1 affecting pancreatic cancer by regulating Hippo-YAP signaling. *Journal of Cellular Physiology*, *233*(8), 5805–5814. DOI: 10.1002/jcp.26357

Chapter 2
Microorganisms Involved in Pancreatic Cancer

P. Saranraj
https://orcid.org/0000-0002-5052-6532
Department of Microbiology, Sacred Heart College, Tirupattur, India

L. Charlie Jelura
Department of Microbiology, Sacred Heart College, Tirupattur, India

U. Subhalakshmi
Department of Microbiology, Sacred Heart College, Tirupattur, India

ABSTRACT

Pancreatic cancer is among the deadliest of all cancers in the world, for other contributors in addition to its late-stage diagnosis and poor prognosis and limited therapeutic efficacy are the high mortality rate concerning this type of cancer. Recently, new findings from microbiome investigations point toward the mighty role of microorganisms in the initiation of pancreatic carcinogenesis and pancreatic tumors progression while also posing chronic challenges in treatment responsiveness. Traditionally believed to be free of all microbial life, the pancreas is now revealed to host an aberrant microbiome predominantly sourced from the gut and oral cavity, which inflicts large-scale modifications in its microenvironment. Current dysbiosis promotes chronic inflammation, immune evasion, and carcinogenesis. Several pathogenic species such as Helicobacter pylori, Porphyromonas gingivalis, and some members of Proteobacteria are rightly considered causative of increased pancreatic cancer risk through mechanisms that relate mainly to inflammation, immune suppression, and genotoxic metabolites. Together with that, the emergence of intratumoral bacteria is implicated in chemoresistance chiefly due to the bacterial cytosine deaminase-mediated degradation of gemcitabine. In addition, microbial

DOI: 10.4018/979-8-3373-1469-3.ch002

effluents like Lipopolysaccharides (LPSs) and secondary bile acids would induce tumor-promoting NF-κB and TLR4 signaling. The emerging concept of the tumor microbiome also presents an avenue for novel therapeutic approaches.

1. INTRODUCTION

Pancreatic cancer remains one of the most aggressive and difficult-to-treat malignancies. Its poor prognosis stems from multiple factors, including the absence of reliable early diagnostic markers, its tendency to invade nerves and blood vessels at an early stage, rapid disease progression, and frequent spread to distant organs. Additionally, pancreatic cancer often recurs after surgery, responds poorly to chemotherapy and radiation, and has a high rate of metastasis. Despite decades of advancements in treatments such as targeted therapy, surgery, and chemotherapy, the five-year survival rate remains dismally low at just 9% (Zhang et al., 2018). Genetic mutations in *KRAS*, *TP53*, and *BRCA* have been linked to pancreatic cancer development. While newer techniques like endoscopic ultrasound and ultrasound-guided fine-needle aspiration offer hope for earlier detection, further research is still needed to discover more effective biomarkers and improve early diagnosis rates (Kamisawa et al., 2016).

Anticancer action by modifying the Tumour Immunological Environment, but it can be directly carcinogenic by causing a state of inflammation. Both the induction of cancer and other diseases are affected differently by interactions between microorganisms that are proximal to or distant from tumour tissue. As per research, the microbiome composition is different based on the type of tumour and most of the bacteria in the tumour are intracellular and reside in cancer and immune cells (Nejman et al., 2020). This holds true for Pancreatic cancer as well. As per recent research, bacteria may have a role to play in some Gastrointestinal malignancies. Recent research indicates that the local microbiota within the pancreas may be mirrored in the specific bacterial environment of the pancreatic cyst fluid sample. Pancreatic cancer tissue is colonized by higher numbers of microorganisms, such as bacteria and fungi, than pancreatic tissue. Their presence affects the prognosis and treatment response of pancreatic cancer as well as stimulating the incidence and advancement of the disease (Riquelme et al., 2019). The bacterial groups observed, the normal pancreas showed a proportionally higher abundance of the genus *Brevibacterium* from the order *Chlamydiales* when compared to tissues from pancreatic cancer (PDAC) patients. The very existence of these microbes in a healthy organ raises important questions about their potential function in maintaining pancreatic health.

This relationship may be linked to a broader defense mechanism. In the gut, a key part of our innate immune protection comes from antimicrobial peptides (AMPs), which are primarily produced by Paneth cells. Research suggests the pancreas likely contributes to and strengthens this defensive network (Pushalkar et al., 2018). In fact, these pancreatic AMPs constitute a significant portion—roughly 10%—of the proteins found in pancreatic juice, with digestive enzymes making up the remainder. A fascinating feedback loop exists between these pancreatic peptides and the gut's microbial community. The intestinal microbiota can influence the pancreas's production of AMPs, which in turn helps regulate immune cells within the pancreas itself. Conversely, the AMPs delivered into the digestive tract via pancreatic secretions can alter the composition of the gut microbiome and modulate the local immune environment there (Ahuja et al., 2017)

The interaction among the gut microbiota metabolites forms a network capable of influencing some host behaviour. Microbes produce glycoproteins and fibres from meals such acetic, propionic and butyric acid, known as Short Chain Fatty Acids (SCFAs), during digestion and fermentation and metabolization of protein. For instance, the way SCFA behaves in the colon could affect the synthesis of Glucagon-like peptide-1 (GLP-1), which controls the release of hormones in the pancreas. Enteric microbes and acetogens like *Blautia hydrogenotrophica, Firmicutes* and *Bacteroidetes* produce acetate across the acetyl-CoA, the lactate and the succinate pathways, respectively (Marroncini et al., 2024). *Firmicutes*, including *Eubacterium rectale, Faecalibacterium prausnitzii, Ruminococcus bromii*, and *Eubacterium hallii* can produce butyrate and these bacteria are capable of making the fermentation of resistant starch (Morrison and Preston, 2016 ; Kimura et al., 2020).

The specific roles that short-chain fatty acid (SCFA) receptors play within the pancreas are still not fully understood. Emerging evidence, primarily from mouse studies, indicates that when SCFAs bind to the FFA2 receptor, they can stimulate the liver to produce more glucose while simultaneously lowering circulating insulin levels. A separate receptor, FFA3, appears to exert an inhibitory effect on insulin secretion from pancreatic beta cells. This suppression is likely mediated through the receptor's connection to intracellular Gi protein pathways.

This creates a nuanced regulatory system: the activation of the FFA2 receptor can promote insulin production via one signaling route (Gq/11), while the activation of the FFA3 receptor can inhibit it via another (Gi). Beyond their direct effects on the pancreas, SCFAs also contribute to metabolic health by helping to manage the gut's bacterial ecosystem and fortify the intestinal lining. By strengthening this barrier, SCFAs help prevent a condition known as metabolic endotoxemia—often associated with obesity, a "leaky gut," insulin resistance, and excess fat accumulation (Priyadarshini et al., 2015).

Due to its close anatomical connection to the digestive system, the pancreatic duct presents a potential entry route for microbiota from the esophagus, stomach, duodenum, or biliary tract to reach the pancreas. However, alternative pathways are also possible, including the migration of oral or gut bacteria via the lymphatic system or the bloodstream. Research suggests that even in healthy individuals, minuscule amounts of microbes may occasionally be present in the portal blood circulation (Tilg et al., 2022). Evidence for this bacterial translocation is growing. For instance, studies on cats with acute pancreatitis have shown that *E. coli* can cross the colon wall and travel through the blood to infect the pancreas. In humans, genetic analysis of blood from acute pancreatitis patients has also confirmed the presence of bacteria. While this seems to be a significant factor during disease, such transit is likely much more difficult and rare under healthy conditions. Another proposed route involves oral bacteria, such as *Porphyromonas gingivalis*, which may drain from the oral cavity into the lymphatic system before eventually entering the broader circulation (Iwai, 2009).

2. COMPOSITION OF MICROORGANISMS COLONIZED IN PANCREATIC CANCER TISSUE

2.1 Bacterial Colonization in Pancreatic Cancer Tissue

The pancreatic duct, which carries digestive enzymes from the pancreas, joins the common bile duct from the liver to form a single opening known as the major duodenal papilla. This gateway empties into the small intestine (duodenum). Researchers believe this anatomical connection provides a potential pathway for bacteria to travel from the gastrointestinal tract and oral cavity into the pancreas itself. This theory of bacterial migration is supported by observations in other species. For instance, in feline medicine, studies suggest that *Escherichia coli* (*E. coli*) can reach the pancreas by refluxing backwards from the intestines into the pancreatic duct. It is also theorized that bacteria can cross the wall of the colon and enter the systemic circulation, eventually reaching the pancreas.

. The kidneys, gallbladder, and intestines can all pass pathogens onto the pancreas. It is still unclear how germs enter the pancreas, but theories include the oral route, whereby they travel from the lower gastrointestinal tract to the portal circulation or mesenteric lymph nodes (Thomas and Jobin, 2020). The various pathways through which microbes from different parts of the pancreas reach the organ. Scientists have discovered that the community of bacteria in the pancreas looks almost identical to the community in the duodenum, the first section of the small intestine. This is true for both healthy individuals and patients, indicating that bacteria likely move from the gut into the pancreas.

Both pancreatic colonized bacteria and gut microbiota are associated with the development of illness. The human gut microbiome comprised 25% of the human tumour microbiome, as demonstrated by Riquelme et al. (2019), which also identified that the bacterial community of normal adjacent tissues varied from that of tumours, implicating the possibility that the gut microbiota might target-therapy colonize pancreatic tumours. The bacterial composition of pancreatic cancer tissue varies from that of normal pancreatic tissue, according to studies. In 12 pancreatic ductal adenocarcinoma (PDAC) samples, Pushalkar et al. (2018) characterized the multivariate region of the bacterial 16S ribosomal RNA (rRNA) gene. They identified 13 phyla, with Proteus (45%), Bacteroides (31%), and Firmicutes (22%), being relatively common and present in all samples. Although in low numbers, Actinobacteria (1%), however, were present in all samples. *Elizabethkingia* and *Pseudomonas* genera were also highly prevalent. Geller et al. (2017) performed deep sequencing of Polymerase Chain Reaction (PCR) - amplified bacterial 16S rDNA and rRNA Fluorescence *in situ* Hybridization (FISH) with probes for bacterial 16S rRNA in 65 PDAC tumour tissues. The most frequently detected group was the class Gammaproteobacteria, which comprised Enterobacteriaceae and *Pseudomonas*. This demonstrated that the bacteria inhabited the pancreas and were included in the milieu surrounding the pancreatic cancer tumour.

2.2. Fungal Colonization in Pancreatic Cancer Tissue

The contribution of fungal flora towards pancreatic cancer development is a new and uncharted field because intestinal fungi are not too profuse and there is no reference genome well-characterized. Pancreatic cancer occurrence is associated with the migration of particular fungus from the gut to colonize the pancreas. One possible new target for the therapy of pancreatic cancer is the fungal genome. *Candida* infection (CI) can significantly increase both total and individual cancer risks in general, as well as specific ones, as per Chung et al. (2017). Chemicals such as nitrosamines, already established carcinogens responsible for the etiology of mouth cancer, can be formed by *Candida* sp. As reported in an earlier study, *Candida albicans* triggers cancer by promoting an increase in expression of adhesion-molecule molecules and production of cytokines for a Proinflammatory response. Ramirez Garcia et al. (2016) infected the intestines of mice with fungi strains tagged using Green Fluorescent Protein (GFP). Through the 30 minutes, the fungi migrated towards the pancreas, which showed that the intestinal fungi might inhabit the organ. Both animal and human models' pancreatic tumors contained 3,000 more times fungus compared to ordinary pancreatic tissues and comprised multiple species.

For example, Malassezia was the most abundant species in mice pancreas and had a relatively much higher abundance than in the gut. Pathogenic fungus binds to Mannose Binding Lectin (MBL) in Pancreatic Tumour Tissues, which initiates the Complement C3 cascade and promotes Pancreatic cancer development. The liver synthesizes MBL, a soluble lectin of the Innate immune system, which is secreted into the circulation to induce leukocyte phagocytosis of microbes, activate the lectin pathway of complement, and regulate inflammation (Choteau et al., 2016). Tumour microenvironment (TME) has a significant impact on tumorigenesis, development, metastasis, and recurrence. In TME, complement activation is immunomodulatory, and the interaction between cancer cells and the complement system facilitates tumour cell invasion, migration, proliferation, and epithelial-mesenchymal transition. MBL initiates the complement cascade inflammatory immunological response by activating protein C3 in response to the carbohydrate structure produced by Malassezia. Complement activation promotes tumour growth by triggering cell migration and proliferation. Tumour progression can be blocked by knocking down C3aR in cancer cells or eliminating MBL/C3 in the extratumoral environment (Dambuza and Brown, 2019).

2.3. Viral Colonization in Pancreatic Cancer Tissue

Hepatitis B or C virus infection increases the risk of Pancreatic cancer, as indicated by some case-control studies and meta-analyses (Fiorino et al., 2013). However, as indicated by some studies, Hepatitis B and C virus infections do not increase the opportunity of getting Pancreatic cancer (Chang et al., 2014). A Swedish study suggests that HCV infection can be associated with an increased risk of pancreatic cancer. Evidence from China shows that HBsAg-positive carriers and chronic HBV infection are significantly at increased risk of developing Pancreatic cancer. HBV has a demonstrated capacity not only to replicate in pancreatic tissues but to infect the tissues of people who have pancreatic cancer. Pancreatic cancer can occur as a consequence of chronic inflammation precipitated by an HBV infection. The HBx regulatory protein coded by the hepatitis B virus causes viral genome transcription to be induced and leads to chronic metabolic disorders, both of which can possibly lead to the occurrence of pancreatic cancer. The host immune system's efficacy to clear the HBV/HCV is reduced when the DNA of the virus is mixed with infected cell DNA. In spite of the very low level of HBV replication in pancreatic cancer cells, it is impossible to disregard the potential role of the hepatitis virus in both chronic pancreatitis and pancreatic cancer (Jin et al., 2013). The role of the microbiome (bacterial, fungal, and viral communities) in the development and progression of pancreatic cancer is an area of intense research. The mechanisms are complex and can include chronic inflammation, immune modulation, cellular damage, and metabolic effects given in Table 1.

Table 1. Microorganism(s) and Their Proposed Role/Mechanism in Pancreatic Ductal Adenocarcinoma (PDAC)

Microorganism(s)	Type	Proposed Role/Mechanism in PDAC	Reference
Porphyromonas gingivalis Aggregatibacter actinomycetemcomitans	Bacterium (Oral)	**Pathogenesis:** Chronic periodontitis. Oral bacteria may translocate to the pancreas via hematogenous spread, inducing a pro-tumorigenic inflammatory microenvironment.	(Farrell et al., 2012)
Fusobacterium nucleatum	Bacterium (Oral/GI)	**Prognosis:** Associated with worse outcomes. Potential mechanisms include immune suppression via binding to immune checkpoints (e.g., TIGIT) and promoting chemoresistance.	(Mitsuhashi et al., 2015); (Geller et al., 2017)
Helicobacter pylori	Bacterium (Gastric)	**Pathogenesis:** Chronic systemic inflammation and immune response. May also induce hyperglycemia and insulin resistance, known risk factors for PDAC.	(Risch et al., 2014); (Xue et al., 2018)
Oral Microbiome Dysbiosis (e.g., *Leptotrichia*, *Campylobacter*, *Streptococcus*)	Bacterial Community	**Diagnostic Biomarker:** Specific shifts in the composition of oral bacteria may serve as non-invasive biomarkers for detecting PDAC.	(Torres et al., 2015); (Fan et al., 2018)
Gut Microbiome Dysbiosis (e.g., ↑ *Proteobacteria*, *Verrucomicrobia*)	Bacterial Community	**Immunomodulation:** Modulates the systemic and tumor immune microenvironment. Influences response to therapy (e.g., immunotherapy, chemotherapy).	(Riquelme et al., 2019); (Pushalkar et al., 2018)
Malassezia spp.	Fungus	**Tumor Progression:** Promotes oncogenesis by activating the complement cascade via the mannose-binding lectin (MBL) pathway, leading to suppressed anti-tumor immunity.	(Aykut et al., 2019)
Hepatitis B Virus (HBV)	Virus	**Pathogenesis:** Chronic hepatic inflammation and cirrhosis. Potential oncogenic properties of the virus itself (e.g., HBx protein).	(Fiorino et al., 2018); (Ben et al., 2011)

Figure 1. Microorganisms Colonized in Pancreatic Cancer Tissue

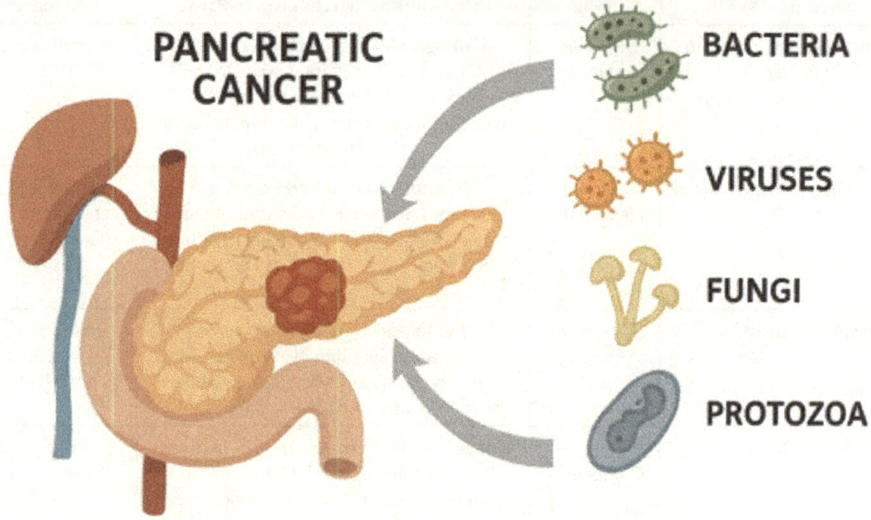

3. PANCREATIC RELATED MICROBE INDUCED INFLAMMATION AND PANCREATIC CANCER

Inflammation triggered by microorganisms is beneficial in defending against pathogens; however, if inflammation persists, it may lead to tissue fibrosis and even carcinogenesis, Microbial induced inflammation leads to tumor development by activating tumor-related inflammatory signaling pathways, including proinflammatory cytokines, Nuclear factor-kappa B (NF-kB), the Toll-like receptor (TLR)/ MyD88 (myeloid differentiation main response gene 88) pathway, and other elements constitute a sophisticated and sensitive network (Ammer Herrmenau et al., 2020). Immune cells like mast cells, dendritic cells, and macrophages, and eosinophils and certain epithelial cells generally exhibit Toll-like receptors (TLRs). They are critical in their role of determining pathogenic chemicals that arise from interior damaged tissue or invasive bacteria and induce inflammation. One mechanism by which microbes that have colonized the pancreas could cause inflammation is by doing this. Lipopolysaccharide (LPS) is a component of the cell wall of Gram-negative bacteria and can be specifically recognized by Toll-like receptor 4 (TLR4), a family member of the Pattern Recognition Receptor (PRR) (Ochi et al., 2012).

The suppression of TLR4 is protective, but the lipopolysaccharide may promote pancreatic carcinogenesis. Pattern Recognition Receptors (PRRs), such as Toll-like receptors (TLRs) located on monocytes or endolysosome membranes, interact with pathogen-related or risk-related molecular patterns to trigger mitogen-related protein kinases (MAPK) kinase-kinase TAK1 (transforming growth factor b activated kinase 1) and IkB (inhibitor of nuclear factor kB) kinase IKK signaling pathway (Kipanyula et al., 2013). Pathogens often secrete cytokines, enhance the pro-inflammatory cell recruitment, and initiate the inflammatory reaction. DNA damage induced by oxidative stress ultimately promotes carcinogenesis, invasion, and metastasis, which affect the responsiveness of the tumor to treatment and other variables (Wei et al., 2019).

Dealing with long-term, smoldering inflammation in the pancreas, a condition known as chronic pancreatitis, is a significant risk factor for developing pancreatic ductal adenocarcinoma (PDAC). This isn't just a local issue; the inflammation creates a state of alarm throughout the entire system, which seems to prime the environment for cancer to initiate. Furthermore, this inflammatory reaction doesn't stop once a tumor appears. Instead, it becomes a key feature of the tumor's immediate surroundings, actively helping the cancer grow and spread to other organs. A key driver of this harmful inflammation can be microbial infections. As highlighted by Wei et al. (2019), these infections are a recognized trigger for the chronic pancreatitis that sets the stage for cancer. The process is often accelerated by genetic factors. For instance, in mouse models, the presence of a mutated KRAS gene—a very common mutation in human PDAC—itself acts as a beacon, drawing immune cells into the pancreas and kicking off the inflammatory process. When you combine this genetic predisposition with other inflammatory stressors, the disease progresses much more rapidly. Research shows that inducing pancreatitis in genetically engineered mice (those with KRAS mutations) for just a single month is enough to trigger the development of precancerous lesions, called Pancreatic Intraepithelial Neoplasia (PanINs). This early stage is critical. It's characterized by a thick, scar-like tissue (fibrosis) and constant inflammatory signals. This chaotic environment doesn't just damage tissue; it actively teaches the emerging cancer cells how to survive, hide from the immune system, and eventually metastasize, as described by Stone and Beatty (2019). Essentially, the body's own desperate attempt to heal through inflammation inadvertently builds a perfect training ground for a deadly cancer.

4. ROLES OF MICROBIOMES IN DEVELOPMENT OF PANCREATIC CANCER (PC)

` While infections are implicated in a significant portion of cancers worldwide, pinpointing a single microbial culprit for pancreatic cancer has proven elusive. Rather than one infectious agent, scientific attention is now focused on the entire ecosystem of microbes—the microbiome—and its collective influence. Investigations suggest that a disruption in the natural balance of this community, particularly changes in the populations of bacteria like *Porphyromonas*, *Neisseria*, and *Fusobacterium*, may be connected to the disease's origin and advancement. A landmark 2019 study led by Riquelme and colleagues offered a profound insight: the types of bacteria living inside the pancreatic tumor itself may predict a patient's fate. The researchers discovered that individuals who survived longer hosted a unique set of microbes, including *Pseudoxanthomonas*, *Streptomyces*, and *Bacillus clausii*, within their tumors. This distinct bacterial signature is so strongly tied to positive outcomes that it is being considered as a potential prognostic tool.

4.1. *Helicobacter pylori* and Pancreatic Cancer (PC)

A period of the past thirty years, growing attention has been paid to the well-known bacterium *Helicobacter pylori*, which colonizes the human stomach. Several earlier researches have tried to link PC presence with *Helicobacter pylori* utilizing serologic and culture-based approaches. The great majority of commensal bacteria, however, cannot be grown, which influences the aim of research on their contribution in Pancreatic illnesses. New techniques, such as next-generation sequencing and metagenomics, have provided a more representative assessment of the microbial community in health and disease and the dynamic interactions between microbiomes and their human hosts (Fraher et al., 2012). To determine whether *Helicobacter pylori* infection was associated with PC. Raderer et al. (1998) used Enzyme-Linked Immunosorbent Assays (ELISA) to analyze IgG antibodies against *Helicobacter pylori* in blood samples from 92 patients with PC, 30 patients with gastric cancer, 35 patients with colorectal cancer, and 27 healthy volunteers. The results showed that 65% of patients with PC and 69% of patients with gastric cancer were sero-positive, compared with only 45% of the other individuals (Raderer et al., 1998). In PC patients, the duodenum revealed higher frequency detection of *Helicobacter pylori* compared to healthy controls. Likewise, additional research confirmed that *Helicobacter pylori* was linked to higher risk of PC in humans by means of meta-analysis. *Helicobacter pylori* may promote the development of PC by causing chronic mucosal inflammation as well as changes in cell proliferation and differentiation (Ding et al., 2010). Several other investigations, meantime, came to the opposite conclusion that *Helicobacter pylori* had no effect on PC. One of the possible reasons for this disparity is that Cytotoxin-associated gene A (Cag-A) positive harms have been the most investigated among the various varieties of *Helicobacter pylori*. Multiple disorders including stomach inflammation and ulceration, cancer of the gastric tract and PC have been connected to Cag-A. However, it remains controversial whether Cag-A-positive or Cag-A-negative strains are associated with PC (Ertz-Archambault et al., 2017).

Scientists believe this blood-type-specific risk may be due to the unique sugar antigens present on the digestive tract lining of non-O individuals. These antigens could make it easier for *H. pylori* bacteria to attach and thrive. While this correlation is clear, the exact biological mechanism behind *H. pylori*'s role in pancreatic cancer is still debated. One theory suggests the infection increases stomach acid production (hyperchlorhydria), which in turn stimulates the pancreas to proliferate excessively. A competing, and seemingly opposite, theory proposes that a chronic *H. pylori* infection damages the stomach lining, leading to reduced acid production (atrophic gastritis and hypochlorhydria). This low-acid environment could allow other bacteria to overgrow, potentially contributing to cancer risk through a different pathway (Blaser, 1992).

5. FUNGI AND VIRUSES IN PANCREATIC CANCER (PC)

Certain research has connected PC development to the growth of fungus and viruses. A prospective cohort research done in Sweden, for instance, found that development of PC was linked to infection with *Candida* sp. in the mouth cavity. Comparably, a different one population-based cohort study conducted in Taiwan revealed that those with *Candida*-infection had a notably greater risk of PC (Chung et al., 2017). Still, the connections between PC and fungal diseases need more research. Hepatitis viruses have somewhat definite functions in triggering the growth of Hepatocellular carcinoma. Still, some data indicated that PC could potentially be linked to hepatitis viruses. While Jin et al. (2013) linked Hepatitis B Virus to chronic pancreatitis, raised serum levels regarding pancreatic enzymes in patients with viral hepatitis. These results show that a possible function of viruses in PC cannot be disregarded and relate to persistent liver disease, chronic pancreatitis and PC (Jin et al., 2013).

6. *FUSOBACTERIUM NUCLEATUM* (FN) ONCOBACTERIUM AND ITS PATHOGENIC MECHANISM IN PANCREATIC CANCER DEVELOPMENT

Fusobacterium nucleatum (Fn) is a common, spindle-shaped bacterium that naturally resides in the human mouth. While it is a normal part of the oral microbiome, it is far from a passive resident. Fn is a master organizer in the complex ecosystem of dental plaque. It acts as a crucial bridge, using specialized adhesion proteins like Fap2 to bind to early colonizers and later invaders, enabling the formation of robust biofilms. In a healthy mouth, this activity is manageable. However, in periodontal disease, Fn's actions become destructive. It directly provokes a strong inflammatory response from the host, triggering the release of signaling molecules (like IL-6 and IL-8) and antimicrobial peptides. This state of chronic inflammation, driven in part by the activation of the NF-κB pathway, creates a damaging environment that can accelerate oral diseases, including carcinogenesis. Furthermore, Fn enhances the virulence of other pathogens, helping them evade the immune system. In immunocompromised individuals, Fn can become an opportunistic invader, escaping the oral cavity to infect sterile sites like root canals.

Beyond its role in oral health, Fn has garnered significant attention in oncology. It is now one of the most studied bacteria linked to cancer, with associations found in cancers of the colon, pancreas, breast, and elsewhere. Although it lives harmlessly in the mouth, Fn possesses the alarming ability to enter the bloodstream and survive the harsh journey through the digestive tract. Its resilience is aided by virulence factors like the FadA protein. Researchers hypothesize that we constantly swallow Fn with our saliva, allowing it to reach the gut. This theory is supported by finding high levels of Fn and FadA in the stool of colorectal cancer patients. Once it translocates, Fn doesn't just stay in the gut; it can disseminate throughout the body via the circulatory system.

Perhaps most remarkably, Fn seems to have a specific homing mechanism for tumors. It uses its Fap2 protein to latch onto a sugar molecule (Gal-GalNAc) that is overly abundant on the surface of many cancer cells. This precise targeting explains why Fn is consistently found enriching the microenvironment of certain tumors, where it is believed to fuel cancer progression by maintaining a state of chronic inflammation and interfering with immune responses.

7. PANCREAS-RELATED MICROBIAL METABOLISM AND PANCREATIC CANCER

The microbial community within a tumor's microenvironment plays a critical role in shaping the local immune response. Through their metabolites, bacteria can directly influence the function and differentiation of immune cells. For instance, certain bacterial byproducts can promote the development of regulatory T-cells, which suppress immune activity, while microbial bile acid metabolites can disrupt the balance of specific gut immune cells. Conversely, some metabolites, like short-chain fatty acids (SCFAs), can have beneficial effects, such as enhancing the memory of cancer-fighting CD8+ T-cells. Overall, these microbial compounds, including palmitoleic acid and SCFAs, can modulate inflammation and tumor growth by controlling the population of regulatory T-cells or reducing the secretion of inflammatory signals like IFN-g (Buchta et al., 2019).

The influence of the microbiome extends to systemic metabolism, where microbiota-induced changes are linked to disorders like diabetes and obesity—both known risk factors for pancreatic cancer (PDAC). Bacteria residing within the pancreatic tumor itself are now recognized as a key component of the tumor microenvironment and a significant contributor to treatment failure. A landmark study by Geller et al. (2017) demonstrated this by showing how bacteria can inactivate a common chemotherapy drug, gemcitabine. These bacteria produce an enzyme called cytidine deaminase (CDDL), which converts the active drug into its ineffective form. Crucially, this chemoresistance can be reversed with antibiotic treatment.

To further understand tumor metabolism, researchers have classified pancreatic cancer cell lines into distinct metabolic subtypes, such as slow-proliferating, glycolytic, and lipogenic, which correlate with known genetic classifications. The interplay between these genetic subtypes and the microbiome's metabolic influence is a vital area for future research. Promisingly, studies have identified early changes in the microbiome that lead to the production of tumor-promoting metabolites, such as elevated serum polyamines in both PDAC patients and mouse models. These findings suggest that profiling these microbial metabolic byproducts could offer a precise and non-invasive strategy for the early detection of pancreatic cancer, potentially improving patient outcomes (Mendez et al., 2020).

8. PANCREATIC CANCER INTRATUMORAL MICROBIOTA

The fascinating quest to connect our body's microbes to pancreatic cancer started with a familiar culprit: *Helicobacter pylori*. Initial research discovered this bacterium, best known for its role in stomach ulcers, present within the pancreatic tumor tissue of a significant number of patients. It was frequently found in those with pancreatic cancer (PDAC) or chronic pancreatitis, yet was absent in healthy individuals, sparking the theory that it could be a contributing factor. This early clue prompted scientists to cast a wider net, leading them directly to the oral microbiome—the diverse community of bacteria in our mouths. Here, the plot thickened. Large-scale studies began to show that people whose mouths harbored certain pathogens, like *Porphyromonas gingivalis* (a key player in gum disease) and *Aggregatibacter actinomycetemcomitans*, faced a measurably higher risk of later developing PDAC.

The connection appears to go even deeper, potentially influencing how the disease manifests in a patient. Researchers have noticed that the particular blend of bacteria present isn't random; it seems to align with specific symptoms a person experiences. For instance, patients who present with jaundice—the yellowing of the skin and eyes—often show a high abundance of the oral bacterium *Prevotella* in their microbiome. Meanwhile, distinct bacterial profiles have been linked to other common symptoms, such as digestive issues like diarrhea and vomiting, or darker urine. This suggests that the microbiome's influence may directly contribute to how the illness is felt by the patient. Recognizing that these gastrointestinal distress signals could be tied to underlying microbial imbalances may encourage earlier medical consultation and improve prognosis. Comprehensive analyses comparing the microbiomes of the mouth, gut, and pancreas in both healthy individuals and PDAC patients reveal distinct patterns. While healthy pancreatic tissue shares similarities with a balanced gut microbiome (featuring phyla like Firmicutes and Proteobacteria and beneficial *Lactobacillus*), cancerous tissue shows a marked decline in these protective species. Instead, it becomes enriched with other bacteria, including *Selenomonas*, *Enterobacter*, *Klebsiella*, and *Prevotella*. The tumor microenvironment itself shows an increase in bacteria like *Capnocytophaga* and *Citrobacter*.

Intriguingly, this bacterial fingerprint isn't just found in full-blown tumors; it's also present in the pancreatic cysts that can eventually become cancerous. Scientists have discovered that the fluid inside a common type of precancerous cyst, known as an IPMN, contains a distinct microbial community. This fluid shows a surprisingly high concentration of bacteria we'd normally expect to find in the mouth, such as *Fusobacterium nucleatum* and *Granulicatella adiacens*. The mere presence of these oral bacteria deep within the pancreas suggests a fascinating and concerning journey—they appear to migrate from their usual home to a new, vulnerable environment. This migration hints that these microbes might be active participants in the very early stages of the disease, potentially helping to nudge a benign cyst toward a more invasive cancer. This discovery underscores the profound and complex link between the bacteria living in and on our bodies and the health of our organs.

9. *FUSOBACTERIUM NUCLEATUM* AND PANCREATIC CANCER PROGNOSIS, THERAPY, AND BIOMARKERS

In a separate study, a team led by Mitsuhashi analyzed tissue samples from 283 individuals diagnosed with pancreatic ductal adenocarcinoma (PDAC). Their goal was to determine if the bacterium *Fusobacterium nucleatum* was present within the tumors and to understand what role, if any, it might play in the progression of the disease. The researchers detected *Fusobacterium* species in nearly 9% of the pancreatic cancer tissue samples. This finding proved to be clinically significant. When they compared survival rates, the data revealed a stark contrast: patients whose tumors harbored this bacterium had a median survival of just over 17 months. This was dramatically shorter than the median survival of almost 33 months seen in patients whose tumors were free of the bacteria, a difference that was statistically significant and pointed to a much poorer prognosis. According to Mitsuhashi et al. (2015), the existence of *Fusobacterium* species may be regarded as a predictive indicator of PC. It was shown that tumours with high levels of *Fusobacterium nucleatum* exhibited resistance to Chemotherapy. The efficacy of these techniques is decreased as a result of the Oncobacterium's interactions with the treatment components or changes in the inflammatory milieu of malignancy. These relationships result in a reduction of the drug's sensitivity (Zhao & Hu, 2020).

The study of Michaud et al. (2007) was the first to show a correlation between the presence of *Fusobacterium* species tumours and the prognosis of Pancreatic cancer in patients who had previously experienced periodontal disease (Michaud et al., 2007). *Fusobacterium* species were more prevalent in pancreatic tail cancer (4/18; 22%) than in body cancer (5/62; 8.0%) or head cancer (16/203; 7.9%), despite the lack of any meaningful correlation. It is still unknown why there are significant *Fusobacterium* species present in pancreatic tail cancer. One possible explanation is that the circulatory supplies of these pancreatic components differ from one another. Additionally, 28% of the surrounding normal tissue contained *Fusobacterium* species-positive malignancy, indicating that the bacterium may contribute to carcinogenesis (Mitsuhashi et al., 2015). The findings of this study could help patients with pancreatic cancer understand important ideas of carcinogenesis and create novel diagnostic and treatment approaches (i.e., eradication). In order to eliminate potential confounding factors, such as disease stage, year of diagnosis, and genetic factors like CpG Island Methylator Phenotype (CIMP) and miRNA expression, Mitsuhashi et al. (2015) adjusted regression analysis results.

Table 2. Microbiome-Targeted Therapeutic Strategies in PC

Clinical Application	Microbiome Source	Microbiome Signature	Potential Use	Reference
Early Detection & Risk Stratification	Oral (Saliva)	↑ *Leptotrichia, Campylobacter*;↓ *Streptococcus, Veillonella*	A non-invasive salivary test to identify high-risk individuals for enhanced screening.	(Fan et al., 2018); (Torres et al., 2015)
Prognostic Assessment	Gut (Stool)	High microbial diversity, specific taxa (e.g., *Pseudobutyrivibrio*)	Predicting long-term survival outcomes following surgical resection of the tumor.	(Riquelme et al., 2019)
Prognostic Assessment	Tumor Tissue	Presence of *Fusobacterium nucleatum*	Identifying patients with more aggressive disease and a likely poorer prognosis.	(Mitsuhashi et al., 2015)
Predicting Treatment Response	Gut (Stool)	Specific bacterial profiles	Predicting efficacy or toxicity of chemotherapy and/or immunotherapy.	(Pushalkar et al., 2018)

The bacterium *Fusobacterium nucleatum* (Fn) is increasingly recognized not just as a passive resident in tumors, but as an active contributor to cancer progression. Its ability to promote genetic mutations, such as high microsatellite instability (MSI), provides a potential explanation for why Fn DNA is so commonly found in malignant tissue and is consistently linked to poorer patient outcomes (Mima et al., 2016). This negative influence is particularly clear in metastatic colon cancer. Research has demonstrated that patients with detectable Fn in their tumors and feces experience significantly worse survival rates and show minimal response to treatment, underscoring its role as a marker for aggressive disease. A revealing contrast has been observed in pancreatic cancer (PDAC). A study by Riquelme et al. (2019) discovered that the composition of the tumor's microbiome itself can predict patient survival. The tumor microbiomes of long-term survivors compared to those who survived for a shorter time. The individuals who lived longer played host to a far richer and more varied community of microbes inside their tumors. A key distinction was the makeup of this community; the long-term survivors' microbiomes were notably enriched with beneficial bacteria such as *Pseudoxanthomonas, Streptomyces, Saccharopolyspora,* and *Bacillus clausii*. This distinct microbial signature is now regarded as a promising prognostic biomarker, indicating a greater potential for long-term survival.

10. CLINICAL APPLICATIONS AND DIAGNOSTIC POTENTIAL

The pancreatic cancer microbiome is rapidly transitioning from a novel finding to a source of tangible clinical applications, offering new avenues for early detection, prognostication, and treatment stratification. The most immediate application lies in non-invasive diagnostics and risk assessment. Notably, a higher degree of gut microbial diversity is predictive of longer survival following surgical resection. Conversely, the presence of specific intratumoral microbes, such as *Fusobacterium nucleatum*, is linked to more aggressive disease and poorer survival, providing a potential tool for stratifying patients into different risk categories at diagnosis. Furthermore, the microbiome is a key modulator of therapy response. Intratumoral bacteria can inactivate chemotherapeutic drugs like gemcitabine, directly contributing to treatment failure, while the gut microbiome shapes the systemic immune landscape, influencing the efficacy of immunotherapy. Analyzing a patient's microbial profile could therefore predict resistance and guide personalized therapeutic decisions, paving the way for adjuvant strategies like selective antibiotics or probiotics to improve treatment outcomes.

Table 3. Clinical Applications and Diagnostic Potential against Pancreatic cancer

Clinical Application	Microbiome Source	Microbiome Signature	Potential Use	Reference
Early Detection & Risk Stratification	Oral (Saliva)	↑ *Leptotrichia, Campylobacter*; ↓ *Streptococcus, Veillonella*	A non-invasive salivary test to identify high-risk individuals for enhanced screening.	(Fan et al., 2018); (Torres et al., 2015)
Prognostic Assessment	Gut (Stool)	High microbial diversity, specific taxa (e.g., *Pseudobutyrivibrio*)	Predicting long-term survival outcomes following surgical resection of the tumor.	(Riquelme et al., 2019)
Prognostic Assessment	Tumor Tissue	Presence of *Fusobacterium nucleatum*	Identifying patients with more aggressive disease and a likely poorer prognosis.	(Mitsuhashi et al., 2015)
Predicting Treatment Response	Gut (Stool)	Specific bacterial profiles	Predicting efficacy or toxicity of chemotherapy and/or immunotherapy.	(Pushalkar et al., 2018)

11. CONCLUSION

In conclusion, the colonization of microorganisms including bacteria, fungi, and viruses within Pancreatic cancer tissue reflects a complex interplay between the host immune system, microbial migration, and the tumor microenvironment. Bacterial communities, especially Proteobacteria and Gammaproteobacteria, show a distinct presence in pancreatic cancer tissues compared to healthy tissues, suggesting their potential involvement in tumor development or progression. Similarly, the presence of fungi such as *Malassezia* and *Candida* species, and their interaction with host immune components like Mannose Binding Lectin, points toward a fungal role in promoting pancreatic carcinogenesis. Moreover, viral agents such as Hepatitis B and C viruses have demonstrated a possible association with increased pancreatic cancer risk, possibly through chronic inflammation and immune modulation. These microbial influences contribute to inflammation-driven tumorigenesis by activating pathways like NF-κB and TLR/MyD88, thereby fostering a pro-tumorigenic environment. While no single microorganism has been definitively established as a direct causative agent of pancreatic cancer, mounting evidence suggests that microbial dysbiosis and host-microbiome interactions are critical factors in pancreatic cancer pathogenesis and may serve as promising targets for diagnosis, prognosis, and therapy.

REFERENCES

Ahuja, M., Schwartz, D. M., Tandon, M., Son, A., Zeng, M., Swaim, W., Eckhaus, M., Hoffman, V., Cui, Y., Xiao, B., Worley, P. F., & Muallem, S. (2017). Orai1-mediated antimicrobial secretion from pancreatic acini shapes the gut microbiome and regulates gut innate immunity. *Cell Metabolism*, *25*(3), 635–646. DOI: 10.1016/j.cmet.2017.02.007

Ammer-Herrmenau, C., Pfisterer, N., Weingarten, M. F. J., & Neesse, A. (2020). The microbiome in pancreatic diseases: Recent advances and future perspectives. *United European Gastroenterology Journal*, *8*(8), 878–885. DOI: 10.1177/2050640620944720

Aykut, B., Pushalkar, S., Chen, R., Li, Q., Abengozar, R., Kim, J. I., Shadaloey, S. A., Wu, D., Preiss, P., Verma, N., Guo, Y., Saxena, A., Vardhan, M., Diskin, B., Wang, W., Leinwand, J., Kurz, E., Kochen Rossi, J. A., Hundeyin, M., & Miller, G. (2019). The fungal mycobiome promotes pancreatic oncogenesis via activation of MBL. *Nature*, *574*(7777), 264–267. DOI: 10.1038/s41586-019-1608-2

Ben, Q., Li, Z., Liu, C., Cai, Q., Yuan, Y., & Wang, K. (2011). Hepatitis B virus status and risk of pancreatic ductal adenocarcinoma: A case-control study from China. *Pancreas*, (5), 675–680. DOI: 10.1097/MPA.0b013e318214f834

Blaser, M. J. (1992). Hypotheses on the pathogenesis and natural history of *Helicobacter pylori* - induced inflammation. *Gastroenterology*, *102*(2), 720–727. DOI: 10.1016/0016-5085(92)90126-J

Buchta, R. C., Feng, T. Y., Azar, F. N., & Rutkowski, M. R. (2019). Impact of the microbiome on cancer progression and response to anti-cancer therapies. *Advances in Cancer Research*, *143*, 255–294. DOI: 10.1016/bs.acr.2019.03.005

Chang, M. C., Chen, C. H., Liang, J. D., Tien, Y. W., Hsu, C., & Wong, J. M. (2014). Hepatitis B and C viruses are not risks for pancreatic adenocarcinoma. *World Journal of Gastroenterology*, *20*(17), 5060–5065. DOI: 10.3748/wjg.v20.i17.5060

Choteau, L., Parny, M., Francois, N., Bertin, B., Fumery, M., Dubuquoy, L., Takahashi, K., Colombel, J.-F., Jouault, T., Poulain, D., Sendid, B., & Jawhara, S. (2016). Role of mannose-binding lectin in intestinal homeostasis and fungal elimination. *Mucosal Immunology*, *9*(3), 767–776. DOI: 10.1038/mi.2015.100

Chung, L. M., Liang, J.-A., Lin, C.-L., Sun, L.-M., & Kao, C.-H. (2017). Cancer risk in patients with candidiasis: A nationwide population-based cohort study. *Oncotarget*, *8*(38), 63562–63573. DOI: 10.18632/oncotarget.18855

Chung, L. M., Liang, J. A., Lin, C. L., Sun, L. M., & Kao, C. H. (2017). Cancer risk in patients with candidiasis: A nationwide population-based cohort study. *Oncotarget*, *8*(38), 63562–63573. DOI: 10.18632/oncotarget.18855

Dambuza, I. M., & Brown, G. D. (2019). Fungi accelerate pancreatic cancer. *Nature*, *574*(7777), 184–185. https://Doi.org/10.1038/d41586-019-02892-y. DOI: 10.1038/d41586-019-02892-y

Ding, S. Z., Goldberg, J. B., & Hatakeyama, M. (2010). Helicobacter pylori infection, oncogenic pathways and epigenetic mechanisms in gastric carcinogenesis. *Future Oncology (London, England)*, *6*(5), 851–862. DOI: 10.2217/fon.10.37

Ertz-Archambault, N., Keim, P., & Von Hoff, D. (2017). Microbiome and pancreatic cancer: A comprehensive topic review of literature. *World Journal of Gastroenterology*, *23*(10), 1899–1908. DOI: 10.3748/wjg.v23.i10.1899

Fan, X., Alekseyenko, A. V., Wu, J., Peters, B. A., Jacobs, E. J., Gapstur, S. M., Purdue, M. P., Abnet, C. C., Stolzenberg-Solomon, R., Miller, G., Ravel, J., Hayes, R. B., & Ahn, J. (2018). Human oral microbiome and prospective risk for pancreatic cancer: A population-based nested case-control study. *Gut*, *67*(1), 120–127. DOI: 10.1136/gutjnl-2016-312580

Fan, X., Alekseyenko, A. V., Wu, J., Peters, B. A., Jacobs, E. J., Gapstur, S. M., Purdue, M. P., Abnet, C. C., Stolzenberg-Solomon, R., Miller, G., Risch, H. A., Visvanathan, K., Hayes, R. B., & Ahn, J. (2018). Human oral microbiome and prospective risk for pancreatic cancer: A population-based nested case-control study. *Gut*, *67*(1), 120–127. DOI: 10.1136/gutjnl-2016-312580

) Farrell, J. J., Zhang, L., Zhou, H., Chia, D., Elashoff, D., Akin, D., Paster, B. J., Joshipura, K., & Wong, D. T. (2012). Variations of oral microbiota are associated with pancreatic diseases including pancreatic cancer. Gut, *61*(4), 582–588. https://doi.org/DOI: 10.1136/gutjnl-2011-300784

Fiorino, S., Bacchi-Reggiani, L., Pontoriero, M., Gallo, C., Chili, E., Masetti, M., Zanini, N., Grondona, A. G., Silvestri, T., Cuppini, A., Jovine, E., & de Biase, D. (2018). Association between Hepatitis B or Hepatitis C Virus Infection and Risk of Pancreatic Adenocarcinoma Development: A Systematic Review and Meta-Analysis. *Pancreatology*, (6), 647–655. DOI: 10.1016/j.pan.2018.05.006

Fiorino, S., Chili, E., Bacchi-Reggiani, L., Masetti, M., Deleonardi, G., Grondona, A. G., Silvestri, T., Magrini, E., Zanini, N., Cuppini, A., Nardi, R., & Jovine, E. (2013). Association between Hepatitis B or Hepatitis C virus infection and risk of pancreatic adenocarcinoma development: A systematic review and meta-analysis. *Pancreatology*, *13*(2), 147–160. DOI: 10.1016/j.pan.2013.01.005

Fraher, M. H., O'Toole, P. W., & Quigley, E. M. (2012). Techniques used to characterize the gut microbiota: A guide for the clinician. *Nature Reviews. Gastroenterology & Hepatology*, *9*(6), 312–322. https:// Doi.org/10.1038/nrgastro.2012.44. DOI: 10.1038/nrgastro.2012.44

Geller, L. T., Barzily-Rokni, M., Danino, T., Jonas, O. H., Shental, N., Nejman, D., Gavert, N., Zwang, Y., Cooper, Z. A., Shee, K., Thaiss, C. A., Reuben, A., Livny, J., Avraham, R., Frederick, D. T., Ligorio, M., Chatman, K., Johnston, S. E., Mosher, C. M., & Straussman, R. (2017). Potential role of intratumor bacteria in mediating tumor resistance to the chemotherapeutic drug gemcitabine. *Science*, *357*(6356), 1156–1160. DOI: 10.1126/science.aah5043

Geller, L. T., Barzily-Rokni, M., Danino, T., Jonas, O. H., Shental, N., Nejman, D., Gavert, N., Zwang, Y., Cooper, Z. A., Shee, K., Thaiss, C. A., Reuben, A., Livny, J., Avraham, R., Frederick, D. T., Ligorio, M., Chatman, K., Johnston, S. E., Mosher, C. M., & Straussman, R. (2017). Potential role of intratumor bacteria in mediating tumor resistance to the chemotherapeutic drug gemcitabine. *Science*, *357*(6356), 1156–1160. DOI: 10.1126/science.aah5043

Iwai, T. (2009). Periodontal bacteremia and various vascular diseases. *Journal of Periodontal Research*, *44*(6), 689–694. DOI: 10.1111/j.1600-0765.2008.01165.x

Jin, Y., Gao, H., Chen, H., Wang, J., Chen, M., Li, G., Wang, L., Gu, J., & Tu, H. (2013). Identification and impact of hepatitis B virus DNA and antigens in pancreatic cancer tissues and adjacent non-cancerous tissues. *Cancer Letters*, *335*(2), 447–454. DOI: 10.1016/j.canlet.2013.03.001

Jin, Y., Gao, H., Chen, H., Wang, J., Chen, M., Li, G., Wang, L., Gu, J., & Tu, H. (2013). Identification and impact of Hepatitis B virus DNA and antigens in pancreatic cancer tissues and adjacent non-cancerous tissues. *Cancer Letters*, *335*(2), 447–454. DOI: 10.1016/j.canlet.2013.03.001

Kamisawa, T., Wood, L. D., Itoi, T., & Takaori, K. (2016). Pancreatic cancer. *Lancet*, *388*(10039), 73–85. DOI: 10.1016/S0140-6736(16)00141-0

Kimura, I., Ichimura, A., Ohue-Kitano, R., & Igarashi, M. (2020). Free fatty acid receptors in health and disease. *Physiological Reviews*, *100*(1), 171–210. DOI: 10.1152/physrev.00041.2018

Kipanyula, M. J., Seke, E. P., Vecchio, L., Farahna, M., Nukenine, E. N., & Nwabo Kamdje, A. H. (2013). Signaling pathways bridging microbial-triggered inflammation and cancer. *Cellular Signalling*, *25*(2), 403–416. DOI: 10.1016/j.cellsig.2012.10.014

Marroncini, G., Naldi, L., Martinelli, S., & Amedei, A. (2024). Gut-liver-pancreas axis crosstalk in health and disease: From the role of microbial metabolites to innovative microbiota manipulating strategies. *Biomedicines, 12*(7), 189–198. DOI: 10.3390/biomedicines12071398

Mendez, R., Kesh, K., Arora, N., Di Martino, L., McAllister, F., Merchant, N., Banerjee, S., & Banerjee, S. (2020). Microbial dysbiosis and polyamine metabolism as predictive markers for early detection of pancreatic cancer. *Carcinogenesis, 41*(5), 561–570. DOI: 10.1093/carcin/bgz116

Michaud, D. S., Joshipura, K., Giovannucci, E., & Fuchs, C. S. (2007). A prospective study of periodontal disease and pancreatic cancer in US male health professionals. *Journal of the National Cancer Institute, 99*(2), 171–175. DOI: 10.1093/jnci/djk021

Mima, K., Nishihara, R., Qian, Z. R., Cao, Y., Sukawa, Y., Nowak, J. A., Yang, J., Dou, R., Masugi, Y., Song, M., Kostic, A. D., Giannakis, M., Bullman, S., Milner, D. A., Baba, H., Giovannucci, E. L., Garraway, L. A., Freeman, G. J., Dranoff, G., & Ogino, S. (2016). *Fusobacterium nucleatum* in colorectal carcinoma tissue and patient prognosis. *Gut, 65*(12), 1973–1980. DOI: 10.1136/gutjnl-2015-310101

Mitsuhashi, K., Nosho, K., Sukawa, Y., Matsunaga, Y., Ito, M., Kurihara, H., Kanno, S., Igarashi, H., Naito, T., Adachi, Y., Tachibana, M., Tanuma, T., Maguchi, H., Shinohara, T., Hasegawa, T., Imamura, M., Kimura, Y., Hirata, K., Maruyama, R., & Ogino, S. (2015). Association of Fusobacterium species in pancreatic cancer tissues with molecular features and prognosis. *Oncotarget, 6*(9), 7209–7220. DOI: 10.18632/oncotarget.3109

Mitsuhashi, K., Nosho, K., Sukawa, Y., Matsunaga, Y., Ito, M., Kurihara, H., Kanno, S., Igarashi, H., Naito, T., Adachi, Y., Tachibana, M., Tanuma, T., Maguchi, H., Shinohara, T., Hasegawa, T., Imamura, M., Kimura, Y., Hirata, K., Maruyama, R., & Shinomura, Y. (2015). Association of *Fusobacterium* species in Pancreatic cancer tissues with molecular features and prognosis. *Oncotarget, 6*(9), 7209–7220. DOI: 10.18632/oncotarget.3109

Morrison, D. J., & Preston, T. (2016). Formation of short chain fatty acids by the gut microbiota and their impact on human metabolism. *Gut Microbes, 7*(3), 189–200. DOI: 10.1080/19490976.2015.1134082

Nejman, D., Livyatan, I., Fuks, G., Gavert, N., Zwang, Y., Geller, L. T., Rotter-Maskowitz, A., Weiser, R., Mallel, G., Gigi, E., Meltser, A., Douglas, G. M., Kamer, I., Gopalakrishnan, V., Dadosh, T., Levin-Zaidman, S., Avnet, S., Atlan, T., Cooper, Z. A., & Straussman, R. (2020). The human tumor microbiome is composed of tumor type-specific intracellular bacteria. *Science*, *368*(6494), 973–980. DOI: 10.1126/science.aay9189

Ochi, A., Nguyen, A. H., Bedrosian, A. S., Mushlin, H. M., Zarbakhsh, S., Barilla, R., Zambirinis, C. P., Fallon, N. C., Rehman, A., Pylayeva-Gupta, Y., Badar, S., Hajdu, C. H., Frey, A. B., Bar-Sagi, D., & Miller, G. (2012). MyD88 inhibition amplifies dendritic cell capacity to promote pancreatic carcinogenesis *via* Th2 cells. *The Journal of Experimental Medicine*, *209*(9), 1671–1687. DOI: 10.1084/jem.20111706

Priyadarshini, M., Villa, S. R., Fuller, M., Wicksteed, B., Mackay, C. R., Alquier, T., Poitout, V., Mancebo, H., Mirmira, R. G., Gilchrist, A., & Layden, B. T. (2015). An acetate-specific GPCR, FFAR2, regulates insulin secretion. *Molecular Endocrinology (Baltimore, Md.)*, *29*(7), 1055–1066. DOI: 10.1210/me.2015-1007

Pushalkar, S., Hundeyin, M., Daley, D., Zambirinis, C. P., Kurz, E., Mishra, A., Mohan, N., Aykut, B., Usyk, M., Torres, L. E., Werba, G., Zhang, K., Guo, Y., Li, Q., Akkad, N., Lall, S., Wadowski, B., Gutierrez, J., Kochen Rossi, J. A., & Miller, G. (2018). The Pancreatic Cancer Microbiome Promotes Oncogenesis by Induction of Innate and Adaptive Immune Suppression. *Cancer Discovery*, *8*(4), 403–416. DOI: 10.1158/2159-8290.CD-17-1134

Pushalkar, S., Hundeyin, M., Daley, D., Zambirinis, C. P., Kurz, E., Mishra, A., Mohan, N., Aykut, B., Usyk, M., Torres, L. E., Werba, G., Zhang, K., Guo, Y., Li, Q., Leopold, N., Chung, M., Robbins, R., Rajurkar, M., Narayanan, R., & Miller, G. (2018). The Pancreatic Cancer Microbiome Promotes Oncogenesis by Induction of Innate and Adaptive Immune Suppression. *Cancer Discovery*, *8*(4), 403–416. DOI: 10.1158/2159-8290.CD-17-1134

Raderer, M., Wrba, F., Kornek, G., Maca, T., Koller, D. Y., Weinlaender, G., Hejna, M., & Scheithauer, W. (1998). Association between helicobacter pylori infection and pancreatic cancer. *Oncology*, *55*(1), 16–19. DOI: 10.1159/000011830

Ramirez-Garcia, A., Rementeria, A., Aguirre-Urizar, J. M., Moragues, M. D., Antoran, A., Pellon, A., Abad-Diaz-de-Cerio, A., & Hernando, F. L. (2016). *Candida albicans* and cancer: Can this yeast induce cancer development or progression? *Critical Reviews in Microbiology*, *42*, 182–193. DOI: 10.3109/1040841X.2014.913004

Riquelme, E., Zhang, Y., Zhang, L., Montiel, M., Zoltan, M., Dong, W., Quesada, P., Sahin, I., Chandra, V., San Lucas, A., Scheet, P., Xu, H., Hanash, S. M., Feng, L., Burks, J. K., Do, K. A., Peterson, C. B., Nejman, D., Tzeng, C. D., & McAllister, F. (2019). Tumor Microbiome Diversity and Composition Influence Pancreatic Cancer Outcomes. *Cell*, *178*(4), 795–806.e12. DOI: 10.1016/j.cell.2019.07.008

Riquelme, E., Zhang, Y., Zhang, L., Montiel, M., Zoltan, M., Dong, W., Quesada, P., Sahin, I., Chandra, V., San Lucas, A., Scheet, P., Xu, H., Hanash, S. M., Feng, L., Burks, J. K., Do, K.-A., Peterson, C. B., Nejman, D., Tzeng, C.-W. D., & McAllister, F. (2019). Tumor Microbiome Diversity and Composition Influence Pancreatic Cancer Outcomes. *Cell*, *178*(4), 795–806. DOI: 10.1016/j.cell.2019.07.008

Risch, H. A., Yu, H., Lu, L., & Kidd, M. S. (2014). Detectable Serum Antibodies to Helicobacter pylori and the CagA Protein Do Not Correlate with Long-Term Risk of Pancreatic Cancer in a Prospective Cohort. *Cancer Epidemiology, Biomarkers & Prevention*, (11), 2461–2464. DOI: 10.1158/1055-9965.EPI-14-0559

Stone, M. L., & Beatty, G. L. (2019). Cellular determinants and therapeutic implications of inflammation in pancreatic cancer. *Pharmacology & Therapeutics*, *201*, 202–213. DOI: 10.1016/j.pharmthera.2019.05.012

Thomas, R. M., & Jobin, C. (2020). Microbiota in pancreatic health and disease: The next frontier in microbiome research. *Nature Reviews. Gastroenterology & Hepatology*, *17*(1), 53–64. DOI: 10.1038/s41575-019-0242-7

Tilg, H., Adolph, T. E., & Trauner, M. (2022). Gut-liver axis: Pathophysiological concepts and clinical implications. *Cell Metabolism*, *34*(11), 1700–1718. DOI: 10.1016/j.cmet.2022.09.017

Torres, P. J., Fletcher, E. M., Gibbons, S. M., Bouvet, M., Doran, K. S., & Kelley, S. T. (2015). Characterization of the salivary microbiome in patients with pancreatic cancer. *PeerJ*, *1373*, e1373. Advance online publication. DOI: 10.7717/peerj.1373

Wei, M. Y., Shi, S., Liang, C., Meng, Q. C., Hua, J., Zhang, Y. Y., Liu, J., Zhang, B., Xu, J., & Yu, X.-J. (2019). The microbiota and microbiome in pancreatic cancer: More influential than expected. *Molecular Cancer*, *18*(1), 97–106. DOI: 10.1186/s12943-019-1008-0

Xue, Y., Xiao, H., Guo, S., Xu, B., Liao, Y., Wu, Y., & Zhang, G. (2018). The association between Helicobacter pylori infection and pancreatic cancer: A meta-analysis. *Journal of Cancer Research and Therapeutics*, *14*, S428–S432. DOI: 10.4103/0973-1482.202888

Zhang, X., Shi, S., Zhang, B., Ni, Q. X., & Xu, J. (2018). Circulating biomarkers for early diagnosis of pancreatic cancer: Facts and hopes. *American Journal of Cancer Research*, *8*, 332–353.

Zhao, K., & Hu, Y. (2020). Microbiome harbored within tumors: A new chance to revisit our understanding of cancer pathogenesis and treatment. *Signal Transduction and Targeted Therapy*, *5*(1), 136–145. DOI: 10.1038/s41392-020-00244-1

Chapter 3
Utilizing the Microbiome as a Preventative or Therapeutic for Pancreatic Cancer

P. Saranraj
https://orcid.org/0000-0002-5052-6532
Department of Microbiology, Sacred Heart College, Tirupattur, India

ABSTRACT

Pancreatic cancer is one of the most fatal tumours, with few therapeutic choices and a low survival rate. This emerging dataset considers the microbiome an essential contributor to the genesis and pathogenesis of pancreatic cancer. The gut and tumor-associated microbiomes can influence pancreatic tumorigenesis primarily through immune regulation, inflammation, and metabolic pathways. Most importantly, dysbiosis, defined as microbial imbalance, has been associated with pancreatic cancer, opening up a potential avenue for prevention and treatment. Probiotic and prebiotic supplementation, faecal microbiota transplantation, and auditory species targeting are some intervention possibilities that can achieve modification of microbiomes for improving immune surveillance, constraining inflammation, and enhancing chemotherapeutics and immunotherapy responses. Furthermore, microbial profiling could be a diagnostic tool in identifying high-risk patients and predicting treatment outcomes. This chapter covers the following aspects: complex interaction between the microbiome and pancreatic cancer, and its application in possible preventive and therapeutic maneuvers against the disease being engineered in the future. New approaches to understanding pancreatic cancer therapy harness microbiota, but the final clinical promise will require further proof. Constraining certain bacteria may enhance the efficacy of traditional chemotherapies and modern immunotherapies

DOI: 10.4018/979-8-3373-1469-3.ch003

such as immune checkpoint inhibitors. Microbial profiling might serve as a new and up-and-coming reliable non-invasive diagnostic tool to screen individuals at high risk for pancreatic cancer and predict therapy outcomes.

1. INTRODUCTION

The connection between microorganisms and cancer has completely resurfaced. Germ theory gained popularity and was extended to encompass carcinogenesis from the end of the nineteenth century, while infectious illnesses were the leading cause of mortality and morbidity. The idea that a bacterium causes cancer was mainly debunked by the middle of the 20th century, which led to a search for genes that modulate cancer. The notion that carcinoma is a communicable disease has received more attention in recent decades. Malignancies of the digestive tract and liver are among the many significantly influenced by microorganisms. Even in cases where germs are not the leading cause of cancer, there may be a complicated interaction between germs and cancer. It is possible that this updated "Germ Theory of Cancer" will enhance and supplement the somatic mutation theory of cancer. Some people with driver mutations may develop cancer due to differences in their microbiota. By altering the microbiome, probiotics and antibiotics may be important in treating cancer. Above all, a better knowledge of the cancer-microbiome axis has implications for developing next-generation immunotherapy due to the close relationship between microorganisms and inflammation in both cancer and bacteria (Rahib et al., 2014).

One of the most dangerous cancers is Pancreatic Ductal Adenocarcinoma (PDAC). It is now the fourth most significant cause of cancer-related deaths globally, and by 2030, it is predicted to rise to the second position. Over the past three decades, a five-year survival rate in general for PDAC patients has stayed relatively steady, spanning between 7% and 9%, despite a moderate improvement in systemic cancer survival rates due to multimodality treatment (Rahib et al., 2014). Pancreatic cancer has a dismal prognosis, even with recent advancements in chemotherapy, surgeries, and radiation techniques. This is especially true when the illness is initially curable. The lack of effective treatments, early recurrence, late-stage presentation, latent metastatic disease at presentation, and the lack of a biomarker that can identify this cancer in its pre-invasive or early stages are the causes of this. Moreover, chronic pancreatitis can increase the risk of patients with PDAC by up to 20 times, making pancreatic inflammation a long-term risk factor (Lowenfels et al., 1993). The poor prognosis is also attributed to the complex biology surrounding the large desmoplastic PDAC tumor microenvironment, which leads to hypovascularity, hypoxia, inadequate drug delivery, and inefficient therapy. Furthermore, success in a PDAC has been difficult, even though immunotherapy has significantly progressed in treating various cancers. Microbes can induce carcinogenesis and have been linked to approximately 10–20% of human cancers. In many solid tumors, their microbiome signature may be linked to survival and responsiveness to treatment, including immunotherapy (Hanahan & Weinberg, 2011).

The fundamental genetic risk factors for pancreatic cancer are still unclear, despite the fact that several of its causes, such as diet, obesity, and smoking, have been identified. BRCA2 (Breast Cancer Gene 2) and other DNA damage repair protein mutations have been linked to PDAC. However, these mutations are only present in 5 – 7% of those affected (Alkassis et al., 2021). Although they make up less than 10% of PNET (Primitive Neuroectodermal Tumors) patients, people with familial disorders such as MEN1, VHL, NF-1, and TSC are more likely to acquire PNET-type tumors. The majority of pancreatic tumors are not discovered until they are in their advanced stages, regardless of the disease's genesis, because of vague symptoms such as back pain and appetite loss that are frequently misinterpreted as other medical conditions (Ro et al., 2013).

To identify cancers, including PC (Pancreatic Cancer), early in the course of the disease, a number of cutting-edge biomarkers and methods have been introduced, including genetic testing, imaging methods, serum biomarkers, and the identification of high-risk premalignant lesions. A continuous ductal system connects the pancreas to the Gastrointestinal Tract (GI). Each of these different GI tract segments' microbiota composition might affect the others, leading to diseases brought on by too prevalent infections. The most popular technique for figuring out the location and diversity of microbial populations in the reservoirs found in the human body is 16S rRNA sequencing. To clarify the functional components of the microbial communities that were taken from the patient, Metagenomic, Metaproteomic, and Metabolomic techniques are used (Liu et al., 2021).

Dysbiosis is characterized by shifts in the taxonomic microbial profiles and the wide range of the microbial community. There is compelling proof that dysbiosis may contribute to the emergence of pancreatic cancer and other GI tract diseases. The role of various microorganisms in the onset or progression of GI tract disorders and neoplasms has been demonstrated using a variety of sequencing techniques (Zhang et al., 2022). Although research on the connection between PC and microbial diversity is still in its early stages, a growing amount of data suggests that PC may be impacted by an interaction involving the microbiome. Naturally, PC should ideally develop as a result of the entry of different bacterial, fungal, and viral species into the digestive tract. This research on the tumor microenvironment and microbiome may ultimately affect therapy effectiveness (Lu et al., 2022).

2. MICROBIOME AND PANCREATIC CANCER: MECHANISTIC INSIGHTS

2.1. Microbial Dysbiosis and Tumorigenesis

Oral health is negatively impacted by the disruption to the oral environmental balance, which results in oral dysbiosis linked to dental conditions, such as periodontal disease and dental caries. In recent years, several epidemiological studies have linked poor dental health to an elevated risk of pancreatic cancer (Ahn et al., 2012). The researchers predicted that oral bacterial status could mediate the association between pancreatic tumor risk and dental condition because microbial balance and activities harm oral health. According to a previous study, a twofold greater risk of PC was linked to elevated blood serum antibody levels for certain oral infections, such as *Porphyromonas gingivalis* (Fan et al. 2018).

High-throughput genetic sequencing was used to evaluate oral bacterial samples directly in order to solve this issue. According to the research, some gram-negative oral bacteria are linked to a threefold increased risk of PC. The person's pancreatic duct was also shown to harbor the bacterium. In a similar vein, recent cohort investigations have demonstrated that PC is more common among those with greater antibodies in circulation against certain oral microorganisms. 405 PC patients had higher levels of ATTC 53978 antibodies against *Porphyromonas gingivalis* than healthy people, according to a 2013 study by Michaud et al. (2013). Patients with a history of dental decay and antibodies in circulation against specific oral pathogenic microbes have been associated with an increased risk of PC, even though a direct correlation between PC and oral bacteria has not yet been shown. *Aggregatibacter actinomycetemcomitans* and *Porphyromonas gingivalis* are recognized keystone oral pathogens that cause tooth loss and periodontitis. According to certain research, this illness raises the chance of PC (Hujoel et al., 2003).

Increased development of periodontal infections, *P. gingivalis* and *A. actinomycetemcomitans*, predisposes to pancreatic cancer. Previous studies showed that *P. gingivalis* bypasses the host immune system by interfering with signaling cascades through receptor degradation and degradation of cytokines. Moreover, scientists had recently demonstrated through experiments that the TLR (Toll-Like Receptors) signaling pathways can be activated by *P. gingivalis* as well as by *A. actinomycetemcomitans*, where TLR activation was one of the leading promoters of PC in experimental animals (Fan et al., 2018). A new study by Barton (2017) indicates a specific change in the cell cycle regulator p53, which is muted by the deletion of arginine, which mainly affects PC patients. This recent finding has proved that this mutation can result from the bacterial Peptide Amine Deaminase (PAD) enzyme, which is usually found in patients suffering from PC. *Porphyromonas gingivalis, Prevotella intermedia, Tannerella forsythia,* and Treponema *denticola* have all revealed activity of their enzymes associated with changing the Pro allele p53Arg72-Pro, which is indeed thought to be a risk factor in patients suffering from PC (Liu et al., 2011).

In contrast, a higher presence of *Fusobacterium* and its species, *Leptotrichia*, is associated with reduced risk for PC. Elsewhere, Olsen et al. (2016) showed that another genus of *Fusobacteria, Alloprevotella*, may pose a risk for PC development. *Leptotrichia* is an opportunistic bacterium that causes a variety of infectious diseases, including endocarditis, pneumonia, bacteremia, osteomyelitis, lung abscess, and periodontitis. Higher levels of blood antibodies against this species suggest the result of an immune response incited by these bacteria. According to some researchers, the immune response generated by these microbes is connected to PC protection (Eribe & Oribe, 2008).

2.2. Immune Modulation by the Microbiome

The immune system is closely associated with the formation and occurrence of tumors, and the impact of microbes on the immune system's functioning is a contentious issue. Using either short-time survival, long-term survival, or control donors, Riquelme et al. (2019) recently performed human fecal microbiota transplantation studies in mice and found that altering the tumor microbiome can influence both tumor immune infiltration and cancer progression (Riquelme et al., 2019). Numerous investigations have revealed that microbiomes have a range of functions inside the body's immune system, including impacts on immunological suppression and development. In the gut lamina propria, the immune system and gut microbiota can interact, and extraintestinal sites have recently shown comparable outcomes. The poor immune systems of germ-free mice were found by Round and Mazmanian (2009) to include hypoplastic lymphatic organs and immune cell defects. However, these mice's immune systems developed after receiving gut microbiome transplants from pathogen-free mice (Round & Mazmanian, 2009). Microbiomes have the ability to activate the immune system by acting as antigens. The immune system is activated when intestinal mucosa damage allows bacteria to pass through the gut lamina propria and reach distant lymphoid organs. However, the human immune system cannot operate without gut microbiota (Iida et al., 2013). In mice with compromised adaptive immunity, $IL22^+$ innate lymphoid cells, Th17 cells, and regulatory T cells mediated responses to gut microbiomes, indicating that the gut microbiome can boost innate immunity. Numerous investigations have demonstrated that specific bacteria, including *Bifidobacterium* species and *Bifidobacterium fragilis*, may be important for the maturation of the immune system. Melanoma, Kidney, Bladder, and Lung Cancer have all shown similar results (Matson et al., 2018).

2.3. Microbial Metabolites and Inflammation

The gut microbiome has a detrimental interaction with pancreatic cancer by producing microbial chemicals that affect inflammation. Crucially, dysbiosis manifests as a disruption in microbiome homeostasis, leading to a pro-inflammatory tumor microenvironment and changed metabolite profiles. While some metabolites, like Lipopolysaccharides (LPS) and secondary bile acids, encourage inflammation, others, like Short-Chain Fatty Acids (SCFAs) like butyrate, have anti-inflammatory properties (Ducreux et al., 2015). Gram-negative bacteria's LPS stimulates TLR4, which starts NF-kappa B signaling and releases pro-inflammatory cytokines that encourage the formation of tumors. Chronic inflammation brought on by bacterial metabolites such as TMAO (Trimethylamine N-oxide) and indole derivatives promotes cancer development. It is interesting to note that they change immune cell activity, leading to T-cell reactions and macrophage polarization that encourage cancer formation. Polyamines, which would boost apoptosis resistance and promote cancer cell proliferation, may be found in other bacterial products. These interactions between cancer cells, metabolites, and gut microbiota worsen chemoresistance and immune evasion, which complicates treatment. Therefore, using probiotics, dietary changes, or specific inhibitors to target microbial metabolites is a possible therapeutic approach. Finding new diagnostics and treatment approaches could improve patient outcomes if the relationship between the microbe metabolites and irritation in pancreatic cancer is better understood (Pei et al., 2019).

3. UTILIZING THE MICROBIOME AS A PREVENTIVE OR THERAPEUTIC FOR PANCREATIC CANCER

3.1. Probiotics and Prebiotics

Probiotics are "live microbes that, when given in sufficient quantities, confer medical advantages on the host". Dietary probiotics are commonly accessible as supplements and functional foods. By modifying immune function and changing gut microbiota composition, probiotics benefit consumers by influencing signaling pathways like MAPK (Mitogen Activated Protein Kinase) and NF-κB (Rahmani et al., 2023). Through in vitro and in vivo testing in a mouse xenograft model, Kita and colleagues (2020) found that ferrichrome derived from the probiotic bacteria Lactobacillus casei inhibits the proliferation of PC cells, particularly those resistant to 5-FU. By activating p53, ferrichrome interrupted the cell cycle and stopped the growth of cancer cells. Following ferrichrome treatment, DNA fragmentation and Poly (ADP-ribose) Polymerase Cleavage suggest that ferrichrome may also cause apoptosis in PC cells. Ferrichrome significantly impacted the expression of mRNAs associated with p53 as well. Ferrichrome generated from probiotics inhibited colorectal and stomach cancer tumors, according to Kita et al. (2020). Ferrichrome and other probiotic-derived chemicals may cause probiotics' tumor-suppressive effects, making them attractive anticancer medications, particularly in refractory and 5-FU-resistant PC (Kita et al., 2020). Chen et al. (2020) investigated the role of *Porphyromonas gingivalis* and probiotics in mice. They found that mice treated with *P. gingivalis* plus probiotics had a lower pancreatic weight than those treated with *P. gingivalis* alone, and that the pancreas expressed significantly fewer genes linked to cancer development. Probiotics reduced and phosphorylated Smad3 expression in KC mice given *P. gingivalis*. Probiotics may be beneficial by lowering cancer cell proliferation and viability and restricting PanIN progression and metastasis. Chen et al. (2020) showed that oral exposure to *P. gingivalis* can hasten the development of PanIN lesions and posited that probiotics could potentially suppress tumor development via blockade of the transforming growth factor-β signaling cascade. A different study conducted by the same authors found that combining gemcitabine and probiotics could decrease serum liver enzymes, vimentin and Ki-67 levels, and grade of pancreatic intraepithelial tumor formation induced in mice. More studies on high-dose probiotic supplementation assessed PanIN alteration and increased liver enzyme levels in blood. It has been shown by Chen et al. (2020) that probiotics may tolerate chemotherapy and increase efficacy for the patient.

The GI bacteria regulate the host's intestinal environment using prebiotics, which are good nutrients for the host. Consuming fiber-rich foods or prebiotics, selectively fermented substances altering the composition and activity of GI microbiota towards the benefit of the host, are two of the most common examples among a variety of dietary strategies to change microbial composition (Gibson et al., 2010). Dietary fibres resistant to digestion, such as resistant starches, generate different prebiotic roles by impacting the community of microbes, increasing the Short Chain Fatty Acids (SCFAs) production, and protecting DNA. RNA-Seq in cancer tissue expression changes in the genes of the carbohydrate metabolic network have been analyzed, with the principal relationship between PC and Resistant Starch (RS) in xenograft mice. Study of the serum samples collected in controls compared to the RS group identified a range of compounds, such as xanthine, hypoxanthine, and inosine, to be lower in the RS group than in the controls (Panebianco et al., 2019). These substances are related to salvage processes and purine metabolism. Most often, high amounts of these are observed in tumor cells as indicators of cancer. In a related study done with xenograft mice, the RS group's miRNA profiles showed that 19 dysregulated miRNAs had been found compared to the controls. With a better prognosis concerning PC associated with high levels of miRNA-375, miRNA-148a-3p, miRNA-125a-5p, and miRNA-200a-3p in the RS group, these miRNAs controlled by RS digestion were found to be connected to oncogenic genes implicated in the development and propagation of cancer (Trivieri et al., 2020). Prebiotics prevent the adhesion of pathogens to epithelial cells. This happens by mimicking Microvillus Glycoconjugates and binding to receptors present on bacterial cells. The broad repertoire of applications for prebiotics is well documented in a number of cancers. However, more research must be done to fully understand its therapeutic potential in the clinical arena concerning pancreatic cancer (Shoaf et al., 2006).

3.2. Microbiome as a Potential Therapeutic Target

Currently, the mainstay treatments for pancreatic cancer include radiation therapy, chemotherapy, and surgery. These adjunctive therapies have a good theoretical basis, but are largely ineffective and detrimental to the patient. Novel approaches like Fecal Microbiota Transplantation, Immunological Modulation, and Personalized Bacteriophage Therapy may serve as alternative options for the currently established therapies. Newer studies have suggested that changing the microbial populations in the pancreatic and gastrointestinal tract may be useful in treating and preventing pancreatic cancer. By identifying specific species that are increased in gastrointestinal neoplasms and then found in other organs too, one can locate encouraging targets for therapy. Immunotherapy, Fecal Microbial Transplantation, Probiotics and Prebiotics, and Antibiotics that alter microbial diversity can modulate either the outcomes of certain malignancies or the development of dysbiosis. Despite scant clinical research on the disease, manipulation of the microbiome has provided a possible alternative therapy for pancreatic cancer (Kashida et al., 2002).

3.3. Microbial Biomarkers for Early Detection

As of right now, there isn't an authorized pancreatic cancer screening program. Better patient outcomes may arise from early diagnosis, which enables Prompt therapy. Because of their poor positive predictive value in individuals who are asymptomatic, serum assays for carbohydrate antigen 19-9 (CA 19-9) are not the best option for screening (Okuda et al., 2022). The tests can be conducted in the clinic since salivary and fecal samples are easier to obtain and less invasive than tissue biopsy specimens from metastatic tumors. The unique microbiota seen in PDAC patients offers new opportunities for the development of diagnostic/screening biomarkers. In order to find bacterial possibilities, Farrell et al. (2012) initially looked into the use of oral microbes as a diagnostic biomarker by comparing the salivary microbiome of ten PDAC patients and ten matched controls (Lu et al., 2022). This was later confirmed in a set of 27 samples with chronic pancreatitis, 28 samples with PDAC, and 28 matched controls. The researchers discovered that the salivary microbiomes of PDAC patients and controls differed significantly. Patients with pancreatic cancer exhibited much lower levels of *Neisseria elongata* and *Streptococcus mitis*, and when these two microbiological biomarkers were combined, they were able to differentiate PDAC patients from healthy people with a sensitivity of 96.4% and a specificity of 82.1%. Additionally, they found that none of the bacterial possibilities from the PDAC study altered significantly in lung cancer when they compared these signs to a HOMIM (Human Oral Microbiome Identification Microarray) profiling analysis in lung cancer. The salivary microbiome of PDAC patients, patients with other illnesses, and healthy individuals was also examined by Torres et al. (2015) (8, 78, and 22 patients, respectively) (Temel et al., 2023). In comparison to the other two groups, the researchers found a significantly higher ratio of *Leptotrichia* to *Porphyromonas* (LP ratio) in the saliva of PDAC patients using high-throughput sequencing. They suggested using the LP ratio as a diagnostic biomarker for PDAC. It is interesting to note that, in contrast to the work by Farrell et al. (2012), the proportions of *Neisseria* and *Streptococcus* did not significantly differ among the patient groups in this inquiry. The authors attributed this to a change in study methodologies. They found that throughout the early stages of PDAC development, the gut microbiota was rich in the bacterial phyla *Proteobacteria* and *Firmicutes*. Due to active metabolic pathways, this was linked to increased serum polyamine levels. Therefore, another non-invasive biomarker for the early detection of PDAC may be the analysis of the metabolism of microbial dysbiosis (Halimi et al., 2021).

4. THERAPEUTIC APPROACHES TARGETING THE MICROBIOME

4.1. Faecal Microbiota Transplantation (FMT)

In order to help control and treat dysbiosis and associated cancers, fecal microbial transplantation has demonstrated remarkable effectiveness against a variety of GI diseases (Chen et al., 2019). Genton et al. (2021) examined the relationship between gut microbiota and immunological and metabolic variables by transplanting the feces of PC patients as well as healthy participants into germ-free mice. They found that mice given FMT from PC patients had reduced visceral fat, although mice in both groups gained the same amount of food and body weight. Other non-metataxonomic factors did not significantly differ between the two groups. PC patients and mice who received their feces as a transplant had higher levels of *Clostridium scindens*, *Clostridium bolteae*, and *Phascolarctobacterium faecium*. Conversely, fewer species of Lachnospiraceae, Coriobacteriaceae, and *Alistipes obesi* were discovered (Genton et al., 2021). Riquelme and colleagues (2018) found that the tumor microbiome of

LTS (Long Term Survival) patients was more alpha-diverse than that of STS (Short Term Survival) patients. Additionally, *Pseudoxanthomonas* sp., *Streptomyces* sp., *Saccharopolyspora* sp., and *Bacillus clausii* were found in the intratumoral microbiome profile of LTS patients. This signal was considered an important prognostic indicator because it predicted long-term survival. Using samples from patients with LTS and STS and healthy controls, Riquelme et al. (2018) conducted mouse FMT experiments to address the role of the microbiota in PDAC. The authors claim that LTS samples were associated with the least tumor growth in mice compared to STS or healthy control donor samples. Animals with tumors from STS became larger than their counterparts receiving FMT with samples from healthy control donors. This indicates that malignant bacteria for PDAC might drive tumor formation, while bacteria from LTS might stop tumor growth (Riquelme et al. 2019).

4.2. Modulating Microbiota to Enhance Chemotherapy and Immunotherapy Responses

The activation or inactivation of particular bacterial species in the stomach may influence drug bioavailability and therapeutic efficacy. Several bacteria can deactivate drugs or transform prodrugs into active forms, leading to reduced effectiveness against cancer cells (Li et al., 2016). The gut microbiota influences drug-related metabolism and disposal, which ascertains their pharmacokinetics and pharmacodynamics. The relationships between immune cells and cancer and the effects of different drugs, such as chemotherapy, have been significant topics of recent studies on PDAC treatment methods. The following section explores the particular mechanisms of microbial digestion and enzyme degradation of chemotherapeutic drugs that can lead to chemotherapy resistance, building on our comprehension of the gut microbiome's role in modulating therapy effectiveness and its influence on drug efficacy, particularly in PDAC (Luo et al., 2024).

In one of the first immunotherapy applications, surgeon-scientist William Coley injected patients with heat-killed *Streptococcal* and *Serratia* organisms ("Coley's toxins"), resulting in immune activation and eventual sarcoma regression. Similarly, *Bacillus* Calmette-Guérin (BCG) has been utilized for bladder cancer immunotherapy for about 50 years. The recent introduction of more specific Immunotherapy in the form of Immune Checkpoint Inhibitors (ICIs) has been a breakthrough in Cancer treatment, earning its discoverers a Nobel Prize and curing cancer in several people. A set of key observations on the Microbiome-mediated effects of ICIs and other Chemo-immunotherapies (Weber, 2014).

The immunotherapeutic effects of low (or "metronomic") dosages of the alkylating drug Cyclophosphamide (CTX) were evident by the mid-2010s. In addition to having potent Th1-inducing properties and working with cancer vaccines, CTX also encourages Th17 cell infiltration into the tumor microenvironment. Th17 cells60, which are crucial for antimicrobial defense, have also recently been found to be produced by bacteria (Liang et al., 2006). These two findings were skillfully coupled by Viaud et al. (2013), who suggested that changes in the gut flora account for CTX's Immunotherapeutic effects. Due to intestinal dysbiosis brought on by CTX therapy, pathogenic Th17 cells (IFN-γ+) are activated, gram-positive bacteria move to lymphoid tissue, and the gut becomes more leaky. Similarly, colon sterilization decreases the effectiveness of CpG-Oligodeoxynucleotide (CpG-ODN) therapy since its immunotherapeutic benefits rely on TNF production by microbiota-primed tumour-associated myeloid cells.

According to preclinical models, the gut microbiota affects how αCTLA-4, αPD-1, and αPDL1 work as immunotherapeutic agents in ICIs. Bacteroides species growth and dysbiosis result from αCTLA-4 therapy in SPF mice. *Burkholderia cepacia, Burkholderia thetaiotaomicron,* and *Burkholderia fragilis* are 'good' bacteria that re-colonize mice fed antibiotics. These bacteria mature dendritic cells and generate an IL12-dependent Th1 response against tumors. *Bifidobacterium* abundance and immunity from tumors are also linked, according to 16S rRNA gene sequencing. In mice, gavage of Bifidobacteria increases the Th1 response and enhances the effectiveness of αPD-L1. More extensive multi-center cohorts from around the globe need to be studied to precisely characterize "good" or "bad" bacteria in cancer immunotherapy. Recent research (Pushalkar et al., 2018) contradicts earlier studies (Sivan et al., 2015) by suggesting that gut microbiota eradication increases the effect of αPD-1-based ICI on pancreatic cancer.

4.3. Targeted Precision Therapies

In the case of Pancreatic Adenocarcinoma (PDAC), targeted precision therapies that target the Tumor Microenvironment (TME) have shown promise, especially when it comes to addressing the epithelial components that are essential for the growth of the cancer and its resistance to therapy. Targeting CAFs (Cancer Associated Fibroblasts) can have beneficial and detrimental effects on patients due to the diverse actions of various CAF subtypes within the TME. Inhibiting the SHH (Sonic Hedgehog Protein) in CAFs is one of the initial attempts (Ho et al., 2020). The results were unclear while acute inhibition increased the amount of medicine that entered tumors, persistent inhibition paradoxically accelerated the growth of cancer, highlighting the technique's potential but obscuring the ideal duration of inhibition. Other strategies, like using Pegylated Recombinant Human Hyaluronidase 20 (PEGPH20) to break down hyaluronic acid produced by CAFs, initially seemed promising for enhancing drug delivery. However, clinical trials failed to yield the anticipated outcomes, preventing additional research in this area (Hosein et al., 2020).

4.3.1. Targeting TME Immune Cells

Immune cell treatments have enormous promise for precisely targeting the TME, except for the stromal matrix. Reducing the expression of GM-CSF (Granulocyte-Macrophage Colony- Stimulating Factor) in malignant epithelial tissue and stromal stem cell-like cancer-associated fibroblasts significantly reduced tumor development and eradicated metastases. According to clinical trials, advanced solid tumors like PDAC can be effectively treated with cabiralizumab, a monoclonal antibody that targets the CSF1R receptor, in combination with nivolumab, a PD1 checkpoint inhibitor (Hosein et al., 2020). Furthermore, blocking the body's own Myc protein significantly reduces pancreatic tumors by preventing Neutrophil and Macrophage penetration. A different method increases CD8 T cell infiltration by transforming macrophages into an immunoenhancing state using CD40 agonists, which are now undergoing clinical research. Patients with a low neutrophil-to-lymphocyte ratio benefit most from the combination of gemcitabine and a CD40 agonist. Galectin-9 is another target; it interacts with macrophage dectin-1 to produce the tumor-promoting M2 phenotype. By increasing $CD4^+$ and $CD8^+$ T-cell activation, blocking galectin-9 limits immunological suppression and, consequently, cancer development. By specifically eliminating Tregs, which are known to restrict immune function, therapeutic regimens that combine small doses of cyclophosphamide and GVAX enhance immune responses to PDAC.

The inhibition of the CSF-1 receptor (CSF-1R), which in animal models successfully lowers TAMs (Tumor Associated Macrophages) and promotes the transcription of PD-L1 and CTLA-4 genes, is the focus of an alternate strategy that uses immunosuppressive cells inside the TME to increase the ratio of $CD8^+$ to $CD4^+$ T cells. Another treatment approach is to regulate chemokines. Myeloid cells have a receptor called CCR2, which attaches to CCL2 to attract TAMs. Results from trials that used CCX872 and PF-04136309 in addition to traditional chemotherapy to reduce CCR2 were inconclusive. In contrast to CXCR2 inhibition, which has the opposite impact, CCR2 blockage decreases monocyte infiltration into tumors, which is linked to a compensatory increase in neutrophil recruitment (Sherman & Beatty, 2023). Therefore, in preclinical PDAC mice, survival is improved by blocking both CCR2 and CXCR2. Lastly, inadequate antigen presentation is another immunologically related obstacle to generating a successful adaptive immune response against PDAC. Compared to most cancers, pancreatic ductal adenocarcinoma tumors contain fewer dendritic cells, and those that do not necessarily have the most favourable profiles for antigen presentation (Hegde et al., 2020).

4.3.2 Targeting Epithelial-to-Mesenchymal Transition

Coming to the transition from Epithelial-Mesenchymal Transition (EMT), it is pertinent to mention that recent data are vague. However, evidence increasingly points to a possibly significant correlation between TME and EMT in pancreatic carcinoma. The ability of cancer cells to pass through the basement membrane and start spreading is aided by the loss of adhesion with other cells in an Epithelial-Mesenchymal Transition (EMT). In mouse models, elevated expression of the markers of EMT was correlated with high levels of IL-6/STAT3 and galectin-1 produced by PSCs, with the induction of nuclear factor erythroid 2 (Nrf2) facilitating such processes (Wu et al., 2017). By enhancing the mobility and invasive nature of cancer cells, the TME also enables metastasis. After leaving the tumor capillaries, these cells may go through the portal veins into the liver and lungs. Several factors support this process. TAMs produce MIP-3α and increase the expression of MMP9. Collagen IV promotes the invasion of pancreatic cancer cells (Campbell et al. 2005). Along with TAMs, CAFs also generate a lot of palladin, which regulates Cdc42 to help alter the ECM. Hypoxia brought on by TME activates HIF1, which activates genes including MMP-2, NF-κB, CX3CR1, LOX, and QSOX1, resulting in invasion and metastasis. Hypoxia in clinical samples activates SHH by a mechanism that is independent of ligands (Goicoechea et al., 2014). In addition to the expression of the previously stated compounds, increasing amounts of galectin-1, HGF, and periostin, as well as components associated with perineural invasion, are released by PSCs in a hypoxic environment, which facilitates the creation of SHH. Lastly, the TME contributes significantly to expanding the premetastatic niche in PDAC, a setting in which primary tumors are primed to stimulate the production of metastases in distant organs. Granulin, which TAMs secrete, induces HSCs to differentiate into myofibroblasts, creating a fibrotic liver environment that encourages the establishment of metastases. Furthermore, the CXCR2 pathway assists in developing pre-metastatic niches, which affect neutrophil and MDSC migration and activation. Finally, TME considerably influences the vital facets of cancer progression, which signifies its relevance in the event of any disease (Eash et al., 2010).

4.3.3. Targeting Exosomes in the TME

Exosomes are known to play important modulatory roles in the pathogenicity of cancer cells. The cancer cells secrete exosomes comprising proteins, lipids, DNA, RNA, and other materials, which are then delivered to target cells, such as TME cells. Exosomes can mediate communication between T cells, B cells, NK cells, DCs, MDSCs, TAMs, CAFs, endothelial cells, and cancer cells (Wu et al., 2024). Since exosomes have a close relationship with TME immune cell modulation, it is clear that they can affect how the tumor reacts to immunotherapy. Exosomes are how PDAC cells interact with CAFs and endothelial cells in vivo. In PDAC, exosomes mediate neo-vascularization since inhibiting exosome production has a repressive effect on angiogenesis. In PDAC, exosomes interact with the thymus, lung, and kidneys (Adem et al., 2024). According to Chen et al. (2020), supporting evidence, a subset of miRNAs generated from CAF-secreted exosomes stimulates PDAC cell growth and migration by triggering signal transduction pathways that control the growth and death of cancer cells. By promoting the growth of more immune cells within the tumor and reversing immunosuppression, the correlation between exosome cargo and TME immune cell regulation offers a possible path toward enhancing the effectiveness of immunotherapy. To suppress the galectin-9/dectin one pathway and induce immunogenic cell death, an exosome-delivery device for bone marrow mesenchymal stem cells has been designed (Chen et al., 2020).

5. FUTURE PERSPECTIVES

5.1. Microbiome-Based Personalized Medicine

Pancreatic Ductal Adenocarcinoma (PDAC) is one of several gastrointestinal disorders that can be treated by altering or reestablishing the gut microbiota. It will investigate whether prebiotics, probiotics, antibiotics, and FMT, which are frequently used to change the gut microbiota, could be used to treat PDAC patients (Rajpoot et al., 2018).

5.1.1 Antibiotic Use and Its Association with PDAC

A detrimental dysbiotic environment can be reversed by antibiotic-induced microbiota reduction. In patients with early-stage gastric cancer, for instance, eliminating *Helicobacter pylori* with an antibiotic combination of amoxicillin and clarithromycin is linked to a decreased risk of metachronous gastric cancer (Choi et al., 2018). Pushalkar et al. (2018) discovered that transplanting feces from PDAC-bearing Pdx1Cre; LSL-KrasG12D; Trp53R172H (KPC) mice negated the anti-tumor effect of bacterial ablation with antibiotics in mouse models. Transferring feces from non-PDAC controls did not result in any noticeable change. Additionally, the researchers discovered that while oral antibiotic treatment slowed the growth of cancers, bulk fecal or select bacterial transfer from PDAC-bearing animals, but not control mice, accelerated the development of tumors (Pushalkar et al., 2018). By stimulating anti-tumor T cells, boosting immune surveillance, and enhancing immunotherapy sensitivity, gut microbiota ablation results in immunogenic remodeling of the cancer microenvironment and tumor growth reduction. In addition to the function of antibiotic chemoprevention in patients with high-risk pancreatic intraepithelial neoplasia, this also suggested the possibility of using antibiotics in combination with ICIs as an enticing strategy for experimental therapeutics in patients with PDAC (Riquelme et al., 2018).

5.1.2. Probiotic Use and Its Association with PDAC

The World Health Organization defines probiotics as "living microbes which, when supplied in adequate quantities, confer beneficial effects on the host". Hill et al. (2014) state that they are most frequently categorized as lactic acid bacteria, especially *Lactobacillus* and *Bifidobacterium* spp. Probiotics are present in fermented foods like kimchi, kombucha, and unfiltered apple cider vinegar, as well as processed meals and dietary supplements including yoghurt, cheese, milk, juices, and smoothies. Through the activation of the innate immune system, reduction of oxidative stress, enhancement of the gut microbiota community, improvement of intestinal barrier function, and modulation of colonization resistance, which inhibits pathogenic bacteria, probiotics have been demonstrated in numerous studies to suppress tumorigenesis (Zhu et al., 2011). Probiotic use in cancer patients, especially those taking immunosuppressive medications, raises safety concerns, nevertheless. Among the dangers are bacterial translocation and systemic invasion, the potential for increasing antibiotic resistance, and the transfer of resistant genes into the local microbiota. By impairing the integrity of the intestinal barrier, dysbiosis of the gut microbiota might increase the probability of bacterial translocation, leading to elevated inflammation and the development of chronic pancreatitis or pancreatic cancer. Probiotics help to stabilize the intestinal barrier, according to several animal studies. In contrast to control patients, Oláh et al. (2002) found that 299 patients with acute pancreatitis who received *Lactobacillus plantarum* through nasojejunal tube feeding experienced a lower rate of pancreatic sepsis and needed fewer surgical procedures (Oláh et al., 2002).

5.1.3. Synbiotics and Postbiotics

Prebiotics and probiotics are combined to create synbiotics. According to a previous study (Motoori et al., 2017), taking symbiotic supplements during neoadjuvant therapy for esophageal cancer improves the gut microbial ecology and reduces chemotherapeutic side effects. The term "postbiotics" refers to chemicals and soluble metabolites produced by gut bacteria that affect host biology. One popular example of a probiotic fermentation product is SCFA. Postbiotics are a safer and more efficient method than consuming live bacteria. In addition to their specific cytotoxicity against tumors, postbiotics can protect the intestinal epithelium. The use of postbiotics in the treatment of cancer is still relatively new. Scientists find it challenging to separate the molecule for therapeutic use and characterize its safety profile in preclinical and clinical settings due to the large variety of metabolites that are available (Rad et al., 2021).

5.1.4. Faecal Microbiota Transplantation (FMT)

Faecal Microbiota Transplantation (FMT) can be given by endoscopy, rectal enema, nasogastric/nasoenteral tube, or consumption of oral fecal capsules. Transplanting fecal microbiota has been shown to be more than 80 – 85% effective in treating recurrent and refractory *Clostridium difficile* infections, but not for any other purpose (Baunwall et al., 2020). The gut microbiota was enabled through FMT to colonize the pancreatic tumor, hence altering the overall bacterial composition of the tumor, as found in-antibiotic-treated by Riquelme et al. (2018). FMT was then found to trigger an immune system activation and anti-tumor response in cancer-bearing mice unlike the FMT involving microflora from STS patients as Riquelme et al. (2019). The tumors of the LTS cohort also exhibited higher diversity and infiltration of CD8+/killer T cells as compared to STS tumors. It would be interesting to see if this work leads to further investigations into the microbiota and FMT treatments for PDAC patients. Although potentially beneficial, FMT has several serious problems, such as the potential for users to get viruses. Therefore, particular emphasis must be put into thorough microbiological screening to mitigate this risk in diseases that are resistant to antibiotics (Cheng et al., 2020).

5.2. Expanding Research on Microbial Profiling and Therapeutic Targets

Important connections between the microbiota and immune response, tumor metabolism, and treatment resistance are emerging in pancreatic cancer. Gut and tumour-associated bacteria have been shown to induce cancer through immunological modulation, microbial metabolites and inflammation. Oncogenic dysbiosis, or imbalance, is associated with elevated aggressiveness and poor prognosis. High-throughput sequencing techniques have facilitated the identification of microbial biomarkers for early diagnosis and targeted intervention. It is predicted that different microbial species will either work in opposition to or in concert to create tumors, making them possible targets for therapy. Consequently, probiotics, antibiotics, or Fecal Microbiota Transplantation (FMT) may be used to regulate the microbiome as a therapeutic adjuvant (Siegel et al., 2021). The goal of the exciting new field of bacteriophage therapy is to reduce the selection pressure on beneficial microbes. From the perspective of human disease, CRISPR-mediated modification of the microbiota may attempt to eradicate diseases while keeping advantageous members. In turn, there is currently a lot of interest in the gut microbiota because of its connection to immunotherapy and chemotherapy responses. Short-chain fatty acids are among the microbial metabolites that are known to be crucial in the microenvironments of pancreatic cancer. Microbial research can benefit from multi-omics analysis and artificial intelligence. Gaining insight into how the immune system and microbiome interact could increase the effectiveness of immunotherapy. Therefore, it is anticipated that personalized microbiome-based treatments may create new therapeutic options for pancreatic cancer. The microbiome is shaped by environmental and nutritional variables, which also affect the risk of cancer. More recent research aims to establish the foundation for precision medicine based on the microbiome. Microbial profiling will change the therapy landscape for pancreatic cancer and assist identify new therapeutic targets (Li et al., 2004).

6. CONCLUSION

The intricate relationship between the microbiome and pancreatic cancer underscores microbial dysbiosis as a critical factor in tumorigenesis, immune modulation, and therapeutic resistance. Oral pathogens like *Porphyromonas gingivalis* and *Aggregatibacter actinomycetemcomitans* drive chronic inflammation and oncogenic signaling via Toll-like receptors (TLRs) and enzymes like Peptide Amine Deaminase (PAD), which alter cell cycle regulators such as p53. Conversely, protective genera like *Fusobacterium* highlight the microbiome's dual role in Pancreatic Cancer (PC) progression. Emerging therapeutic strategies leverage probiotics (e.g., *Lactobacillus casei*), prebiotics, and fecal microbiota transplantation (FMT) to restore microbial equilibrium, enhance chemotherapy efficacy, and modulate immune responses, as evidenced by reduced tumor growth in preclinical models. Microbial metabolites, including Short-chain fatty acids (SCFAs) and LPS, further influence Inflammation and Tumor microenvironments (TME), while salivary and fecal microbial biomarkers offer non-invasive diagnostic potential. Advances in targeting TME components such as Cancer-associated fibroblasts (CAFs), immune checkpoints, and exosomes reveal synergistic opportunities when combined with microbiome modulation. Future directions emphasize personalized microbiome-based therapies, integrating multi-omics, AI-driven profiling, and precision interventions like bacteriophage therapy to overcome chemoresistance and optimize immunotherapy. However, challenges remain in ensuring probiotic safety, standardizing FMT protocols, and translating preclinical findings into clinical practice. Collectively, harnessing the microbiome's mechanistic and therapeutic potential promises to revolutionize pancreatic cancer management, underscoring the need for interdisciplinary research to bridge gaps in understanding and application.

REFERENCES

Adem, B., Bastos, N., Ruivo, C. F., Sousa-Alves, S., Dias, C., Vieira, P. F., Batista, I. A., Cavadas, B., Saur, D., Machado, J. C., Cai, D., & Melo, S. A. (2024). Exosomes define a local and systemic communication network in healthy pancreas and pancreatic ductal adenocarcinoma. *Nature Communications*, *15*(1), 1496–1502. DOI: 10.1038/s41467-024-45753-7

Ahn, J., Segers, S., & Hayes, R. B. (2012). Periodontal disease, *Porphyromonas gingivalis* serum antibody levels and orodigestive cancer mortality. *Carcinogenesis*, *33*(5), 1055–1058. DOI: 10.1093/carcin/bgs112

Alkassis, S., Yazdanpanah, O., & Philip, P. A. (2021). BRCA mutations in pancreatic cancer and progress in their targeting. *Expert Opinion on Therapeutic Targets*, *25*(7), 547–557. DOI: 10.1080/14728222.2021.1957462

Barton, M. K. (2017). Symptoms, cancer-related distress, and overall distress may contribute to racial disparities in the outcomes of patients with early-stage breast cancer. *CA: a Cancer Journal for Clinicians*, *67*(4), 257–258. DOI: 10.3322/caac.21371

Baunwall, S. M. D., Lee, M. M., Eriksen, M. K., Mullish, B. H., Marchesi, J. R., Dahlerup, J. F., & Hvas, C. L. (2020). Faecal microbiota transplantation for recurrent *Clostridioides difficile* infection: An updated systematic review and meta-analysis. *EClinicalMedicine*, *29*, 100642. DOI: 10.1016/j.eclinm.2020.100642

Campbell, A. S., Albo, D., Kimsey, T. F., White, S. L., & Wang, T. N. (2005). Macrophage inflammatory protein-3alpha promotes pancreatic cancer cell invasion. *The Journal of Surgical Research*, *123*(1), 96–101. DOI: 10.1016/j.jss.2004.07.013

Chen, D., Wu, J., Jin, D., Wang, B., & Cao, H. (2019). Fecal microbiota transplantation in cancer management: Current status and perspectives. *International Journal of Cancer*, *145*(8), 2021–2031. DOI: 10.1002/ijc.32003

Chen, S. M., Chieng, W. W., Huang, S. W., Hsu, L. J., & Jan, M. S. (2020). The synergistic tumor growth-inhibitory effect of probiotic *Lactobacillus* on transgenic mouse model of pancreatic cancer treated with gemcitabine. *Scientific Reports*, *10*(1), 20319–20326. DOI: 10.1038/s41598-020-77322-5

Cheng, W. Y., Wu, C. Y., & Yu, J. (2020). The role of gut microbiota in cancer treatment: Friend or foe? *Gut*, *69*(10), 1867–1876. DOI: 10.1136/gutjnl-2020-321153

Choi, I. J., Kook, M.-C., Kim, Y.-I., Cho, S.-J., Lee, J. Y., Kim, C. G., Park, B., & Nam, B. H. (2018). *Helicobacter pylori* therapy for the prevention of metachronous gastric cancer. *The New England Journal of Medicine, 378*(12), 1085–1095. DOI: 10.1056/NEJMoa1708423

Ducreux, M., Cuhna, A. S., Caramella, C., Hollebecque, A., Burtin, P., Goere, D., Seufferlein, T., Haustermans, K., Van Laethem, J. L., Conroy, T., & Arnold, D. (2015). Cancer of the pancreas: ESMO Clinical Practice Guidelines for diagnosis, treatment and follow-up. *Annals of Oncology : Official Journal of the European Society for Medical Oncology, 26*, 56–68. DOI: 10.1093/annonc/mdv295

Eash, K. J., Greenbaum, A. M., Gopalan, P. K., & Link, D. C. (2010). CXCR2 and CXCR4 antagonistically regulate neutrophil trafficking from murine bone marrow. *The Journal of Clinical Investigation, 120*(7), 2423–2431. DOI: 10.1172/JCI41649

Eribe, E. R., & Olsen, I. (2008). *Leptotrichia* species in human infections. *Anaerobe, 14*(3), 131–137. DOI: 10.1016/j.anaerobe.2008.04.004

Fan, X., Alekseyenko, A. V., Wu, J., Peters, B. A., Jacobs, E. J., Gapstur, S. M., Purdue, M. P., Abnet, C. C., Stolzenberg-Solomon, R., Miller, G., Ravel, J., Hayes, R. B., & Ahn, J. (2018). Human oral microbiome and prospective risk for pancreatic cancer: A population-based nested case-control study. *Gut, 67*(1), 120–127. DOI: 10.1136/gutjnl-2016-312580

Farrell, J. J., Zhang, L., Zhou, H., Chia, D., Elashoff, D., Akin, D., Paster, B. J., Joshipura, K., & Wong, D. T. W. (2012). Variations of oral microbiota are associated with pancreatic diseases including pancreatic cancer. *Gut, 61*(4), 582–588. DOI: 10.1136/gutjnl-2011-300784

Genton, L., Lazarevic, V., Stojanovic, O., Spiljar, M., Djaafar, S., Koessler, T., Dutoit, V., Gaïa, N., Mareschal, J., Macpherson, A. J., Herrmann, F., Trajkovski, M., & Schrenzel, J. (2021). Metataxonomic and metabolic impact of fecal microbiota transplantation from patients with pancreatic cancer into germ-free mice: A pilot study. *Frontiers in Cellular and Infection Microbiology, 11*, 752889. DOI: 10.3389/fcimb.2021.752889

Gibson, G. R., Scott, K. P., Rastall, R. A., Tuohy, K. M., Hotchkiss, A., Dubert-Ferrandon, A., Gareau, M., Murphy, E. F., Saulnier, D., Loh, G., Macfarlane, S., Delzenne, N., Ringel, Y., Kozianowski, G., Dickmann, R., Lenoir-Wijnkoop, I., Walker, C., & Buddington, R. (2010). Dietary prebiotics: Current status and new definition. *Food Science and Technology Bulletin, 7*(1), 1–19. DOI: 10.1616/1476-2137.15880

Goicoechea, S. M., Garcia-Mata, R., Staub, J., Valdivia, A., Sharek, L., McCulloch, C. G., Hwang, R. F., Urrutia, R., Yeh, J. J., Kim, H. J., & Otey, C. A. (2014). Palladin promotes invasion of pancreatic cancer cells by enhancing invadopodia formation in cancer-associated fibroblasts. *Oncogene, 33*(10), 1265–1273. DOI: 10.1038/onc.2013.68

Halimi, A., Gabarrini, G., Sobkowiak, M. J., Ateeb, Z., Davanian, H., Gaiser, R. A., Arnelo, U., Valente, R., Wong, A. Y. W., Moro, C. F., Del Chiaro, M., Özenci, V., & Sällberg Chen, M. (2021). Isolation of pancreatic microbiota from cystic precursors of pancreatic cancer with intracellular growth and DNA-damaging properties. *Gut Microbes, 13*(1), 1983101. DOI: 10.1080/19490976.2021.1983101

Hanahan, D., & Weinberg, R. A. (2011). Hallmarks of cancer: The next generation. *Cell, 144*(5), 646–674. DOI: 10.1016/j.cell.2011.02.013

Hegde, S., Krisnawan, V. E., Herzog, B. H., Zuo, C., Breden, M. A., Knolhoff, B. L., Hogg, G. D., Tang, J. P., Baer, J. M., Mpoy, C., Lee, K. B., Alexander, K. A., Rogers, B. E., Murphy, K. M., Hawkins, W. G., Fields, R. C., DeSelm, C. J., Schwarz, J. K., & DeNardo, D. G. (2020). Dendritic cell paucity leads to dysfunctional immune surveillance in pancreatic cancer. *Cancer Cell, 37*(3), 289–307. DOI: 10.1016/j.ccell.2020.02.008

Hill, C., Guarner, F., Reid, G., Gibson, G. R., Merenstein, D. J., Pot, B., Morelli, L., Canani, R. B., Flint, H. J., Salminen, S., Calder, P. C., & Sanders, M. E. (2014). Expert consensus document: The International Scientific Association for Probiotics and Prebiotics consensus statement on the scope and appropriate use of the term probiotic. *Nature Reviews. Gastroenterology & Hepatology, 11*(8), 506–514. DOI: 10.1038/nrgastro.2014.66

Ho, W. J., Jaffee, E. M., & Zheng, L. (2020). The tumour microenvironment in pancreatic cancer clinical challenges and opportunities. *Nature Reviews. Clinical Oncology, 17*(9), 527–540. DOI: 10.1038/s41571-020-0363-5

Hosein, A. N., Brekken, R. A., & Maitra, A. (2020). Pancreatic cancer stroma: An update on therapeutic targeting strategies. *Nature Reviews. Gastroenterology & Hepatology, 17*(8), 487–505. DOI: 10.1038/s41575-020-0300-1

Hujoel, P. P., Drangsholt, M., Spiekerman, C., & Weiss, N. S. (2003). An exploration of the periodontitis–cancer association. *Annals of Epidemiology, 13*(5), 312–316. DOI: 10.1016/S1047-2797(02)00425-8

Iida, N., Dzutsev, A., Stewart, C. A., Smith, L., Bouladoux, N., Weingarten, R. A., Molina, D. A., Salcedo, R., Back, T., Cramer, S., Dai, R.-M., Kiu, H., Cardone, M., Naik, S., Patri, A. K., Wang, E., Marincola, F. M., Frank, K. M., Belkaid, Y., & Goldszmid, R. S. (2013). Commensal bacteria control cancer response to therapy by modulating the tumor microenvironment. *Science*, *342*(6161), 967–970. DOI: 10.1126/science.1240527

Kashida, Y., Sasaki, Y. F., Ohsawa, K. I., Yokohama, N., Takahashi, A., & Watanabe, T. (2002). Mechanistic study on flumequine hepatocarcinogenicity focusing on DNA damage in mice. *Toxicological Sciences*, *69*(2), 317–321. DOI: 10.1093/toxsci/69.2.317

Kita, A., Fujiya, M., Konishi, H., Tanaka, H., Kashima, S., Iwama, T., Ijiri, M., Murakami, Y., Takauji, S., Goto, T., Sakatani, A., Ando, K., Ueno, N., Ogawa, N., & Okumura, T. (2020). Probiotic-derived ferrichrome inhibits the growth of refractory pancreatic cancer cells. *International Journal of Oncology*, *57*(3), 721–732. DOI: 10.3892/ijo.2020.5096

Li, D., Xie, K., Wolff, R., & Abbruzzese, J. L. (2004). Pancreatic cancer. *Lancet*, *363*(9414), 1049–1057. DOI: 10.1016/S0140-6736(04)15841-8

Li, H., He, J., & Jia, W. (2016). The influence of gut microbiota on drug metabolism and toxicity. *Expert Opinion on Drug Metabolism & Toxicology*, *12*(1), 31–40. DOI: 10.1517/17425255.2016.1121234

Liang, S. C., Tan, X. Y., Luxenberg, D. P., Karim, R., Dunussi-Joannopoulos, K., Collins, M., & Fouser, L. A. (2006). Interleukin (IL)-22 and IL-17 are co-expressed by Th17 cells and cooperatively enhance expression of antimicrobial peptides. *The Journal of Experimental Medicine*, *203*(10), 2271–2279. DOI: 10.1084/jem.20061308

Liu, J., Liu, C., & Yue, J. (2021). Radiotherapy and the gut microbiome: Facts and fiction. *Radiation Oncology (London, England)*, *16*(1), 9–17. DOI: 10.1186/s13014-020-01735-9

Liu, L., Wang, K., Zhu, Z. M., & Shao, J. H. (2011). Associations between P53 Arg72Pro and development of digestive tract cancers: A meta-analysis. *Archives of Medical Research*, *42*(1), 60–69. DOI: 10.1016/j.arcmed.2011.01.008

Lowenfels, A. B., Maisonneuve, P., Cavallini, G., Ammann, R. W., Lankisch, P. G., Andersen, J. R., Dimagno, E. P., Andrén-Sandberg, A., & Domellöf, L. (1993). Pancreatitis and the risk of pancreatic cancer. *The New England Journal of Medicine*, *328*(20), 1433–1437. DOI: 10.1056/NEJM199305203282001

Lu, Y., Yuan, X., Wang, M., He, Z., Li, H., Wang, J., & Li, Q. (2022). Gut microbiota influence immunotherapy responses: Mechanisms and therapeutic strategies. *Journal of Hematology & Oncology, 15*(1), 47–56. DOI: 10.1186/s13045-022-01273-9

Luo, W., Wen, T., & Qu, X. (2024). Tumor immune microenvironment-based therapies in pancreatic ductal adenocarcinoma: Time to update the concept. *Journal of Experimental & Clinical Cancer Research : CR, 43*(1), 1–32. DOI: 10.1186/s13046-024-02835-x

Matson, V., Fessler, J., Bao, R., Chongsuwat, T., Zha, Y., Alegre, M.-L., Luke, J. J., & Gajewski, T. F. (2018). The commensal microbiome is associated with anti-PD-1 efficacy in metastatic melanoma patients. *Science, 359*(6371), 104–108. DOI: 10.1126/science.aao3290

Michaud, D. S., Izard, J., Wilhelm-Benartzi, C. S., You, D. H., Grote, V. A., Tjonneland, A., Dahm, C. C., Overvad, K., Jenab, M., Fedirko, V., Boutron-Ruault, M. C., Clavel-Chapelon, F., Racine, A., Kaaks, R., Boeing, H., Foerster, J., Trichopoulou, A., Lagiou, P., Trichopoulos, D., & Riboli, E. (2013). Plasma antibodies to oral bacteria and risk of pancreatic cancer in a large European prospective cohort study. *Gut, 62*(12), 1764–1770. DOI: 10.1136/gutjnl-2012-303006

Motoori, M., Yano, M., Miyata, H., Sugimura, K., Saito, T., Omori, T., Fujiwara, Y., Miyoshi, N., Akita, H., Gotoh, K., Takahashi, H., Kobayashi, S., Noura, S., Ohue, M., Asahara, T., Nomoto, K., Ishikawa, O., & Sakon, M. (2017). Randomized study of the effect of synbiotics during neoadjuvant chemotherapy on adverse events in esophageal cancer patients. *Clinical Nutrition (Edinburgh, Lothian), 36*(1), 93–99. DOI: 10.1016/j.clnu.2015.11.008

Okuda, S., Hirose, Y., Takihara, H., Okuda, A., Ling, Y., Tajima, Y., Shimada, Y., Ichikawa, H., Takizawa, K., Sakata, J., & Wakai, T. (2022). Unveiling microbiome profiles in human inner body fluids and tumor tissues with pancreatic or biliary tract cancer. *Scientific Reports, 12*(1), 8766–8775. DOI: 10.1038/s41598-022-12658-8

Oláh, A., Belágyi, T., Issekutz, Á., Gamal, M. E., & Bengmark, S. (2002). Randomized clinical trial of specific *Lactobacillus* and fibre supplement to early enteral nutrition in patients with acute pancreatitis. *British Journal of Surgery, 89*(9), 1103–1107. DOI: 10.1046/j.1365-2168.2002.02189.x

Olsen, I., Taubman, M. A., & Singhrao, S. K. (2016). *Porphyromonas gingivalis* suppresses adaptive immunity in periodontitis, atherosclerosis, and Alzheimer's disease. *Journal of Oral Microbiology, 8*(1), 33029–33036. DOI: 10.3402/jom.v8.33029

Panebianco, C., Villani, A., & Pazienza, V. (2019). High levels of prebiotic resistant starch in diet modulate gene expression and metabolomic profile in pancreatic cancer xenograft mice. *Nutrients*, *11*(4), 709–717. DOI: 10.3390/nu11040709

Pei, X., Song, F., & Wang, Z. (2019). Emerging incidence trends and application of curative treatments of pancreatic cancer in the USA. *Medicine*, *98*(51), e17175. DOI: 10.1097/MD.0000000000017175

Pushalkar, S., Hundeyin, M., Daley, D., Zambirinis, C. P., Kurz, E., Mishra, A., Mohan, N., Aykut, B., Usyk, M., Torres, L. E., Werba, G., Zhang, K., Guo, Y., Li, Q., Akkad, N., Lall, S., Wadowski, B., Gutierrez, J., Kochen Rossi, J. A., & Miller, G. (2018). The pancreatic cancer microbiome promotes oncogenesis by induction of innate and adaptive immune suppression. *Cancer Discovery*, *8*(4), 403–416. DOI: 10.1158/2159-8290.CD-17-1134

Rad, A. H., Maleki, L. A., Kafil, H. S., Zavoshti, H. F., & Abbasi, A. (2021). Postbiotics as promising tools for cancer adjuvant therapy. *Advanced Pharmaceutical Bulletin*, *11*(1), 1–5. DOI: 10.34172/apb.2021.001

Rahib, L., Smith, B. D., Aizenberg, R., Rosenzweig, A. B., Fleshman, J. M., & Matrisian, L. M. (2014). Projecting cancer incidence and deaths to 2030: The unexpected burden of thyroid, liver, and pancreas cancers in the United States. *Cancer Research*, *74*(11), 2913–2921. DOI: 10.1158/0008-5472.CAN-14-0155

Rahmani, N., Pourali, G., Hosseini, N., Fiuji, H., Maftooh, M., Hassanian, S. M., Ferns, G. A., Khazaei, M., & Avan, A. (2023). Probiotics as a therapeutic approach in colorectal cancer. *Current Cancer Drug Targets*, *23*(10), 764–777. DOI: 10.2174/1568009623666230413081513

Rajpoot, M., Sharma, A. K., Sharma, A., & Gupta, G. K. (2018). Understanding the microbiome: Emerging biomarkers for exploiting the microbiota for personalized medicine against cancer. *Seminars in Cancer Biology*, *52*, 1–8. DOI: 10.1016/j.semcancer.2018.02.003

Riquelme, E., Maitra, A., & McAllister, F. (2018). Immunotherapy for pancreatic cancer: More than just a gut feeling. *Cancer Discovery*, *8*(4), 386–388. DOI: 10.1158/2159-8290.CD-18-0123

Riquelme, E., Zhang, Y., Zhang, L., Jenq, R., Wargo, J., Montiel, M., Zoltan, M., Dong, W., & Quesada, P. (2019). Tumor microbiome diversity and composition influence pancreatic cancer outcomes. *Cell*, *178*(4), 795–806. DOI: 10.1016/j.cell.2019.07.008

Ro, C., Chai, W., Yu, V. E., & Yu, R. (2013). Pancreatic neuroendocrine tumors: Biology, diagnosis, and treatment. *Chinese Journal of Cancer*, *32*(6), 312–324. DOI: 10.5732/cjc.012.10295

Round, J. L., & Mazmanian, S. K. (2009). The gut microbiota shapes intestinal immune responses during health and disease. *Nature Reviews. Immunology*, *9*(5), 313–323. DOI: 10.1038/nri2515

Sherman, M. H., & Beatty, G. L. (2023). Tumor microenvironment in pancreatic cancer pathogenesis and therapeutic resistance. *Annual Review of Pathology*, *18*(1), 123–148. DOI: 10.1146/annurev-pathmechdis-031621-024600

Shoaf, K., Mulvey, G. L., Armstrong, G. D., & Hutkins, R. W. (2006). Prebiotic galacto-oligosaccharides reduce adherence of entero-pathogenic *Escherichia coli* to tissue culture cells. *Infection and Immunity*, *74*(12), 6920–6928. DOI: 10.1128/IAI.01030-06

Siegel, R. L., Miller, K. D., Fuchs, H. E., & Jemal, A. (2021). Cancer statistics, 2021. *CA: a Cancer Journal for Clinicians*, *71*(1), 7–33. DOI: 10.3322/caac.21654

Sivan, A., Corrales, L., Hubert, N., Williams, J. B., Aquino-Michaels, K., Earley, Z. M., Benyamin, F. W., Man Lei, Y., Jabri, B., Alegre, M.-L., Chang, E. B., & Gajewski, T. F. (2015). Commensal *Bifidobacterium* promotes antitumor immunity and facilitates anti–PD-L1 efficacy. *Science*, *350*(6264), 1084–1089. DOI: 10.1126/science.aac4255

Temel, H. Y., Kaymak, Ö., Kaplan, S., Bahcivanci, B., Gkoutos, G. V., & Acharjee, A. (2023). Role of microbiota and microbiota derived short-chain fatty acids in PDAC. *Cancer Medicine*, *12*(5), 5661–5675. DOI: 10.1002/cam4.5323

Torres, P. J., Fletcher, E. M., Gibbons, S. M., Bouvet, M., Doran, K. S., & Kelley, S. T. (2015). Characterization of the salivary microbiome in patients with pancreatic cancer. *PeerJ*, *3*, e1373. DOI: 10.7717/peerj.1373

Trivieri, N., Panebianco, C., Villani, A., Pracella, R., Latiano, T. P., Perri, F., Binda, E., & Pazienza, V. (2020). High levels of prebiotic resistant starch in diet modulate a specific pattern of miRNAs expression profile associated with a better overall survival in pancreatic cancer. *Biomolecules*, *11*(1), 26–38. DOI: 10.3390/biom11010026

Viaud, S., Saccheri, F., Mignot, G., Yamazaki, T., Daillère, R., Hannani, D., Enot, D. P., Pfirschke, C., Engblom, C., Pittet, M. J., Schlitzer, A., Ginhoux, F., Apetoh, L., Chachaty, E., Woerther, P.-L., Eberl, G., Bérard, M., Ecobichon, C., Clermont, D., & Zitvogel, L. (2013). The intestinal microbiota modulates the anticancer immune effects of cyclophosphamide. *Science*, *342*(6161), 971–976. DOI: 10.1126/science.1240537

Weber, J. S. (2014). Current perspectives on immunotherapy. *Seminars in Oncology*, *41*(5), S14–S29. DOI: 10.1053/j.seminoncol.2014.09.003

Wu, Y., Han, W., Dong, H., Liu, X., & Su, X. (2024). The rising roles of exosomes in the tumor microenvironment reprogramming and cancer immunotherapy. *MedComm*, *5*(4), e541–e550. DOI: 10.1002/mco2.541

Wu, Y. S., Chung, I., Wong, W. F., Masamune, A., Sim, M. S., & Looi, C. Y. (2017). Paracrine IL-6 signaling mediates the effects of pancreatic stellate cells on epithelial-mesenchymal transition via Stat3/Nrf2 pathway in pancreatic cancer cells. *Biochimica et Biophysica Acta (BBA) -. Biochimica et Biophysica Acta. G, General Subjects*, *1861*(2), 296–306. DOI: 10.1016/j.bbagen.2016.10.006

Zhang, T., Gao, G., Sakandar, H. A., Kwok, L.-Y., & Sun, Z. (2022). Gut dysbiosis in pancreatic diseases: A causative factor and a novel therapeutic target. *Frontiers in Nutrition*, *9*, 814269. DOI: 10.3389/fnut.2022.814269

Zhu, Y., Luo, T. M., Jobin, C., & Young, H. A. (2011). Gut microbiota and probiotics in colon tumorigenesis. *Cancer Letters*, *309*(2), 119–127. DOI: 10.1016/j.canlet.2011.06.004

Chapter 4
Role of Nanotechnology in Pancreatic Cancer

B. Lokeshwari
https://orcid.org/0009-0005-6612-5134
Department of Microbiology, Sacred Heart College, Tirupattur, India

M. Divya
Department of Microbiology, Sacred Heart College, Tirupattur, India

U. Subhalakshmi
Department of Microbiology, Sacred Heart College, Tirupattur, India

P. Prakathi
Department of Microbiology, Sacred Heart College, Tirupattur, India

ABSTRACT

Pancreatic Cancer (PC) has a five-year survival rate of fewer than 5% due to its late-stage diagnosis, poor prognosis, and significant resistance to traditional therapy. Nanotechnology has become a game-changer, providing novel medicinal and diagnostic approaches to address these issues. Since pancreatic tumours have extensive stromal barriers, this allows for precision targeting of cancer cells, reduces off-target effects, and improves drug delivery systems. In order to increase the effectiveness of treatment, nanoparticles, including metallic, lipid, and polymeric varieties, are essential. Gold, quantum dots, and superparamagnetic iron oxide are examples of nanoparticles that improve the sensitivity and specificity of early tumour detection in diagnostics. Advanced nanocarriers, like liposomes and polymeric nanoparticles, are used therapeutically to encapsulate RNA interference inhibitors and chemotherapeutic drugs (like gemcitabine and paclitaxel), enhancing their pharmacokinetics, stability, and bioavailability. When coupled to nanoparticles, targeting ligands like

DOI: 10.4018/979-8-3373-1469-3.ch004

peptides and antibodies improve selectivity for cancer cells, and stimuli-responsive systems enable regulated drug release that is triggered by the tumour microenvironment (e.g., pH, enzymes). Key resistance mechanisms like as hypoimmunogenicity, stromal desmoplasia, altered drug transport, and cancer stem cell survival are also addressed by nanotechnology. Artificial intelligence also speeds up the design of nanoparticles, improves delivery, and makes customised treatment plans possible. Despite its potential, issues with stability, large-scale manufacturing, and possible toxicity need to be resolved in order to speed up clinical translation. With early diagnosis, focused therapy, and better treatment results, nanotechnology has the potential to completely transform PC management.

1. INTRODUCTION

Pancreatic cancer, which affects men more frequently than women, is a major cause of death as well as one of the most prevalent types of cancer. It has a survival rate of fewer than 5% after five years. The disease known as Pancreatic Cancer (PC) is extremely aggressive and almost always fatal. According to Kamisawa et al. (2016), Ductal Adenocarcinoma is the most prevalent form of Pancreatic Cancer, and it starts in the exocrine connective tissue that produces enzymes. The location of the tumour in the pancreas may have an impact on how the symptoms manifest clinically (Ducreux et al., 2015). Nearly 65% of PC tumours affect the Pancreatic neck and Skull; because of bile obstruction, patients usually present with Jaundice and Epigastric pain (Tempero et al., 2019).

Pancreatic cancer can occasionally manifest as a multi-differentiated tumour (2%), in the tail area (10%), or even inside the digestive tract (15%). Patients may also have late-onset Type 2 diabetes, stomach pain, and weight loss (Gheorghe et al., 2020). About 95% of all exocrine-originating pancreatic cancer subtypes are Pancreatic Adeno Carcinomas (PDAC). Acinar and cystadenocarcinoma cells are less prevalent. Five per cent of PC patients have endocrine tumours, including Neuroendocrine Tumours (PNET) (Hackeng et al., 2016). Drug resistance is an important contributor to the poor prognosis of pancreatic cancer, which can be inherent (natural) or acquired (as a result of pharmacological therapy) (Binenbaum et al., 2015).

PDAC and other pancreatic neoplasms are solid tumours made up of a close extracellular matrix, normal cells such as fibroblasts, and a near-stromal milieu of cancerous cells. Drug penetration is hampered by the arrangement's proximity. Drugs can permeate through the malignant stroma, and the tight tumour stroma usually makes it difficult for the pharmacological molecules to distinguish between healthy and malignant cells (Sofuni et al., 2005). Growth hormone-stimulated stromal desmoplastic processes cause the Pancreatic Stellate Cells (PSC) to release collagen, hyaluronic acid, and other extracellular matrix components. Primary stem cells reduce cellular vascularity, leading to hypoxia and stromal fibrosis. The stromal barrier of PSC tightens blood arteries and raises interstitial fluid pressure, which inhibits the passive transfer of chemotherapeutic medicines and ultimately results in treatment failure (Erkan et al., 2012). Using nanotechnology to deliver medications to particular parts of the body is one economical way to treat diseases and other ailments.

Nanomedicine is one promising approach that is quickly being used to change the way PC is treated (El-Zahaby et al., 2018). According to Ali et al. (2020), generally speaking, nanoparticles are described as having a minimum of one dimension between 1 and 100 nm and spanning a variety of platforms with varying chemical, physical, and material components. About tumour cells, nanoparticles may also be tailored for a certain drug to improve picture quality and lessen side effects linked to Current Chemotherapy. The gastrointestinal absorption of a drug or imaging contrast formulation can raise the potential efficacy per dosage. Using passive or active targeting to administer drugs or imaging contrast materials, successful nanoparticles must be built with components that are specifically suited to a disease's physiological barrier, as well as nano-engineered components for particle extravasation, aggregation, and tumour penetration. To make the treatment more effective for pancreatic cancer, various nanoparticles, such as metallic, lipid, and polymeric ones, have been produced (Santos Rebelo et al., 2018).

2. THERAPY RESISTANCE IN USING NANOPARTICLE-BASED PANCREATIC CANCER

Nanotechnology can successfully counteract certain resistance characteristics of pancreatic tumours, predisposing patients to treatment. Many of the treatment modalities, including chemotherapy, radiation therapy, and molecularly targeted agents, have been unable to manage Pancreatic tumours. Intrinsic as well as extrinsic properties of the malignant cell population from the neighbouring microenvironment are accountable for the multifactorial complexity of the PC recalcitrant condition (Schober et al., 2014). These may already exist before the start of therapy, or they may emerge following the early phase of treatment, sensitivity and primary resistance mechanisms, respectively.

Figure 1. Mechanisms of Therapy Resistance in Nanoparticle-Based Pancreatic Cancer

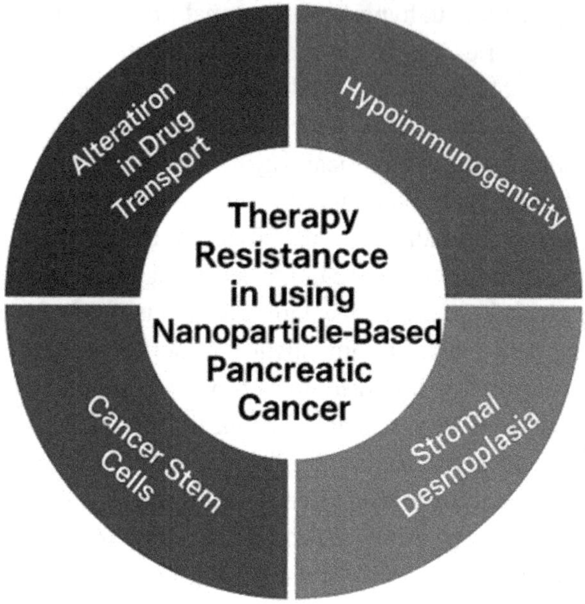

2.1. Alterations in Drug Transport

Gemcitabine's initial treatment may be particularly affected by impaired drug absorption and rapid drug efflux, the most prevalent chemoresistance mechanism in PC. Because gemcitabine is hydrophilic and has a hard time diffusing across cell membranes' lipid bilayer, nucleoside transporters are necessary for its intracellular uptake. In patients treated with gemcitabine for pancreatic cancer, downregulation of hENT1 nucleoside transporters has been associated with a poorer survival rate. Expression of nucleoside transporters is required for the efficient utilisation of drug formulation in nanoparticles in the resistance process, which includes processes such as clathrin-mediated endocytosis and micropinocytosis (Rennick et al., 2021).

Nanoparticle packing may improve drug intracellular uptake, as illustrated by increased tumour cytotoxicity of nano-encapsulated gemcitabine relative to free drug. Chemoresistance to the illness can be caused by changes in transmembrane efflux pump expression and function, similar to uptake transporters. Drug ejection by cells is done through the A triphosphate-binding Cassette (ABC), which has P-glycoprotein multidrug resistance proteins and breast cancer resistance proteins (Robey et al., 2018). These proteins restrict the intracellular drug pool and the therapeutic effect by excluding molecules from crossing the lipid bilayer and making it easier to move molecules out into the extracellular space.

Nanoparticle-based drug delivery systems are very effective because efflux pumps cannot easily detect them. In several models, the adverse correlation between the efficacy of photodynamic treatment and ABCG2 expression was thwarted by the photosensitizer included in polymeric nanoparticles (Roh et al., 2017). In addition, nanoparticles have been employed to deliver therapies capable of altering the expression and function of membrane transporters (Wang et al., 2021). A hENT1-encoding DNA plasmid is encapsulated within PC cells to induce expression of the uptake transporter. Chemosensitizers, which modulate bidirectional drug passage through the cell membrane, and standard-of-care drugs, e.g., gemcitabine, are combined in dual-loaded nanoparticles to treat pancreatic cancer.

2.2. Hypoimmunogenicity

Pancreatic Cancer (PC) is known to possess a "cold" immune system, which significantly reduces the demand for sophisticated Immuno-oncology (IO) treatments like Pancreatic Cancer Inhibitors. This contrasts with other "hot" cancers like lung cancer and melanoma. Chemotherapy that is capable of inducing Immunogenic Cell Death (ICD) enhances Cancer Immunity (Liu et al., 2021). Doxorubicin and Oxaliplatin polymeric nanoformulations have been shown to enhance the expression of Damage-Associated Molecular Patterns (DAMPs) and Mature Dendritic Cells, and stimulate Adaptive Immune Elements downstream in PC models (Zhao et al., 2016).

Both of the nanoformulations were effectively employed as a component of a preventative vaccine strategy and suppressed the growth of established Pan02 allografts. Vaccine-based approaches to PC have only partially exploited Nanotechnology until now. Nanotechnology can significantly amplify the Immunostimulatory capacity of Vaccines and is an emerging solution to Hypoimmunogenicity (Banerjee et al., 2019). Nanoparticles may also be with materials having Adjuvants (Lebre et al., 2018), ideally targeting Antigen-Presenting Cells actively or passively and averting the breakdown of unstable Vaccine ingredients such as Peptides and Nucleic acids (Lorkowski et al., 2021).

2.3. Stromal Desmoplasia

Up to 90% of the entire tumour mass could be desmoplasia, or the growth of a thick fibrotic stroma (Christenson et al., 2020). Highly impenetrable networks regarding Extra Cellular Matrix (ECM), proteins collagen, fibronectin, and hyaluronan surround non-neoplastic subsets of cells. These components are targets for therapeutic approaches based on nanomedicine since they provide drug resistance through several physical and biological processes.

2.3.1. Physical Barriers

Pancreatic tumours with their inherent hypervascularity sometimes cause poor perfusion, therefore affecting drug delivery. Unchecked cancer cell proliferation in a localised tissue area causes too much strain and compressive pressures that collapse and cause most of the vasculature to be non-functional. As the tumour's lymphatics fail to drain, plasma leaks from hyperpermeable capillaries, and interstitial pressure rises. Numerous components of drug transport, such as extravasation across the endothelium, injection into the tumour, and transit through the interstitial space, contribute to these deviations in drug resistance to therapy. As Vennin et al. (2018) have revealed, the stroma offers the possibility for improved treatment penetrance of pancreatic cancer.

Through the production of Extracellular Matrix (ECM) components, fibroblasts, particularly their Pancreatic Stellate Cell (PSC) progenitors, have emerged as desirable candidates for the central role in the desmoplastic reaction. These cells are latent at homeostatic levels during pancreatic carcinogenesis but are triggered by paracrine and contact-mediated signals from cancer cells and other stromal components. Nano-inspired strategies for suppressing PSC and fibroblast activity have been demonstrated by several mechanisms, including lipid regulations (Hossen et al., 2019), downregulation of Wnt 16 (Cun et al., 2019), reconstituting relaxing or TRAIL expression (Hu et al., 2019), and inhibition of PI3K or MAPK (Saha et al., 2016). Nano-formulated inhibitors aiming at both routes have been shown in PC models to downregulate PSC and fibroblast activation markers.

The efficacy and administration of Chemotherapeutics is their Mardhian et al. (2020). The pH differential of the stroma preserves the outermost areas while selectively damaging the inner core by releasing medicines micro-encased in acidic environments. Designed to solve the vasculature, the PC microenvironment physical barriers seek to re-establish intertumoral drug perfusion and vascular patency (Cao et al., 2021). Although the hyperpermeability of young vasculature may help medication penetration to solid tumours, the endothelial lining of PC arteries is often rather high in coverage with pericytes. The cells can seal vascular fenestrations that stop medications from reaching the tumour bed from the blood in Pancreatic cancer.

Transforming Growth Factor (TGF) Signalling is the essential pathway mediating pericyte contacts with endothelial cells, according to Zonneville et al. (2018); hence, blocking this process could improve cancer medication delivery. The complexation of a TGF-inhibitor to mesoporous silica nanoparticles (Meng et al., 2013) can disturb the colocalization of endothelial cells and pericytes. Pre-treatment of pancreatic BxPC-3 xenografts with nanoparticles slowed down tumour growth, and a subsequently applied nanoformulation of gemcitabine penetrated better. Reduced toxicity along with the later enhanced capacity to bypass this chemo-resistant nature, shown by comparisons of free and nano-manufactured medicines.

2.3.2. Biological Barriers

The complex biological connections between stromal components and the neoplastic epithelium produced extra resistance to these treatments. Fibroblasts and lymphoid and myeloid immune cells are stromal cells. Many advances in molecular communication and cross-talk among these cells have shown their importance in cancer growth and therapy resistance (Huber et al., 2020). They also help create the immunosuppressive PC microenvironment, which can reduce IO therapy sensitivity. Nanotechnology has made numerous therapeutic methods for stromal cell biology modification more accessible (Bejarano et al., 2021). When immune suppression of surveillance in the pancreatic cancer microenvironment, fibroblasts can resist therapy in addition to desmoplasia growth. Nanoparticles encapsulated in liposomes contain plasmid DNA expressing a high-affinity CXCL12-binding extracellular protein to restore anti-tumour immunity. This formulation sequestered CXCL12 and produced considerable CD8+ T-cell infiltration that preconditioned tumours for checkpoint inhibition utilising a code-livered PDL1 trap in Orthotopic KPC allografts.

The limited efficacy of non-encapsulated combination trap therapy indicated that nanotechnology dramatically minimises PC immunotherapy resistance. By limiting tumour-PSC interaction via the CXCL12/CXCR4 axis, these nanoparticles produced several immunostimulatory events: They included CD8+ T cell recruitment and M2 macrophage reduction. The tumour microenvironment becomes immunogenic, making PC more susceptible to IO therapies like checkpoint inhibitors. Macrophages adopt the power source pro-tumour M2-like phenotype during pancreatic carcinogenesis, which modifies their surface markers and secretes immune-suppressing signals. To restore anti-tumour immunity, macrophages are re-educated via TLR agonism and kinase inhibition to induce M1-like polarisation. Using this sensitivity and producing environmentally sensitive nanoparticles should assist in selectively delivering M1 polarising chemicals to macrophages (Zhou et al., 2021).

PEG is a protective covering that keeps cells intact in the bloodstream until they reach the tumour (Han et al., 2018). The pancreatic cancer stroma also contains regulatory lymphocytes (T-cells) and myeloid-derived suppressor cells. Though rare, they can contribute disproportionately to drug resistance by inhibiting dendritic cell function, M2 macrophages, and T-cell anergy to satisfy tumours' immune escape (Jang et al., 2017). Direct targeting of such cell subsets has not been fully studied, but other nano-based techniques that generated positive results in PC models of nanomedicine have shown alterations in their tumour morphology (Lu et al., 2017).

2.4. Cancer Stem Cells

The unique ability of CSCs to self-renew and differentiate into mature progeny distinguishes them from a small pool of tumour-resident pluripotent cells. Additionally, they exhibit a phenotype that is incredibly durable to many different therapeutic approaches. CSCs are thought to be important targets for long-term tumour therapy because they have been identified as the main causes of oncogenesis. Targeting CSCs has developed methods for creating nanomedicines that disrupt the biology of CSCs. Some of these a polymeric nanoformulations since the naturally occurring xanthonoid mango tin's poor water solubility renders it inappropriate for usage as a free entity (Verma et al., 2016). Additionally, there was no sign of metastatic hepatic nodules, and the tumour load had decreased. Copper oxide nanoparticles (Benguigui et al., 2019) and superparamagnetic iron oxide nanoparticles coupled with curcumin or a leptin inhibitor are two other nanopreparations that have been demonstrated to lessen stem-like characteristics in PC models. To increase the selectivity of CSC targeting, several formulations have been altered using ligands that bind to CSC surface markers such as CD44 and CD133 (Nigam Joshi et al., 2017).

3. ROLE OF ARTIFICIAL INTELLIGENCE AND MACHINE LEARNING IN ADVANCING NANOTECHNOLOGY FOR PANCREATIC CANCER

The integration of Artificial Intelligence (AI) and Machine Learning (ML) is fundamentally revolutionizing the application of nanotechnology in pancreatic cancer (PC), offering a paradigm shift from traditional, often empirical, approaches to a data-driven, predictive, and highly precise discipline that accelerates progress across the entire spectrum of nanomedicine, from rational drug design and optimized delivery to enhanced diagnostics and personalized treatment strategies. In the realm of nanoparticle design and discovery, AI algorithms, particularly deep learning models, can analyze vast and complex datasets encompassing material science, chemistry, and biology to predict the optimal physicochemical properties such as size, shape, surface charge, and composition of novel nanocarriers (e.g., polymeric nanoparticles, liposomes, solid lipid nanoparticles) for specific chemotherapeutic agents like gemcitabine or paclitaxel, thereby overcoming intrinsic limitations of poor solubility and stability that plague many conventional drugs (Ali et al., 2020; Pearce et al., 2012); these models can simulate molecular interactions between a drug candidate and a proposed nanocarrier material, predicting encapsulation efficiency, loading capacity, and release kinetics with remarkable accuracy, which drastically reduces the need for costly and time-consuming trial-and-error experimentation in the lab.

Furthermore, ML-driven generative models are now being employed to *de novo* design entirely new nanoparticle constructs and targeting ligands, exploring a chemical space far beyond human intuition to create highly specific molecules that can, for instance, better bind to overexpressed receptors on PC cells such as uPAR or target specific markers on cancer stem cells (CD44, CD133) to mitigate therapy resistance and recurrence (Nigam Joshi et al., 2017; Verma et al., 2016). Beyond design, AI plays a critical role in optimizing nanoparticle delivery and overcoming physiological barriers, a paramount challenge in PC due to its dense, hypoxic, and highly fibrotic stroma that severely limits drug perfusion and promotes resistance (Erkan et al., 2012; Provenzano & Hingorani, 2013); by analyzing high-resolution medical imaging (CT, MRI) of tumors, ML algorithms can map the unique and heterogeneous tumor microenvironment (TME) of individual patients, identifying regions of high stromal density, vascular leakage, and interstitial fluid pressure to inform the design of nanoparticles with tailored penetration capabilities (Vennin et al., 2018).

Predictive models can determine the ideal nanoparticle size to navigate the compressed vasculature or suggest surface modifications (e.g., with enzymes like PEGPH20 that degrade hyaluronic acid) to locally disrupt the stromal barrier and enhance nanoparticle accumulation, a strategy that has shown promise in pre-clinical models (Von Hoff et al., 2011; Cao et al., 2021); moreover, reinforcement learning algorithms can model the complex pharmacokinetics and biodistribution of nanoparticles in silico, forecasting how a nanoparticle of a given design will travel through the bloodstream, evade the immune system, extravasate into the tumor, and ultimately penetrate the stromal matrix to reach the cancer cells, thereby enabling the virtual screening of thousands of nanoparticle variants to identify those with the highest predicted tumor bioavailability and lowest off-target toxicity before a single synthesis is attempted (Petros & DeSimone, 2010). In diagnostics and early detection, AI-powered nano-diagnostics are creating a new frontier for identifying PC at its earliest, most treatable stages by enabling the ultra-sensitive analysis of liquid biopsies; nanoparticles functionalized to capture rare circulating tumor cells (CTCs), exosomes, or specific proteins can be used in concert with AI algorithms that analyze complex, multiplexed biomarker data from these captures, detecting subtle, cancer-specific signatures that are imperceptible to conventional assays, thus facilitating a panel-based diagnostic approach that significantly improves accuracy over single biomarkers (Malhotra et al., 2012; Chikkaveeraiah et al., 2012).

These ML models can integrate data from nano-sensors based on quantum dots, gold nanoparticles, or nanowires to identify patterns indicative of early neoplasia, even in cases of paraneoplastic diabetes which often precedes overt cancer symptoms, by correlating nascent cancer biomarkers with markers of β-cell dysfunction, thereby stratifying high-risk patients and enabling earlier intervention (Gheorghe et al., 2020). Perhaps most transformative is the role of AI in personalising nanomedicine treatments, where ML models can integrate a patient's multi-omic data (genomics, proteomics, transcriptomics) with data on nanoparticle performance to recommend the most effective nanotherapy regimen to a liposomal formulation of irinotecan, a polymeric nanoparticle carrying a siRNA against HIF1α to overcome hypoxia-induced resistance, or an immunostimulatory nano-vaccine designed to reverse the immunosuppressive TME (Zhao et al., 2015; Lorkowski et al., 2021; Bejarano et al., 2021). This approach allows for the selection of nanocarriers and payloads that are precisely tailored to overcome the unique resistance mechanisms, be they related to drug transport alterations, stromal desmoplasia, or hypoimmunogenicity present in an individual's tumour, moving beyond the one-size-fits-all model of traditional chemotherapy (Schober et al., 2014).

AI is indispensable in accelerating clinical translation and manufacturing, where AI-driven automation and quality control systems can monitor and control the complex synthesis, purification, and scale-up processes of therapeutic nanoparticles, ensuring batch-to-batch consistency, high yield, and reproducible efficacy that are critical for regulatory approval and clinical adoption, while also optimizing clinical trial design by identifying patient subpopulations most likely to respond to a novel nanotherapy based on their historical data and biomarker profiles, thus making trials more efficient and increasing their chances of success (Blanco et al., 2011). The convergence of AI and nanotechnology is not merely an incremental improvement but a fundamental force multiplier, creating a powerful feedback loop where nanotechnologies generate rich, high-dimensional biological data and AI provides the computational power to interpret it, learn from it, and generate actionable insights, thereby propelling the field towards a future of intelligent, adaptive, and truly personalized nanomedicines capable of tackling the formidable challenge of pancreatic cancer with unprecedented precision and efficacy.

4. NANO-DIAGNOSTICS FOR THE EARLY DETECTION OF PANCREATIC CANCER

Early detection and good treatment of pancreatic cancer may improve overall patient survival since most patients who survive the disease for five years or more have tolerable disease at diagnosis and are suitable candidates for curative resection. Furthermore, the heterogeneity and stromal complexity within the tumour milieu limit the potential biomarkers of pancreatic cancer. The simultaneous detection of a panel of biomarkers could be required for early diagnosis of pancreatic tumours in an attempt to increase accuracy relative to individual biomarkers. More rapid, precise, cost-effective, and more reliable with lower limits of detection biomarker detection systems. The application of cancer diagnostics could undergo a full revolution thanks to nano-diagnostic platforms (Malhotra et al., 2012).

To improve their sensitivity towards the electrochemical identification of cancer biomarkers, certain electrochemical immunosensors have additionally included the fields of nanotechnology, like magnetic particles, small particles of gold, quantum dots, and carbon nanotubes (Chikkaveeraiah et al., 2012). With detection limits many orders of magnitude lower than the clinically significant levels for diagnostic use, the nanowire biosensors facilitate rapid and accurate determination of the ovarian cancer biomarkers insulin-like growth factor-II and cancer antigen-125 in direct measurement of human whole blood from a mere fingerprick. Through the application of nanoporous alumina membranes to microfabricated silicon platforms, nano monitors allow rapid, label-free, and highly specific analysis of pancreatic cancer cell lysate glycans.

These biosensors could be utilised to diagnose pancreatic cancer in the clinic by identifying transmembrane glycoproteins such as mucins, which regulate tumour growth and metastasis and are produced on pancreatic cancer cells. Nano-diagnostics may help diagnose pancreatic cancer-related paraneoplastic diabetes early. Diabetes or Hyperglycemia can appear two to three years before Pancreatic Cancer and affect up to 85% of individuals. Therefore, a large patient population might evaluate the diagnostic capability of nano-diagnostics combining early cancer markers with β-cell malfunction markers (El-Zahaby et al., 2018). Cancer detection, prevention, and diagnosis are possible with nano-diagnostics. Biomarker identification may be more sensitive using nano-diagnostic platforms and small sample quantities. Nano-diagnostics for cancer biomarker identification's multiplexity, increased sensitivity, and specificity could be used to monitor patient response to treatment or detect early recurrences that conventional assays cannot detect.

5. NANOMEDICINES AS THERAPEUTICS FOR PANCREATIC CANCER

In many pre-clinical cancer models, liposome-surfaced nanoparticles and nanomaterials produced by polymers have been largely utilised. Such nanoparticles have already proven to hold high promise as extremely effective drug delivery systems for chemotherapy drugs or RNA interference (RNAi) inhibitors, and are currently in the process of being tested in human clinical trials (Blanco et al., 2011).

Figure 2. Nanomedicine-Based Therapeutic Approaches for Pancreatic Cancer

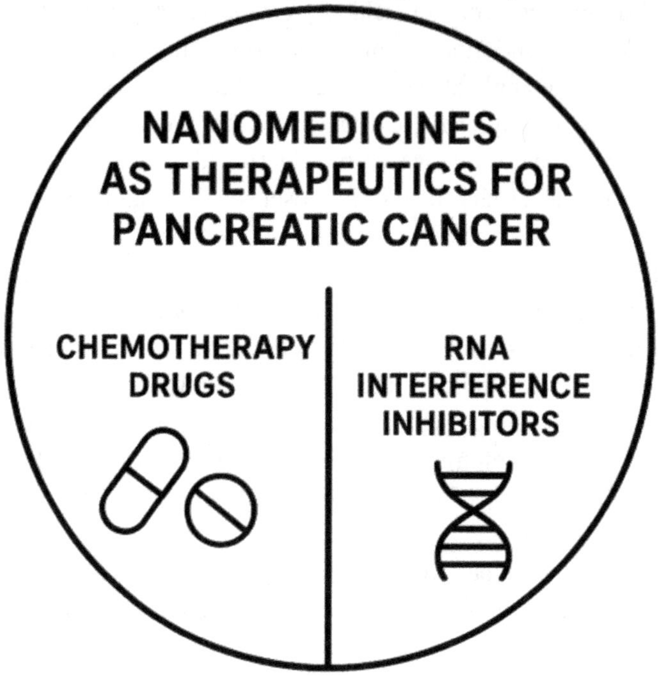

5.1. Chemotherapy Drugs

Many chemotherapeutic medicines have poor pharmacokinetics, off-target effects, and tumour absorption. Nanotechnology for chemotherapeutic drug delivery. Smart nanoparticle design for chemotherapeutic drug administration improves drug solubility, stability, and half-life (Pearce et al., 2012). Chemotherapy-encapsulated nanoparticles bypass most tumour cells' surface multi-drug-resistant efflux pumps. In 1995, the FDA authorised "Doxil" as the first nanoparticle drug. Liposomes containing doxorubicin are called Doxil. Around 100 nm in diameter. A tiny amount of polyethene glycol (PEG)-lipid was added to the liposome to reduce nanoparticle clearance from the circulation and prolong plasma doxorubicin half-life, increasing tumour bioavailability. Doxorubicin in liposomes improves tumour absorption, anti-cancer activity, and systemic off-target toxicity. Doxil treats platinum-resistant ovarian cancer. Nanoparticle gemcitabine for chemotherapy (Leamon et al., 2013).

Vincent et al. (2011) say gemcitabine is the preferred treatment for metastatic or incurable pancreatic cancer. Nanoparticles are used as the medication's delivery vehicle to circumvent some of the mechanisms that make gemcitabine susceptible in pancreatic cancer cells and optimise its distribution to pancreatic tumours. Overexpression of the ribonucleotide reductase subunit M1 in pancreatic cancer cells can be exploited to overcome resistance with a nanoparticle containing gemcitabine [4-(N) stearoyl gemcitabine] (GemC18). Pancreatic cancer cells and blood arteries around the tumour stroma have higher uPAR receptor levels. Gemcitabine was coupled to agentic IONPs using a lysosomal cleavable tetrapeptide linker. Nanoparticles and gemcitabine inhibited orthotopically xenografted mice pancreatic tumour growth and allowed MRI to detect any leftover tumours. Nanotechnology is also being developed to improve the administration and use of additional chemotherapy medications that could be given alongside gemcitabine or as a secondary treatment for pancreatic tumours.

The tumour microenvironment was the only place these nanoparticles were designed to slowly release their contents. This medication may decrease the progression of early-stage pancreatic cancer. Another nanoparticle-conjugated chemotherapeutic drug, albumin-bound paclitaxel (Nab-paclitaxel or Abraxane® (Abraxis Bioscience), has garnered attention. When given alone or with gemcitabine, nab-paclitaxel depletes pancreatic stroma in pancreatic cancer xenograft animal models. Intertumoral gemcitabine concentration increased 2.8 times after stroma ablation (Von Hoff et al., 2011). A recent Phase III MPACT trial improved metastatic pancreatic cancer patients' median survival to 8.5 months from 6.7 months with Gemcitabine alone. Nab-paclitaxel and gemcitabine were used to dissolve paclitaxel, reducing Cremophor-related toxicities like neutropenia and neuropathy and allowing patients to tolerate higher doses (Ma and Hidalgo, 2013). Enzymatic medication PEGPH20 targets Hyaluronic Acid (HA), a key component of Pancreatic Cancer's desmoplastic stroma. Nanotechnology can transport medications directly to tumour cells and therapeutically target tumour stroma to deplete and normalise tumour vascularity, making it a promising novel pancreatic cancer treatment.

5.2.RNA Interference Inhibitors

Selectivity, safety, and efficacy in overcoming multidrug resistance seem to give new hope beyond systemic drug administration with RNA interference (RNAi) therapeutic techniques. If an RNA target sequence is generated, RNA interference (RNAi) can eliminate all mRNA. They now study how short-interfering RNAs (siRNAs) can efficiently lower target gene expression in organisms and cell cultures. The RNA-Induced Silencing Complex (RISC) in the cell's cytoplasm coordinates mRNA cleavage with a complementary siRNA sequence. Artificial siRNAs can stimulate the cell's natural process. As a potent gene therapy, the approach can decrease genes connected to human illnesses, including cancer. Schroeder et al. (2010) developed nanoparticles that self-assemble on siRNA and protect it from degradation.

The non-toxic nanoparticle-siRNA complexes lowered apo B for 11 days. SNALPs have also been used to transport siRNA to silence a gene that promotes invasive hepatocellular cancer in an orthotopic mouse model. Nanoparticle-siRNA complexes reduced pancreatic cancer cell HER-2 expression, making them gemcitabine-sensitive. Human clinical trials are underway to assess the safety and efficacy of systemic siRNA delivery utilising modified nanoparticles for cancer therapy. A TfR-targeting cyclodextrin-nanoparticle (CALAA-01) was utilised to inject systemic siRNA into solid tumour patients in a phase I trial (Davis et al., 2010). CALAA-01, a siRNA-nanoparticle compound, reduced RRM2 in malignant melanoma patients. The ALN-VSP nanoparticle-siRNA combination was successful and well tolerated every two weeks for 23 months (Tabernero et al., 2013).

6. NANO-BASED DRUG DELIVERY SYSTEMS FOR PANCREATIC CANCER TREATMENT

Gene delivery, pathotropic nanoparticles, micellar nanoparticles, liposomal nanoparticles (Au et al., 2016), and albumin-conjugated paclitaxel nanoparticles. Pancreatic cancer treatment uses inhibition-based RNA. This treatment is promising as a substitute for traditional ones because of its specificity, toxicity, and ability to overcome pharmacological sensitivity. Nanoparticle-delivered siRNA protects pancreatic cancer against breakdown and immune system clearance, providing direct and indirect immunomodulation alternatives. Direct immunomodulation occurs when nanoparticles physically engage with immune cells to activate and activate them. Nanoparticles carry Immune-Stimulating Substances like Cytokines or Antigens to boost the immune system's defences against pancreatic cancer cells. Nanoparticles targeting the tumour microenvironment can indirectly affect the immune system. These systems guide therapeutic chemicals to immunosuppressive cells such as T-cells, Dendritic cells, and Antibody receptors to lower immunological checkpoints and boost anticancer immune responses (Jindal et al., 2021).

Figure 3. Nano-Based Drug Delivery Systems for Pancreatic Cancer Treatment

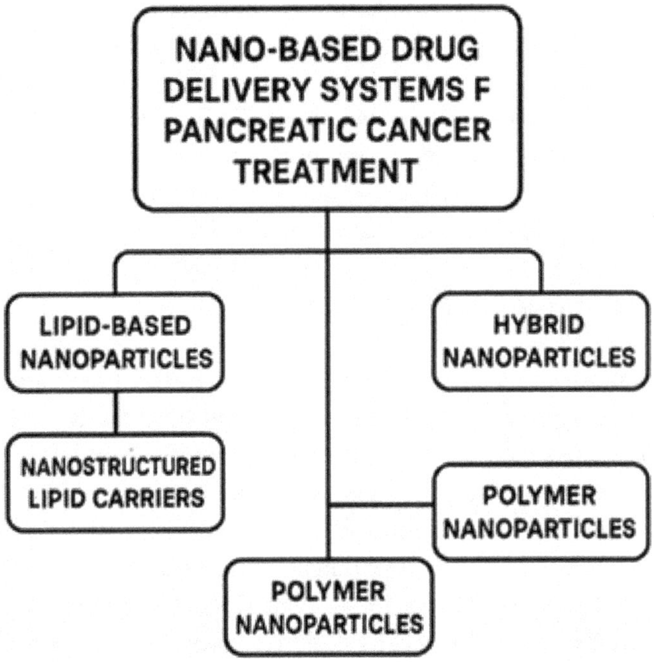

6.1. Lipid-Based Nanoparticles

Liposomes are the most frequently used of the numerous lipid-derived nanocarriers. Liposomes are round, colloidal particles that support the delivery of both water-soluble and insoluble substances and provide precision targeting flexibility (Judge et al., 2009). Their low stability, especially in aqueous dispersion and upon storage for long durations, high cost, low cargo, and immediate release are certain disadvantages. They are not used exclusively as lipid-based nanoparticle types, and others are on the rise as well.

6.2. Solid Lipid Nanoparticles

Solid lipid nanoparticles (SLN) are more stable and release less because they include a solid lipid or a combination of solid lipids at room and body temperature. Encapsulating aspirin with curcumin. In nanocarriers with 85 and 69% encapsulation efficiency and 150 and 250 nm particle diameters. Human pancreatic cancer cell lines MIA PC-2 and Panc-1 were tested for apoptosis and survival. SLN morphology with GEM incorporated showed cytotoxic effects on primary pancreatic cell lines (PPCL-46) and pancreatic cancer cell lines (MiaPC-2).

SLN structures were made using poloxamer 188, polysorbate 80, and glyceryl monostearate. Multifunctional drug delivery systems for diverse routes, SLNs improve pancreatic cancer therapy's efficacy and safety (Rana, 2007). Lipidic compounds, which are common in SLNs, undergo physicochemical changes to form a denser and organised matrix, but they also change shape, which can trigger drug release during storage. Slowed or hindered crystallisation may also lower medication payload.

6.3. Nanostructured Lipid Carriers

Spherical Nanostructured Lipid Carriers (NLCs) encapsulate pharmaceuticals in a liquid-solid matrix. When incompatible liquid and solid lipids mix, NLC forms. This creates new lipid matrix topologies that increase matrix defects and loading capacity without compromising formulation stability. Zhao et al. (2015) developed lipid-based nanoparticles to systemically distribute cancer cell miRNA expression vectors. Besides releasing GEM and Baicalein, prodrug-based, hyaluronic acid-coated NLCs fight pancreatic cancer. They coated NLC with hyaluronic acid (HA), which may connect to most cancer cells' high receptors. Afterwards, BCL and GEM were injected into the NLC centre. NLCs increase loading capacity and formulation stability by integrating liquid lipid into the solid matrix.

6.4. Hybrid Nanoparticles

"Lipid-polymer hybrid nanoparticles" are polymeric nanoparticles with a single- or two-layer lipid shell around a polymeric core. The lipid layer is stable, biocompatible, and protective, whereas the cationic polymeric core holds siRNA and medication (Zhao et al., 2015). Apoprotein B siRNA was given to non-human primates in altered liposomes. GEM becomes more resistant to pancreatic cancer therapies when HIF1a siRNA (si-HIF1a) is co-delivered by a lipid-polymer hybrid nanoparticle. Nanoparticle aggregation, serum si-HIF1a stability, and GEM leakage were prevented by the polymer core's PEGylated lipid bilayer. SiRNA distribution uses cationic lipid polymers, which bind to genes, leak endosomes, and pass through cell membranes without injury. Cationic lipid polymers bind negatively charged siRNA via ionic interactions. Despite enzymatic breakdown, self-assembled lipoplexes increase siRNA release from the endosomal/lysosomal compartment, endocytosis, and cytosolic storage (Lin et al., 2022).

New pancreatic cancer treatments combine hybrid nanoparticles and siRNA. Paclitaxel was encapsulated in an albumin nanoparticle and attached to a modified thermosensitive liposome to improve its penetration into pancreatic ductal adenocarcinoma, which has a significant tumour stroma. Paclitaxel was better retained in solid tumours because of the liposome formulation. In addition, photothermal IR-780 was included. The IR-780 enlarged the tumour interstitial space when photothermal therapy and nanoparticle administration were combined, making drug release from modified liposomes easier (Yu et al., 2020). A hybrid nanoparticle enhanced pancreatic cancer prognosis by boosting therapeutic penetration through dense tumour stroma and medication stability and protection through lipid-polymer coating. The cationic lipid polymers were promising siRNA transfection agents, while paclitaxel and a photothermal agent increased drug release and therapeutic effect.

6.5. Polymer Nanoparticles

Normal polymer nanoparticles are biocompatible, biodegradable, and non-toxic. The main natural polymers include alginate, albumin, gelatin, and chitosan. Polyesters like PCL, PLA, and molecules cannot be polymerised in situ, but synthetic polymers can be used. Matrix-based (nanospheres) and vesicular polymeric nanoparticles exist. Medical nanocapsules are hollow and surrounded by a polymer membrane (Barenholz, 2012). Drug nanospheres are supplied using a polymer matrix. Dendrimers, micelles, and conjugated pharmaceuticals are polymer nanostructures beyond nanoparticles.

7. TOXICITY CONCERNS IN NANOPARTICLE DELIVERY SYSTEMS

The toxicity associated with this type of delivery mechanism might be due to the size, composition, or payload of the nanoparticles. The smaller particles that have the same chemical and crystal structure as larger ones, more hazards. They can easily penetrate biological barriers and reach target organs because of their small size. Furthermore, the smaller nanoparticles are capable of damaging intact cell membranes, inducing severe immunological responses, and crossing the blood-brain barrier. The balance of toxicity and therapeutic efficacy is imperative (Bahadar et al., 2016). Since the charge of the toxicity and accumulation of nanoparticles is also influenced by their surface charge, this must be considered. Because it inhibits undesirable particle aggregation that modifies their physicochemical properties, such as dispersion, surface-to-volume ratio, and surface activity, a zeta potential value greater than 30 mV is ideal. These alterations could result in macrophage clearance, vascular/lymphatic obstruction, inflammation, or toxicity. Sometimes, material encapsulation might result in increased ROS production, which can lead to DNA alterations.

Cationic liposomal nanoparticles can interact with serum proteins, lipoproteins, and the extracellular matrix, resulting in oxidative stress and/or aggregation that may cause harm to non-target tissue (Lv et al., 2006). Due to their inherent metallic character and high surface area to size, metallic nanoparticles have the tendency to aggregate in solution and have low charge at physiological pH. In addition to harming fetal development by crossing the placenta, gold nanoparticles cause reactive oxygen to be produced and trigger the start of autoimmunity (Chang, 2010). Due to their minute size (1–2 nm), these gold nanoparticles are even more dangerous for both normal and cancerous human cells. Conversely, larger gold nanoparticles (4.8–12 nm) are less toxic to normal cells but highly toxic to cancer cells. The drug that these nanoparticles transport is toxic at the cellular level using changing membrane potential, enhancing ROS generation at the mitochondrial level, inducing autophagy, or altering gene expression (Ryu et al., 2014). Though gemcitabine and erlotinib are commonly utilised to treat pancreatic cancer, they are extremely dangerous.

8. ADVANTAGES AND DISADVANTAGES OF NANO-BASED DRUG DELIVERY SYSTEMS

Nanomedicine uses nanobiotechnology to deliver medication. Nanobiotechnologies are also being considered for nano surgery. This technology could improve medical diagnosis, treatment, and nanoscale system injection (Li et al., 2020). Compared to classical treatments, nanomedicine for pancreatic cancer has fewer systemic toxicities due to ligand conjugation on nanoparticles, controlled and sustained drug release, less administration since local drug time and concentration are improved, greater tumour penetration within the tumour microenvironment, and passive tumour accumulation due to the permeability and retention effect. Nanomedicine and tumour formation skills can slow pancreatic cancer's high metastatic rate. Interventions at different cancer metastasis levels can alter different aspects of the process.

Cancer stem cells, which produce primary metastases, are targeted to control metastasis. Drug delivery and nanoparticle distribution improve with tumour site remodelling. The solid tumour's stroma makes the EPR effect useless for nanoparticle penetration in this malignancy. Blocking oncogenic exosomes may reduce niche development and metastasis. Nanocarriers are 100–10,000 times smaller than human cells. Due to the enhanced EPR effect, they passively target pancreatic tumour cells and are stable in physiological conditions. They bound to cancer cells and entered blood arteries based on size (Gianella et al., 2011). Their non-physiological chemical surface can precipitate, touch, and harm cells. Proteins, polysaccharides, and modified polyesters are natural or polymer-based nanoparticles with several applications and a potential future in targeted chemotherapy.

Monoclonal Antibodies (MA), which are used in oncological therapy, can target tumour cells (Heinz et al., 2017). Nanostructured materials are made from nanoparticles with specific shapes or characteristics. These substances are non-polymers, like carbon nanotubes and metal nanoparticles and polymers like dendrimers and micelles. Paclitaxel, an antitumor chemotherapy drug for solid tumours like pancreatic cancer, is ineffective due to its low water solubility. It was also tested in albumin-based formulations, ultrasonically responsive nano-emulsions, and mixed micelles. Many nanostructures are being used to transport medications to boost half-life, stability, and drug accumulation at their intended surfaces.

9. FUTURE PERSPECTIVES

In oncology, nanoparticles are widely used because of their various benefits. Nanoparticles' medication delivery potential drives their usage in cancer treatment. Encapsulating drugs in nanoparticles can overcome several of their problems, including enzymatic or metabolic degradation, poor water solubility, poor pharmacokinetics, and high toxicity. Cancer therapy sometimes includes mixing drugs with distinct pharmacologies, which may make dosage and tumour distribution more challenging to control at synergistic ratios. Petros & DeSimone (2010) suggest co-formulation utilising a single nanoparticle platform to integrate the pharmacokinetics and biodistribution of each medication. Nanoparticles' capacity to exploit undifferentiated tumour tissues' "leaky" vasculature and underdeveloped lymphatics can improve tumour medicine administration. These properties allow "passive" nanoparticle accumulation in tumours, causing the "Enhanced Permeability and Retention (EPR) effect," which deposits payloads preferentially at the target location.

Functionalizing nanoparticle surfaces with peptides and antibodies improves tumour retention. In many receptor–ligand pairs, "active" targeting engages nanoparticles with tumour cells. The creation of "smart" nanoparticles that release their payload upon activation has increased tumour medication distribution control. X-ray irradiation, ultrasound, and external light have been the most common stimuli. Endogenous drug release can be achieved by creating nanoparticles that react to pH, redox, hypoxia, or enzymes (Elgogary et al., 2016).

Metallic nanoparticles' thermal and radiosensitising properties make them popular therapies. Metallic nanoparticles are highly valued despite their contrast enhancement potential for imaging and diagnostic applications.

Polymers can make nanoparticles that release cargo under regulated conditions and meet specifications. Because polylactic-co-glycolic acid (PLGA) contains biodegradable ester groups, its breakdown rate depends on its monomer ratio (Ding et al., 2020). PLGA with a 50:50 monomeric ratio hydrolyses faster than grades with larger quantities of either component. Changes in polymer type can affect nanoencapsulated drug release kinetics. A "stealth" layer of hydrophilic polymers can protect nanoparticles from the immune system's detection as foreign elements. Most modern nanoformulations contain polyethene glycol (PEG), which helps here. Nanoparticle design and application are versatile due to these and other materials' unique features (Lin et al., 2018).

10. CONCLUSION

In conclusion, nanotechnology heralds a transformative era in the management of pancreatic cancer (PC), offering innovative solutions to overcome the formidable challenges posed by its late diagnosis, aggressive nature, and profound therapy resistance. In nanoscale materials, researchers have developed advanced diagnostic and therapeutic platforms that significantly enhance early detection, improve drug delivery, and enable precise targeting of cancer cells and their supportive stroma. Nanoparticles, including metallic, lipid, polymeric, and hybrid systems, facilitate the encapsulation of chemotherapeutic agents, RNA interference inhibitors, and immunomodulators, thereby improving drug stability, bioavailability, and pharmacokinetics while minimising systemic toxicity. The application of nano-diagnostics, such as functionalized nanoparticles for capturing circulating tumour cells or exosomes, coupled with artificial intelligence for data analysis, allows for ultrasensitive, multiplexed biomarker detection, promising earlier and more accurate diagnosis. Furthermore, nanomedicine addresses key mechanisms of therapy resistance, including altered drug transport, stromal desmoplasia, hypoimmunogenicity, and cancer stem cell persistence through tailored strategies such as stimuli-responsive drug release, stromal remodelling, and immune microenvironment reprogramming. Despite these advancements, challenges remain in ensuring the clinical translation of nanotherapeutics, particularly concerning large-scale manufacturing reproducibility, long-term stability, and potential nanotoxicity, which must be rigorously addressed through continued research and regulatory pathways. The integration of artificial intelligence and machine learning further amplifies the potential of nanotechnology by enabling predictive modelling for nanoparticle design, personalised treatment regimens based on multi-omic data, and optimisation of clinical trial designs, thereby accelerating the development of intelligent, adaptive nanomedicines. The convergence of nanotechnology with emerging fields such as immuno-oncology, gene editing, and personalised medicine holds immense potential for revolutionising PC treatment, ultimately moving towards this devastating disease can be managed with unprecedented precision, efficacy, and improved patient outcomes. The evolution of nanobiotechnology not only enhances our therapeutic arsenal but also the pancreatic cancer biology.

11. REFERENCES

Ali, E. S., Sharker, S. M., Islam, M. T., Khan, I. N., Shaw, S., Rahman, A., Uddin, S. J., Shill, M. C., Rehman, S., Das, N., Ahmad, S., Shilpi, J. A., Tripathi, S., Mishra, S. K., & Mubarak, M. S. (2020). Targeting cancer cells with nanotherapeutics and nanodiagnostics: Current status and future perspectives. *Seminars in Cancer Biology*, *69*, 52–68. DOI: 10.1016/j.semcancer.2020.01.011 PMID: 32014609

Au, M., Emeto, T. I., Power, J., Vangaveti, V. N., & Lai, H. (2016). Emerging therapeutic potential of nanoparticles in pancreatic cancer: A systematic review of clinical trials. *Biomedicines*, *4*(3), 20. DOI: 10.3390/biomedicines4030020 PMID: 28536387

Bahadar, H., Maqbool, F., Niaz, K., & Abdollahi, M. (2016). Toxicity of nanoparticles and an overview of current experimental models. *Iranian Biomedical Journal*, *20*(1), 1–11. DOI: 10.22045/ibj.2016.01 PMID: 26286636

Banerjee, K., Gautam, S. K., Kshirsagar, P., Ross, K. A., Spagnol, G., Sorgen, P., Wannemuehler, M. J., Narasimhan, B., Solheim, J. C., Kumar, S., Batra, S. K., & Jain, M. (2019). Amphiphilic polyanhydride-based recombinant MUC4β-nanovaccine activates dendritic cells. *Genes & Cancer*, *10*(1-2), 52–62. DOI: 10.18632/genesandcancer.189 PMID: 31258832

Barenholz, Y. (2012). Doxil® - The first FDA-approved nanodrug: Lessons learned. *Journal of Controlled Release*, *160*(2), 117–134. DOI: 10.1016/j.jconrel.2012.03.020 PMID: 22484195

Bejarano, L., Jordão, M. J., & Joyce, J. A. (2021). Therapeutic targeting of the tumour microenvironment. *Cancer Discovery*, *11*(4), 933–959. DOI: 10.1158/2159-8290.CD-20-1808 PMID: 33811125

Benguigui, M., Weitz, I. S., Timaner, M., Kan, T., Shechter, D., Perlman, O., Sivan, S., Raviv, Z., Azhari, H., & Shaked, Y. (2019). Copper oxide nanoparticles inhibit pancreatic tumour growth primarily by targeting tumour-initiating cells. *Scientific Reports*, *9*(1), 12613. DOI: 10.1038/s41598-019-48959-8 PMID: 31471546

Binenbaum, Y., Na'ara, S., & Gil, Z. (2015). Gemcitabine resistance in pancreatic ductal adenocarcinoma. *Drug Resistance Updates*, *23*, 55–68. DOI: 10.1016/j.drup.2015.10.002 PMID: 26690340

Blanco, E., Hsiao, A., Mann, A. P., Landry, M. G., Meric-Bernstam, F., & Ferrari, M. (2011). Nanomedicine in cancer therapy: Innovative trends and prospects. *Cancer Science*, *102*(7), 1247–1252. DOI: 10.1111/j.1349-7006.2011.01941.x PMID: 21447010

Cao, J., Yang, P., Wang, P., Xu, S., Cheng, Y., Qian, K., Xu, M., Sheng, D., Li, Y., Wei, Y., & Zhang, Q. (2021). 'Adhesion and release' nanoparticle-mediated efficient inhibition of platelet activation disrupts endothelial barriers for enhanced drug delivery in tumours. *Biomaterials, 269*, 120620. DOI: 10.1016/j.biomaterials.2020.120620 PMID: 33421709

Chang, C. (2010). The immune effects of naturally occurring and synthetic nanoparticles. *Journal of Autoimmunity, 34*(3), J234–J246. DOI: 10.1016/j.jaut.2009.11.009 PMID: 19995678

Chikkaveeraiah, B. V., Bhirde, A. A., Morgan, N. Y., Eden, H. S., & Chen, X. (2012). Electrochemical immune sensors for the detection of cancer protein biomarkers. *ACS Nano, 6*(8), 6546–6561. DOI: 10.1021/nn3023969 PMID: 22835068

Christenson, E. S., Jaffee, E., & Azad, N. S. (2020). Current and emerging therapies for patients with advanced pancreatic ductal adenocarcinoma: A bright future. *The Lancet. Oncology, 21*(5), e135–e145. DOI: 10.1016/S1470-2045(19)30795-8 PMID: 32135117

Cun, X., Chen, J., Li, M., He, X., Tang, X., Guo, R., Deng, M., Li, M., Zhang, Z., & He, Q. (2019). Tumour-associated fibroblast-targeted regulation and deep tumour delivery of chemotherapeutic drugs with a multifunctional size-switchable nanoparticle. *ACS Applied Materials & Interfaces, 11*(44), 39545–39559. DOI: 10.1021/acsami.9b13957 PMID: 31617997

Davis, M. E., Zuckerman, J. E., Choi, C. H. J., Seligson, D., Tolcher, A., Alabi, C. A., Yen, Y., Heidel, J. D., & Ribas, A. (2010). Evidence of RNAi in humans from systemically administered siRNA via targeted nanoparticles. *Nature, 464*(7291), 1067–1070. DOI: 10.1038/nature08956 PMID: 20305636

Ding, Y., Xu, H., Xu, C., Tong, Z., Zhang, S., Bai, Y., Chen, Y., Xu, Q., Zhou, L., Ding, H., Sun, Z., Yan, S., Mao, Z., & Wang, W. (2020). A nanomedicine fabricated from gold nanoparticles-decorated metal–organic framework for cascade chemo/chemodynamic cancer therapy. *Advancement of Science, 7*(17), 2001060. DOI: 10.1002/advs.202001060 PMID: 32995124

Ducreux, M., Cuhna, A. S., Caramella, C., Hollebecque, A., Burtin, P., Goéré, D., Seufferlein, T., Haustermans, K., Van Laethem, J.-L., Conroy, T., & Arnold, D. (2015). Cancer of the pancreas: ESMO Clinical Practice Guidelines for diagnosis, treatment and follow-up. *Annals of Oncology : Official Journal of the European Society for Medical Oncology, 26*(suppl5), v56–v68. DOI: 10.1093/annonc/mdv295 PMID: 26314780

El-Zahaby, S. A., Elnaggar, Y. S. R., & Abdallah, O. Y. (2018). Reviewing two decades of nanomedicine implementations in targeted treatment and diagnosis of pancreatic cancer: An emphasis on state-of-the-art. *Journal of Controlled Release, 293*, 21–35. DOI: 10.1016/j.jconrel.2018.11.013 PMID: 30445002

Elgogary, A., Xu, Q., Poore, B., Alt, J., Zimmermann, S. C., Zhao, L., Fu, J., Chen, B., Xia, S., Liu, Y., Neisser, M., Nguyen, C., Lee, R., Park, J. K., Reyes, J., Hartung, T., Rojas, C., & Alexander, R. K. Yuan, & Hanes, J. (2016). Combination therapy with BPTES nanoparticles and metformin targets the metabolic heterogeneity of pancreatic cancer. *Proceedings of the National Academy of Sciences, 113*(36), E5328–E5336. https://doi.org/DOI: 10.1073/pnas.1611406113

Erkan, M., Hausmann, S., Michalski, C. W., Fingerle, A. A., Dobritz, M., Kleeff, J., & Friess, H. (2012). The role of stroma in pancreatic cancer: Diagnostic and therapeutic implications. *Nature Reviews. Gastroenterology & Hepatology, 9*(8), 454–467. DOI: 10.1038/nrgastro.2012.115 PMID: 22710569

Gheorghe, G., Bungau, S., Ilie, M., Behl, T., Vesa, C. M., Brisc, C., Bacalbasa, N., Turi, V., Costache, R. S., & Diaconu, C. C. (2020). Early diagnosis of pancreatic cancer: The key to survival. *Diagnostics (Basel), 10*(11), 869. DOI: 10.3390/diagnostics10110869 PMID: 33114412

Gianella, A., Jarzyna, P. A., Mani, V., Ramachandran, S., Calcagno, C., Tang, J., Kann, B., Dijk, W. J. R., Thijssen, V. L., Griffioen, A. W., Storm, G., Fayad, Z. A., & Mulder, W. J. M. (2011). Multifunctional nanoemulsion platform for imaging-guided therapy evaluated in experimental cancer. *ACS Nano, 5*(6), 4422–4433. DOI: 10.1021/nn103336a PMID: 21557611

Hackeng, W. M., Hruban, R. H., Offerhaus, G. J. A., & Brosens, L. A. A. (2016). Surgical and molecular pathology of pancreatic neoplasms. *Diagnostic Pathology, 11*(1), 47. DOI: 10.1186/s13000-016-0497-z PMID: 27267993

Han, X., Li, Y., Xu, Y., Zhao, X., Zhang, Y., Yang, X., Wang, Y., Zhao, R., Anderson, G. J., Zhao, Y., & Nie, G. (2018). Reversal of pancreatic desmoplasia by re-educating stellate cells with a tumour microenvironment-activated nanosystem. *Nature Communications, 9*(1), 3390. DOI: 10.1038/s41467-018-05906-x PMID: 30139933

Heinz, H., Pramanik, C., Heinz, O., Ding, Y., Mishra, R. K., Marchon, D., Flatt, R. J., Estrela-Lopis, I., Llop, J., Moya, S., & Ziolo, R. F. (2017). Nanoparticle decoration with surfactants: Molecular interactions, assembly, and applications. *Surface Science Reports, 72*(1), 1–58. DOI: 10.1016/j.surfrep.2017.02.001

Hossen, N., Rao, G., Dey, A., Robertson, J. D., Bhattacharya, R., & Mukherjee, P. (2019). Gold nanoparticle transforms activated cancer-associated fibroblasts to quiescence. *ACS Applied Materials & Interfaces*, *11*(30), 26060–26068. DOI: 10.1021/acsami.9b03313 PMID: 31117437

Hu, M., Wang, Y., Xu, L., An, S., Tang, Y., Zhou, X., Li, J., Liu, R., Dan, H., & Huang, L. (2019). Relaxin gene delivery mitigates liver metastasis and synergises with checkpoint therapy. *Nature Communications*, *10*(1), 2993. DOI: 10.1038/s41467-019-10893-8 PMID: 31278269

Huber, M., Brehm, C. U., Gress, T. M., Buchholz, M., Alhamwe, B. A., von Strandmann, E. P., Slater, E. P., Bartsch, J. W., Bauer, C., & Lauth, M. (2020). The immune microenvironment in pancreatic cancer. *International Journal of Molecular Sciences*, *21*(19), 7307. DOI: 10.3390/ijms21197307 PMID: 33022971

Jang, J.-E., Hajdu, C. H., Liot, C., Miller, G., Dustin, M. L., & Bar-Sagi, D. (2017). Crosstalk between regulatory T cells and tumour-associated dendritic cells negates anti-tumour immunity in pancreatic cancer. *Cell Reports*, *20*(3), 558–571. DOI: 10.1016/j.celrep.2017.06.062 PMID: 28723561

Jindal, A., Sarkar, S., & Alam, A. (2021). Nanomaterials-mediated immunomodulation for cancer therapeutics. *Frontiers in Chemistry*, *9*, 629635. DOI: 10.3389/fchem.2021.629635 PMID: 33708759

Judge, A. D., Robbins, M., Tavakoli, I., Levi, J., Hu, L., Fronda, A., Ambegia, E., McClintock, K., & MacLachlan, I. (2009). Confirming the RNAi-mediated mechanism of action of siRNA-based cancer therapeutics in mice. *The Journal of Clinical Investigation*, *119*(3), 661–673. DOI: 10.1172/JCI37515 PMID: 19229107

Kamisawa, T., Wood, L. D., Itoi, T., & Takaori, K. (2016). Pancreatic cancer. *Lancet*, *388*(10039), 73–85. DOI: 10.1016/S0140-6736(16)00141-0 PMID: 26830752

Leamon, C. P., Lovejoy, C. D., & Nguyen, B. (2013). Patient selection and targeted treatment in the management of platinum-resistant ovarian cancer. *Pharmacogenomics and Personalized Medicine*, *6*, 113–125. DOI: 10.2147/PGPM.S24943 PMID: 24109193

Lebre, F., de Lima, M. P., Lavelle, E., & Borges, O. (2018). Mechanistic study of the adjuvant effect of chitosan-aluminium nanoparticles. *International Journal of Pharmaceutics*, *552*(1-2), 7–15. DOI: 10.1016/j.ijpharm.2018.09.044 PMID: 30244149

Li, Y. J., Wu, J. Y., Wang, J. M., Xiang, D. X., & Jia, Y. B. (2020). Emerging nanomedicine-based strategies for preventing metastasis of pancreatic cancer. *Journal of Controlled Release*, *320*, 105–111. DOI: 10.1016/j.jconrel.2020.01.041 PMID: 31978441

Lin, H. J., Liang, T. L., Chang, Y. Y., Liu, D. Z., Fan, J. Y., Roffler, S. R., & Lin, S. Y. (2022). Development of irinotecan liposome armed with dual-target anti-epidermal growth factor receptor and anti-fibroblast activation protein-specific antibody for pancreatic cancer treatment. *Pharmaceutics*, *14*(6), 1202. DOI: 10.3390/pharmaceutics14061202 PMID: 35745775

Lin, L., Fan, Y., Gao, F., Jin, L., Li, D., Sun, W., Li, F., Qin, P., Shi, Q., Shi, X., & Du, L. (2018). UTMD promoted the delivery of dendrimer-entrapped gold nanoparticles for pancreatic cancer therapy. *Theranostics*, *8*(7), 1923–1939. DOI: 10.7150/thno.22834 PMID: 29556365

Liu, X., Jiang, J., Liao, Y. P., Tang, I., Zheng, E., Qiu, W., Lin, M., Wang, X., Ji, Y., Mei, K. C., & Nel, A. E. (2021). Combination chemo-immunotherapy for pancreatic cancer using the immunogenic effects of an irinotecan silicasome nanocarrier plus anti-PD-1. *Advancement of Science*, *8*(6), 2002147. DOI: 10.1002/advs.202002147 PMID: 33747719

Lorkowski, M. E., Atukorale, P. U., Bielecki, P. A., Tong, K. H., Covarrubias, G., Zhang, Y., Loutrianakis, G., Moon, T. J., Santulli, A. R., Becicka, W. M., & Karathanasis, E. (2021). Immunostimulatory nanoparticle incorporating two immune agonists for the treatment of pancreatic tumours. *Journal of Controlled Release*, *330*, 1095–1105. DOI: 10.1016/j.jconrel.2020.11.014 PMID: 33188827

Lu, J., Liu, X., Liao, Y. P., Salazar, F., Sun, B., Jiang, W., Chang, C. H., Jiang, J., Wang, X., Wu, A. M., & Nel, A. E. (2017). Nano-enabled pancreas cancer immunotherapy using immunogenic cell death and reversing immunosuppression. *Nature Communications*, *8*(1), 1811. DOI: 10.1038/s41467-017-01651-9 PMID: 29180759

Lv, H., Zhang, S., Wang, B., Cui, S., & Yan, J. (2006). Toxicity of cationic lipids and cationic polymers in gene delivery. *Journal of Controlled Release*, *114*(1), 100–109. DOI: 10.1016/j.jconrel.2006.04.014 PMID: 16831482

Ma, W. W., & Hidalgo, M. (2013). The winning formulation: The development of paclitaxel in pancreatic cancer. *Clinical Cancer Research*, *19*(22), 5572–5579. DOI: 10.1158/1078-0432.CCR-13-1356 PMID: 23918602

Malhotra, R., Patel, V., Chikkaveeraiah, B. V., Munge, B. S., Cheong, S. C., Zain, R. B., Abraham, M. T., Dey, D. K., Gutkind, J. S., & Rusling, J. F. (2012). Ultrasensitive detection of cancer biomarkers in the clinic by use of a nanostructured microfluidic array. *Analytical Chemistry*, *84*(14), 6249–6255. DOI: 10.1021/ac301392g PMID: 22697359

Mardhian, D. F., Vrynas, A., Storm, G., Bansal, R., & Prakash, J. (2020). FGF2-engineered SPIONs attenuate tumour stroma and potentiate the effect of chemotherapy in a 3D heterospheroidal model of pancreatic tumour. *Nanotheranostics*, *4*(1), 26–39. DOI: 10.7150/ntno.38092 PMID: 31911892

Meng, H., Zhao, Y., Dong, J., Xue, M., Lin, Y. S., Ji, Z., Mai, W. X., Zhang, H., Chang, C. H., Brinker, C. J., Zink, J. I., & Nel, A. E. (2013). Two-wave nanotherapy to target the stroma and optimise gemcitabine delivery to a human pancreatic cancer model in mice. *ACS Nano*, *7*(12), 10048–10065. DOI: 10.1021/nn404083m PMID: 24295225

Nigam Joshi, P., Agawane, S., Athalye, M. C., Jadhav, V., Sarkar, D., & Prakash, R. (2017). Multifunctional inulin-tethered silver-graphene quantum dots nanotheranostic module for pancreatic cancer therapy. *Materials Science and Engineering C*, *78*, 1203–1211. DOI: 10.1016/j.msec.2017.03.176 PMID: 28575959

Pearce, T. R., Shroff, K., & Kokkoli, E. (2012). Peptide-targeted lipid nanoparticles for anticancer drug delivery. *Advanced Materials*, *24*(28), 3803–3822. DOI: 10.1002/adma.201200832 PMID: 22674563

Petros, R. A., & DeSimone, J. M. (2010). Strategies in the design of nanoparticles for therapeutic applications. *Nature Reviews. Drug Discovery*, *9*(8), 615–627. DOI: 10.1038/nrd2591 PMID: 20616808

Provenzano, P. P., & Hingorani, S. R. (2013). Hyaluronan, fluid pressure, and stromal resistance in pancreatic cancer. *British Journal of Cancer*, *108*(1), 1–8. DOI: 10.1038/bjc.2012.569 PMID: 23299539

Rana, T. M. (2007). Illuminating the silence: Understanding the structure and function of small RNAs. *Nature Reviews. Molecular Cell Biology*, *8*(1), 23–36. DOI: 10.1038/nrm2085 PMID: 17183358

Rennick, J. J., Johnston, A. P. R., & Parton, R. G. (2021). Key principles and methods for studying the endocytosis of biological and nanoparticle therapeutics. *Nature Nanotechnology*, *16*(3), 266–276. DOI: 10.1038/s41565-021-00858-8 PMID: 33712737

Robey, R. W., Pluchino, K. M., Hall, M. D., Fojo, A. T., Bates, S. E., & Gottesman, M. M. (2018). Revisiting the role of ABC transporters in multidrug-resistant cancer. *Nature Reviews. Cancer, 18*(7), 452–464. DOI: 10.1038/s41568-018-0005-8 PMID: 29643473

Roh, Y. J., Kim, J. H., Kim, I. W., Na, K., Park, J. M., & Choi, M. G. (2017). Photodynamic therapy using photosensitizer-encapsulated polymeric nanoparticles to overcome ATP-binding cassette transporter subfamily G2 function in pancreatic cancer. *Molecular Cancer Therapeutics, 16*(7), 1487–1496. DOI: 10.1158/1535-7163.MCT-16-0642 PMID: 28416605

Ryu, J. H., Lee, S., Son, S., Kim, S. H., Leary, J. F., Choi, K., & Kwon, I. C. (2014). Theranostic nanoparticles for future personalised medicine. *Journal of Controlled Release, 190*, 477–484. DOI: 10.1016/j.jconrel.2014.04.027 PMID: 24780269

Saha, S., Xiong, X., Chakraborty, P. K., Shameer, K., Arvizo, R. R., Kudgus, R. A., Dwivedi, S. K. D., Hossen, M. N., Gillies, E. M., Robertson, J. D., & Mukherjee, P. (2016). Gold nanoparticle reprograms pancreatic tumour microenvironment and inhibits tumour growth. *ACS Nano, 10*(12), 10636–10651. DOI: 10.1021/acsnano.6b02231 PMID: 27758098

Santos-Rebelo, A., Garcia, C., Eleutério, C., Bastos, A., Coelho, S. C., Coelho, M. A. N., Molpeceres, J., Viana, A. S., Ascensão, L., & Pinto, J. F. (2018). Development of Parvifloron D-loaded smart nanoparticles to target pancreatic cancer. *Pharmaceutics, 10*(4), 216. DOI: 10.3390/pharmaceutics10040216 PMID: 30400382

Schober, M., Jesenofsky, R., Faissner, R., Weidenauer, C., Hagmann, W., Michl, P., Heuchel, R. L., Haas, S. L., & Löhr, J. M. (2014). Desmoplasia and chemoresistance in pancreatic cancer. *Cancers (Basel), 6*(4), 2137–2154. DOI: 10.3390/cancers6042137 PMID: 25337831

Schroeder, A., Levins, C. G., Cortez, C., Langer, R., & Anderson, D. G. (2010). Lipid-based nanotherapeutics for siRNA delivery. *Journal of Internal Medicine, 267*(1), 9–21. DOI: 10.1111/j.1365-2796.2009.02189.x PMID: 20059641

Sofuni, A., Iijima, H., Moriyasu, F., Nakayama, D., Shimizu, M., Nakamura, K., Itokawa, F., & Itoi, T. (2005). Differential diagnosis of pancreatic tumours using ultrasound contrast imaging. *Journal of Gastroenterology, 40*(5), 518–525. DOI: 10.1007/s00535-005-1578-z PMID: 15942718

Tabernero, J., Shapiro, G. I., Lorusso, P. M., Cervantes, A., Schwartz, G. K., Weiss, G. J., Paz-Ares, L., Cho, D. C., Infante, J. R., Alsina, M., Gounder, M. M., Falzone, R., Harrop, J., White, A. C. S., Toudjarska, I., Bumcrot, D., Meyers, R. E., Hinkle, G., Svrzikapa, N., & de Sauvage, F. J. (2013). First-in-human trial of an RNA interference therapeutic targeting VEGF and KSP in cancer patients with liver involvement. *Cancer Discovery*, *3*(4), 406–417. DOI: 10.1158/2159-8290.CD-12-0429 PMID: 23358650

Tempero, M. A., Malafa, M. P., Chiorean, E. G., Czito, B., Scaife, C., Narang, A. K., Bartholomew, M. J., & Bekaii-Saab, T. (2019). Pancreatic Adenocarcinoma, Version 1.2019. *Journal of the National Comprehensive Cancer Network : JNCCN*, *17*(3), 202–210. DOI: 10.6004/jnccn.2019.0014 PMID: 30865919

Vennin, C., Murphy, K. J., Morton, J. P., Cox, T. R., Pajic, M., & Timpson, P. (2018). Reshaping the tumour stroma for treatment of pancreatic cancer. *Gastroenterology*, *154*(4), 820–838. DOI: 10.1053/j.gastro.2017.11.280 PMID: 29287624

Verma, R. K., Yu, W., Shrivastava, A., Shankar, S., & Srivastava, R. K. (2016). α-Mangostin-encapsulated PLGA nanoparticles inhibit pancreatic carcinogenesis by targeting cancer stem cells in human, and transgenic (KrasG12D, and KrasG12D/tp53R270H) mice. *Scientific Reports*, *6*(1), 32743. DOI: 10.1038/srep32743 PMID: 27624879

Vincent, A., Herman, J., Schulick, R., Hruban, R. H., & Goggins, M. (2011). Pancreatic cancer. *Lancet*, *378*(9791), 607–620. DOI: 10.1016/S0140-6736(10)62307-0 PMID: 21620466

Von Hoff, D. D., Ramanathan, R. K., Borad, M. J., Laheru, D. A., Smith, L. S., Wood, T. E., Korn, R. L., Desai, N., Trieu, V., Iglesias, J. L., Zhang, H., Soon-Shiong, P., Shi, T., Rajeshkumar, N. V., Maitra, A., & Hidalgo, M. (2011). Gemcitabine plus nab-paclitaxel is an active regimen in patients with advanced pancreatic cancer: A phase I/II trial. *Journal of Clinical Oncology*, *29*(34), 4548–4554. DOI: 10.1200/JCO.2011.36.5742 PMID: 21969517

Wang, H., Liang, Y., Yin, Y., Zhang, J., Su, W., White, A. M., Jiang, B., Xu, J., Zhang, Y., Stewart, S., & Li, Y. (2021). Carbon nano-onion-mediated dual targeting of P-selectin and P-glycoprotein to overcome cancer drug resistance. *Nature Communications*, *12*(1), 312. DOI: 10.1038/s41467-020-20588-0 PMID: 33436622

Yu, Q., Qiu, Y., Li, J., Tang, X., Wang, X., Cun, X., Xu, S., Liu, Y., Li, M., Zhang, Z., & He, Q. (2020). Targeting cancer-associated fibroblast by dual-responsive lipid-albumin nanoparticles to enhance drug perfusion for pancreatic tumour therapy. *Journal of Controlled Release*, *321*, 564–575. DOI: 10.1016/j.jconrel.2020.02.040 PMID: 32112854

Zhao, X., Li, F., Li, Y., Wang, H., Ren, H., Chen, J., Nie, G., & Hao, J. (2015). Co-delivery of HIF1α siRNA and gemcitabine via biocompatible lipid-polymer hybrid nanoparticles for effective treatment of pancreatic cancer. *Biomaterials*, *46*, 13–25. DOI: 10.1016/j.biomaterials.2014.12.028 PMID: 25678112

Zhao, X., Yang, K., Zhao, R., Ji, T., Wang, X., Yang, X., Zhang, Y., Cheng, K., Liu, S., Hao, J., Ren, H., & Nie, G. (2016). Inducing enhanced immunogenic cell death with nanocarrier-based drug delivery systems for pancreatic cancer therapy. *Biomaterials*, *102*, 187–197. DOI: 10.1016/j.biomaterials.2016.06.032 PMID: 27343466

Zhou, W., Zhou, Y., Chen, X., Ning, T., Chen, H., Guo, Q., Zhang, Y., Liu, P., Zhang, Y., Li, C., & Zhang, Z. (2021). Pancreatic cancer-targeting exosomes for enhancing immunotherapy and reprogramming tumour microenvironment. *Biomaterials*, *268*, 120546. DOI: 10.1016/j.biomaterials.2020.120546 PMID: 33253966

Zonneville, J., Safina, A., Truskinovsky, A. M., Arteaga, C. L., & Bakin, A. V. (2018). TGF-β signalling promotes tumour vasculature by enhancing the pericyte-endothelium association. *BMC Cancer*, *18*(1), 670. DOI: 10.1186/s12885-018-4587-z PMID: 29921235

Chapter 5

Microbiome Immunomodulatory Responses Offer Therapeutic Potential Against Pancreatic Cancer

M. Divya
Department of Microbiology, Sacred Heart College, Tirupattur, India

R. Nisha
Department of Microbiology, Sacred Heart College, Tirupattur, India

Yuvalakshmi Logesan
https://orcid.org/0009-0005-4579-1170
Department of Microbiology, Sacred Heart College, Tirupattur, India

ABSTRACT

The neoplasm that develops in the pancreas is called pancreatic tissue cancer. According to recent research, the gut microbiota affects both the immune response and the effectiveness of treatment for PDAC. One tumor microenvironment that is extremely immunosuppressive is Pancreatic ductal adenocarcinoma (PDAC). By controlling both systemic and local immune responses, the microorganisms have a significant impact on oncogenesis, which in turn affects tumor growth and the effectiveness of treatment. The effectiveness of immunotherapy and chemotherapy may be impacted by the way some bacteria alter the activity of cytotoxic T cells and other immune components. Research indicates that the immune response can be shifted in favor of tumor suppression by modifying the microbiome through

DOI: 10.4018/979-8-3373-1469-3.ch005

procedures like fecal microbiota transplantation. Modified immunological profiles have been connected to dysbiosis or imbalance in microbial populations, which could improve treatment results. The significance of microbial communities in cancer control is further highlighted by the fact that medications that deplete the microbiome can trigger anti-cancer immune responses. These discoveries open the door to novel treatments that target the microbiota to improve the effectiveness of pancreatic cancer treatment.

1. INTRODUCTION

Pancreatic cancer is the fifth most common cause of cancer-related fatalities in developed countries, resulting in the deaths of 260,000 individuals each year. 5-year survival is reduced to 6% by aggressiveness and delayed start. Prognostic factors that make pancreatic cancer the most refractory malignant tumor include the lack of early diagnostic markers, early neurovascular development, rapid deaths, extensive metastases to multiple organs, high postoperative recurrence and metastatic spread rates, poor response to chemoradiotherapy, and other factors. New cancer development and treatment targets include the human microbiome. It can induce cancer by changing the Tumour Immunological Microenvironment and producing inflammation (Schawkat et al., 2020). Microorganism interactions near or far from Tumour tissues increase malignancy and illness. As in healthy Pancreatic tissue, Bacteria and Fungi colonise malignant tissue. Their presence accelerates Pancreatic cancer growth and influences prognosis and treatment (Zhang et al., 2018) Immune system participation in cancer start and dissemination. Both the natural and adaptive immune responses fight cancer. The immune system needs Cytotoxic T cells (CD8), T helper-1 (Th1) cells, and Mature Dendritic cell type (DCs), pro-inflammatory stimulated macrophages (M1), and NK cells to fight cancer (Timmer et al., 2021). Cancer cells manipulate and avoid immune responses. The cancer cells use contact-dependent components like PD-L1 expression, IL-10, TGF-b, and VEGF secretion, and MHC class I peptide presentation interference to alter the immune system and prevent effector immune cell detection. MHC class I affects NK cell cytotoxic function, receptor activation, numbers, and proliferation to help cancer cells avoid identification and destruction (Amieva and Peek, 2016). Cancer cells modulate local and systemic immunity, causing Tumour development and Immunosuppression. New cancer development and prevention targets include the human microbiome. It can induce cancer by changing the Tumour immunological microenvironment and producing inflammation (Schawkat et al., 2020). Microorganism interactions near or far from Tumour tissues increase malignancy and illness. As in healthy Pancreatic tissue, bacteria and fungi colonise malignant tissue. Their presence accelerates

Pancreatic cancer growth and influences prognosis and treatment (Zhang et al., 2018). Immune system participation in cancer start and dissemination. Both the natural and adaptive immune mechanisms fight cancer. The immune system needs cytotoxic CD8 T cells, T helper-1 (Th1) cells, mature dendritic cells (DCs), pro-inflammatory activated macrophages (M1), and NK cells to fight cancer (Timmer et al., 2021). Cancer cells manipulate and avoid immune responses. Cancer cells use contact-dependent factors like PD-L1 expression, IL-10, TGF-b, and VEGF secretion, and MHC class I peptide presentation interference to alter the immune system and prevent effector immune cell detection. MHC class I affects NK cell cytotoxic function, receptor activation, numbers, and proliferation to help cancer cells avoid identification and destruction (Amieva and Peek, 2016). Cancer cells modulate local and systemic immunity, causing Tumour development and immunosuppression.

Many individuals have chronic disease, and only early-stage instances can be operated on. The combination of chemotherapy is the conventional treatment for advanced illness, although its toxicity restricts treatment length and results vary (Durack and Lynch, 2019). Pancreatic cancer patients have not responded well to single-agent immunotherapy, even when combined with chemotherapy and additional immunotherapies. Pancreas cancer immunotherapy may fail due to the highly suppressive Tumour microenvironment. Investigations are underway into the role of different microorganisms in cancer. According to Biesel et al., (2025)infectious infections may cause 7–20% of malignancies worldwide. Several gastrointestinal malignancies are linked to the microbiome. The bacterium *Helicobacter pylori* as its role in stomach cancer pathobiology are the best examples. Most bacteria affect immunity and metabolism in the GI tract by interacting with host cells. Microbial α-diversity measures the number of organisms in a sample (Ahn et al., 2013). Cancer patients, include colorectal, breast, or Pancreatic cancer, showed reduced gut microbial α-diversity compared to healthy controls. Melanoma patients that respond to immunotherapy have a larger gut microbial α-diversity than non-responders (Zhang et al., 2018). Multiple diagnostic methods, including positron emission tomography, endoscopic ultrasonography, magnetic resonance imaging, and multi-detector CT, are used to screen for PC (Karpiński, 2019). Certain oral bacteria can cause cancer. Several of these microorganisms are linked to PC, colorectal cancer, and OSCC (Park et al., 2021). Type 2 diabetes, obesity, smoking, chronic pancreatitis, and pathogenic microorganisms all contribute to Pancreatic cancer. In addition, Helicobacter pylori in addition to variable kinds of ABO blood can cause Pancreatic cancer (Bracci, 2017). In addition to obesity, autoimmune Pancreas inflammation and Cardiovascular disease, bacteria contribute to lung, colorectal, esophageal, & Hepatocellular Carcinoma. Poor oral health, a history of periodontal disease, and an imbalance in the gut microbiota may all raise the risk of Pancreatic cancer. The microbial ecology determines Pancreatic cancer progression or reversal. The nitrosamine exposure, inflammatory processes, innate as well as adaptive immune suppression, & Tumour environment modifications may also be involved (Thomas and Jobin, 2020). Potential oral, intestinal, *Helicobacter pylori*, and intratumor bacteria signalling pathways linked to Pancreatic cancer growth and spread.

2. MICROBIAL ASSOCIATION WITH PANCREATIC CANCER

2.1 Microbes colonization in Pancreatic cancer tissues

The Pancreatic and hepatic ducts form the common bile duct, which leads to the major duodenum nipple. Pancreatic tissue bacteria travel from the mouth and GI tract through the duct. Cats' colons can reflux *E. coli* into their circulation and Pancreatic ducts. The kidney, gallbladder, and colon can transfer germs to the Pancreas (Vogtmann et al., 2020). Oral bacteria from the lower gastrointestinal tract can reach the portal circulation or mesenteric lymph glands of the Pancreas. Disease development is influenced by Pancreatic and intestinal bacteria. The gut microbiota made nearly 25% of the human cancer microbiome and differed from normal surrounding tissues, indicating that it can colonise Pancreatic Tumours. Research shows that Pancreatic cancer tissue has different microorganisms than healthy tissue. The most common gammaproteobacteria in Pancreatic cancer tissues, *Enterobacteriaceae* and *Pseudomonas* sp, imply they invaded the organ and were part of the Tumour microenvironment. Pancreatic cancer is linked to oral microbial makeup (Maekawa et al., 2018). With pancreatitis, oral bacteria can enter the Pancreatic. Pancreatic and oral microbiome are similar. Oral *Clostridium sp* are found in normal Pancreatic tissues. Bile promotes Pancreatic bacterial colonisation. In a research on chronic pancreatitis and Pancreatic cancer, *Enterococcal* DNA was identified in 29 Pancreatic juice samples taken using drainage tubes after pancreatectomy from 20 Pancreatic cancer patients and 16 duodenal or bile duct cancer patients. Pancreatic cancer and chronic pancreatitis patients have *Enterococcus* and *Enterobacter* species in their bile and tissue. The microbiota is affected by liver disease and bile duct occlusion. PC-induced liver damage alters gut flora and homeostasis. *Escherichia coli* may damage Pancreatic microbiota(Fig-1). Common bile duct stents may affect duodenal flora. Proton pump inhibitors and other therapies may alter the Pancreatic colonised microbiome, raising Pancreatic cancer risk (Brusselaers et al., 2020).

The role of intestinal fungus in Pancreatic cancer is unknown due to their low abundance and absence of a well-characterized referring genome. Pancreatic cancer is linked to intestinal fungal colonisation. A new Pancreatic cancer therapeutic target may be the Fungal genome. Candida infection (CI) considerably raises cancer risk (Chung et al., 2017). *Candida nitrosamines* cause mouth cancer. Within 30 minutes, the intestinal fungus colonised the Pancreas. Pancreatic Tumours in humans and rats have 3,000 times more fungus than healthy tissues and have several forms. Cancer development, metastasis, and recurrence are all affected by the Tumour microenvironment. TME complement activation modulates the immune system and promotes cancer cell proliferation, migration, invasion, and Epithelial-mesenchymal transition (Afshar-Kharghan, 2017). Fungus flora may detect early cancer.

Hepatitis C and Hepatitis B virus infection increased Pancreatic cancer risk in case-control or meta-analyses. demonstrating Hepatitis B and C do not cause cancer of the Pancreas (Stasiewicz et al., 2021). People with HBsAg or acute Hepatitis B infection are at risk for Pancreatic cancer. In 1980, HBV patients' Pancreatic juice had HBcAg in the plasma of Pancreatic acinar cells. Chronic inflammation from HBV infection can cause Pancreatic cancer. The Hepatitis B virus's regulatory HBx protein increases viral genome transcription and causes metabolic problems that may lead to cancer in the Pancreas. Hepatitis virus can cause severe pancreatitis and cancer, yet Pancreatic cancer cells inhibit HBV replication (Cruz et al., 2024).

Figure 1. Microbial Colonization in PC tissues

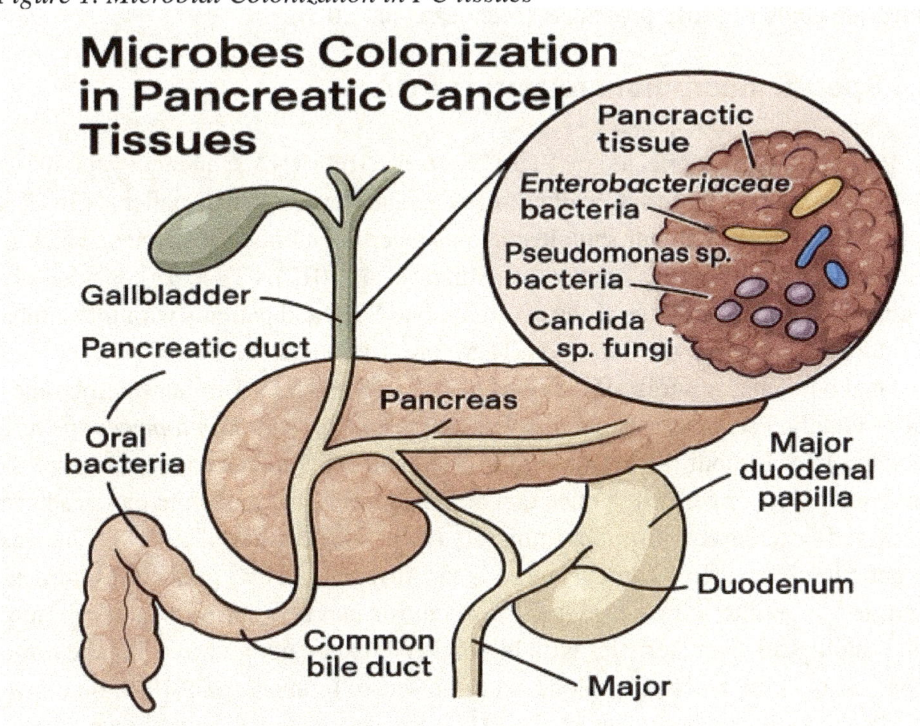

2.3 Interaction between Pancreatic cancer cells and tumor-associated Neutrophils

Tumour microenvironment microbial metabolites alter immune cell division and function. Certain bacteria create compounds that boost regulatory T cell production. Microbial bile acids affect gut RORg regulating T cell regulation (Song et al., 2020). Microbe-produced short-chain acids improve CD8+ T cell memory. Bacterial metabolites decrease inflammation and prevent Tumours by regulating the immune system. Diabetes and obesity, mediated by microbiome-induced metabolism alterations, worsen PDAC. Siddiqui et al., (2025) shown that Pancreas colonisation bacteria in the PDAC is a Tumour a microenvironment may mediate treatment resistance. Nucleoside analogue gemcitabine treats bladder, breast, lung, and Pancreatic cancer. Metabolomics revealed lipogenic, Glycolytic, and slow-proliferating Pancreatic cell lines. We found a substantial Metabolic-Collisson's subtype association. how Microbiota-Metabolic influences affect PDAC genetic subtypes. Early carcinogenesis is strongly linked to host chemicals that induce cancer and microbial alterations. A precise, noninvasive technique for early PDAC detection could improve prognosis (Mendez et al., 2020).

2.4 Specific microbiota related to PDA

Patient survival is affected by PDAC bacteria. 16S rRNA sequencing classified DNA from bacteria from surgically resected tissue from 68 PDAC patients (36 LTS and 32 STS). Each Tumour sample contains a certain number of species, which is part of microbiota alpha diversity (Kurilshikov et al., 2017). LTS had a considerably higher Tumour microbiome alpha diversity than STS, and patients with high alpha variation have longer overall survival. Therefore, Tumour alpha diversity may predict survival outcomes in surgically excised PDAC LTS and STS Tumour microbiomes differ greatly. *Pseudomonas* sp, *Saccharopolyspora* sp, and *Streptomyces* sp were found in LTS Tumour tissues, but not in STS patients. Patients with healthy intestinal microbiota or germ-free mice that obtained faeces from treating patients have increased systemic & anti-tumor immunity (Gopalakrishnan et al., 2018). Changes in gut microbiota affect Tumour microbiota. Advanced PDAC patients' excrement were fed to antibiotic-treated mice. PC diagnosis can be improved by combining microbiological characteristics with biomarkers that are not invasive like the urine biomarkers being researched along with the serum biomarker CA19-9, that have PC detection limitations (Chen et al., 2022). Numerous studies have shown the relevance of gut and Tumour microbiota in Pancreatic cancer. Microbiome diversity may predict PDAC survival and guide treatment.

3. IMMUNOMODULATORY RESPONSE IN PANCREATIC CANCER - 3

3.1 Immune cells and PDAC

Pancreatic cancer immune cells reduce inflammation. The Tumour microenvironment has more CD4+CD25+FoxP3+ cells. Tregs prevent autoimmunity by releasing CTLA-4 and releasing IL-10 and TGF-b. Pancreatic cancer patients had increased blood Tregs and Tumours. Low Tregs to in circulation a year on resection improve survival, but Tregs at the Tumour site are connected to advanced disease presentation, worse surgical resection rates, and lower post-resection survival. Treg cells increase while CD8+ receptors decrease. Tregs are a possible Pancreatic cancer target. Immature myeloid cells impair both adaptive and innate immune systems as MDSCs. In Immunology, they generate reactive oxygen species, restrict T cell homing to lymph nodes, express large quantities of arginase, which depletes T cell protein synthesis amino acid L-arginine, and sequester T cell activation amino acid cysteine. These factors suppress effector T and NK cell activity and promote Treg formation. MDSC-induced Immune suppression caused premalignant Tumours to become Pancreatic cancer in mice (Lekan & Weiner, 2024). Pancreatic cancer patients had higher MDSC levels, that are connected to Treg cell counts & IL-13, than healthy controls. Pancreatic cancer is poorly predicted by elevated MDSC levels. Many cancer predictions are worsened by TAM invasion. TGF-b and IL-10 from the Tumour microenvironment transform M1 (pro-inflammatory or traditionally activated) macrophages to M2 (anti-inflammatory or alternatively activated). The Cytokines promote blood vessel development, matrix transforming, Tumour metastasis, and Adaptive immunity suppression. TAMs affect the immune system via expressing PD-L1 or secreting IL-10 and TGF-b. Pancreatic cancer Tumours have high TAMs. M2 split TAMs are related with a poorer outcome in Pancreatic cancer (Sivakumar et al., 2025).

3.2 Interaction of Immune system to Pancreatic cancer

Pancreatic cancer microenvironment includes immunological infiltration. The extracellular matrix's proteins, tumor-associated fibroblasts, the Vasculature are also crucial. An strong desmoplastic stroma reaction promotes carcinogenesis and treatment resistance in Pancreatic cancer. CAFs stimulate Tumour progression via immune system interactions. CAFs attract TAMs in the Tumour microenvironment via NF-kbeta, encouraging proliferation and fibrosis. CAFs also decrease effector T cells and block TNF-a & IFN-c activation with FAP-a. Due to its overexpression on Pancreatic cancer stroma and cells, monoclonal antibodies against FAP-a are being produced (Ge et al., 2021). Later-discussed CD40 agonists affect TAMs and CAFs as given Fig 2.

Figure 2. Immune System Dynamics in Pancreatic Cancer

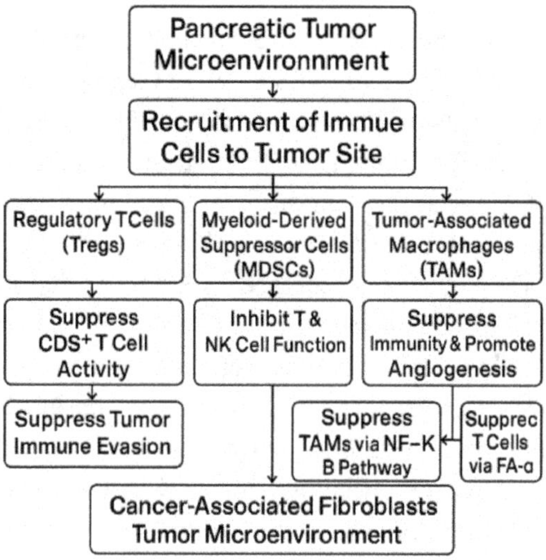

3.4 Impact of microbiome in immunotherapy and chemotherapy

Many immunotherapeutic methods are being tested in clinical studies. We will deplete Treg, increase tumor-specific cytotoxic T cells, disrupt co-stimulatory and inhibitory receptors and ligands, and vaccinate T cells (Siveen and Kuttan 2009). Table 1.

Table 1. Comparative review of Antigen used and its Concomitant Therapy

Type of Vaccine	Antigen Targeted	Co-administered Treatment	Key Results	Reference
Recombinant protein	K-ras mutant	Gemcitabine, Yeast	2.4 months OS improvement	**(Mantovani et al., 2008)**
Recombinant protein	K-ras mutant	Gemcitabine	Ongoing	**(Riquelme et al., 2019)**
Viral vector-expressing gene	CEA, MUC-1	TRICOM, GM-CSF	No OS advantage	**(Hamada et al., 2019)**

continued on following page

Table 1. Continued

Type of Vaccine	Antigen Targeted	Co-administered Treatment	Key Results	Reference
Genetically created, lethally irradiated allogeneic Tumour.	Whole Tumour	Cyclophosphamide, Cetuximab	Trial completed; Primary results not formally published	**(Zhang et al., 2018)**
Listeria vector weakened	Mesothelin and entire Tumour	Adjuvant radiation/ Chemotherapy	Developed delayed hypersensitive and DTH was linked to longer survival.	**(Jemal et al., 2011)**

4. THREPTIC IMPLANTS FOR PANCREATIC CANCER

4.1 FMT as a Therapeutic strategies - 4

A PDAC animal model was produced by placing human fecal microbial transplantation (hFMT) in mice that had orthotopic cancer cell implantation. Gut-pancreatic cancer microbial cross-talk was demonstrated by the overlap between this donor's gut microbiota and 25% of the typical human PDAC microbial composition, but not with the surrounding normal tissue. These mice readily spread human intestinal microbes, as demonstrated by forty (Shi et al., 2012). The Tumour microbiota of humanised microbial mice changed after donor transplantation. While long-term PDAC survivors produced the strongest reversal and Tumour growth, healthy controls produced slower Tumour growth and a smaller TME immune suppression reversal than short-term survivors. Antibiotics or Cytotoxic T cell reduction eliminated this impact after transplant. Thus, hFMT improved PDAC Tumours by altering the immune system and gut/tumor microbial axis. showing that FMT can modulate immune activation, gut and Tumour microbiotas, and outcomes, making it ideal for use with immunotherapy and chemotherapy for Pancreatic cancer or other cancers (Yamamura and Sonoshita 2025). Other clinical trials use FMT to treat autoimmune, inflammatory, and metabolic illnesses and prevent *Clostridioides difficile* infections. FMT is becoming a popular cancer treatment. Several early-phase clinical trials are studying hFMT's effects on cancer therapy responses and toxicity. FMT needs clinical trials to prove its safety and efficacy in changing the human Pancreas Tumour microbiome and improving immune response to increase survival.

4.2 Immunotherapy and Radiotherapy

Cancer is known for evading immune surveillance. Tumours elude identification and death by escaping the host's immunological monitoring. Radiation may alert the immune system to cancer cell antigens. Ionising radiation can produce based alteration, single-strand break, and double-strand break (Paparo et al., 2020). Many neoantigens that boost immune surveillance may come from radiation-induced DNA changes. Radiation may increase cancer cell MHC expression to present Tumour antigen to deadly T lymphocytes. The T-cell receptor must engage with peptide-bound MHC molecules to activate. Tumours often downregulate MHC-I to avoid immune recognition. Radiation may boost cancer cell MHC-I expression, making them visible to cytotoxic T lymphocytes. Finally, radiation primes tumor-specific T lymphocytes by causing antigen-presenting cells to phagocytose injured Tumour cells. Radiation causes malignant cells to produce DAMP or translocate calreticulin to the cell membrane for phagocytosis. This immune cell death process releases HMGB1 and ATP, helping dendritic cells and macrophages phagocytose cancer cells (Balázs et al., 2019). Radiation seems to improve immune modulation with immune checkpoint blockers (Fig 3).

Figure 3. Radiotherapy and Immunotherapy in Cancer Defense

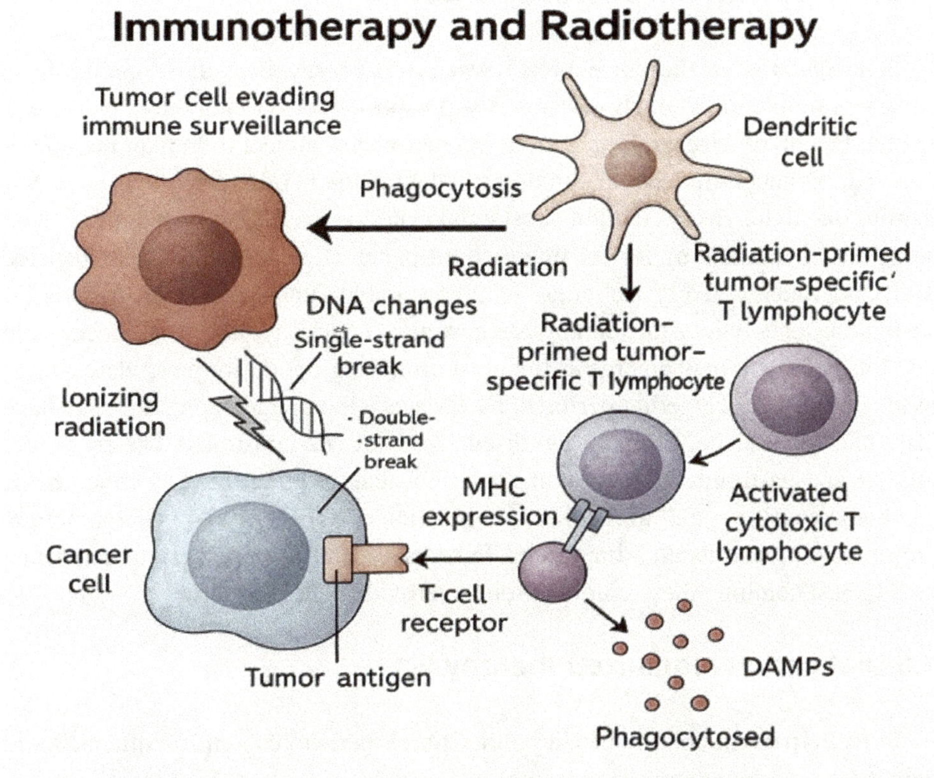

4.3 Intensity modulated Radiation therapy (IMRT)

IMRT, a popular radiation planning and delivery technology, uses several radiation beams to deliver a conformal dose to the target while sparing neighbouring normal organs (Wu et al., 2021). Before IMRT, 3D conformal irradiation (3D-CRT) was used. The 3D-CRT target (where all beams connect) was dosed with three or four beams. IMRT uses seven to nine beams to spread low dosage scatter and provide a more typical quantity to the target. IMRT can "Dose paint." A big advantage over 3D-CRT. IMRT can be used for SBRT (3–6 fractions) or longer radiation courses (15–28 fractions). IMRT beats longer radiation courses. They tolerate adjacent stomach and small intestine structures (Caccialanza et al., 2016). However, IMRT increases Tumour dose while respecting healthy tissue dose limits.

4.4 Potential applications of microorganisms in the treatment of Pancreatic ancer

Investigations on the correlation between microorganisms and tumours have advanced significantly, likely offering new prospects for the treatment of pancreatic cancer. Oncolytic viruses, which are microorganisms subject to human manipulation, exhibit uncertain clinical outcomes in the treatment of pancreatic cancer. Numerous oncolytic viruses exhibit substantial synergistic effects when administered alongside chemotherapy for the treatment of pancreatic cancer. It is also justified to decide which delivery technique is most suitable. Numerous clinical trials investigating oncolytic viral therapy are currently underway, and it is conceivable that this treatment may emerge as the most promising option for pancreatic cancer in the near future. Targeting pertinent bacteria as a therapeutic approach may have distinct impacts since, as our earlier discussions have demonstrated, bacteria in the tumour and gastrointestinal system may significantly affect the effectiveness of chemotherapy(Lu et al., 2021). The combination of antibiotics and chemotherapy presents both benefits and drawbacks. Further research is necessary to determine how to best combine these combinations to provide better outcomes.

4.5 Diet and personalized therapy 9-1

Early PC patients need dietary support. Clinical nutritionists and dietitians should help patients as therapeutic team members (Caccialanza et al., 2020). Cancer patients need preoperative dietetics counsel to avoid preoperative weight loss, malnutrition, and postoperative problems. Nutritional aid begins with an expert exam using authorised equipment at diagnosis and during therapy. Mini Nutritional Assessment (MNA), malnutrition Screening Tool (MST), Nutritional Risk Screening 2002 (NRS 2002), & Malnutrition Universal Screening Tool are recommended. Once nutrition risk is established, clinical nutritionists should initiate a nutritional therapy strategy for cancer patients (Kim et al., 2019). The nutritional intervention must match the planned oncological treatment, clinical condition, diet, and Tumour site.

Table 2. Mechanisms of Oncological treatment

Targeted Mechanism	Targeted Pathway
Targeting DNA Repair Deficiency	PARP, ATM, ATR, DNA-PK
Targeting Epigenetic Alterations	HDACs and HATs, Bromodomain proteins
Inhibiting Oncogenic Signaling Pathways	The EGFR, HER2, FAK, and BTK

continued on following page

Table 2. Continued

Targeted Mechanism	Targeted Pathway
Targeting the Tumor Microenvironment & Metabolism	Hedgehog pathway, VEGF
Harnessing the Immune System	Mutated KRAS peptides, Survivin peptides (T-cell responses)

Nutritional supplements may affect gut microbiota. ONS should prevent and treat malnutrition. A study on ONS for Pancreatic & bile duct cancer patients receiving chemotherapy found that daily energy, carbohydrates, fats, and proteins consumption rose significantly after eight weeks and longer. Following the first chemotherapy cycle, the ONS group had a larger weight, mass without fat, muscle and bone weight, cell mass, and fat mass than the non-ONS group (Natto et al., 2024). If stool function is normal but the patient cannot get enough energy from oral sources, whole and integral Enteral Nutrition (EN) should be considered. If symptoms (such as nausea, vomiting, or diarrhoea) or patient refusal prevent EN, Parenteral Nutrition (PN) is needed. Reefing syndrome in extremely malnourished patients can be avoided by progressively increasing dietary energy while monitoring clinical and metabolic stability (Kaźmierczak-Siedlecka et al., 2020).

5. FUTURE DIRECTIONS AND CHALLENGES

5.1 Addressing the knowledge gap

Chronic, Acute, or Recurring Pancreatitis is expensive and deadly. Despite promising early treatments, no medications are approved to treat chronic inflammation, exocrine nor endocrine dysfunction, and neoplasia (Mendez et al., 2020). The National Institute of Diabetes, Digestive, or Kidney Diseases seminars revealed many gaps in our understanding of Pancreatic inflammatory disease pathways. These workshops stressed the significance of developing and testing pharmaceutical targets to change pancreatitis' course. Fibrosis, chronic or acute Pancreatic inflammation, and gene mutation reversal are therapy targets (Kamarajah et al., 2025).

5.2 Emerging Technologies

SDCT, MDCT, or MRI/MRCP are first-line treatments for solid Pancreatic Tumours. EUS can clarify initial results or provide further tissue confirmation for T staging. EUS is better than MRI or CT scans for local T stage of vascular invasion in non-metastatic Pancreatic Adenocarcinoma patients (Jamal & Khan, 2025). CT and MRI find distant metastases better. The Neuroendocrine status of the suspected Tumour determines the optimum imaging approach for localisation and detection. Since cross-sectional imaging cannot show regional extension, EUS and other kinds of imaging are complementary in solid Pancreatic cancer patients (Kolbeinsson et al., 2023). Multiple imaging modalities predict resectability better preoperatively. As FDG-PET, PET/MDCT, along with echo-enhanced ultrasound become more accessible, Pancreatic exocrine cancer treatment will grow.

5.3 Intellectual conundrums and Possibility of Pancreatic cancer therapy using targeted treatments

PC has a high molecular diversity, with the possibility for several genetic variations and signalling pathway activation states to exist within tumors and within the same patient. Since the pharmaceutical targets now available are somewhat limited, it is challenging to identify a universal target or therapeutic approach for targeted therapy that can be applied to all patients (Hirooka et al., 2022). The complexity and resilience of these targets have hindered the development of targeted medicines, even though certain genetic abnormalities, such as TP53 and KRAS, are common in pancreatic cancer. Significant resistance to targeted therapy is exhibited by pancreatic cancer; even in cases where initial treatment is successful, the tumor may gradually develop resistance over time. This results in a shorter duration of focused treatment efficacy and a shorter patient survival time. The effectiveness of treatment is significantly impacted by the microenvironment of pancreatic cancer (Zhou et al., 2025). Inflammatory reactions and fibrosis around the tumor may limit medication delivery and effectiveness, which would lower the efficacy of treatment. The evaluation of the clinical efficacy and safety of novel targeted therapy is further complicated by the aggressive nature of pancreatic cancer and its delayed diagnosis, which make it difficult to recruit sufficient patient populations for clinical studies.

6. CONCLUSION

A highly immunosuppressive tumor microenvironment (TME), delayed diagnosis, and poor survival rates make pancreatic ductal adenocarcinoma (PDAC) one of the most deadly cancers. Due to the limited efficacy of the previous emphasis on cytotoxic chemotherapy and direct tumor targeting, a paradigm shift in treatment approach is required. One promising and novel way to rewire the immunosuppressive PDAC TME and get past treatment resistance is by targeted microbiota alteration. There are several different ways that the microbiome specifically influences people. First of all, microbial dysbiosis is not merely a bystander but an active participant in oncogenesis. It is characterized by a loss of overall diversity and an enrichment of particular pathogenic taxa, such as Pseudomonas sp. in short-term survival or Enterobacteriaceae and fungus within the tumor. These microbes can directly promote chronic inflammation, produce carcinogenic metabolites like nitrosamines, and suppress local immune surveillance. The most promising clinical application of this knowledge lies in combining microbiome modulation with established therapies. The evidence for fecal microbiota transplantation (FMT) from long-term survivors is particularly potent. Humanized mouse models demonstrate that FMT can effectively transfer a protective microbial community, leading to TME reprogramming, enhanced anti-tumor immunity, and significant tumor growth inhibition. This provides a clear, mechanistic rationale for deploying FMT as an adjunct to immunotherapy and chemotherapy. Similarly, the interaction with radiotherapy is critical; the microbiome may influence the abscopal effect and the efficacy of radiation-induced immunogenic cell death, suggesting that microbiome status should be a consideration in radiation planning. However, translating these preclinical insights into clinical practice faces significant challenges that define the future research agenda. The microbiome is a fundamental component of pancreatic cancer biology. Its targeted modulation is no longer a theoretical concept but an emerging therapeutic pillar. By dismantling the immunosuppressive barriers erected by the tumor and its resident microbes, we can potentially unlock the full potential of existing and future therapies. The path forward requires a concerted, interdisciplinary effort from microbiologists, immunologists, and oncologists to conduct rigorous clinical trials that will definitively establish microbiome-based strategies as a standard, life-extending component of pancreatic cancer care. The challenge is immense, but the potential to finally alter the relentless trajectory of this disease makes it a pursuit of utmost importance.

7. REFERENCES

Afshar-Kharghan, V. (2017). The role of the complement system in cancer. *The Journal of Clinical Investigation*, *127*(3), 780–789. DOI: 10.1172/JCI90962

Ahn, J., Sinha, R., Pei, Z., Dominianni, C., Wu, J., Shi, J., Goedert, J. J., Hayes, R. B., & Yang, L. (2013). Human gut microbiome and risk for colorectal cancer. *Journal of the National Cancer Institute*, *105*(24), 1907–1911. DOI: 10.1093/jnci/djt300

. Amieva, M., & Peek, R. M., Jr. (2016). Pathobiology of *Helicobacter pylori*–induced gastric cancer. *Gastroenterology, 150*(1), 64 78. https://doi.org/DOI: 10.1053/j.gastro.2015.09.004

Balázs, K., Kis, E., Badie, C., Bogdándi, E. N., Candéias, S., Cruz Garcia, L., & Sáfrány, G. (2019). Radiotherapy-induced changes in the systemic immune and inflammation parameters of head and neck cancer patients. *Cancers (Basel)*, *11*(9), 1324. DOI: 10.3390/cancers11091324

Biesel, E. A., Sundheimer, J., Badr, M. T., Posadas-Cantera, S., Chikhladze, S., Fichtner-Feigl, S., & Wittel, U. A. (2025). Microbiological colonization of the pancreatic tumor affects postoperative complications and outcome after pancreatic surgery. *Frontiers in Cellular and Infection Microbiology*, *15*, 1521952. DOI: 10.3389/fcimb.2025.1521952

Bracci, P. M. (2017). Oral health and the oral microbiome in pancreatic cancer: An overview of epidemiological studies. *Cancer Journal (Sudbury, Mass.)*, *23*(6), 310–314. DOI: 10.1097/PPO.0000000000000287

Brusselaers, N., Sadr-Azodi, O., & Engstrand, L. (2020). Long-term proton pump inhibitor usage and the association with pancreatic cancer in Sweden. *Journal of Gastroenterology*, *55*(4), 453–461. DOI: 10.1007/s00535-019-01652-z

Caccialanza, R., Lobascio, F., Brugnatelli, S., & Pedrazzoli, P. (2020). Nutritional support in pancreatic cancer. *Cancer*, *126*(8), 1810–1811. DOI: 10.1002/cncr.32713

Caccialanza, R., Pedrazzoli, P., Cereda, E., Gavazzi, C., Pinto, C., Paccagnella, A., Beretta, G. D., Nardi, M., Laviano, A., & Zagonel, V. (2016). Nutritional support in cancer patients: A position paper from the Italian Society of Medical Oncology (AIOM) and the Italian Society of Artificial Nutrition and Metabolism (SINPE). *Journal of Cancer*, *7*(2), 131–135. DOI: 10.7150/jca.13818

Chen, Z., Zhang, S., Dong, S., Xu, H., & Zhou, W. (2022). Association of the microbiota and pancreatic cancer: Opportunities and limitations. *Frontiers in Immunology*, *13*, 844401. DOI: 10.3389/fimmu.2022.844401

Chung, L. M., Liang, J. A., Lin, C. L., Sun, L. M., & Kao, C. H. (2017). Cancer risk in patients with candidiasis: A nationwide population-based cohort study. *Oncotarget*, *8*(38), 63562–63573. DOI: 10.18632/oncotarget.18855

Cruz, M. S., Tintelnot, J., & Gagliani, N. (2024). Roles of microbiota in pancreatic cancer development and treatment. *Gut Microbes*, *16*(1), 2320280. DOI: 10.1080/19490976.2024.2320280

Durack, J., & Lynch, S. V. (2019). The gut microbiome: Relationships with disease and opportunities for therapy. *The Journal of Experimental Medicine*, *216*(1), 20–40. DOI: 10.1084/jem.20180448

Ge, Y., Wang, X., Guo, Y., Yan, J., Abuduwaili, A., Aximujiang, K., Yan, J., & Wu, M. (2021). Gut microbiota influence tumor development and Alter interactions with the human immune system. *Journal of Experimental & Clinical Cancer Research : CR*, *40*(1), 42. DOI: 10.1186/s13046-021-01845-6

Gopalakrishnan, V., Spencer, C. N., Nezi, L., Reuben, A., Andrews, M. C., Karpinets, T. V., & Wargo, J. A. (2018). Gut microbiome modulates response to anti–PD-1 immunotherapy in melanoma patients. *Science*, *359*(6371), 97–103. DOI: 10.1126/science.aan4236

Hamada, T., Nowak, J. A., Milner, D. J.Jr, Song, M. Y., & Ogino, S. J. (2019). Integration of microbiology, molecular pathology, and epidemiology: A new paradigm to explore the pathogenesis of microbiome-driven neoplasms. *The Journal of Pathology*, *247*(5), 615–628. DOI: 10.1002/path.5236

Hirooka, Y., Kasuya, H., Ishikawa, T., Kawashima, H., Ohno, E., Villalobos, I. B., Naoe, Y., Ichinose, T., Koyama, N., Tanaka, M., Kodera, Y., & Goto, H. (2022). A Phase I clinical trial of EUS-guided intratumoral injection of the oncolytic virus, HF10 for unresectable locally advanced pancreatic cancer. *BMC Cancer*, *18*(1), 596. DOI: 10.1186/s12885-018-4453-z

Jamal, M. H., & Khan, M. N. (2025). Developments in pancreatic cancer emerging therapies, diagnostic methods, and epidemiology. *Pathology, Research and Practice*, *156012*, 156012. Advance online publication. DOI: 10.1016/j.prp.2025.156012

Jemal, A., Bray, F., Center, M. M., Ferlay, J., Ward, E., & Forman, D. (2011). Global cancer statistics. *CA: a Cancer Journal for Clinicians*, *61*(2), 69–90. DOI: 10.3322/caac.20107

Kamarajah, S. K., Gopalan, V., Khan, Z., Baker, D. M., Lucas, A., Hawkins, D., Munnelly, S., Hollyman, M., Magill, L., & Lee, M. J. (2025). Gaps and uncertainties in the management of acute pancreatitis: A scoping review and quality assessment of clinical practice guidelines. *EClinicalMedicine*, *84*, 103216. Advance online publication. DOI: 10.1016/j.eclinm.2025.103216

Karpiński, T. M. (2019). Role of oral microbiota in cancer development. *Microorganisms*, *7*(1), 20. DOI: 10.3390/microorganisms7010020

Kaźmierczak-Siedlecka, K., Dvořák, A., Folwarski, M., Daca, A., Przewłócka, K., & Makarewicz, W. (2020). Fungal gut microbiota dysbiosis and its role in colorectal, oral, and pancreatic carcinogenesis. *Cancers (Basel)*, *12*(5), 1326. DOI: 10.3390/cancers12051326

Kim, S. H., Lee, S. M., Jeung, H. C., Lee, I. J., Park, J. S., Song, M., Lee, D. K., & Lee, S.-M. (2019). The effect of nutrition intervention with oral nutritional supplements on pancreatic and bile duct cancer patients undergoing chemotherapy. *Nutrients*, *11*(6), 1145. DOI: 10.3390/nu11051145

Kolbeinsson, H. M., Chandana, S., Wright, G. P., & Chung, M. (2023). Pancreatic cancer: A review of current treatment and novel therapies. *Journal of Investigative Surgery*, *36*(1), 2129884. DOI: 10.1080/08941939.2022.2129884

Kurilshikov, A., Wijmenga, C., Fu, J., & Zhernakova, A. (2017). Host genetics and gut microbiome: Challenges and perspectives. *Trends in Immunology*, *38*(9), 633–647. DOI: 10.1016/j.it.2017.06.003

Lekan, A. A., & Weiner, L. M. (2024). The role of chemokines in orchestrating the immune response to pancreatic ductal adenocarcinoma. *Cancers (Basel)*, *16*(3), 559. DOI: 10.3390/cancers16030559

Li, J., Liu, J., Zhou, Z., Wu, R., Chen, X., Yu, C., Stockwell, B., Kroemer, G., Kang, R., & Tang, D. (2023). Tumor-specific GPX4 degradation enhances ferroptosis-initiated antitumor immune response in mouse models of pancreatic cancer. *Science Translational Medicine*, *15*(720), eadg3049. DOI: 10.1126/scitranslmed.adg3049

Lu, S. Y., Hua, J., Xu, J., Wei, M. Y., Liang, C., Meng, Q. C., Liu, J., Zhang, B., Wang, W., Yu, X.-J., & Shi, S. (2021). Microorganisms in chemotherapy for pancreatic cancer: An overview of current research and future directions. *International Journal of Biological Sciences*, *17*(10), 2666–2682. DOI: 10.7150/ijbs.59117

Maekawa, T., Fukaya, R., Takamatsu, S., Itoyama, S., Fukuoka, T., Yamada, M., Hata, T., Nagaoka, S., Kawamoto, K., Eguchi, H., Murata, K., Kumada, T., Ito, T., Tanemura, M., Fujimoto, K., Tomita, Y., Tobe, T., Kamada, Y., & Miyoshi, E. (2018). Possible involvement of *Enterococcus* infection in the pathogenesis of chronic pancreatitis and cancer. *Biochemical and Biophysical Research Communications*, *506*(4), 962–969. DOI: 10.1016/j.bbrc.2018.10.169

Mantovani, A., Allavena, P., Sica, A., & Balkwill, F. (2008). Cancer-related inflammation. *Nature*, *454*(7203), 436–444. DOI: 10.1038/nature07205

Mendez, R., Kesh, K., Arora, N., Di Martino, L., McAllister, F., Merchant, N., Banerjee, S., & Banerjee, S. (2020). Microbial dysbiosis and polyamine metabolism as predictive markers for early detection of pancreatic cancer. *Carcinogenesis*, *41*(5), 561–570. DOI: 10.1093/carcin/bgz116

. Natto, H. A., Sahoo, D., & Muneera, N. (2024). Benefits of personalized diet, nutrition, and exercise programs for cancer survivors. *International Journal of Trends in OncoScience*, 12-22.

Paparo, L., Tripodi, L., Bruno, C., D'Agostino, L., Di Costanzo, M., Cosenza, L., & Nocerino, R. (2020). Protective action of *Bacillus clausii* probiotic strains in an in vitro model of rotavirus infection. *Scientific Reports*, *10*(1), 12636. DOI: 10.1038/s41598-020-69533-7

Park, W., Chawla, A., & O'Reilly, E. M. (2021). Pancreatic cancer: A review. *Journal of the American Medical Association*, *326*(9), 851–862. DOI: 10.1001/jama.2021.13027

Riquelme, E., Zhang, Y., Zhang, L., Montiel, M., Zoltan, M., Dong, W., Quesada, P., Sahin, I., Chandra, V., San Lucas, A., Scheet, P., Xu, H., Hanash, S. M., Feng, L., Burks, J. K., Do, K.-A., Peterson, C. B., Nejman, D., Tzeng, C.-W. D., & McAllister, F. (2019). Tumor microbiome diversity and composition influence pancreatic cancer outcomes. *Cell*, *178*(4), 795–806. DOI: 10.1016/j.cell.2019.07.008

Schawkat, K., Manning, M. A., Glickman, J. N., & Mortele, K. J. (2020). Pancreatic ductal adenocarcinoma and its variants: Pearls and perils. *Radiographics*, *40*(1), 121–140. DOI: 10.1148/rg.2020190184

Shi, M., Yu, D. H., Chen, Y., Zhao, C. Y., Zhang, J., Liu, Q. H., & Zhu, M. H. (2012). Expression of fibroblast activation protein in human pancreatic adenocarcinoma and its clinicopathological significance. *World Journal of Gastroenterology*, *18*(8), 840–846. DOI: 10.3748/wjg.v18.i8.840

Siddiqui, Z. R., Rahman, S., Verma, N., Srivastava, A., Jahan, N., Mohanty, S., & Suman, S. (2025). Gut–Oral microbial Dysbiosis: A correlated ecosystem. *Advanced Gut & Microbiome Research, 2025*(1), 7351229. DOI: 10.1155/agm3/7351229

Sivakumar, S., Jainarayanan, A., Arbe-Barnes, E., Sharma, P. K., Leathlobhair, M. N., Amin, S., Reiss, D. J., Heij, L., Hegde, S., Magen, A., Tucci, F., Sun, B., Wu, S., Anand, N. M., Slawinski, H., Revale, S., Nassiri, I., Webber, J., Hoeltzel, G. D., & Bashford-Rogers, R. (2025). Distinct immune cell infiltration patterns in pancreatic ductal adenocarcinoma (PDAC) exhibit divergent immune cell selection and immunosuppressive mechanisms. *Nature Communications, 16*(1), 1397. DOI: 10.1038/s41467-024-55424-2

Siveen, K. S., & Kuttan, G. (2009). Role of macrophages in tumour progression. *Immunology Letters, 123*(2), 97–102. DOI: 10.1016/j.imlet.2009.02.011

Song, X., Sun, X., Oh, S. F., Wu, M., Zhang, Y., Zheng, W., Geva-Zatorsky, N., Jupp, R., Mathis, D., Benoist, C., & Kasper, D. L. (2020). Microbial bile acid metabolites modulate gut RORγ^+ regulatory T cell homeostasis. *Nature, 577*(7790), 410–415. DOI: 10.1038/s41586-019-1865-0

Stasiewicz, M., Kwaśniewski, M., & Karpiński, T. M. (2021). Microbial associations with pancreatic cancer: A new frontier in biomarkers. *Cancers (Basel), 13*(15), 3784. DOI: 10.3390/cancers13153784

Thomas, R. M., & Jobin, C. (2020). Microbiota in pancreatic health and disease: The next frontier in microbiome research. *Nature Reviews. Gastroenterology & Hepatology, 17*(1), 53–64. DOI: 10.1038/s41575-019-0242-7

Timmer, F. E., Geboers, B., Nieuwenhuizen, S., Dijkstra, M., Schouten, E. A., Puijk, R. S., de Vries, J. J. J., van den Tol, M. P., Bruynzeel, A. M. E., Streppel, M. M., Wilmink, J. W., van der Vliet, H. J., Meijerink, M. R., Scheffer, H. J., & de Gruijl, T. D. (2021). Pancreatic cancer and immunotherapy: A clinical overview. *Cancers (Basel), 13*(16), 4138. DOI: 10.3390/cancers13164138

Vogtmann, E., Han, Y., Caporaso, J. G., Bokulich, N., Mohamadkhani, A., Moayyed-kazemi, A., & Pourshams, A. (2020). Oral microbial community composition is associated with pancreatic cancer: A case-control study in Iran. *Cancer Medicine, 9*(2), 797–806. DOI: 10.1002/cam4.2660

Wu, M., Liu, J., Wu, S., Xie, H., Wang, Y., Zhang, J., & Zhang, Y. (2021). Systemic immune activation and responses of irradiation to different metastatic sites combined with immunotherapy in advanced non-small cell lung cancer. *Frontiers in Immunology, 12*, 803247. DOI: 10.3389/fimmu.2021.803247

Yamamura, R., & Sonoshita, M. (2025). Fecal microbiota transplantation as a novel therapeutic strategy for pancreatic cancer. *Translational and Regulatory Sciences*, *7*(1), 37–45. DOI: 10.33611/trs.2025-003

Zhang, L., Sanagapalli, S., & Stoita, A. (2018). Challenges in diagnosis of pancreatic cancer. *World Journal of Gastroenterology*, *24*(19), 2047–2060. DOI: 10.3748/wjg.v24.i19.2047

Zhang, X., Shi, S., Zhang, B., Ni, Q. X., & Xu, J. (2018). Circulating biomarkers for early diagnosis of pancreatic cancer: Facts and hopes. *American Journal of Cancer Research*, *8*, 332–353. DOI: 10.7150/ijbs.31083

Zhou, X., Wang, X., Yang, S., & Huang, Z. (2025). Advances in immunotherapy and targeted therapy for pancreatic cancer. *Oncology and Translational Medicine*, *11*(2), 81–91. DOI: 10.1097/ot9.0000000000000074

Chapter 6
Standard Treatments of Pancreatic Cancer and Their Limitations

Shraddha Devarshi
https://orcid.org/0000-0002-6725-8917
School of Pharmacy, Indira University, Pune, India

Tejal Bele
https://orcid.org/0000-0002-4170-6232
School of Pharmacy, Indira University, India

Amruta P. Walvekar
https://orcid.org/0000-0001-7262-8380
School of Pharmacy, Indira University, Pune, India

Pallavi Chouhan
https://orcid.org/0000-0001-8755-3422
School of Pharmacy, Indira University, Pune, India

Rutuja Kamble
https://orcid.org/0000-0002-7919-7197
School of Pharmacy, Indira University, Pune, India

ABSTRACT

Pancreatic cancer is significant global issue due to high death rates, aggressive progression, and poor prognosis. The current treatments include surgical resection, chemotherapy, radiotherapy, and targeted therapies. Surgical resection offers the only potential for cure but is feasible in less than 20% of patients due to late-stage diagnosis. Chemotherapy regimens have improved survival modestly but are often

DOI: 10.4018/979-8-3373-1469-3.ch006

limited by toxicity and chemoresistance. Radiotherapy is primarily used for local control in unresectable disease but has limited impact on overall survival. Targeted therapies and immunotherapies have shown minimal efficacy due to the highly desmoplastic and immunosuppressive tumor microenvironment. Moreover, the heterogeneity of pancreatic tumors and the paucity of predictive biomarkers complicate the personalization of treatment strategies. These limitations underscore the urgent need for novel therapeutic approaches, early detection methods, and biomarker-driven clinical trials to enhance treatment efficacy and improve patient outcomes.

INTRODUCTION

Pancreatic cancer also known as pancreatic ductal adenocarcinoma (PDAC), is a deadly cancer and is significant global issue due to high death rates and delay in diagnosis. In United States, it ranks as fourth leading cause of death (Klein, 2021) (Afghani & Klein, 2022) (Muratović & Nikolić, 2023) (Ilic & Ilic, 2022) (Hu et al., 2021) (Xiang et al., 2023). In 2020, there were approximately 495,773 new cases and 466,003 deaths from pancreatic cancer worldwide, with the highest incidence and mortality rates observed in the Western Pacific Region (Ilic & Ilic, 2022). The age-standardized incidence rates (ASRs) for pancreatic cancer are highest in the European Region, while the lowest rates are reported in the South-East Asia Region (Ilic & Ilic, 2022). Given the aggressive nature of disease, multi-modality treatment approach is paramount to improve patient outcomes (Crippa et al., 2017). Table no.1 shows various risk factors for Pancreatic cancer.

Table 1. Risk Factors for Pancreatic cancer.

Modifiable Risk Factors	Non-Modifiable Risk Factors	Socioeconomic and Environmental Factors
Smoking	Age	Socioeconomic Status
Obesity	Gender	Environmental Exposures
Diabetes Mellitus	Genetic Predisposition	Healthcare Access and Utilization
Alcohol Consumption		

SURGICAL TREATMENT

The only potential curative treatment option if surgical resection. Although, main limiting factor is that only small portion of patients (10-20%) are eligible at the time of diagnosis. This low percentage is due to the aggressive nature of the disease, often manifesting only after substantial progression. (Garcia-Sampedro et al., 2021)

The common surgical techniques available are:

1.Pancreaticoduodenectomy (Whipple Procedure):

This surgery entails the removal of the pancreas' head, the duodenum, the gallbladder, and part of the stomach. Pylorus-preserving pancreaticoduodenectomy (PPPD) is advantageous over traditional Whipple procedure as it has shorter operation duration and reduced blood loss, however, associated with higher incidences of delayed gastric emptying (DGE). DGE can delay post-operative recovery in patients (Symeonidis et al., 2023) (Alonso et al., 2024). Whipple procedure along with arterial resection (AR) has its own set of disadvantages and therefore has to be reserved for selected patients. Post-operative fistula and haemorrhage are common in Whipple procedure, with higher chances in AR (Abdelmohsin et al., 2024).

2. Distal Pancreatectomy:

This procedure involves extracting the pancreas' tail and body, frequently along with the spleen. The chances of occurrence of postoperative pancreatic fistulas (POPFs) is between 30-60% which increases risk of morbidity, mortality and prolong hospilization. Postpancreatectomy Acute Pancreatitis (PPAP) can occur in 3.9% can cause mortality in severe cases. (Moussa et al., 2024) (Bannone et al., 2023).

3. Total Pancreatectomy:

This involves removal of the entire pancreas, although it is rarely recommended due to severe long-term complications such as endocrine, exocrine insufficiencies, and pancreatic fistula (Jabłońska et al., 2021), (Boone, 2024). This technique has 32% morbidity and 5% mortality (Chen & Lin, 2023).

Even with noteworthy advancement in surgical techniques and improved perioperative care, the survival rate for patients undergoing resection is very low (Robatel & Schenk, 2022).

Surgical Challenges and Limitations

The pancreas's complex location, surrounded by vital organs and blood vessels like the portal vein, superior mesenteric artery, and celiac axis, highly complicates surgical resection. Due to the delicate nature of these surrounding organs, requires careful precision, increasing the risk of vascular injury, bleeding and damage to organs. Surgical procedures are difficult to perform in locally advanced disease due high vascular encroachment. Procedures involving vascular resection, including portal vein resection, present considerable technical difficulty and heightened morbidity and mortality risks (Ravikumar et al., 2014). The role of arterial resection remains a subject of debate, as its oncologic benefit must be weighed against the substantial risks involved.

The difficulty in accurately visualizing pancreatic tumors, especially on conventional imaging modalities (Lewis et al., 2023), presents another significant limitation. This lack of clear visualization can lead to incomplete resection, increasing the risk of local recurrence. The development of more advanced imaging techniques, such as magnetic resonance imaging (MRI) with real-time tracking capabilities, is crucial for improving surgical planning and minimizing the risk of incomplete resection. The use of intraoperative ultrasound (IOUS) and other advanced imaging technologies during surgery can further enhance the accuracy of tumor resection (Lewis et al., 2023).

ADJUVANT AND NEOADJUVANT THERAPIES

Adjuvant therapies: It plays a significant role in management of resectable pancreatic cancer, particularly in early stage. Although, the effectiveness is limited in advanced stage.

Adjuvant chemotherapy has shown improved overall survival in patients with early-stage (I and II) pancreatic cancer, with notable differences in recurrence-free survival observed in stage I patients. (Li et al., 2023)

The mFOLFIRINOX regimen is the current standard of care for fit patients, demonstrating significant survival benefits. Following agents are commonly used in adjuvant therapies: (Conroy et al., 2023) (Mann et al., 2023).

Figure 1.

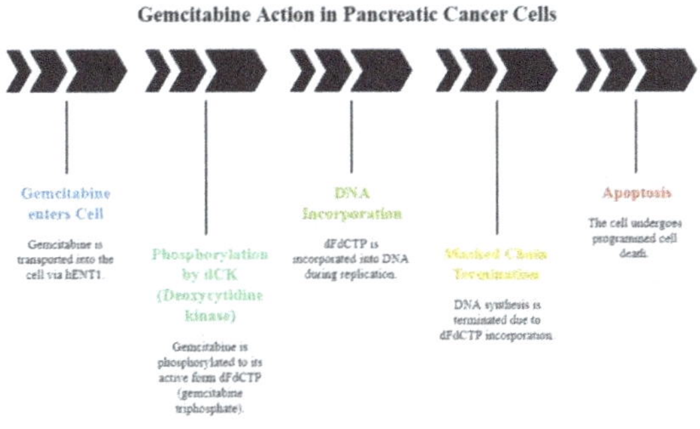

1. Gemcitabine: A nucleoside analogue, helps to to target residual cancer cell post-operatively. It has shown to reduce risk of recurrence & improve overall survival. (Fig no.1 shows the mechanism of action of gemcitabine)
2. 5-Flurouracil (5-FU): In a Phase II trial it was combined with portal vein infusion along with mitomycin C and cisplatin followed by Gemcitabine shown improved benefits (Minoru Kitago et al., 2024).
3. FOLFIRINOX: It is combination of 5-Flurouracil (5-FU), leucovorin, irinotecan, and oxaliplatin. The PRODIGE trial showed improved overall survival in resectable pancreatic cancer as compared to monotherapy (Cecchini et al., 2024).
4. Capecitabine: The ESPAC-4 trial specifically highlighted the survival benefits of gemcitabine plus capecitabine, establishing it as a recommended regimen in clinical practice (Mann et al., 2023) (Biagi et al., 2023).

However, in advanced-stage pancreatic cancer, adjuvant chemotherapy does not substantially improve recurrence-free or overall survival, suggesting the need for alternative treatment strategies (Li et al., 2023). Factors such as early disease recurrence, prolonged recovery, and patient age contribute to the underutilization of adjuvant therapies (Conroy et al., 2023). Newer treatment option such as immunotherapy and nanotechnology are being explored to overcome the limitation of conventional therapies (Zheng et al., 2024) (Alam & Dhoundiyal, 2023).

Neoadjuvant therapy: It is preferred in borderline resectable or locally advanced pancreatic cancer before surgical approach. It includes chemotherapy, radiation or combination of both. The main purpose of this therapy is shrinking the size of tumor, improving resection margins, eradicting metastatic cells, and identifying patients who are less likely to benefit from surgical resection. Chemotherapy include

FOLFIRINOX and Gemcitabine –based combinations. Studies have shown that FOLFIRINOX leads to higher R0 while there is no difference in overall survival in both treatment groups (Dhamija K et al., 2025).

Chemoradiation aims to prevent spread of tumor and reduce positive margin. However, recent studies shows mixed results regarding its impact on survival (Paisey & Bateman, 2024) (Bryant et al., 2024).

The identification of patients appropriate for neoadjuvant therapies is challenging, as majority patients present with advanced disease where its use is limited. (Něměček, R., & Eid, M. (2024). The role of neoadjuvant treatment in localized pancreatic cancer. Determining patients who will benefit from this therapy is complex as prognostic factors may influence clinical outcomes.

SYSTEMIC THERAPY FOR ADVANCED/ METASTATIC PANCREATIC CANCER

The basic treatment approach for advanced or metastatic pancreatic cancer patients remains systemic chemotherapy. Systemic therapy provides the primary intervention for advanced pancreatic cancer because of the malignancy's aggressive behavior (Ettrich & Seufferlein, 2021). Advancements in chemotherapy treatment methods and supportive care strategies have not resolved the critical barriers involving natural treatment resistance in addition to drug resistance development and unfavorable treatment side effects together with pancreatic cancer's biological diversity. (Fig no. 2 shows the cancer therapies spectrum based on directness of tumor attack)

Figure 2. Objectives of Systemic Therapy

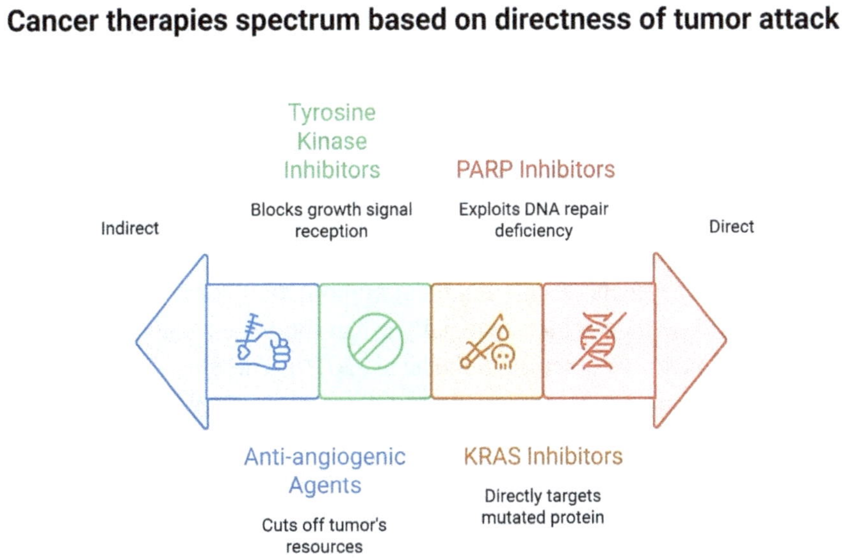

Survival enhancement through disease progression control stands as the principal purpose for using systemic therapy in pancreatic cancer treatments. Chemotherapy stands as the main treatment option for advanced pancreatic cancer patients because surgical removal becomes impossible at this stage. The role of systemic therapy in pancreatic cancer treatment includes reducing associated cancer symptoms like intractable pain, obstructive jaundice and cachexia to improve patients' quality of life (Lideståhl et al., 2006). The cytostatic and cytotoxic actions of systemic chemotherapy help prevent malignant cell dissemination which in turn protects physical functioning and avoids disease-related complications.

Efficacious Chemotherapy Regimens

Many tested chemotherapy combinations exist to treat advanced pancreatic cancer patients. Gemcitabine monotherapy represents the historical standard first-line therapy because it fights cancer cells through two actions: DNA replication blockage and quick cell apoptosis in fast-growing tumors. The survival benefits from single-agent gemcitabine therapy remain limited, which drives medical professionals to consider alternative combination treatments (Gresham et al., 2014).

Gemcitabine combined with nab-paclitaxel represents a key breakthrough in pancreatic cancer therapy. Studies indicate that using gemcitabine combined with nab-paclitaxel provides patients and doctors with improved overall survival and progression-free survival results beyond using gemcitabine independently. The drug delivery of nab-paclitaxel becomes more effective inside tumors since it breaks through stromal desmoplasia to enhance toxicity toward neoplastic cells (Wainberg et al., 2020).

FOLFIRINOX demonstrates better survival benefits than single-agent gemcitabine specifically in patients with good performance status using its composition of folinic acid (leucovorin), 5-fluorouracil (5-FU), irinotecan, and oxaliplatin. FOLFIRINOX performs its action through simultaneous disruption against three cellular processes: DNA synthesis and topoisomerase DNA repair function and mitotic progression. Stronger anti-cancer effects of this treatment combination come at the expense of increased toxic side effects which especially affect the patient's neutrophil counts, intestinal health, and nerve function (Suker et al., 2016). Therefore, patient selection demands strict criteria and doctors must provide close supportive care.

NALIRIFOX represents a new and effective treatment option when nanoliposomal irinotecan is used together with 5-FU and leucovorin for advanced disease patients. Nanoliposomal delivery systems improve drug absorption and sustained distribution into the bloodstream, enhancing therapeutic effects and possibly reducing adverse effects (Nichetti et al., 2024).

Limitations and Challenges of Systemic Therapy

The improvement of chemotherapeutic regimens for pancreatic cancer treatment has not solved the numerous challenging obstacles present in systemic therapy. The most substantial barrier to these regimens is their extreme toxicity levels. Multiple patients develop serious adverse side effects from chemotherapeutic treatment that cause suppressed bone marrow function along with liver damage and mouth sores and nerve damage which deteriorate patients' quality of life and may lead to dose adjustments and stoppage of therapy (Chakrabarti et al., 2022).

Pancreatic cancer faces an additional major challenge from drug-resistant outcomes. Pancreatic cancer tumors grow within an environment that demonstrates multiple forms of heterogeneity and durability as well as multiple resistance pathways that develop. Dense stromal fibrosis together with hypoxic tumor niches as well as an immunosuppressive environment, makes it possible for cancer cells to escape cytotoxic effects leading to therapeutic failure and disease progression.

The extended survival offered by chemotherapy lasts only temporarily although it brings limited benefit since patient's experience survival periods that extend to months instead of years. The current situation highlights the necessity for innovative treatments to generate longer-lasting beneficial patient outcomes (Palumbo et al., 2013).

The reason for suboptimal systemic treatment outcomes is the lack of reliable predictive biomarkers. Pancreatic cancer lacks adequate biomarkers primarily because it does not benefit from molecular profiling techniques for therapy selection. Predictive biomarkers that undergo successful identification and validation methods will enable better patient care by letting healthcare providers provide personalized treatments that should enhance outcomes.

Pancreatic cancer has proven difficult for targeted therapies to succeed because of the numerous complex genetic alterations found in the disease (Bazeed et al., 2022). The broad application of targeted therapy remains limited by the lack of uniform genetic mutations that can be treated with specific inhibitors even though inhibitors for BRCA-mutated tumors have obtained encouraging results.

IMMUNOTHERAPY IN PANCREATIC CANCER

The immune system of a patient functions as the target of immunotherapy to detect and destroy cancer cells. The novel treatment method has changed how we treat different cancers although it shows minimal success in treating pancreatic cancer because of the dense immunotoxic conditions in the region (Foley et al., 2016). Numerous immunotherapeutic approaches are currently being studied despite their limited impact on pancreatic cancer treatment.

Immune Checkpoint Inhibitors

The immune checkpoint inhibitors (ICIs) including anti-PD-1 and anti-CTLA-4 monoclonal antibodies have proven effective for treating malignancies of melanoma and non-small cell lung cancer. The therapeutic compounds restore suppressed immunity while amplifying tumor-killing functions of T-cells. Alternatively, the use of immune checkpoint inhibitors as standalone treatments has produced limited results in pancreatic cancer because the disease creates obstacles to immune cell infiltration through desmoplastic stroma formation (Johansson et al., 2016). Clinical researchers currently pursue multiple trials that combine ICIs with chemotherapy and radiation along with additional immune-modulating agents to reinforce their therapeutic effectiveness.

Cancer Vaccines

Vaccine treatment for cancer includes a mechanism to show tumor-associated antigens to antigen-presenting cells (APCs) which results in the formation of cytotoxic T lymphocytes (CTLs) capable of fighting malignancies. Researchers study three types of vaccine platforms such as peptide-based, dendritic cell-based and viral vector-based vaccines for pancreatic cancer applications (Salman et al., 2013).

Adoptive Cell Therapy

The adoptive cell therapy (ACT) procedure adjusts and grows immune cells outside the body to make them more effective against tumors. The therapeutic value of CAR T-cell treatments in hematologic malignancies has proven effective. Still, researchers have struggled to apply it to solid tumors because of poor T-cell infiltration combined with heterogeneous tumor antigens. Research teams work to develop methods that will enhance T-cell duration in the body along with their movement capabilities and their capacity to penetrate tumors for greater pancreatic cancer treatment outcomes.

TARGETED THERAPY IN PANCREATIC CANCER

Pancreatic ductal adenocarcinoma (PDAC) represents the primary pancreatic cancer type and possesses remarkable aggressiveness while usually being detected when the disease has spread widely through the body (Seicean, 2015). PDAC requires new therapeutic strategies because traditional treatments, including surgery and chemotherapy together with radiation therapy, demonstrate constrained success.

The most common genetic defect in pancreatic ductal adenocarcinoma (PDAC) takes place through KRAS (Kirsten rat sarcoma viral oncogene homolog) mutations, which affect 90%–95% of all cases. Uncontrolled cell growth and survival together with treatment resistance occur because of KRAS mutations, thus making KRAS an essential genetic target for pancreatic cancer (Luo, 2021). The highly effective role of KRAS in tumor advancement has historically made it an "undruggable" target because of its tight GTP connection and unavailable binding sites. Recent breakthroughs in drug research have produced KRAS G12C inhibitors that include sotorasib and adagrasib as new therapeutic options.

Experimental research on PDAC KRAS G12C mutations is ongoing despite their limited occurrence (1%–3% of cases) as opposed to NSCLC and colorectal cancer because of earlier success in treating these cancers with these inhibitors. The research data from preclinical evaluations together with early clinical trials indicate that sotorasib (AMG 510) produces limited beneficial outcomes when used to treat pancreatic cancer patients whose tumors possess KRAS G12C mutations through achieving stabilization of disease along with some minor response outcomes (Zeitouni et al., 2016). Doctors consider adagrasib (MRTX849) a promising treatment for pancreatic cancer because laboratory tests demonstrate elevated potency and extended KRAS inhibition compared to sotorasib (AMG 510).

The use of KRAS inhibitors encounters multiple barriers when treating pancreatic cancer. The treatment impact of G12C-specific inhibitors remains limited because PDAC predominantly presents mutations of KRAS G12D (45%) or KRAS G12V (35%). Pancreatic tumors can bypass KRAS inhibitor resistance through two different mechanisms: tumor cells acquire alternative pathways and develop new mutations to activate them.

PARP Inhibitors

Olaparib represents a PARP inhibitor that produces clinical advantages within patients bearing germline mutations of the BRCA1 or BRCA2 genes. PARP inhibitors function through enzyme-blocking activities since PARP enzymes prove essential for fixing DNA damage (Zhu et al., 2020). PARP-dependent DNA repair serves as a crucial pathway for cancer cells with BRCA mutations because their homologous recombination pathway remains dysfunctional.

The inhibition of PARP activity by these drugs causes DNA damage to build up which leads to synthetic lethality and death of cancer cells. The Food and Drug Administration has approved Olaparib treatment for metastatic pancreatic cancer patients who possess BRCA mutations after responding to platinum-based first-line chemotherapy.

The application of PARP inhibitors shows promise but the therapy exists only for specific patient groups along with ongoing resistance mechanism challenges. Scientists continue investigations about using immune checkpoint inhibitors and additional DNA damage response inhibitors with PARP inhibitors to expand therapeutic options.

EGFR Inhibitors

Pancreatic cancer frequently displays increased expression of epidermal growth factor receptor (EGFR) which leads to critical functions in tumor expansion and cell replication and cancer cell endurance. Medical experts have investigated this specific pathway as a possible therapeutic solution. The targeted therapy erlotinib works as an EGFR tyrosine kinase inhibitor and received approval for pancreatic cancer treatment with gemcitabine (Walsh et al., 2012).

The single-agent use of EGFR inhibitors provides limited therapeutic advantages since it leads to a minor survival benefit. The ineffectiveness of these treatments results from various pathways that signal redundantly as well as from diverse cancer cell types and defense strategies by the cancer cells. Scientists currently investigate multiple therapy approaches to combine EGFR inhibitors either with targeted treatments or chemotherapy regimens or immunotherapy strategies to provide better outcomes in pancreatic cancer patients.

Hedgehog Pathway Inhibitors

Hedgehog (Hh) signaling serves as a major factor in pancreatic cancer advancement through creation of dense stromal tissue that impedes medication delivery to cancer cells. Medical professionals developed Hedgehog inhibitors including vismodegib and sonidegib as a means to intervene with this signaling pathway while attempting to both split tumor-stroma complexes and boost medicine penetration (Onishi, 2014).

Studies of Hedgehog inhibitors in pancreatic cancer treatment have led to disappointing results because these drugs produced minimal impact on patient survival duration. The failure of Hedgehog pathway inhibition occurs due to a side effect of altered stromal-tumor communications that speeds up tumor growth. Clinical research now combines Hedgehog inhibitors with chemotherapy and immune checkpoint inhibitors as well as stromal-targeted agents to enhance patient response.

The success of targeted therapies in pancreatic cancer treatment faces barriers from drug resistance as well as tumor heterogeneity together with a complicated microenvironment of the disease.

Pancreatic cancer treatment using targeted therapy faces multiple operational barriers that hinder its success. The inability to effectively treat pancreatic cancer arises mainly from tumor complexity in addition to resistance formation and insufficient diagnostic probes for appropriate drug choices.

Treatment of pancreatic cancer faces considerable obstacles due to low numbers of treatable targets available. Pancreatic cancer presents a highly heterogeneous mutationally complex profile through which other malignancies differ because it contains few actionable therapeutic targets. Pancreatic tumors contain various drug-resistant mutations which restrict doctors from developing new effective treatments for patients.

Drug resistance presents a significant challenge that decreases the extended duration of effectiveness of targeted therapy. Pancreatic cancer cells adapt through several resistance mechanisms that include obtaining secondary mutations to escape drug effectiveness and by activating alternative signaling routes as well as modifying drug processing and release. Research toward combination therapy as well as second-generation inhibitors becomes crucial because treatment failure and disease progression occur when cells develop resistance.

Pancreatic tumors are hindered by heterogeneity through their existence of numerous genetically distinct cancer cell subpopulations. Various types of tumor cells that exist in a single patient present a challenge in developing specific medication because different cancer cells inside the same individual might react differently to anticancer drugs. The dense stromal nature of pancreatic tumors creates difficulties for targeted agents to reach their targets because it makes drug delivery challenging and less effective.

STROMAL TARGETING THERAPIES IN PANCREATIC CANCER

Pancreatic cancer develops a thick stromal microenvironment that severely impacts drug resistance together with immune evasion and tumor advancement. A physical and biochemical barrier exists within the stroma which is composed of fibroblasts and extracellular matrix parts along with immune cells that prevent chemotherapy and targeted treatments from reaching their targets. Stromal targeting therapies are developed to break down the protective barrier while increasing medication transport so patients gain improved clinical results.

Drugs deliver better into pancreatic tumors through the enzyme activity of hyaluronidase that degrades hyaluronic acid (HA) which transforms the pancreatic tumor stroma. Pancreatic ductal adenocarcinoma (PDAC) tumors have dense extracellular tissue that leads to elevated interstitial fluid pressure which interferes with blood circulation and hindering the performance of chemotherapeutic agents. Medical research has examined PEGylated recombinant hyaluronidase (PEGPH20) as a chemotherapy additive for better tumor blood flow and drug transport. The productive trial results for HA-high tumors in clinical studies did not advance the treatment due to elevated toxicity levels, which produced thromboembolic events (Neesse et al., 2015).

FAK inhibitors work by suppressing signaling mechanisms that sustain pancreatic cancer stromal cells while also controlling fibrosis development and immune suppression in the disease. As a non-receptor tyrosine kinase, FAK executes vital functions to support tumor-stroma relationships which boost cancer cell development and protect oncological resistance and limit immune cell activities (Jiang et al., 2019). Too much activity of FAK activity exists in pancreatic ductal adenocarcinoma cells leading to a dense stromal microenvironment that blocks drug delivery and prevents immune cells from functioning effectively. These therapeutic approaches block FAK to help decrease the amount of fibrosis alongside increasing immune cell entry and better chemotherapy effectiveness.

Limitations of Stromal Targeting Therapies

1. Potential for Off-Target Effects: The administration of stromal targeting therapies might unintentionally harm normal tissue structures which could produce harmful side effects.
2. Complex Stromal Interactions: Rupturing the tumor stroma could create unforeseen side effects by altering functions which both support tumors and control their growth.
3. Lack of Predictive Biomarkers: There is a lack of reliable biomarkers to identify patients who would benefit the most from stromal-targeting approaches, making it challenging to implement personalized treatment strategies (Hosein et al., 2020).
4. Therapeutic Resistance and Variability: The diverse characteristics of pancreatic cancer stromal tissue create inconsistent responses among patients when using stromal-targeting drugs.
5. Drug Delivery Challenges: The objective of stromal targeting treatments to enhance drug penetration may trigger unwanted alterations of tumor microenvironment that reduce therapeutic effectiveness.

Table no.2 shows the summary of all the innovative therapies for pancreatic cancer.

Table 2. Summary of innovative therapies for pancreatic cancer.

Therapy	Type/Target	Description	Mechanism of Action
PARP Inhibitors (e.g., Olaparib)	Targeted Therapy	Used in patients with BRCA1/2 mutations	Inhibit PARP enzyme involved in DNA repair, leading to cancer cell death
Immunotherapy (e.g., Immune Checkpoint Inhibitors – Nivolumab, Pembrolizumab)	Immunotherapy	Stimulates the immune system to attack cancer cells	Blocks PD-1/PD-L1 or CTLA-4 pathways to enhance T-cell response
CAR-T Cell Therapy (e.g., targeting Mesothelin)	Cell-based Immunotherapy	Genetically modified T-cells to recognize and kill cancer cells	Engineered T-cells target tumor-associated antigen like mesothelin
Oncolytic Viruses (e.g., Reolysin, Pelareorep)	Viral Therapy	Viruses that selectively infect and kill cancer cells	Replicate within tumors, causing cell lysis and immune activation
Cancer Vaccines (e.g., GVAX, CRS-207)	Immunotherapy	Stimulate the body to recognize and attack pancreatic cancer cells	Induce immune response against tumor-associated antigens
Stroma-Targeting Agents (e.g., PEGPH20)	Stromal Modulators	Break down tumor stroma to improve drug delivery	Degrades hyaluronic acid in the stroma, enhancing chemotherapy penetration

continued on following page

Table 2. Continued

Therapy	Type/Target	Description	Mechanism of Action
Tyrosine Kinase Inhibitors (e.g., Erlotinib)	Targeted Therapy	Inhibit EGFR signaling in cancer cells	Block tyrosine kinase activity required for tumor growth
KRAS G12C Inhibitors (e.g., Sotorasib)	Targeted Therapy	Target KRAS mutations common in pancreatic cancer	Binds and inhibits mutant KRAS protein
Microbiome Modulators	Adjunct Therapy	Modify gut or tumor microbiota to enhance treatment	Aims to alter immune environment and drug response
Organoid-Guided Personalized Therapy	Precision Medicine	Uses patient-derived tumor organoids to test drug sensitivity	Enables individualized therapy by screening drug response ex vivo

Novel Chemotherapeutic Agents and Combinations in Pancreatic Cancer

Pancreatic cancer represents a difficult-to-treat malignancy therefore researchers actively explore new chemotherapeutic agents and drug combinations to enhance pancreatic cancer treatment results. The main research priority targets the creation of new drugs and seeks better ways to combine medications and better methods for drug delivery to achieve improved results for patients.

1. Developing New Drugs

Cancer research requires the creation of new chemotherapeutic agents that use different action mechanisms. Traditional cancer treatments with gemcitabine and fluorouracil (5-FU) show limited effects because they encounter resistance together with heterogeneous tumor populations. Researchers examine emerging cytotoxic agents to help cancer cells survive and maintain healthy tissue integrity. DNA-reactive agents and metabolic inhibitors along with prodrugs represent promising pancreatic cancer treatment strategies because of their ability to exploit cancer-specific DNA repair defects and activate dynamically within tumor locations relative to normal cells. The medical sector is now closer to achieving better targeted cancer treatment methods.

2. Optimizing Drug Combinations

Multiple agents currently undergo investigation as potential treatments for pancreatic cancer because this aggressive disease resists standard chemotherapy methods. Strategies include:

- The simultaneous use of chemotherapy drugs with targeted therapy approaches cancer cells from various angles. Researchers have achieved positive results from combining gemcitabine with PARP inhibitors in BRCA-mutated tumor treatment (Chi et al., 2021).
- The combination of chemotherapy with immune checkpoint inhibitor drugs through immunochemotherapy brings greater enhancement to the cancer-fighting capabilities of the immune system.
- The combined use of FOLFIRINOX treatment with 5-FU, leucovorin, irinotecan, and oxaliplatin and gemcitabine and nab-paclitaxel has proven better at improving patient survival rates than using individual therapies

3. Improving Drug Delivery

Drug penetration remains a primary treatment challenge in pancreatic cancer because dense stromal tissue creates barriers around tumors. Researchers are working on innovative ways to enhance drug delivery and increase therapeutic concentration within the tumor:

- Nanoparticles serve as drug carriers which provide stability to medications and improve penetration and help control drug delivery directly to tumors.
- The usage of hyaluronidase enzymes enables the breakdown of extracellular material and decreases interstitial pressure thus enhancing drug penetration through tissues.

Limitations of Novel Chemotherapeutic Approaches

1. Toxicity

New chemotherapeutic agents designed for enhanced treatment effectiveness bring unpredictable toxicity elements that obstruct their practical use in medical settings. Drugs designed to target specific pathways create severe side effects for normal tissue cells because they trigger gastrointestinal problems and destroy bone marrow and cause damage to organs. Prolonged administration of combination therapies becomes difficult because higher toxicity levels occur as a result of their enhanced tumor-killing properties. The necessary treatment of these side effects requires both precise medication dosage adjustment and supportive medical interventions for protecting patients from harm (Robatel & Schenk, 2022).

2. Drug Resistance

The production of new chemotherapy agents faces substantial difficulties because of drug resistance development. Pancreatic cancer cells demonstrate a strong capacity to adapt which enables them to resist chemotherapy through genetic mutations as well as enhanced drug expulsion and alternative survival pathway activations. The development of drug resistance leads to the demise of effectiveness for both new and promising chemotherapy agents. Scientists investigate combination treatments together with alternating drug protocols and resistance mechanism targeting strategies to enhance lasting results from new therapeutic agents (Long et al., 2011).

3. Clinical Trial Design

The clinical implementation of chemotherapeutic agents needs well-designed trials yet the process involves multiple barriers. The recruitment of patients becomes challenging because pancreatic cancer operates swiftly and patients possess a short time between diagnosis and intervention opportunity. Medical research along with several trial stages is essential to discover proper drug dosages and combination protocols while also developing predictors of patient treatment response through biomarkers (Kolbeinsson et al., 2022). Clinical tests become harder to design because pancreatic tumors show various subtypes which could respond differently to identically applied treatments. The development of effective treatments requires adaptive trial approaches alongside biomarker assessments for patient screening and international connections in clinical research to quicken treatment discovery efforts.

Chimeric Antigen Receptor T-cell (CAR-T) therapy:

This is novel technique which involves genetically modifying T-cells so that they can express receptors that target specific tumour-associated antigens (TAAs), to identify and destroy them. As most of the pancreatic cancer are diagnosed in advanced stages, where the conventional therapies have limited role (Garcia-Sampedro et al., 2021). They act through various pathways such as, perforin and granzyme, to induce programmed cell death in pancreatic cancer cells while immune response is elicited through cytokine secretion. Various studies are ongoing to evaluate the effectiveness of CAR-T therapy in pancreatic cancer and identify the TAAs. (Czaplicka et al., 2024). There is a potential to combine existing therapies with the CAR-T therapy (J Blanquicett & Aguirre, 2021). The survival and function can get affected by the heterogeneous and complex nature of pancreatic tumor which poses a major challenge to this therapy (Leroux & Konstantinidou, 2021).

While CAR-T therapy offers a novel treatment option for managing pancreatic cancer, however, further studies need to be conducted to understand the full potential of the therapy.

PALLIATIVE CARE AND SUPPORTIVE MEASURES IN PANCREATIC CANCER

Pancreatic cancer produces significant pain symptoms because the tumor destroys nearby nerves and tissue structures. Controlling pain in pancreatic cancer patients requires opioid analgesics alongside nerve blocks and the treatment of neuropathic pain with antidepressants and anticonvulsant medications. Patients with pancreatic cancer frequently benefit from interventional treatments which include radiotherapy together with palliative surgeries which help decrease pain levels and make patients more comfortable.

1. Pain Management

Pancreatic cancer produces significant pain symptoms because the tumor destroys nearby nerves and tissue structures. Effective pain management includes opioid medications alongside celiac plexus block procedures and practices both opioid and neuromodulatory drugs for treating neuropathic symptoms (Conroy et al., 2016). The medical procedures of radiotherapy along with palliative surgeries enable healthcare providers to help patients experience reduced pain and improved comfort.

2. Symptom Control

Several additional symptoms like nausea and vomiting along with fatigue and jaundice and depression create serious deterioration in patient quality of life. The main treatments for these symptoms include antiemetic drugs and appetite stimulants and corticosteroids along with antidepressant medications. The performance of endoscopic or surgical procedures through biliary stenting enables relief of obstructive jaundice to promote better patient health.

3. Nutritional Support

Pancreatic cancer patients typically experience weight loss along with malnutrition because their tumors cause digestive enzyme deficiency and metabolic dysfunction. The support of proper nutrition includes prescribing pancreatic enzyme replacement therapy (PERT) combined with dietary adjustments for patients whose malnutrition requires either enteral or parenteral nourishment. The preservation of nutrition promotes strength maintenance while it builds tolerance to treatments as well as it improves general life quality.

4. Psychosocial Support

The diagnosis of pancreatic cancer produces emotional distress which affects both patients and their family members. Support organizations that offer counseling and support groups together with palliative care services function as crucial interventions to manage the anxiety and depression while helping patients cope. By providing complete caregiver resources patients gain both professional medical care together with strengthened emotional ability to handle their disease path.

The future of standard treatment for pancreatic cancer is poised for significant advancements, driven by innovations in early detection, personalized medicine, and novel therapeutic approaches. Despite the current low 5-year survival rate, ongoing research and clinical trials are paving the way for more effective interventions. The integration of molecular profiling, targeted therapies, and advanced surgical techniques are central to these developments, offering hope for improved patient outcomes. Below are key areas of focus for the future of pancreatic cancer treatment.

Future advancement of Standard Treatment for Pancreatic Cancer:

A contributing factor to high mortality is delayed diagnosis or detection of disease in advanced stage. Developing screening tools and biomarker can help tackle this issue effectively (Liu et al., 2022). Newer therapies like Targeted therapies and Immunotherapies are emerging with better safety and efficacy profile (Stec et al., 2024). Additionally, advancement in surgical technique has led to better resection rates. Surgical techniques such as laparoscopic and robotic assisted are minimally invasive although the benefits over chemotherapy is under investigation (Yang, 2023) In the ongoing clinical trials, therapeutic efficacy of irreversible electroporation (IRE) and other ablative therapies are under investigation. Also, the efficacy of Transarterial therapies is being evaluated for managing pancreatic cancer (Narayanan et al., 2020) Even though advancement in treatment options are being explored, there are various challenges which needs to be addressed like diagnostic techniques for early detection, adverse effects of chemotherapy, risk of complication post-surgical intervention. However, with continued research and clinical trials, attempts to improve treatment outcomes and quality of patients is underway.

CONCLUSION

Pancreatic cancer remains a formidable challenge in oncology, characterized by a dismal prognosis and limited treatment options. Despite significant advancements in our understanding of the disease and the development of novel therapeutic strategies, the limitations of current treatment modalities highlight the urgent need for continued research and innovation. A multidisciplinary approach, incorporating advanced imaging techniques, molecular profiling, personalized medicine, and innovative drug delivery systems, is crucial for improving patient outcomes. The integration of nanotechnology, advanced radiotherapy techniques, and novel immunotherapies offers exciting possibilities for overcoming the limitations of current treatments and improving the lives of patients with pancreatic cancer. The ultimate goal is to transform pancreatic cancer from a devastating and often incurable disease into a manageable and potentially curable condition. Continued investment in research, focused on identifying novel biomarkers, understanding the intricate mechanisms of chemoresistance and immune evasion, and developing more effective and personalized therapeutic approaches, is essential to achieving this goal.

REFERENCES

Abdelmohsin, O., Russell, T. B., Labib, P. L., & Aroori, S. (2024). SP4.3 - Pancreatoduodenectomy for malignancy with concomitant arterial resection: Results from the Recurrence After Whipple's (RAW) study. *British Journal of Surgery, 111*(Supplement_8), znae197.043. Advance online publication. DOI: 10.1093/bjs/znae197.043

Afghani, E., & Klein, A. P. (2022). Pancreatic Adenocarcinoma. *Hematology/Oncology Clinics of North America, 36*(5), 879–895. DOI: 10.1016/j.hoc.2022.07.002 PMID: 36154788

Aftab Alam, M., & Dhoundiyal, S. (2023). Overcoming the Limitations of Therapeutic Strategies to Combat Pancreatic Cancer Using Nanotechnology. *Current Cancer Drug Targets, 23*(9), 697–717. Advance online publication. DOI: 10.2174/1568009623666230329085618 PMID: 36999420

Alonso, I. J., Quinto, A. M., Maestro, O. C., Murillo, L. A., Conde, P. R., Fernández, C. F., & Romero, C. J. (2024). Duodenopancreatectomía cefálica tipo Whipple versus duodenopancreatectomía con preservación pilórica. Estudio retrospectivo. *Cirugía Española, 102*(5), 265–274. DOI: 10.1016/j.ciresp.2024.02.005 PMID: 38493929

Bannone, E., Romandini, E., Kleive, D., Marchegiani, G., Gilg, S., Sahakyan, M. A., Ghorbani, P., Perri, G., Sparrelid, E., Labori, K. J., & Salvia, R. (2023). Postpancreatectomy Acute Pancreatitis (PPAP) after Distal Pancreatectomy: A Tri-institutional International Cohort Study. *HPB : The Official Journal of the International Hepato Pancreato Biliary Association, 25*, S230–S231. DOI: 10.1016/j.hpb.2023.07.079

Bazeed, A. Y., Day, C. M., & Garg, S. (2022). Pancreatic Cancer: Challenges and Opportunities in Locoregional Therapies. *Cancers (Basel), 14*(17), 4257. DOI: 10.3390/cancers14174257 PMID: 36077794

Biagi, J. J., Cosby, R., Bahl, M., Elfiki, T., Goodwin, R., Hallet, J., Hirmiz, K., & Mahmud, A. (2023). Adjuvant Chemotherapy and Radiotherapy in Resected Pancreatic Ductal Adenocarcinoma: A Systematic Review and Clinical Practice Guideline. *Current Oncology (Toronto, Ont.), 30*(7), 6575–6586. DOI: 10.3390/curroncol30070482 PMID: 37504342

Blanquicett, J, C., & E. Aguirre, L. (. (2021). Therapeutic Advances for Pancreatic Cancer: A Slow and Challenging Feat that Continues to Evolve. *Acta Scientific Gastrointestinal Disorders, 4*(7), 50–52. DOI: 10.31080/ASGIS.2021.04.0268 PMID: 34414366

Boone, B. A. (2024). Employing Advanced Technology to Reduce Postoperative Pancreatic Fistula. *Annals of Surgery Open : Perspectives of Surgical History, Education, and Clinical Approaches*, *5*(1), e373–e373. DOI: 10.1097/AS9.0000000000000373 PMID: 38883937

Bryant, J. M., Nakashima, J., Khatri, V. M., Sinnamon, A. J., Denbo, J. W., Hodul, P., Malafa, M., Hoffe, S., & Frakes, J. M. (2024). The Evolving Role of Neoadjuvant Radiation Therapy in Pancreatic Adenocarcinoma. *Journal of Clinical Medicine*, *13*(22), 6800–6800. DOI: 10.3390/jcm13226800 PMID: 39597944

Cecchini, M., Salem, R. R., Robert, M., Czerniak, S., Blaha, O., Zelterman, D., Rajaei, M., Townsend, J. P., Cai, G., Chowdhury, S., Yugawa, D., Tseng, R., Mejia Arbelaez, C., Jiao, J., Shroyer, K., Thumar, J., Kortmansky, J., Zaheer, W., Fischbach, N., & Lacy, J. (2024). Perioperative Modified FOLFIRINOX for Resectable Pancreatic Cancer: A Nonrandomized Controlled Trial. *JAMA Oncology*, *10*(8), 1027. Advance online publication. DOI: 10.1001/jamaoncol.2024.1575 PMID: 38900452

Chakrabarti, S., Kamgar, M., & Mahipal, A. (2022). Systemic Therapy of Metastatic Pancreatic Adenocarcinoma: Current Status, Challenges, and Opportunities. *Cancers (Basel)*, *14*(11), 2588. DOI: 10.3390/cancers14112588 PMID: 35681565

Chen, Z., & Lin, Y. (2023). A commentary on "Minimally invasive versus open total pancreatectomy: A systematic review and meta-analysis.". *International Journal of Surgery*, *110*(1), 600–601. DOI: 10.1097/JS9.0000000000000770 PMID: 37738018

Chi, J., Chung, S. Y., Parakrama, R., Fayyaz, F., Jose, J., & Saif, M. W. (2021). The role of PARP inhibitors in BRCA mutated pancreatic cancer. *Therapeutic Advances in Gastroenterology*, *14*, 175628482110148. DOI: 10.1177/17562848211014818 PMID: 34025781

Conroy, T., Bachet, J.-B., Ayav, A., Huguet, F., Lambert, A., Caramella, C., Maréchal, R., Van Laethem, J.-L., & Ducreux, M. (2016). Current standards and new innovative approaches for treatment of pancreatic cancer. *European Journal of Cancer*, *57*, 10–22. DOI: 10.1016/j.ejca.2015.12.026 PMID: 26851397

Conroy, T., Pfeiffer, P., Vilgrain, V., Lamarca, A., Seufferlein, T., O'Reilly, E. M., Hackert, T., Golan, T., Prager, G., Haustermans, K., Vogel, A., & Ducreux, M. (2023). Pancreatic cancer: ESMO Clinical Practice Guideline for diagnosis, treatment and follow-up†. *Annals of Oncology : Official Journal of the European Society for Medical Oncology*, *34*(11), 987–1002. Advance online publication. DOI: 10.1016/j.annonc.2023.08.009 PMID: 37678671

Crippa, S., Piccioli, A., Guarneri, G., Longo, E., & Falconi, M. (2017). Pancreatic ductal adenocarcinoma in 2017: Time to change the therapeutic algorithm? *Endoscopic Ultrasound*, *6*(9), S62–S65. DOI: 10.4103/eus.eus_61_17 PMID: 29387691

Czaplicka, A., Lachota, M., Pączek, L., Zagożdżon, R., & Kaleta, B. (2024). Chimeric Antigen Receptor T Cell Therapy for Pancreatic Cancer: A Review of Current Evidence. *Cells*, *13*(1), 101. DOI: 10.3390/cells13010101 PMID: 38201305

Dhamija, K., Awuah, K.-F. B., Marwaha, A., Kharoud, H., & Monga, D. K. (2025). Neoadjuvant therapy in borderline resectable and resectable pancreatic cancer. *Journal of Clinical Oncology*, *43*(4, suppl), 735–735. DOI: 10.1200/JCO.2025.43.4_suppl.735

Ettrich, T. J., & Seufferlein, T. (2021). Systemic Therapy for Metastatic Pancreatic Cancer. *Current Treatment Options in Oncology*, *22*(11), 106. Advance online publication. DOI: 10.1007/s11864-021-00895-4 PMID: 34665339

Foley, K., Kim, V., Jaffee, E., & Zheng, L. (2016). Current progress in immunotherapy for pancreatic cancer. *Cancer Letters*, *381*(1), 244–251. DOI: 10.1016/j.canlet.2015.12.020 PMID: 26723878

Garcia-Sampedro, A., Gaggia, G., Ney, A., Mahamed, I., & Acedo, P. (2021). The State-of-the-Art of Phase II/III Clinical Trials for Targeted Pancreatic Cancer Therapies. *Journal of Clinical Medicine*, *10*(4), 566–566. DOI: 10.3390/jcm10040566 PMID: 33546207

Gresham, G. K., Wells, G. A., Gill, S., Cameron, C., & Jonker, D. J. (2014). Chemotherapy regimens for advanced pancreatic cancer: A systematic review and network meta-analysis. *BMC Cancer*, *14*(1), 471. Advance online publication. DOI: 10.1186/1471-2407-14-471 PMID: 24972449

Hosein, A. N., Brekken, R. A., & Maitra, A. (2020). Pancreatic cancer stroma: An update on therapeutic targeting strategies. *Nature Reviews. Gastroenterology & Hepatology*, *17*(8), 487–505. DOI: 10.1038/s41575-020-0300-1 PMID: 32393771

Hu, J.-X., Zhao, C.-F., Chen, W.-B., Liu, Q.-C., Li, Q.-W., Lin, Y.-Y., & Gao, F. (2021). Pancreatic cancer: A review of epidemiology, trend, and risk factors. *World Journal of Gastroenterology*, *27*(27), 4298–4321. DOI: 10.3748/wjg.v27.i27.4298 PMID: 34366606

Ilic, I., & Ilic, M. (2022). International patterns in incidence and mortality trends of pancreatic cancer in the last three decades: A joinpoint regression analysis. *World Journal of Gastroenterology*, *28*(32), 4698–4715. DOI: 10.3748/wjg.v28.i32.4698 PMID: 36157927

Jabłońska, B., Pawlicki, K., & Mrowiec, S. (2021). Associations between Nutritional and Immune Status and Clinicopathologic Factors in Patients with Pancreatic Cancer: A Comprehensive Analysis. *Cancers (Basel)*, *13*(20), 5041. DOI: 10.3390/cancers13205041 PMID: 34680194

Jiang, H., Liu, X., Knolhoff, B. L., Hegde, S., Lee, K. B., Jiang, H., Fields, R. C., Pachter, J. A., Lim, K.-H., & DeNardo, D. G. (2019). Development of resistance to FAK inhibition in pancreatic cancer is linked to stromal depletion. *Gut*, *69*(1), 122–132. DOI: 10.1136/gutjnl-2018-317424 PMID: 31076405

Johansson, H., Andersson, R., Bauden, M., Hammes, S., Holdenrieder, S., & Ansari, D. (2016). Immune checkpoint therapy for pancreatic cancer. *World Journal of Gastroenterology*, *22*(43), 9457. DOI: 10.3748/wjg.v22.i43.9457 PMID: 27920468

Kitago, M., Endo, Y., Aiura, K., Takigawa, Y., Tani, N., Matsui, J., Suzuki, K., Nishiyama, R., Nakano, Y., Abe, Y., Yagi, H., Shinoda, M., Itano, O., Tanabe, M., & Kitagawa, Y. (2024). Adjuvant 5-fluorouracil and portal vein infusion chemotherapy followed by gemcitabine for pancreatic cancer. *Cancer Medicine*, *13*(14), e7459. Advance online publication. DOI: 10.1002/cam4.7459 PMID: 39030993

Klein, A. P. (2021). Pancreatic cancer epidemiology: Understanding the role of lifestyle and inherited risk factors. *Nature Reviews. Gastroenterology & Hepatology*, *18*(7), 493–502. DOI: 10.1038/s41575-021-00457-x PMID: 34002083

Kolbeinsson, H. M., Chandana, S., Wright, G. P., & Chung, M. (2022). Pancreatic Cancer: A Review of Current Treatment and Novel Therapies. *Journal of Investigative Surgery*, *36*(1), 1–11. DOI: 10.1080/08941939.2022.2129884 PMID: 36191926

Leroux, C., & Konstantinidou, G. (2021). Targeted Therapies for Pancreatic Cancer: Overview of Current Treatments and New Opportunities for Personalized Oncology. *Cancers (Basel)*, *13*(4), 799. DOI: 10.3390/cancers13040799 PMID: 33672917

Lewis, B., Guta, A., Shin, J., Ji, Z., Kim, J. S., & Kim, T. (2023). Evaluating motion of pancreatic tumors and anatomical surrogates using cine MRI in 0.35T MRgRT under free breathing conditions. *Journal of Applied Clinical Medical Physics*, *24*(6), e13930. Advance online publication. DOI: 10.1002/acm2.13930 PMID: 37073428

Li, X., Zhou, E., Dong, X., Zhao, C., Han, Y., Cui, B., & Lin, X. (2023). Adjuvant chemotherapy in pancreatic cancer at different AJCC stages: A propensity score matching analysis. *European Journal of Medical Research*, *28*(1), 606. Advance online publication. DOI: 10.1186/s40001-023-01572-y PMID: 38115156

Lideståhl, A., Permert, J., Linder, S., Bylund, H., Edsborg, N., & Lind, P. (2006). Efficacy of systemic therapy in advanced pancreatic carcinoma. *Acta Oncologica, 45*(2), 136–143. DOI: 10.1080/02841860500537861 PMID: 16546858

Liu, L., Wang, W. Q., & Lou, W. H. (2022). [Ten directions for improving clinical therapeutic effect of pancreatic cancer in the future]. *PubMed, 60*(1), 10–16. DOI: 10.3760/cma.j.cn112139-20211109-00525 PMID: 34954940

Long, J., Zhang, Y., Yu, X., Yang, J., LeBrun, D. G., Chen, C., Yao, Q., & Li, M. (2011). Overcoming drug resistance in pancreatic cancer. *Expert Opinion on Therapeutic Targets, 15*(7), 817–828. DOI: 10.1517/14728222.2011.566216 PMID: 21391891

Luo, J. (2021). KRAS mutation in pancreatic cancer. *Seminars in Oncology, 48*(1), 10–18. DOI: 10.1053/j.seminoncol.2021.02.003 PMID: 33676749

Mann, K., Jones, R. P., Ghaneh, P., & Neoptolemos, J. P. (2023). Adjuvant Chemotherapy in Pancreatic Cancer. In *Pancreas* (pp. 1143–1152). Lippincott Williams & Wilkins., DOI: 10.1002/9781119876007.ch148

Moussa, A. S. A., Hafez, A. H. A., Aziz, A. A. R. A., & Rayan, M. T. (2024). Open distal pancreatectomy stump closure by linear stapling versus continuous suturing: A retrospective–prospective comparative study. *The Egyptian Journal of Surgery, 43*(2), 413–420. DOI: 10.4103/ejs.ejs_298_23

Muratović, B., & Nikolić, A. (2023). Epidemiology of pancreatic cancer. *Zdravstvena Zastita, 52*(4), 36–49. DOI: 10.5937/zdravzast52-47366

Narayanan, G., Ucar, A., Gandhi, R. T., Nasiri, A., Inampudi, P., Wilson, N. M., & Asbun, H. J. (2020). Emerging Ablative and Transarterial Therapies for Pancreatic Cancer. *Digestive Disease Interventions, 04*(04), 389–394. DOI: 10.1055/s-0040-1721415

Neesse, A., Algül, H., Tuveson, D. A., & Gress, T. M. (2015). Stromal biology and therapy in pancreatic cancer: A changing paradigm. *Gut, 64*(9), 1476–1484. DOI: 10.1136/gutjnl-2015-309304 PMID: 25994217

Němeček, R., & Eid, M. (2024). The role of neoadjuvant treatment in localized pancreatic cancer. *Rozhledy v Chirurgii, 103*(11), 429–436. DOI: 10.48095/ccrvch2024429 PMID: 39645401

Nichetti, F., Rota, S., Ambrosini, P., Pircher, C., Gusmaroli, E., Droz Dit Busset, M., Pusceddu, S., Sposito, C., Coppa, J., Morano, F., Pietrantonio, F., Di Bartolomeo, M., Mariani, L., Mazzaferro, V., de Braud, F., & Niger, M. (2024). NALIRIFOX, FOLFIRINOX, and Gemcitabine With Nab-Paclitaxel as First-Line Chemotherapy for Metastatic Pancreatic Cancer: A Systematic Review and Meta-Analysis. *JAMA Network Open*, *7*(1), e2350756. DOI: 10.1001/jamanetworkopen.2023.50756 PMID: 38190183

Onishi, H. (2014). Hedgehog signaling pathway as a new therapeutic target in pancreatic cancer. *World Journal of Gastroenterology*, *20*(9), 2335. DOI: 10.3748/wjg.v20.i9.2335 PMID: 24605030

Paisey, S. A., & Bateman, A. R. (2024). Neoadjuvant chemoradiotherapy for pancreatic cancer. *CRC Press EBooks*, 71–82. DOI: 10.1201/9781003579755-9

Palumbo, M. O., Kavan, P., Miller, W. H., Panasci, L., Assouline, S., Johnson, N., Cohen, V., Patenaude, F., Pollak, M., Jagoe, R. T., & Batist, G. (2013). Systemic cancer therapy: Achievements and challenges that lie ahead. *Frontiers in Pharmacology*, *4*. Advance online publication. DOI: 10.3389/fphar.2013.00057 PMID: 23675348

Ravikumar, R., Sabin, C., Hilal, M. A., Bramhall, S., White, S., Wigmore, S., Imber, C. J., & Fusai, G. (2014). Portal Vein Resection in Borderline Resectable Pancreatic Cancer: A United Kingdom Multicenter Study. *Journal of the American College of Surgeons*, *218*(3), 401–411. DOI: 10.1016/j.jamcollsurg.2013.11.017 PMID: 24484730

Robatel, S., & Schenk, M. (2022). Current Limitations and Novel Perspectives in Pancreatic Cancer Treatment. *Cancers (Basel)*, *14*(4), 985. DOI: 10.3390/cancers14040985 PMID: 35205732

Salman, B., Zhou, D., Jaffee, E. M., Edil, B. H., & Zheng, L. (2013). Vaccine therapy for pancreatic cancer. *OncoImmunology*, *2*(12), e26662. DOI: 10.4161/onci.26662 PMID: 24498551

Seicean, A. (2015). New targeted therapies in pancreatic cancer. *World Journal of Gastroenterology*, *21*(20), 6127. DOI: 10.3748/wjg.v21.i20.6127 PMID: 26034349

Stec, W. M., Kudas, Z., Górka, M., Wojtkiewicz, A., Piekarska, M., & Szerej, K. (2024). Advancements in Pancreatic Cancer Treatment: A Comprehensive Review of Current Therapies and Future Directions. *Quality in Sport*, *27*, 54941. DOI: 10.12775/QS.2024.27.54941

Suker, M., Beumer, B. R., Sadot, E., Marthey, L., Faris, J. E., Mellon, E. A., El-Rayes, B. F., Wang-Gillam, A., Lacy, J., Hosein, P. J., Moorcraft, S. Y., Conroy, T., Hohla, F., Allen, P., Taieb, J., Hong, T. S., Shridhar, R., Chau, I., van Eijck, C. H., & Koerkamp, B. G. (2016). FOLFIRINOX for locally advanced pancreatic cancer: A systematic review and patient-level meta-analysis. *The Lancet. Oncology*, *17*(6), 801–810. DOI: 10.1016/S1470-2045(16)00172-8 PMID: 27160474

Symeonidis, D., Zacharoulis, D., Kissa, L., Samara, A. A., Petsa, E., & Tepetes, K. (2023). From Classic Whipple to Pylorus Preserving Pancreaticoduodenectomy and Ultimately to Pylorus Resecting - Stomach Preserving Pancreaticoduodenectomy. *Revue de Chirurgie*, *118*(4), 335. DOI: 10.21614/chirurgia.2023.v.118.i.4.p.335 PMID: 37697996

Wainberg, Z. A., Hochster, H. S., Kim, E. J., George, B., Kaylan, A., Chiorean, E. G., Waterhouse, D. M., Guiterrez, M., Parikh, A., Jain, R., Carrizosa, D. R., Soliman, H. H., Lila, T., Reiss, D. J., Pierce, D. W., Bhore, R., Banerjee, S., Lyons, L., Louis, C. U., & O'Dwyer, P. J. (2020). Open-label, Phase I Study of Nivolumab Combined with *nab*-Paclitaxel Plus Gemcitabine in Advanced Pancreatic Cancer. *Clinical Cancer Research*, *26*(18), 4814–4822. DOI: 10.1158/1078-0432.CCR-20-0099 PMID: 32554514

Walsh, N., Kennedy, S., Larkin, A., Corkery, B., O'Driscoll, L., Clynes, M., Crown, J., & O'Donovan, N. (2012). EGFR and HER2 inhibition in pancreatic cancer. *Investigational New Drugs*, *31*(3), 558–566. DOI: 10.1007/s10637-012-9891-x PMID: 23076814

Xiang, X., Chen, X., He, Y., Wang, Y., Xia, W., Ye, S., Wang, S., Xiao, Y., Li, Q., Wang, X., Luo, W., & Li, J. (2023). Pancreatic cancer challenge in 52 Asian countries: Age-centric insights and the role of modifiable risk factors (1990-2019). *Frontiers in Oncology*, *13*, 1271370. Advance online publication. DOI: 10.3389/fonc.2023.1271370 PMID: 37849795

Yang, Y. M. (2023). [Current surgical concepts and future perspectives in the treatment of pancreatic cancer]. *PubMed*, *61*(1), 1–6. DOI: 10.3760/cma.j.cn112139-20221021-00453 PMID: 36603876

Zeitouni, D., Pylayeva-Gupta, Y., Der, C., & Bryant, K. (2016). KRAS Mutant Pancreatic Cancer: No Lone Path to an Effective Treatment. *Cancers (Basel)*, *8*(4), 45. DOI: 10.3390/cancers8040045 PMID: 27096871

Zheng, R., Liu, X., Zhang, Y., Liu, Y., Wang, Y., Guo, S., Jin, X., Zhang, J., Guan, Y., & Liu, Y. (2024). Frontiers and future of immunotherapy for pancreatic cancer: From molecular mechanisms to clinical application. *Frontiers in Immunology*, *15*, 1383978. Advance online publication. DOI: 10.3389/fimmu.2024.1383978 PMID: 38756774

Zhu, H., Wei, M., Xu, J., Hua, J., Liang, C., Meng, Q., Zhang, Y., Liu, J., Zhang, B., Yu, X., & Shi, S. (2020). PARP inhibitors in pancreatic cancer: Molecular mechanisms and clinical applications. *Molecular Cancer*, *19*(1), 49. Advance online publication. DOI: 10.1186/s12943-020-01167-9 PMID: 32122376

Chapter 7
Combination Therapies Against Pancreatic Cancer for Enhancing Treatment Effectiveness

N. Usha
Department of Microbiology, Sacred Heart College, Tirupattur, India

K. Gayathri
https://orcid.org/0009-0007-3786-2009
Department of Microbiology, Sacred Heart College, Tirupattur, India

B. Lokeshwari
https://orcid.org/0009-0005-6612-5134
Department of Microbiology, Sacred Heart College, Tirupattur, India

L. Yuvalakshmi
https://orcid.org/0009-0005-4579-1170
Department of Microbiology, Sacred Heart College, Tirupattur, India

ABSTRACT

Pancreatic Cancer (PC) remains one of the deadliest cancers with an extremely high mortality rate, and the number of cases is expected to steadily increase with time. There have been ongoing efforts to employ novel approaches to combat PC in order to improve treatment efficacy and mitigate cytotoxicity. A potential remedy for treatment difficulties, the combination cancer-targeting and gene-silencing strategy has demonstrated better results in terms of patient survival rates and quality of life. It specifically addresses a number of barriers to reduce tumor metastasis and recurrence and to ease delivery issues. Even while siRNA, a kind of a single strand

DOI: 10.4018/979-8-3373-1469-3.ch007

nucleic acid with excellent binding capacity and specificity that targets molecules, has emerged as a promising PC tactic in recent years, it can disrupt the expression of several genes. Molecular targeted therapy, photothermal treatment combined with gene therapy and immunotherapy for pancreatic cancer. Immunotherapies, which include CD40 against CCR2 inhibitors, macrophage-targeted medicines, and cytotoxicity are examples of new and developing treatments for pancreatic cancer. treatments that target T lymphocytes. Despite numerous challenges, efforts to understand the variety of pancreatic tumors are progressing. The secret to effectively treating this fatal illness will be combining immunological and conventional targeting. However, recent developments have led to improved outcomes and have changed practice in the past decade and future perspectives. This paper summarises combination therapies and enhancing the treatment effectiveness against pancreatic cancer that brought us to where we are today, along with emerging therapies.

1. INTRODUCTION

The equivalent of 8.2 million people worldwide passed away from malignant neoplasms each year, and estimates suggest that number will rise to 12 million by 2030. With a 5-year-end life expectancy rate of less than 9%, pancreatic cancer (PC) was identified as one of the most malignant and deadly oncologic pathologies among these cancers (Rawla et al., 2019).The global prevalence of pancreatic cancer was 1–10 cases per 100,000 people worldwide, and it was significantly more common in men living in industrialised areas (Ryan et al., 2014).Numerous risk factors that can be changed or eliminated in epidemiological studies, such as germline alterations (e.g., in the genes for BRCA1, BRCA2, or CDKN2A), obesity, type 2 diabetes, tobacco use, prolonged pancreatitis, and a hypercaloric diet that includes an excessive amount of dietary fats and refined carbohydrates. With this typical late-stage diagnosis, which restricted the availability and effectiveness of curative treatment options, PC was thought to have a severe clinical prognosis (Wolfgang et al., 2013).

The asymptomatic progression of pancreatic cancer in its early stages made treatment very difficult. Early and reliable diagnosis is made more difficult by the fact that individuals with early-stage PC usually present with ambiguous or non-specific clinical symptoms, such as minor gastrointestinal issues or exhaustion. Gastrointestinal symptoms, such as dyspepsia (also known as burning sensations), feeling sick, emesis (nausea), cachexia (voluntarily acquired weight loss linked to metabolic failure), and epigastric or upper abdomen pain, were frequently observed in advanced stages of pancreatic cancer. The main causes of PC's poor prognosis were its high potential for metastasis and quick systemic dispersion, which sped up the course of the disease and made the majority of systemic treatment plans essentially useless (Fatima et al., 2022).

Radiation therapy, responsible for cytotoxic treatment with chemotherapy, and surgical removal were the standard treatment strategies for PC. The main surgical strategy was pancreatic oduodenectomy, sometimes known as the "Whipple procedure". Effectiveness of various therapeutic approaches was limited, especially for patients with metastatic or locally advanced illness. This stromal architecture exacerbated disease resistance to traditional therapies by acting as a major barrier to therapeutic administration and response (Du et al., 2018).

The conventional therapeutic approaches have not significantly raised long-term survival rates in recent decades. Only 15% to 25% of patients even undergoing surgery showed positive clinical outcomes, highlighting the urgent need for innovative treatment approaches. In order to improve therapy specificity and patient outcomes, emerging therapeutic treatments placed a strong emphasis on targeting tumour metabolism, oncogenic signalling pathways, and the tumour microenvironment. Targeted molecular therapies are among the cutting-edge treatment approaches, and they have shown significant effectiveness recently (Du et al., 2018).

Targeted therapies, specific to traditional chemotherapeutic medicines, target certain patient subgroups according to the genomic and phenotypic features of their cancers. Using Small Interfering RNA (siRNA), which is made up of 19–23 base-paired double-stranded RNA molecules, is one potential strategy. By using the RNA interference mechanism, siRNA can selectively suppress the expression of particular genes. The large molecular size, strong hydrophilia, and negative-charged surface of this substance, which limit its membrane permeability, siRNA has poor cellular internalisation, which has hampered its clinical applicability. The siRNA is quickly removed from the bloodstream and is extremely vulnerable to enzymatic breakdown in serum (Singh et al., 2022).

Combinatory regimens are frequently used in cancer treatment to reduce systemic toxicity. Injected chemotherapeutic drugs with cell-destination compounds like aptamers and siRNA is a particularly promising approach. Aptamers are oligonucleotides made of single-strand RNA or DNA that are 25 to 60 nucleotides long. They can attach to molecular targets, including tumor markers or receptors on the cell surface that are too many on malignant cells, with a high level of specificity and affinity for three-dimensional shapes. Treatments utilizing siRNA and aptamers, along with metabolomic technologies, have emerged as efficient tools for enhancing the understanding of Cancer Cell Biology (Yin et al., 2015).

Finding the small-molecule metabolites produced by metabolic processes in tumor cells was the aim of metabolomics. One of these new ideas, spatial metabolomics, was able to pinpoint the exact chemical attributes and locations of chemicals in tissue samples. By defining defensive chemicals, the metabolic the phenotype and biochemical processes, spatial metabolomics provided comprehensive high-resolution imaging analysis of the metabolic framework of cancerous tissues in contrast to normal epithelial cells (Yin et al., 2015).

Conventional bulk measurement techniques, which consolidated cellular responses from entire tissue samples, frequently overlooked the intrinsic heterogeneity and functional variability present within specific tissue compartments. Nevertheless, spatial metabolomic approaches circumvented these constraints by providing a more localized understanding of tissue-specific metabolism. These findings demonstrated that neoplastic cells exhibited unique metabolic reprogramming, encompassing alterations that promoted advancement, dissemination, and cellular survival. The advancement of equipment has enabled researchers to identify and measure metabolic activities linked to the metastatic cascade. The use of physical metabolomics to find biomarkers linked to cancer development and tumor growth is becoming more common. In the study of biological tissues and vital organs, the combination of spatial detail and metabolism analysis using matrix-assisted laser treatment desorption-ionization mass-spectrum imaging (MALDI-MSI) proved to be highly effective. A notable work integrated MALDI-MSI with high-quality spatial metabolomics, utilizing Multi-Cellular Tumor Spheroids (MCTS) in an animal in vitro model (Wolfgang et al., 2013).

This method effectively uncovered working chemical fingerprints of cancer cells, including increased oxidation of fatty acids, heightened phosphate-dependent adrenergic metabolic processes, and the de novo synthesis of phosphodiesterase. These fingerprints were important for the tumor to grow and stay alive. These metabolomic methods make it easier to find cells that are cancerous by showing higher amounts of important enzymes that control metabolism. It was specifically demonstrated that several enzymes, including the enzyme fatty acid synthase (FASN), choline kinase alpha (CHKA), cytoplasmic phospholipase A2 (cPLA2), and a substance identified as miR-181a-5p-glutaminase (GLS), were significantly upregulated in malignant tissues. After surgically removing tumors from patients with pancreatic carcinoma (PC), normal pancreatic tissues were examined for metabolic markers associated with tumor cell proliferation and metastasis. Additionally, it was demonstrated that metabolomic insights improved therapeutic outcomes when integrated with siRNA/aptamer-based treatment and chemotherapy. This combination technique made cancer cells more adaptable to chemotherapy and helped the two treatments work better together (Spring et al., 2016).

People are interested in new combinatorial medicines, notably those that involve aptamers, siRNA, and metabolomic technologies. These strategies aimed to enhance patient outcomes, augment pharmacological selectivity, and surmount therapeutic resistance. Even though there has been a lot of development, there are still problems with improving delivery techniques, dealing with resistance pathways, and better integrating metabolism into clinical procedures for customized treatment and finding biomarkers (Soo et al., 2012).

2. SIRNA MEDIATED CHEMOTHERAPY

When diagnosed with pancreatic cancer (PC), the majority of patients are in a very advanced stage of the disease and frequently have metastases. After diagnosis, their chances of survival are not good. PC is a highly lethal and deadly cancer that happens very seldom but kills a lot of people. The disease's early asymptomatic progression, which hindered timely diagnosis and led to a severe presentation, was the primary factor contributing to this unfavorable prognosis. Even with major improvements in treatment modalities, PC's natural resistance to chemotherapy and its capacity to expand to other body sections were still the main reasons for low survival rates, with a typical survival time of a year or fewer. Late-stage diagnosis worsened these conditions, rendering therapeutic interventions such surgical resection infeasible (Collins & Wertman, 2006). PC continued to be a significant barrier to treatment. Chemotherapy, radiation therapy, and tumor excision surgery were typical elements of routine treatment protocols (Hanaf-Bojd et al., 2016). Only those with a limited illness suitable for surgical intervention may get the sole potentially curative treatment, which involved an operation for excision of the tumor that was cancerous. The TNM categorization system was used for directing medical therapy for prostate cancer, which was mostly based on the disease stage upon diagnosis. It assessed tumor size (T), involvement of lymph nodes in the region (N), and the possibility of metastasis dissemination (M). This staging method gave us important information for making treatment strategies and figuring out what the future holds (Butt et al., 2016). Adjuvant chemotherapy, radiation treatment, and surgical resection were often utilized to treat individuals with sickness in its early stages. Chemotherapy was the major treatment for advanced-stage PC. It was largely used to control symptoms and help people live longer. The average survival time for gemcitabine, which and other standard chemotherapy treatments was just four to nine months, which was not good. These disadvantages underscored the urgent necessity for innovative therapeutic strategies to combat the malignant biological conduct and chemotherapy-resistant characteristics of pancreatic cancer (Khder et al., 2016).

Among the most popular therapies for pancreatic cancer were chemotherapy combination regimens, such as modified chemotherapy and nab-paclitaxel. However, these treatments' high levels of toxicity frequently made clinical administration challenging. The resistant mechanism that pancreatic cancer cells exhibit has come to light due to the limited capacity of conventional treatments to significantly improve survival. For example, gemcitabine, an EGFR (epithelial growth factor receptor) blocker, showed some beneficial properties but did not produce curative effects (Ahmed et al., 2022). Drug resistance is a chronic problem, necessitating continued research into new treatment modalities such immunological and chemotherapy combinations, molecule-by- targeted medications, and biological substance therapies. Antitumor effects may be enhanced by these treatments by tackling the molecular reasons of resistance. In an effort to enhance patient outcomes, a number of research assessed the effectiveness of combining the medication gemcitabine with biologic treatments such aptamers as & tiny messenger RNA (siRNA), cytotoxic medicines, or molecularly targeted therapy. The clinical importance of the data was limited, despite meta-analyses showing moderate survival advantages when aptamers or siRNA were introduced into therapies for chronic pancreatic cancer are based on gemcitabine. The significance of alternate and more efficient treatment methods is demonstrated by the fact that other chemotherapy drugs, such as the combination of cape & S-1 (5-fluorouracil derivatives), just slightly improved therapeutic outcomes (Geier et al., 2020).

The 5-fluorouracil, leucovorin, irinotecan, & oxaliplatin chemotherapy treatment outperformed gemcitabine monotherapy in clinical studies, particularly in those who could tolerate the toxicities. A severe toxicity profile limited its use to physically healthy patients, disqualifying old or fragile patients from treatment eligibility despite its strong survival advantages (Zhang et al., 2021). A promising substitute is intra-arterial chemotherapy, which minimises systemic damage while delivering greater quantities of chemotherapeutic drugs directly to the tumour. However, procedural and logistical constraints limited its broad clinical usefulness. Worldwide survival rates for cancer of the pancreas have remained relatively unchanged over the past ten years despite the accessibility of numerous therapeutic approaches, which points to the urgent need for new and improved treatments that can address the aggressive and chemoresistant nature of the disease (Wang et al., 2021).

Treatment for pancreatic cancer that has spread may be significantly improved by recent developments in molecularly targeted therapeutics, such as small interfering RNA (siRNA) and aptamers, along with nanocarrier-based systems. In an effort to make treatment plans more effective and raise overall survival rates, these therapies concentrated on particular biochemical pathways or enhanced the delivery of chemotherapy medications to cancerous cells. But the problem of increased toxicity persisted, especially when these methods were used in conjunction with traditional chemotherapeutic medicines, underscoring the necessity of striking an equilibrium between patient safety and therapeutic efficacy (Robatel & Schenk, 2022).

Combining developments in molecular science, immunotherapy, which stands for drug delivery technologies, with combination therapies that target several aspects of tumour biology has become a viable approach to enhance pancreatic cancer clinical treatment. To overcome the enormous obstacles that came with such an aggressive and extremely deadly cancer, the care of pancreatic cancer in the future required a diverse and integrated strategy that made use of cutting-edge technologies to develop safer and more effective therapeutic approaches (Jain et al., 2017).

3. PHOTO THERMAL THERAPY

Nanotechnology-based photothermal therapy (PTT) presented encouraging solutions for the treatment of pancreatic cancer. The different ways that photothermal therapy and other therapies for pancreatic cancer can be combined (Plana et al., 2022). A new approach to treating pancreatic cancer was made possible by photothermal therapy, which, when paired with other treatments like irradiation, not only reduced the tumours' susceptibility to radiation but also raised their oxygen content and controlled the tumour microenvironment. Polymer nano-radiopharmaceutical photothermal effects counteracted the Epithelial-Mesenchymal Transition (EMT), inhibited tumour stem cell growth, and decreased the adverse effects of radiopharmaceutical medications (Mishra et al., 2014). A photothermal-based nanoparticle consisting of anti-urokinase plasminogen stimulating activating receptors (uPAR), polyethylene glycol (PEG), and indocyanine green-modified golden tiny capsules enhanced the median survival rate of complete ablation by 25% in a single intervention when paired with Iodine-125 (^{125}I) Interstitial a fluid Brachytherapy (IBT-^{125}I). Nano-enzymes with photothermal characteristics caused localised thermal reactions, reduced glutathione (GSH) and eventually caused tumour cells to undergo apoptosis and ferroptosis when exposed to laser radiation (Amjad et al., 2015).Within the tumour microenvironment, the laser enhanced the catalytic potential and photothermal effect of nano-enzymes. In an acidic Tumour Microenvironment (TME), a new double-enzyme-like active nanoenzyme showed efficacious pancreatic tumour cell death, eradicated tumour cells, and Photo Dynamic Treatment (PDT) created reactive oxygen species, transformed energy from photons into particles of oxygen, and created oxidative stress responses using photosensitisers. A Comprehensive Nuclear-Test-Ban Treaty photosensitising drug with aggregation-induced emission properties was created to address the problems of hypoxic and heat shock protein impediment in pancreatic tumour phototherapy (Lin et al., 2013).An amphiphilic polymer combined with an epidermal growth factor receptor (EGFR)-targeted polypeptide was used to create this drug, which greatly reduced tumour growth and successfully visualised pancreatic cancer. Photodynamic treatment and photothermal therapy, guided by confocal laser endoscopy, were used to treat PDAC, also known as pancreatic ductal a utilizing a novel platform based on gold nanoclusters (Kolemen et al., 2016). Table 1 shows how pancreatic cancer can be treated with a combination of chemotherapy and photothermal therapy drugs.

Table 1. Integration of Photothermal Therapy with Chemotherapy Drugs for Pancreatic Cancer

Therapeutic Regimen	Reagents for Photo thermal Therapeutic Applications	Type of Pancreatic Cancer	Combined Benefits	References
Camptothecin	Indocyanine Green	PC	Killed tumor cells	Neoptolemos et al.(2004)
Abraxane	Indocyanine green	PDAC	Reduced the number of CAFs	Xie et al.(2020)
Bortezomib +Cyclosporine	IR-820	PC	Induced tumor cell apoptosis	Evans et al.(2008)
Paclitaxel	Poly dopamine	PC	Induced tumor cell apoptosis	Ferrone et al.(2015)
Gemcitabine +Bortezomib	PEGylated thermo sensitive lipids	PC	Improved the internalization of cancer cells	Xu et al.(2022)
Gemcitabine +IGF1	Black TiO_2 Nanoparticles (808 nm near infrared irradiation)	PDAC	Overcame the Drug Resistance	Murphy et al. (2018)
DOX +Zwitterionic chitosan	Gold-graphene oxide (808 nm NIR laser irradiation)	PC	Enhanced anti-tumor efficacy	Banstola et al. (2019)
Gemcitabine	CTh	PDAC	Inhibited the growth of PDAC tumors	Thapa et al.(2017)
Paclitaxel	IR-780	PDAC	Killed tumor cells	Teng et al.(2020)
Gemcitabine	Gold nanoparticles (808 nm NIR laser irradiation)	PC	Broke the interstitial barrier	Zhan et al.(2020)

3.1. Photothermal Therapy Combined with Gene therapy

The K-Ras mutation proved a common finding in pancreatic cancer patients and an important target for treatment. A gene treatment aimed at the G12V mutation of K-Ras was developed alongside a synergistic therapeutic approach utilizing reduced oxidized graphene covered with gold nanostars and interconnected with folic acid (Yin et al., 2017). In murine models of pancreatic cancer, the combination of genetic counseling and photothermal treatment exhibited a substantial anti-cancer impact (Yang et al., 2019). We simultaneously transported HDAC1 and K-Ras siRNAs using multipurpose single-layer oxidized carbon nanosheets, which made gene silencing very effective. This method showed a lot of promise for fighting pancreatic cancer when used with near-infrared laser heating (Morrison et al., 2018).

The photothermal impact from the laser irradiation controlled how the drugs spread, making them work better. This nanocompound has demonstrated a synergistic anticancer effect when siRNA inhibited oncogenic signaling pathways and a drug called induced apoptosis. A subsequent study examined further nanotechnology-based devices targeting K-Ras mutations. Therapeutic compounds were effectively delivered using graphene-based delivery devices that also produced localized photo-thermal effects that enhanced anti-tumor efficacy (Zhao et al., 2019). Nanostructures functionalized with tumor-targeting agents, such as folic acid, significantly enhanced selective binding to cells of pancreatic cancer while minimizing off-target effects. Preclinical investigations have shown that using these kinds of nano receivers to control the release of siRNA and chemotherapy drugs works well in both in vitro as well as vivo settings. One extremely effective treatment for pancreatic cancer is photothermal therapy in conjunction with gene therapy that has a good chance of working even when other treatments don't. In addition to helping therapeutic drugs breakdown down, the photothermal action of laser irradiation altered the tumor microenvironment, increasing the susceptibility of cancer cells to gene silencing. Preclinical experiments in animals showed that this combination method reduced systemic toxicity and increased treatment effectiveness (Zhou et al., 2018).

In another work, gold nanostars functionalised with vitamin folic acid and linked with siRNA aiming at the G12V mutations of K-Ras were evaluated. These nanostructures used a combination process of photothermal disintegration and gene silencing to accurately ablate tumours when subjected to laser light. In animal models of pancreatic cancer, the combination therapy successfully prevented tumour growth and increased survival. Similarly, graphene oxide-based nanosheets capable of co-delivery of siRNAs and small therapeutic molecules showed strong anti-cancer effects when coupled with near-infrared photothermal treatment. K-Ras expression was downregulated by siRNA-mediated gene silencing, and the photothermal effect compromised cancer cell membranes, so enhancing the therapeutic drug absorption (Feig et al., 2012). Biodegradable nanocarriers allow siRNAs targeted at K-Ras and chemotherapeutic medicines to be administered simultaneously. Photothermal activation made possible by graphene quantum dots as carriers provided fine control over drug release. This method activated the microscopic complex site-specifically utilising laser irradiation, therefore reducing off-target effects and maximising the therapeutic efficacy. With siRNA blocking K-Ras-driven carcinogenic pathways and doxorubicin promoting death, doxorubicin and siRNA co-delivery revealed synergistic effects (Stromnes et al., 2014).

Pancreatic cancer treatments incorporated multifunctional nanomaterials to address critical problems, including tumour heterogeneity and drug resistance. For instance, folic acid-functionalised miniature carriers especially targeted pancreatic cancer cells that overexpressed folate receptors. Through reducing the buildup of therapeutic molecules in healthy tissues, this targeted treatment assisted in reducing systemic unfavorable effects. When combined with photothermal treatment, these nanocarriers helped preclinical mice reduce their tumours and lower recurrence rates (Ino et al., 2013). Photodynamic Rehabilitation (PDT) was incorporated as a supplementary strategy to gene and photothermal treatment options in order to improve therapeutic treatments even further. Photodynamic medicines deposited onto nanocarriers generated Reactive Oxygen Species (ROS) upon laser activation, hence improving the anti-cancer properties of the combined treatment (Beatty et al., 2013).

Preclinical studies brought attention to the transformative possibilities of nanotechnology-based pancreatic cancer therapies. By concentrating on the K-Ras modification and using the complementary advantages associated with suppression of genes, photothermal treatment, and chemotherapy administration, these strategies offer a good approach to increase patient outcomes. The exact production of nano complexes by laser irradiation enabled the experimental conversion of nanomedicine-based interventions for pancreatic cancer to be made practicable, hence lowering systemic toxicity and enabling governed therapeutic transportation (Jaaks et al., 2022).

3.2. Photothermal Therapy Combined with Immunotherapy

Pancreatic cancer has been found to be treatable with immunotherapy, which comprises modified T cell therapies, immunological checkpoint inhibitors, and therapeutic vaccinations. Still, issues including immunological responses and cytokine release syndrome abound (Cunningham et al., 2006). Immunotherapy and complementary therapeutic techniques may be able to alter immune responses against tumour cells, increasing the effectiveness of treatment. In preclinical models, 75% of subcutaneous tumours in mice treated with photothermal therapy and local immunological adjuvant for pancreatic cancer completely disappeared. This was followed by a notable rise in T-populations of cells and the development of tumour-specific immune memories. Furthermore, imiquimod-loaded 1,2-distearoyl-sn-glycero-3-phosphoethanolamine-poly (DSPE-PEG) and indocyanine green-functionalised opaque ferric oxide nanoparticles, accompanied by ion-assisted MRI-guided Interventional Photo Radiation Therapy Ipswich Touch Test (IpTT), generated strong anti-tumour immune responses and enabled the targeted destruction of immunogenic cells (Murphy et al., 2018).Furthermore, when paired with laser irradiation, poly-dopamine (DP)-coated N/PGEM/DP-5 and N/PGEM/DP-16 nanoparticles, which contained gemcitabine and NLG919, respectively, and had a significant DP coating, showed a remarkable improvement in the suppression of pancreatic cancer progression (Barbour et al., 2020).

Pancreatic cancer has been found to be treatable with immunotherapy, which comprises modified T cell therapies, immunological checkpoint inhibitors, and therapeutic vaccinations. Still, issues including immunological responses and cytokine release syndrome abound (Cunningham et al., 2006). Immunotherapy and complementary therapeutic techniques may be able to alter immune responses against tumour cells, increasing the effectiveness of treatment. In preclinical models, 75% of subcutaneous tumours in mice treated with photothermal therapy and local immunological adjuvant for pancreatic cancer completely disappeared. This was followed by a notable rise in T-populations of cells and the development of tumour-specific immune memories. The ion-assisted MRI-guided Interventional Illustration Radiation Therapy Ipswich Touch Test (IpTT), paired with imiquimod-loaded 1,2-distearoyl-sn-glycero-3-phosphoethanolamine-poly (DSPE-PEG) and indocyanine green-functionalized opaque ferric oxide nanoparticles, elicited robust anti-tumor immune responses and enabled the targeted destruction of immunogenic cells (Murphy et al., 2018). Moreover, in conjunction with laser treatment, poly-dopamine (DP)-coated N/PGEM/DP-5 as well N/PGEM/DP-16 nanoparticles, and these incorporated gemcitabine and NLG919, as well as exhibited a substantial DP coating, demonstrated a considerable enhancement in the inhibition of pancreatic cancer progression (Barbour et al., 2020).

4. NEW AND EMERGING TREATMENTS

A complicated interaction between the malignant pancreas tumor's internal cellular traits and external environmental signals governed its behavior. Mutations and genetic alterations that facilitate unregulated cell proliferation, provide resistance to apoptosis, and enhance the likelihood of The main element influencing the possible carcinogenicity of malignant mitochondria is metastasis. These genetic alterations enabled cancer cells to flourish, disseminate into adjacent tissues, and advance the trajectory of the disease. The Tumour Microenvironment (TME), a key external factor, had a big effect on how the tumor acted. Every one of the many intracellular and extracellular elements that comprised the TME helped to define the pathogenic features of the cancer (Groot Koerkamp et al., 2017). Two key stromal compartments, biological components, fibroblasts and myofibroblasts, maintained and changed the distribution matrix that cells formed Electronic Control Module (ECM). The structural support and modulation of cell signalling pathways of the ECM affected cancer cell motility, invasion, and metastases. Participating in angiogenesis, endothelial cells and other vascular cells allow the quickly growing cancer to get blood flow (Dalmasso et al., 2022). The sometimes faulty newly produced vasculature made therapeutic efforts more challenging and resulted in inadequate drug delivery and tumour hypoxia. Dendritic cells, T cells, and macrophages, The growth of the cancer was influenced by the immune cells present throughout Total Mesorectal Excision (TME) in two ways. Although those immune cells could potentially possess anti-tumour properties, the TME frequently reduced or altered their activity, therefore enabling cancer cells to evade immune monitoring. The ECM itself was absolutely vital in encouraging the spread of cancer. Its composition, including components like collagen and fibronectin, could dynamically change in response to interactions between malignant tumour cells and epithelial components, therefore promoting the movement and spread of cancerous cells.

The TME had a lot of growth factors, inflammatory chemicals, and other soluble molecules that let the stromal and cancer cells talk to each other. These drugs affected the growth of cancer and the body's ability to fight it off by modulating fibrosis, immune responses, and inflammation. These were interleukins, tumor necrosis factor (TNF), as well as converting growth factor-beta (TGF-β). Ultimately, the host microenvironment significantly influenced the biology of pancreatic cancer tumors, alongside the intrinsic characteristics of the cancer cells. The invasive and invasive character of pancreatic cancer, which is influenced by the intricate interactions amongst the malignant cells and the surrounding stroma, made treatment techniques difficult. To make personalized drugs that can change the TME and improve the health of people with pancreatic cancer, we need to understand these complicated interactions very well (Siegel et al., 2019).

4.1. Immunotherapy

The immunosuppressive tumor microenvironment (TME) of pancreas cancer was one of the most talked-about things that affected how the cancer grew and how well it responded to chemotherapy. This setting made it very hard for tumors to avoid the immune system and for treatments to work. Preclinical research indicated that immune-mediated and inflammatory cells constituted approximately fifty percent of the tumor cell mass in carcinoma of the pancreas, markedly expediting the disease's growth. Still, the immune system in this environment was better at suppressing than stimulating. The tumor microenvironment (TME) was distinguished by a significant presence of macrophages, myeloid-derived suppressor cells (MDSCs), as well T-cell regulatory cells (Song et al., 2015). These cells came together to establish an immune Prevention Conditions that made it harder for effective immune systems against tumors to start. However, there was a glaring absence of cytotoxic T-cells are necessary for the direct destruction of cancerous cells. One of the main reasons why pancreatic cancer developed and spread was this imbalance in the populations of lymphocytes. The immunosuppressive qualities of the TME allowed tumor cells to evade immune surveillance, allowing for continued tumor development and spread. The humoral immune responses that target cancer antigens like mucin MUC-1 and mesothelin have a clear correlation with the outcome of pancreatic cancer. Although these antigens might elicit a body reaction that could help identify and eradicate the tumour, the highly suppressed TME frequently reduced the overall efficacy of this response (Nussbaum et al., 2016).

The pancreatic cancer patients have shown better clinical outcomes when intratumoral lymphocytes that are cytotoxic and assistance T cells are present. Although these cells were essential in producing a strong anti-tumour immune response, their efficacy was usually hampered by the hostile TME environment. The prognosis was much influenced by the way immunological checkpoint regulators, including programmed death-1 (PD-1) ligand, were expressed in the tumour. Successful inhibition of immune activity and promotion of immune avoidance caused by the tumour helps the PD-1 and ligand cooperate to create tolerance to antibodies (Chua & Saxel, 2010). Tregs reduced anti-tumour immunity; hence, their growth within the tumour was usually connected to worse clinical results. Furthermore, shown is the negative link between the percentage of Tregs to cells with regard to prognosis; a higher ratio indicates a more suppressed immune milieu and less effective therapeutic treatments. To tackle these problems, To strengthen the immune system's defenses against pancreatic cancer tumors, a number of treatment strategies have been studied.

The intratumoral concentration of Treg cells also greatly affected these strategies aimed at either reducing the patient's prognosis. These immunosuppressive cells compromised the body's ability to mount a successful immune response against tumour immunity suppression or to increase immune responses to support more effective targeting and destruction of cancer cells by so restricting the production and function of the interest or immune system cells, which includes cytotoxic T-cells. One such approach was immune checkpoint inhibitors, developed to prevent the use of inhibitory signals by tumours avoiding immune detection. Targeting immunological checkpoint proteins such as PD-1 or its ligand, these medicines sought to restore immune system functioning and enhance its capacity to find and combat cancerous cells. Another strategy was the development of immunisations targeting specific tumour antigens, such as mesothelin and MUC-1. The purpose of these vaccines was to prepare the body's defenses to identify and specifically target cancer cells. Additionally, several modified T cell therapies, such as Chimeric Antigen Receptor (CAR) T cell treatment, have been investigated as a means to boost the efficacy of cytotoxic memory T cells targeted specifically for pancreatic cancer cells. By genetically altering a patient's own lymphocytes to express sensors that identified particular tumour-associated antigens, CAR T-cell therapies enhanced the lymphocytes' capacity to destroy tumour cells. The distinct immunosuppressive features of pancreatic cancer called TME remained major obstacles to the effectiveness of these treatments, despite their encouraging experimental and early clinical research. A multifaceted method that combines adoptive T cell treatments, tumour-specific vaccinations, and immune checkpoint inhibition has shown promise in enhancing anti-tumour immunity and disrupting immunological tolerance.

4.2. Macrophage – Targeted Therapies

A member of the superfamily of tumor necrosis factor receptors, CD40 controlled inflammatory processes and cancer-related fibrosis in addition to influencing T-cell activation. Preclinical data suggested that CD40 activation could elicit T-cell responses against tumors. In a clinical trial for metastatic pancreatic cancer, the administration of gemcitabine and the anti-CD40 antagonist antibody CP-870,893 resulted in responses associated with tumor-infiltrating macrophages rather than lymphocyte infiltration (Cunningham et al., 2009). The reduction of the tumour stroma was mechanistically linked to the macrophages' activity linked to the tumour (TAMs) and the subsequent production of a cytotoxic macrophage phenotype. TAM suppression via chemokine (C-C motif) or colony-stimulating factor-1 receptor Antagonism of receptor 2 enhanced anti-tumor T-cell responses and chemotherapeutic effectiveness in other preclinical models. The development of successful macrophage-targeted immunotherapy was crucial to promoting anti-stromal and anti-cancer behaviour at the same time because of the dual pro- and tumor-fighting effects of TAMs. Despite the lack of long-term outcome data, combination therapy showed a favourable safety record, with a 52% success rate in 23 evaluable patients (Hosein et al., 2013).

4.3. Cytotoxic T-Lymphocytes Targeted Therapies

Through the specially designed reduction of inhibitory suppressor cells derived from myeloid cells (Myeloid-Derived Suppressor Cells (MDSC)) and triggering of autologous CD8+ T cells using adoptive T cell treatments, vaccines against cancer, or Interferon (IFNs), an immunologically reactive environment was induced. Checkpoint blockade drugs that target cytotoxic T-lymphocyte-associated protein 4 (CTLA-4), indole amine 2,3-dioxygenase (IDO), programmed cell death ligand-1 (PD-L1), and programmed cell death 1 (PD-1) were also used in this strategy. Clinical trials employing checkpoint blockade drugs by myself, including PD-L1 & CTLA-4 inhibiting agents, have not shown considerable benefit in pancreatic cancer due to the possibly restricted neoantigenic potential of this disease type. Checkpoint blockade inhibitors have been actively investigated in combination with tumour vaccines, agents that target immunosuppressive cell populations like regulatory T cells (Treg) and MDSC, chemotherapy, or radiation therapy (Robinson et al., 2003).

Pilot investigations using cytokine-induced T cells showed that they were safe in recurrent pancreatic cancer, having an eleven-month Progression-Free Survival

(PFS) period and an overall survival of 27 weeks, which were equivalent to second-line chemotherapeutic regimens. Furthermore, T-cell genetic engineering has demonstrated promise in developing immunotherapeutic approaches for pancreatic cancer by increasing the levels of expression and efficacy of tumour-antigen-specific antibodies or making those resistant to inhibitory signals. In order to activate the adaptive immune system's reaction and induce the production of potent cytotoxic T-lymphocytes, vaccines against cancer have been developed to encourage the development of mature dendritic cell populations for their presentation of certain tumour antigens. Numerous cancer vaccine strategies have been used to study pancreatic cancer, including whole-cell vaccines that overexpress a specific epitope, peptide-based vaccinations, and DNA vaccines, which embed DNA encoding an antigen of interest into a vector for tumor cell uptake. Using two human allograft pancreatic cell lines with malignancy (HAPa1 and HAPa2), Algen pantucel-L is an irradiation mixture that has been genetically altered for expressing the animal's enzyme α-1, 3-Galactosyl Transferase Enzyme (α-GT). Several whole-cell vaccines have shown promise in the treatment of pancreatic cancer, including this one. Although α Gal epitope is not normally expressed by humans, they do have a significant quantity of anti-α Gal antibody (Smeenk et al., 2007). Algen pantucel-L vaccination causes "hyperacute rejection" against the allograft vaccine cells by activation of complement and cytotoxicity that is Antibody-Dependent Cellular Cytotoxicity (ADCC). The immune system is activated similarly to transplant rejection when exposed to the entire antigen repertoire of the vaccination cells. The adjuvant usage of algen pantucel-L in conjunction with gemcitabine as Phase II studies evaluated 5-fluorouracil (5-FU)-based radiotherapy and chemotherapy following pancreatic cancer surgery; the drug was well tolerated, as well as the 1-year unaffected-by-disease rate of survival was 62%. The 1-year surviving rate of 86% was favorable when compared to the adjuvant RTOG-9704, and this had a 6-9% 1-year survival rate. A 96% 1-year rate of survival was attained with higher vaccine doses (three hundred million cells/dose). According to biomarker analyses, patients who produced another anti-calreticulin antibody response or an anti-membrane restricted recombined mesothelin response (Tarannum et al., 2022).

5. FUTURE PERSPECTIVES

It was established that pancreatic cancer was a highly aggressive tumour that presented difficult treatment options. Although surgical excision was still the most common treatment option, its effectiveness had not significantly increased over time. Drug resistance frequently constrained the effectiveness of chemotherapy, despite its initial use as a treatment. This is a dense tumour stroma and tumour heterogeneity.

Nanomaterials have demonstrated promise in overcoming biological limitations related to medication delivery in various fields of medical research. In order to enable accurate targeted therapy and controlled release, nano-drug delivery platforms were created aimed at cancer cells and hypoxic tumour micro environments. The only nanomedicine currently The FDA-approved albumin-bound paclitaxel is being used in clinical trials for pancreatic cancer treatment in cases of metastatic pancreatic cancer. One promising approach to improving treatment efficacy was the creation of pharmaceutical drug delivery mechanisms based on nano biotechnology. With the use of nanotechnology or tiny antibody fragments, molecularly modified medications and nanomaterials have shown promise in improving outcomes for pancreatic cancer patients (Cao et al., 2019).Furthermore, significant progress in pancreatic cancer treatment was made via aptamer-functionalised nanomaterials. Alternative molecular targets and innovative nano-drug delivery methods were actively investigated to optimise treatment regimens, even if some molecularly targeted medicines were still in clinical trials. This helped to enhance individualised therapy options for pancreatic cancer. Despite being a potentially effective cancer treatment method, photothermal therapy (PTT) its efficacy was restricted by the light's limited ability to penetrate tissue, especially for deep-seated tumours. Beyond superficial tissue layers, imaging-guided localised regional interventional PTT has become a unique treatment approach for pancreatic cancer. Furthermore, major advancements were created to treat pancreatic cancer possible by combining PTT with immunotherapy treatment, gene therapy, and nanoenzymes. However, treating problems with the tumor stroma as well as hypoxia in the tumor microenvironment remained important, and continued innovation was expected to drive future advancements in the medical management of pancreatic cancer and biotechnology advances as well as the interconnected integration of biology, materials science, pharmacology, and medicine. These developments would ultimately benefit a larger patient population (Elzoghby et al., 2012).

5.1 Neoadjuvant Therapy

Neoadjuvant or intraoperative therapy is a novel treatment strategy for pancreatic cancer, particularly for detachable and localized unresectable cancers and tumours that are borderline resectable. For several decades, there was a lack of data of excellent quality through randomised controlled trials (RCTs) within the adjuvant context owing to challenges with study preparation and patient recruitment. The first randomized trial of neoadjuvant chemoradiotherapy for pancreatic cancer was prematurely terminated due to low patient enrollment. Numerous Phase III randomized trials were underway to gather valuable data regarding this approach. The NEOPAC study, for instance, contrasted the medication gemcitabine with neoadjuvant gemcitabine–oxaliplatin following adjuvant gemcitabine. On the other hand, the National University of Educational Planning and Administration (NEO-PA) experiment looked at neoadjuvant chemoradiotherapy vs upfront surgery. The previously Preoperative Chemoradiotherapy vs Immediate Surgery for Pancreatic Cancer (PREOPANC) study also investigated these approaches for pancreatic cancer that was both resectable and marginally resectable (Garcia-Sampedro et al., 2021).

For patients with possibly treatable pancreatic tumors, the European Study Association for the Study of Pancreatic Cancer - Trial 5F (ESPAC-5F) trial evaluated urgent surgery, gemcitabine–capecitabine, preparatory chemoradiotherapy, as well as a four-arm design.

In a Phase II/III randomized controlled trial (NCT014587) that compare adjuvant treatment with chemotherapy and electromagnetic radiation therapy with gemcitabine, which against neoadjuvant radio therapy and chemotherapy combined with gemcitabine, the interim report in the abstract indicated an average survival duration of 23 weeks for neoadjuvant treatment, in contrast to eleven months for the latter following early surgery. Interestingly, adjuvant chemotherapy and radiation were shown to be unsuccessful, and even when compared to patients with advanced locally or metastatic illness receiving conventional adjuvant therapy, the average length of stay in the upfront surgery sample was much shorter than anticipated for this patient population. In the neoadjuvant situation, chemotherapy replaced chemoradiotherapy with the introduction of more powerful chemotherapeutic regimens, especially FOLFIRINOX. Afterwards, some centers reported significant reconstruction Although 50% of the tumors initially remained undetectable due to distant metastases, rates of up to 60% in regionally advanced, unresectable cases administered the neoadjuvant FOLFIRINOX were observed. Crucially, imaging did not always indicate a response to treatment, which highlights the need for interdisciplinary consultation and personalised advice regarding surgical exploration (Rubinsky et al., 2007). These included the ability to target tissues efficiently, made possible by intact tumour perfusion, to treat any possible micro metastases hat were presents point of surgery. It has also been demonstrated to be more well-tolerated than adjuvant chemotherapy in other malignancies, which has raised completion rates. Individuals with locally advanced and borderline removable Pancreatic Ducts Adenocarcinoma (PDAC) as well as those with resectable tumors have been enrolled in numerous clinical trials in recent years. The information from the National Oncology Database was analysed in relation to resectable PDAC, comparing patients with early-stage PDAC who received resection and had chemotherapy of any kind or at any time to those who did not (Tangutoori et al., 2016). Though the removal rates are low are lower are lower in the neo-adjuvantction (66% vs. 81.3%), a meta-analysis of 3,484 patients suffering from resectable and possibly selectable sickness who received any kind of neo-adjuvant regimen alongside or without radiation therapies found an insignificant overall survival advantage in those acquiring neo-adjuvant medicine (18.8 vs. 14.8 months). According to these theories, certain patients with localised advanced PDAC may experience aggressive disease development and find that resection is not beneficial. For patients with intermediate or locally advanced cancer, the current National Comprehensive Cancer Network (NCCN) guidelines suggested neoadjuvant therapy, with gemcitabine combined with the combination of n as the preferred medicines (Ychou et al., 2003).

5.2. Hepatic Artery Infusion Therapy

A catheter was placed into the gastroduodenal artery as part of Hepatic Artery Infusion (HAI) therapy which supplies the liver's hepatic arterial vasculature, to deliver chemotherapy directly into the liver. Increased hepatic chemotherapeutic drug concentration and decreased systemic toxicity were two benefits of HAI. The advantages of HAI treatment for colorectal cancer that had spread to the liver had long been known. HAI has been utilized as an adjuvant in a few minor studies for progressive pancreatic ductal adenocarcinoma, with varying degrees of therapeutic efficacy. In their non-randomised trial, Wang et al. contrasted 43 individuals who received adjunct 2-cycle HAI treatment following 4-cycle systemic therapy with 44 individuals received 5-FU plus adjuvant systemic gemcitabine alone. The 5-year lifespan probability (danger ratio [HR] 0.60) as the liver metastasis-free morbidity (HR 0.50) were significantly higher in the HAI group, despite the fact that the 5-year free-of-illnesses rates of survival were the same in the two groups. HAI chemotherapy had a 54% 4-year rate of longevity and a 53% 3-year survival rate in the adjuvant context. Six out of seven individuals (85%) reacted to the brief research on patients who experienced hepatic recurrence after resection. A Phase 2 trial employing floxuridine-based HAI immunotherapy was actively seeking participants for those with liver metastases following PDAC surgery (NCT03856658) (Boone et al., 2013).

5.3. Immuno and Targeted Systemic Therapy

The development of PDAC therapies has undergone a paradigm shift in the last ten years, fuelled by developments in bioinformatics and next-generation sequencing technology. These developments made it easier to find driver mutations and abnormal signalling pathways in PDAC, which in turn helped identify new treatment targets. About 25% of PDAC patients have somatic or germline mutations in the homologous recombination repair (HRR) genes (including ATM, BAP1, BARD1, BLM, BRIP1, CHEK2, FAM175A, FANCA, FANCC, NBN, RAD50, RAD51, RAD51C, and RTEL1) and DNA Damage Repair (DDR) pathway (which includes BRCA1, BRCA2, and PALB2). Whole genome and exosome sequencing as a whole identified a greater percentage of sufferers with homology-recombination deficiency (HRD) (24–44%) than gene-level centre or targeted NGS (14.5–16.5%), according to a recent meta-analysis that comprised six studies with 21,842 PDAC patients (Gjertsen et al., 2001).

KRAS is being actively investigated as a potential therapeutic target (NCT03608631, NCT01676259). This reaction persisted for more than half a year. A thorough list of significant active KRAS-targeting experiments was supplied. Because the tumour microenvironment (TME) is immunosuppressive, PDAC has historically demonstrated a limited response to immunotherapy. About 2% of PDAC patients had mismatch correction deficiency with microsatellite instability (MSI-H). Pembrolizumab was approved as a tumor-agnostic treatment for those with advanced cancers who had MSI-H status as a result of the KEYNOTE-158 research. With one complete reaction, a response objective ratio of 18%, and an average length of recovery of 13.4 months, the 22 patients with d MMR/MSI-H and progressive PDAC who were assessed in this study showed encouraging responses. Owing to PDAC's immunologically "cold" character, a number of research projects have concentrated on boosting immune activity by activating innate lymphocytes or by causing inflammation in the TME, which makes it easier to attract cytotoxic T cells. In a recent study, a pancreatic cancer mouse model was injected with non-disease-causing *Listeria* bacteria that carried a gene expressing tetanus toxin (Panni et al., 2014).

The effects of gemcitabine and paclitaxel in combination with durvalumab (PDL-1 inhibitor) & AZD0171 (anti-LIF1 monoclonal antibodies antibody) were assessed in an open-label Phase 2 clinical research (NCT04999969). Immunological alternative responses indicators that were evaluated included tumor mutant burdens (TMB), PDL-1 communication, & T-cell response signatures. Twelve PDAC patients who had progressed on therapy based on platinum and PARP inhibitors and exhibited microbial line Homology-Recombination Deficiency (HRD) alterations, including BRCA1, BRCA2, RAD51C, RAD51D, and ATM, were included in the small cohort research. Given that germline damages to DNA (DDR) variants in genes result in genomic instability and higher TMB, it was hypothesized that patients with certain DDR mutations may benefit therapeutically from immunotherapy. For four cycles, these patients received ipilimumab and nivolumab, and then nivolumab alone. The Disease Control Rate (DCR) was 58%, while the overall rate of response was 42%. Four patients (two with BRCA1, one with BRCA2, and one with RAD51C) had Complete Responses (CR), whereas one patient (with BRCA1) showed Partial Responses (PR). After two years, three out of the four patients who achieved CR stopped receiving medication. Next-Generation Sequencing (NGS) was also used to pinpoint the genetic drivers of tumours and inform the choice of targeted treatment.Tropomyosin Receptor Kinase (TRK) was one target that was found. Based on phase I trials and case series, TRK inhibitors like larotrectinib and entrectinib have been included in PDAC therapy regimens as second-line medicines, despite the fact that the occurrence of TRK fusions in PDAC is uncommon (about 0.5%) (Pino et al., 2009).

6. CONCLUSION

Treatment for pancreatic carcinoma is still challenging clinically. Significant progress has been achieved in recent years to improve patient outcomes, even though it will probably grow into the second leading cause of cancer-related deaths in the upcoming decade. Improvements in perioperative care and the creation of more potent adjuvant medicines, which significantly increase survival—a 30% This success has been attributed in part to adjuvant therapy and the observed up to 5-year survival rate following tumor removal. Additionally, a sizable portion of patients (up to 50% or more) have locally advanced, incurable malignancies or those with tumors that are just marginally resectable have responded favorably to surgical procedures following neoadjuvant therapy regimens. The management of metastatic pancreas cancer has seen significant advancements after a period of stagnation, especially with the use of combined medicines that, in ideal circumstances, virtually double median survival. Additionally, individuals with a satisfactory performance status who have disease progression after first-line treatment now have options for second-line therapy that are supported by research. Numerous difficulties remained, and At every patient stage, the general outcome for pancreas cancer remained bleak. Anti-angiogenic treatment and EGFR inhibition were noteworthy instances. Likewise, early attempts to take advantage of the hypoxic microenvironment or target the tumour stroma were unsuccessful. The great molecular heterogeneity of pancreatic cancer and its associated stromal and inflammatory elements may have contributed to these setbacks by affecting medication accessibility, metabolism, and signalling pathways. Additionally, treatment for pancreatic cancer has not advanced despite the fact that immunotherapies have shown promise in treating other human tumour types and have shown promise in treating this illness. This is because the immune response is still a highly complicated regulatory network. Significant progress has been made in understanding the intricate molecular composition of pancreatic cancer and its unique microenvironment. In order to build personalised medicine for pancreatic cancer, the issue now was to apply this information to clinical practice by determining which patient subgroups benefit from particular therapy. This strategy required interdisciplinary cooperation and the creation of innovative trial designs. Future work would need to concentrate on identifying patient subpopulations for certain medicines that were both easily accessible and deliverable, while assessing this approach through carefully planned, economically viable clinical trials.

7. REFERENCES

Ahmed, S., Hasan, M. N., Altass, H. M., Bera, A., Alsantali, R., Pan, N., Alzahrani, A. Y. A., Bagchi, D., Al-Fahemi, J. H., Khder, A. S., & Pal, S. K. (2022). Tetracycline encapsulated in Au nanoparticle-decorated ZnO nanohybrids for enhanced antibacterial activity. *ACS Applied Nano Materials*, *5*(3), 4484–4492. DOI: 10.1021/acsanm.2c00655

Amjad, M. W., Amin, M., Katas, H., Butt, A., Kesharwani, P., & Iyer, A. (2015). In vivo antitumor activity of folate-conjugated cholic acid-polyethylenimine micelles for the codelivery of doxorubicin and siRNA to colorectal adenocarcinomas. *Molecular Pharmaceutics*, *12*(11), 4247–4258. DOI: 10.1021/acs.molpharmaceut.5b00827 PMID: 26567518

Banstola, A., Pham, T. T., Jeong, J. H., & Yook, S. (2019). Polydopamine-tailored paclitaxel-loaded polymeric microspheres with adhered NIR-controllable gold nanoparticles for chemo-phototherapy of pancreatic cancer. *Drug Delivery*, *26*(1), 629–640. DOI: 10.1080/10717544.2019.1628118 PMID: 31237149

Barbour, A., Samra, J., Haghighi, K. S., Donoghoe, M. W., Burge, M., Harris, M. T., Chua, Y. J., Mitchell, J., O'Rourke, N., Chan, H., Gebski, V. J., Gananadha, S., Croagh, D. G., Kench, J. G., & Goldstein, D. (2020). The AGITG GAP study: A phase II study of perioperative gemcitabine and nab-paclitaxel for resectable pancreas cancer. *Annals of Surgical Oncology*, *27*(7), 2506–2515. DOI: 10.1245/s10434-020-08205-2 PMID: 31997125

Beatty, G., Torigian, D., Chiorean, E., Saboury, B., Brothers, A., Alavi, A., Troxel, A. B., Sun, W., Teitelbaum, U. R., Vonderheide, R. H., & O'Dwyer, P. J. (2013). A phase I study of an agonist CD40 monoclonal antibody (CP-870,893) in combination with gemcitabine in patients with advanced pancreatic ductal adenocarcinoma. *Clinical Cancer Research*, *19*(22), 6286–6295. DOI: 10.1158/1078-0432.CCR-13-1320 PMID: 23983255

Boone, B. A., Steve, J., Krasinskas, A. M., Zureikat, A. H., Lembersky, B. C., Gibson, M. K., Stoller, R. G., Zeh, H. J., & Bahary, N. (2013). Outcomes with FOLFIRINOX for borderline resectable and locally unresectable pancreatic cancer. *Journal of Surgical Oncology*, *108*(4), 236–241. DOI: 10.1002/jso.23392 PMID: 23955427

Butt, A. M., Amin, M., Katas, H., Abdul Murad, N. A., Jamal, R., & Kesharwani, P. (2016). Doxorubicin and siRNA codelivery via chitosan-coated pH-responsive mixed micellar polyplexes for enhanced cancer therapy in multidrug-resistant tumors. *Molecular Pharmaceutics*, *13*(2), 4179–4190. DOI: 10.1021/acs.molpharmaceut.6b00776 PMID: 27934479

Cao, X., Hu, Y., Luo, S., Wang, Y., Gong, T., Sun, X., Fu, Y., & Zhang, Z. (2019). Neutrophil-mimicking therapeutic nanoparticles for targeted chemotherapy of pancreatic carcinoma. *Acta Pharmaceutica Sinica. B*, *9*(3), 575–589. DOI: 10.1016/j.apsb.2018.12.009 PMID: 31193785

Chua, T. C., & Saxena, A. (2010). Extended pancreaticoduodenectomy with vascular resection for pancreatic cancer: A systematic review. *Journal of Gastrointestinal Surgery*, *14*(9), 1442–1452. DOI: 10.1007/s11605-009-1129-7 PMID: 20379794

Collins, I., & Workman, P. (2006). New approaches to molecular cancer therapeutics. *Nature Chemical Biology*, *2*(12), 689–700. DOI: 10.1038/nchembio840 PMID: 17108987

Cunningham, D., Allum, W., Stenning, S. P., Thompson, J. N., Van de Velde, C. J. H., Nicolson, M., Scarffe, J. H., Lofts, F. J., Falk, S. J., Iveson, T. J., Smith, D. B., Langley, R. E., Verma, M., Weeden, S., & Chua, Y. J. (2006). Perioperative chemotherapy versus surgery alone for resectable gastroesophageal cancer. *The New England Journal of Medicine*, *355*(1), 11–20. DOI: 10.1056/NEJMoa055531 PMID: 16822992

Cunningham, D., Chau, I., Stocken, D. D., Valle, J. W., Smith, D., Steward, W., Harper, P. G., Dunn, J., Tudur-Smith, C., West, J., Falk, S., Crellin, A., Adab, F., Thompson, J., Leonard, P., Ostrowski, J., Eatock, M., Scheithauer, W., Herrmann, R., & Neoptolemos, J. P. (2009). Phase III randomized comparison of gemcitabine versus gemcitabine plus capecitabine in patients with advanced pancreatic cancer. *Journal of Clinical Oncology*, *27*(33), 5513–5518. DOI: 10.1200/JCO.2009.24.2446 PMID: 19858379

Dalmasso, B., Puccini, A., Catalano, F., Borea, R., Iaia, M. L., Bruno, W., Fornarini, G., Sciallero, S., Rebuzzi, S. E., & Ghiorzo, P. (2022). Beyond BRCA: The emerging significance of DNA damage response and personalized treatment in pancreatic and prostate cancer patients. *International Journal of Molecular Sciences*, *23*(9), 4709–4710. DOI: 10.3390/ijms23094709 PMID: 35563100

Du, C., Qi, Y., Zhang, Y., Wang, Y., Zhao, X., Min, H., Han, X., Lang, J., Qin, H., Shi, Q., Zhang, Z., Tian, X., Anderson, G. J., Zhao, Y., Nie, G., & Yang, Y. (2018). Epidermal growth factor receptor-targeting peptide nanoparticles simultaneously deliver gemcitabine and olaparib to treat pancreatic cancer with breast cancer 2 (BRCA2) mutation. *ACS Nano*, *12*(11), 10785–10796. DOI: 10.1021/acsnano.8b01573 PMID: 30407790

Elzoghby, A. O., Samy, W. M., & Elgindy, N. A. (2012). Albumin-based nanoparticles as potential controlled release drug delivery systems. *Journal of Controlled Release*, *157*(2), 168–182. DOI: 10.1016/j.jconrel.2011.07.031 PMID: 21839127

Evans, D. B., Varadhachary, G. R., Crane, C. H., Sun, C. C., Lee, J. E., Pisters, P. W. T., Vauthey, J.-N., Wang, H., Cleary, K. R., Staerkel, G. A., Charnsangavej, C., Lano, E. A., Ho, L., Lenzi, R., Abbruzzese, J. L., & Wolff, R. A. (2008). Preoperative gemcitabine-based chemoradiation for patients with resectable adenocarcinoma of the pancreatic head. *Journal of Clinical Oncology*, *26*(21), 3496–3502. DOI: 10.1200/JCO.2007.15.8634 PMID: 18640930

Fatima, M., Abourehab, M. A. S., Aggarwal, G., Jain, G. K., Sahebkar, A., & Kesharwani, P. (2022). Advancement of cell-penetrating peptides in combating triple-negative breast cancer. *Drug Discovery Today*, *27*(11), 103353. DOI: 10.1016/j.drudis.2022.103353 PMID: 36099963

Feig, C., Gopinathan, A., Neesse, A., Chan, D., Cook, N., & Tuveson, D. (2012). The pancreas cancer microenvironment. *Clinical Cancer Research*, *18*(16), 4266–4276. DOI: 10.1158/1078-0432.CCR-11-3114 PMID: 22896693

Ferrone, C. R., Marchegiani, G., Hong, T. S., Ryan, D. P., Deshpande, V., McDonnell, E. I., Sabbatino, F., Santos, D. D., Allen, J. N., Blaszkowsky, L. S., Clark, J. W., Faris, J. E., Goyal, L., Kwak, E. L., Murphy, J. E., Ting, D. T., Wo, J. Y., Zhu, A. X., Warshaw, A. L., & Castillo, C. F. (2015). Radiological and surgical implications of neoadjuvant treatment with FOLFIRINOX for locally advanced and borderline resectable pancreatic cancer. *Annals of Surgery*, *261*(1), 12–17. DOI: 10.1097/SLA.0000000000000867 PMID: 25599322

Garcia-Sampedro, A., Gaggia, G., Ney, A., Mahamed, I., & Acedo, P. (2021). The State-of-the-Art of Phase II/III Clinical Trials for Targeted Pancreatic Cancer Therapies. *Journal of Clinical Medicine*, *10*(4), 566–556. DOI: 10.3390/jcm10040566 PMID: 33546207

Geier, B., Sogin, E. M., Michellod, D., Janda, M., Kompauer, M., Spengler, B., Dubilier, N., & Liebeke, M. (2020). Spatial metabolomics of in situ host–microbe interactions at the micrometre scale. *Nature Microbiology*, *5*(3), 498–510. DOI: 10.1038/s41564-019-0664-6 PMID: 32015496

Gjertsen, M. K., Buanes, T., & Rosseland, A. R. (2001). Intradermal ras peptide vaccination with granulocyte-macrophage colony-stimulating factor as adjuvant: Clinical and immunological responses in patients with pancreatic adenocarcinoma. *International Journal of Cancer*, *92*(3), 441–450. DOI: 10.1002/ijc.1205 PMID: 11291084

Groot Koerkamp, B., Sadot, E., Kemeny, N., Gönen, M., Leal, J. N., Allen, P. J., Cercek, A., DeMatteo, R. P., Kingham, T. P., Jarnagin, W. R., & D'Angelica, M. I. (2017). Perioperative hepatic arterial infusion pump chemotherapy is associated with longer survival after resection of colorectal liver metastases: A propensity score analysis. *Journal of Clinical Oncology*, *35*(17), 1938–1944. DOI: 10.1200/JCO.2016.71.8346 PMID: 28426374

Hanaf-Bojd, M. Y., Ansari, L., & Malaekeh-Nikouei, B. (2016). Codelivery of anticancer drugs and siRNA by mesoporous silica nanoparticles. *Therapeutic Delivery*, *7*(9), 649–655. DOI: 10.4155/tde-2016-0045 PMID: 27582236

Hosein, P. J., de Lima Lopes, G., Pastorini, V. H., Gomez, C., Macintyre, J., Zayas, G., Reis, I., Montero, A. J., Merchan, J. R., & Rocha Lima, C. M. (2013). A phase II trial of nab-Paclitaxel as second-line therapy in patients with advanced pancreatic cancer. *American Journal of Clinical Oncology*, *36*(2), 151–156. DOI: 10.1097/COC.0b013e3182436e8c PMID: 22307213

Ino, Y., Yamazaki-Itoh, R., Shimada, K., Iwasaki, M., Kosuge, T., Kanai, Y., & Hiraoka, N. (2013). Immune cell infiltration as an indicator of the immune microenvironment of pancreatic cancer. *British Journal of Cancer*, *108*(4), 914–923. DOI: 10.1038/bjc.2013.32 PMID: 23385730

Jaaks, P., Coker, E. A., Vis, D. J., Edwards, O., Carpenter, E. F., Leto, S. M., Dwane, L., Sassi, F., Lightfoot, H., Barthorpe, S., van der Meer, D., Yang, W., Beck, A., Mironenko, T., Hall, C., Hall, J., Mali, I., Richardson, L., Tolley, C., & Garnett, M. J. (2022). Effective drug combinations in breast, colon and pancreatic cancer cells. *Nature*, *603*(7899), 166–173. DOI: 10.1038/s41586-022-04437-2 PMID: 35197630

Jain, A., Jain, A., Parajuli, P., Mishra, V., Ghoshal, G., Singh, B., Shivhare, U. S., Katare, O. P., & Kesharwani, P. (2017). Recent advances in galactose-engineered nanocarriers for the site-specific delivery of siRNA and anticancer drugs. *Drug Discovery Today*, *23*(5), 960–973. DOI: 10.1016/j.drudis.2017.11.003 PMID: 29129804

Khder, A., Ashour, S., Altass, H., & Khairou, K. S. (2016). Pd nanoparticles supported on iron oxide nanorods for CO oxidation: Effect of preparation method. *Journal of Environmental Chemical Engineering*, *4*(1), 4794–4800. DOI: 10.1016/j.jece.2016.10.019

Kolemen, S., Ozdemir, T., Lee, D., Kim, G. M., Karatas, T., Yoon, J., & Akkaya, E. U. (2016). Remote-controlled release of singlet oxygen by the plasmonic heating of endoperoxide-modified gold nanorods: Towards a paradigm change in photodynamic therapy. *Angewandte Chemie International Edition*, *55*(11), 3606–3610. DOI: 10.1002/anie.201510064 PMID: 26845734

Lin, G., Hu, R., Law, W. C., Chen, C.-K., Wang, Y., Li Chin, H., Nguyen, Q. T., Lai, C. K., Yoon, H. S., Wang, X., Xu, G., Ye, L., Cheng, C., & Yong, K.-T. (2013). Biodegradable nanocapsules as siRNA carriers for mutant K-Ras gene silencing of human pancreatic carcinoma cells. *Small*, *9*(16), 2757–2763. DOI: 10.1002/smll.201201716 PMID: 23427041

Mishra, V., Kesharwani, P., & Jain, N. K. (2014). siRNA nanotherapeutics: A Trojan horse approach against HIV. *Drug Discovery Today*, *19*(12), 1913–1920. DOI: 10.1016/j.drudis.2014.09.019 PMID: 25281591

Morrison, A., Byrne, K., & Vonderheide, R. (2018). Immunotherapy and prevention of pancreatic cancer. *Trends in Cancer*, *4*(6), 418–428. DOI: 10.1016/j.trecan.2018.04.001 PMID: 29860986

Murphy, J., Wo, J., Ryan, D., Jiang, W., Yeap, B. Y., Drapek, L. C., Blaszkowsky, L. S., Kwak, E. L., Allen, J. N., Clark, J. W., Faris, J. E., Zhu, A. X., Goyal, L., Lillemoe, K. D., DeLaney, T. F., Fernández-del Castillo, C., Ferrone, C. R., & Hong, T. S. (2018). Total neoadjuvant therapy with FOLFIRINOX followed by individualized chemoradiotherapy for borderline resectable pancreatic adenocarcinoma: A phase 2 clinical trial. *JAMA Oncology*, *4*(7), 963–969. DOI: 10.1001/jamaoncol.2018.0329 PMID: 29800971

Murphy, J. E., Wo, J. Y., Ryan, D. P., Jiang, W., Yeap, B. Y., Drapek, L. C., Blaszkowsky, L. S., Kwak, E. L., Allen, J. N., Clark, J. W., Faris, J. E., Zhu, A. X., Goyal, L., Lillemoe, K. D., DeLaney, T. F., Fernández-del Castillo, C., Ferrone, C. R., & Hong, T. S. (2018). Total neoadjuvant therapy with FOLFIRINOX followed by individualized chemoradiotherapy for borderline resectable pancreatic adenocarcinoma: A phase 2 clinical trial. *JAMA Oncology*, *4*(7), 963–969. DOI: 10.1001/jamaoncol.2018.0329 PMID: 29800971

Neoptolemos, J., Stocken, D., Friess, H., Bassi, C., Dunn, J. A., Hickey, H., Beger, H., Fernandez-Cruz, L., Dervenis, C., Lacaine, F., Falconi, M., Pederzoli, P., Pap, A., Spooner, D., Kerr, D. J., & Büchler, M. W. (2004). A randomized trial of chemoradiotherapy and chemotherapy after resection of pancreatic cancer. *The New England Journal of Medicine*, *350*(12), 1200–1210. DOI: 10.1056/NEJMoa032295 PMID: 15028824

Nussbaum, D. P., Adam, M. A., Youngwirth, L. M., Ganapathi, A. M., Roman, S. A., Tyler, D. S., Sosa, J. A., & Blazer, D. G.III. (2016). Minimally invasive pancreaticoduodenectomy does not improve use or time to initiation of adjuvant chemotherapy for patients with pancreatic adenocarcinoma. *Annals of Surgical Oncology*, *23*(3), 1026–1033. DOI: 10.1245/s10434-015-4937-x PMID: 26542590

Panni, R. Z., Sanford, D. E., Belt, B. A., Mitchem, J. B., Worley, L. A., Goetz, B. D., Mukherjee, P., Wang-Gillam, A., Link, D. C., DeNardo, D. G., Goedegebuure, S. P., & Linehan, D. C. (2014). Tumor-induced STAT3 activation in monocytic myeloid-derived suppressor cells enhances stemness and mesenchymal properties in human pancreatic cancer. *Cancer Immunology, Immunotherapy : CII*, *63*(5), 513–528. DOI: 10.1007/s00262-014-1527-x PMID: 24652403

Pino, M. S., Milella, M., Gelibter, A., Sperduti, I., De Marco, S., Nuzzo, C., Bria, E., Carpanese, L., Ruggeri, E. M., Carlini, P., & Cognetti, F. (2009). Capecitabine and celecoxib as second-line treatment of advanced pancreatic and biliary tract cancers. *Oncology*, *76*(4), 254–261. DOI: 10.1159/000205388 PMID: 19246950

Plana, D., Palmer, A. C., & Sorger, P. K. (2022). Independent drug action in combination therapy: Implications for precision oncology. *Cancer Discovery*, *12*(3), 606–624. DOI: 10.1158/2159-8290.CD-21-0212 PMID: 34983746

Rawla, P., Sunkara, T., & Gaduputi, V. (2019). Epidemiology of pancreatic cancer: Global trends, etiology and risk factors. *World Journal of Oncology*, *10*(1), 10–27. DOI: 10.14740/wjon1166 PMID: 30834048

Robatel, S., & Schenk, M. (2022). Current limitations and novel perspectives in pancreatic cancer treatment. *Cancers (Basel)*, *14*(4), 985–986. DOI: 10.3390/cancers14040985 PMID: 35205732

Robinson, K., Lambiase, L., Li, J., Monteiro, C., & Schiff, M. (2003). Fatal cholestatic liver failure associated with gemcitabine therapy. *Digestive Diseases and Sciences*, *48*(9), 1804–1808. DOI: 10.1023/A:1025415616592 PMID: 14561005

Rubinsky, B., Onik, G., & Mikus, P. (2007). Irreversible electroporation: A new ablation modality - clinical implications. *Technology in Cancer Research & Treatment*, *6*(1), 37–48. DOI: 10.1177/153303460700600106 PMID: 17241099

Ryan, D. P., Hong, T. S., & Bardeesy, N. (2014). Pancreatic adenocarcinoma. *The New England Journal of Medicine*, *371*(11), 1039–1049. DOI: 10.1056/NEJMra1404198 PMID: 25207767

Siegel, R. L., Miller, K. D., & Jemal, A. (2019). Cancer statistics. *CA: a Cancer Journal for Clinicians*, *69*(1), 7–34. DOI: 10.3322/caac.21551 PMID: 30620402

Singh, V., Sheikh, A., Abourehab, M. A. S., & Kesharwani, P. (2022). Dostarlimab as a miracle drug: Rising hope against cancer treatment. *Biosensors (Basel)*, *12*(8), 617. DOI: 10.3390/bios12080617 PMID: 36005013

Smeenk, H. G., van Eijck, C. H. J., Hop, W., Erdmann, J., Tran, K. C. K., Debois, M., van Cutsem, E., van Dekken, H., Klinkenbijl, J. H., & Jeekel, J. (2007). Long-term survival and metastatic pattern of pancreatic and periampullary cancer after adjuvant chemoradiation or observation: Long-term results of EORTC trial 40891. *Annals of Surgery, 246*(5), 734–740. DOI: 10.1097/SLA.0b013e318156eef3 PMID: 17968163

Song, K. B., Kim, S. C., Hwang, D. W., Lee, J. H., Lee, D. J., Lee, J. W., Park, K.-M., & Lee, Y.-J. (2015). Matched case-control analysis comparing laparoscopic and open pylorus-preserving pancreaticoduodenectomy in patients with periampullary tumors. *Annals of Surgery, 262*(1), 146–155. DOI: 10.1097/SLA.0000000000001079 PMID: 25563866

Soo, R. A., Yong, W. P., & Innocenti, F. (2012). Systemic therapies for pancreatic cancer—The role of pharmacogenetics. *Current Drug Targets, 13*(6), 811–828. DOI: 10.2174/138945012800564068 PMID: 22458528

Spring, B. Q., Bryan Sears, R., Zheng, L. Z., Mai, Z., Watanabe, R., Sherwood, M. E., Schoenfeld, D. A., Pogue, B. W., Pereira, S. P., Villa, E., & Hasan, T. (2016). A photoactivatable multi-inhibitor nanoliposome for tumour control and simultaneous inhibition of treatment escape pathways. *Nature Nanotechnology, 11*(4), 378–387. DOI: 10.1038/nnano.2015.311 PMID: 26780659

Stromnes, I., Brockenbrough, J., Izeradjene, K., Carlson, M. A., Cuevas, C., Simmons, R. M., Greenberg, P. D., & Hingorani, S. R. (2014). Targeted depletion of an MDSC subset unmasks pancreatic ductal adenocarcinoma to adaptive immunity. *Gut, 63*(11), 1769–1781. DOI: 10.1136/gutjnl-2013-306271 PMID: 24555999

Tangutoori, S., Spring, B. Q., Mai, Z., Palanisami, A., Mensah, L. B., & Hasan, T. (2016). Simultaneous delivery of cytotoxic and biologic therapeutics using nanophotoactivatable liposomes enhances treatment efficacy in a mouse model of pancreatic cancer. *Nanomedicine (London), 12*(1), 223–234. DOI: 10.1016/j.nano.2015.08.007 PMID: 26390832

Tarannum, M., Holtzman, K., Dréau, D., Mukherjee, P., & Vivero-Escoto, J. L. (2022). Nanoparticle combination for precise stroma modulation and improved delivery for pancreatic cancer. *Journal of Controlled Release, 347*(1), 425–434. DOI: 10.1016/j.jconrel.2022.05.019 PMID: 35569588

Teng, T., Lin, R., Lin, Z., Ke, K., Lin, X., Pan, M., Zhang, D., & Huang, H. (2020). Photothermal augment stromal disrupting effects for enhanced Abraxane synergy chemotherapy in pancreatic cancer PDX model. *Biomaterials Science, 8*(12), 3278–3285. DOI: 10.1039/D0BM00549E PMID: 32355947

Thapa, R. K., Nguyen, H. T., Gautam, M., Shrestha, A., Lee, E. S., Ku, S. K., Choi, H.-G., Yong, C. S., & Kim, J. O. (2017). Hydrophobic binding peptide-conjugated hybrid lipid-mesoporous silica nanoparticles for effective chemo-photothermal therapy of pancreatic cancer. *Drug Delivery*, *24*(1), 1690–1702. DOI: 10.1080/10717544.2017.1396382 PMID: 29098877

Wang, S., Zheng, Y., Yang, F., Zhu, L., Zhu, X., Wang, Z., Wu, X.-L., Zhou, C.-H., Yan, J.-Y., Hu, B.-Y., Kong, B., Fu, D.-L., Bruns, C., Zhao, Y., Qin, L.-X., & Dong, Q.-Z. (2021). The molecular biology of pancreatic adenocarcinoma: Translational challenges and clinical perspectives. *Signal Transduction and Targeted Therapy*, *6*(1), 1–23. DOI: 10.1038/s41392-021-00659-4 PMID: 34219130

Wolfgang, C. L., Herman, J. M., Laheru, D. A., Klein, A. P., Erdek, M. A., Fishman, E. K., & Hruban, R. H. (2013). Recent progress in pancreatic cancer. *CA: a Cancer Journal for Clinicians*, *63*(5), 318–348. DOI: 10.3322/caac.21190 PMID: 23856911

Xie, Y., Hang, Y., Wang, Y., Sleightholm, R., Prajapati, D. R., Bader, J., Yu, A., Tang, W., Jaramillo, L., Li, J., Singh, R. K., & Oupický, D. (2020). Stromal modulation and treatment of metastatic pancreatic cancer with local intraperitoneal triple miRNA/siRNA nanotherapy. *ACS Nano*, *14*(1), 255–271. DOI: 10.1021/acsnano.9b03978 PMID: 31927946

Xu, K., Jin, L., Xu, L., Zhu, Y., Hong, L., Pan, C., Li, Y., Yao, J., Zou, R., Tang, W., Wang, J., Wu, A., & Ren, W. (2022). IGF1 receptor-targeted black TiO2 nanoprobes for MRI-guided synergetic photothermal-chemotherapy in drug resistant pancreatic tumor. *Journal of Nanobiotechnology*, *20*(1), 315–316. DOI: 10.1186/s12951-022-01525-3 PMID: 35794573

Yang, C., Chan, K., Xu, G., Yin, M., Lin, G., Wang, X., Lin, W.-J., Birowosuto, M. D., Zeng, S., Ogi, T., Okuyama, K., Permatasari, F. A., Iskandar, F., Chen, C.-K., & Yong, K.-T. (2019). Biodegradable polymer-coated multifunctional graphene quantum dots for light-triggered synergetic therapy of pancreatic cancer. *ACS Applied Materials & Interfaces*, *11*(3), 2768–2781. DOI: 10.1021/acsami.8b16168 PMID: 30589254

Ychou, M., Conroy, T., Seitz, J. F., Gourgou, S., Hua, A., Mery-Mignard, D., & Kramar, A. (2003). An open phase I study assessing the feasibility of the triple combination: Oxaliplatin plus irinotecan plus leucovorin/5-fluorouracil every 2 weeks in patients with advanced solid tumors. *Annals of Oncology : Official Journal of the European Society for Medical Oncology*, *14*(3), 481–489. DOI: 10.1093/annonc/mdg119 PMID: 12598357

Yin, F., Hu, K., Chen, Y., Yu, M., Wang, D., Wang, Q., Yong, K.-T., Lu, F., Liang, Y., & Li, Z. (2017). siRNA delivery with PEGylated graphene oxide nanosheets for combined photothermal and gene therapy for pancreatic cancer. *Theranostics*, *7*(5), 1133–1148. DOI: 10.7150/thno.17841 PMID: 28435453

Yin, F., Yang, C., Wang, Q., Zeng, S., Hu, R., Lin, G., Tian, J., Hu, S., Lan, R. F., Yoon, H. S., Lu, F., Wang, K., & Yong, K.-T. (2015). A light-driven therapy of pancreatic adenocarcinoma using gold nanorods-based nanocarriers for co-delivery of doxorubicin and siRNA. *Theranostics*, *5*(8), 818–833. DOI: 10.7150/thno.11335 PMID: 26000055

Zhan, X., Nie, X., Gao, F., Zhang, C., You, Y.-Z., & Yu, Y. (2020). An NIR-activated polymeric nanoplatform with ROS- and temperature-sensitivity for combined photothermal therapy and chemotherapy of pancreatic cancer. *Biomaterials Science*, *8*(21), 5931–5940. DOI: 10.1039/D0BM01324B PMID: 32966381

Zhang, Z., Gao, S., Xu, Y., & Zhao, C. (2021). Regulation of ABCG2 expression by Wnt5a through FZD7 in human pancreatic cancer cells. *Molecular Medicine Reports*, *23*(1), 1–11. DOI: 10.3892/mmr.2020.11690 PMID: 33200805

Zhao, Z., Zheng, L., Chen, W., Weng, W., Song, J., & Ji, J. (2019). Delivery strategies of cancer immunotherapy: Recent advances and future perspectives. *Journal of Hematology & Oncology*, *12*(1), 126–127. DOI: 10.1186/s13045-019-0817-3 PMID: 31779642

Zhou, F., Yang, J., Zhang, Y., Liu, M., Lang, M. L., Li, M., & Chen, W. R. (2018). Local phototherapy synergizes with immunoadjuvant for treatment of pancreatic cancer through induced immunogenic tumor vaccine. *Clinical Cancer Research*, *24*(21), 5335–5346. DOI: 10.1158/1078-0432.CCR-18-1126 PMID: 30068705

Chapter 8
Adjuvants and Their Role in the Treatment of Pancreatic Cancer

K. Kesavardhini
Department of Microbiology, Sacred Heart College, Tirupattur, India

A. Sabina Banu
Department of Microbiology, Sacred Heart College, Tirupattur, India

P. Saranraj
https://orcid.org/0000-0002-5052-6532
Department of Microbiology, Sacred Heart College, Tirupattur, India

ABSTRACT

Pancreatic cancer is one of the most aggressive and lethal malignancies, characterized by poor prognosis and limited therapeutic options. Despite advancements in surgical techniques and systemic therapies, the five-year survival rate remains dismal. Adjuvant has emerged as crucial components in the multidisciplinary treatment approach for pancreatic cancer, offering the potential to enhance therapeutic efficacy and improve patient outcomes. Adjuvants, substances that enhance the effects of primary therapies, play a pivotal role in the management of pancreatic cancer. These include Chemotherapy, Radiotherapy, Immunotherapy, and Targeted agents, Radiotherapy, often used as an Adjuvant to Systemic treatments, provides local control by targeting Residual cancer cells in the tumor bed. Additionally, advancements in Immunotherapy including Immune inhibitors and Cancer vaccines overcoming the Immune-suppressive tumor Microenvironment of Pancreatic Cancer. Targeted therapies, focusing on Mutations and DNA damage repair. Moreover, the integration of precision medicine and biomarker-driven approaches is refining the

DOI: 10.4018/979-8-3373-1469-3.ch008

use of Adjuvants, enabling personalized treatment strategies. Challenges remain, including resistance to therapy, toxicity, and the heterogeneity of pancreatic tumors. In conclusion, adjuvants are integral to the contemporary management of pancreatic cancer, providing a pathway to improved survival and quality of life transforming the therapeutic application of this disease.

1. INTRODUCTION

Pancreatic cancer, an aggressive form of cancer characterized by late diagnosis and poor prognosis, generally refers to Pancreatic Ductal Adenocarcinoma (PDAC) that has the highest metastatic capacity and resistance against conventional treatment, admiring the name of one of the deadliest cancers. Adjuvant therapy is a type of therapy given after surgical resection to eliminate micro metastatic disease, decrease chances of recurrence, and improve overall survival (Bray et al., 2018). The modalities already established in the treatment of pancreatic cancer in the adjuvant setting include Chemotherapy, Radiation Therapy, Targeted Therapy, and Immunotherapy with a reasonable scientific rationale for prolonging survival and delaying recurrence. Chemotherapy (particularly Gemcitabine and Fluorouracil-based regimens) forms the cornerstone of Adjuvant treatment and trials including the ESPAC-4 trial have demonstrated an association with improved survival and combination Chemotherapy (such as gemcitabine and capecitabine). More recently, modified FOLFIRINOX consisting of 5-fluorouracil, leucovorin, irinotecan, and oxaliplatin had been the trial for superior to Gemcitabine monotherapy with respect to overall survival.

The role of Adjuvant Chemoradiotherapy remains controversial, with some phase 3 trials showing no survival benefit, although it may benefit select high-risk patients with positive surgical margins. The emergence of Targeted therapies, such as KRAS inhibitors specifically for the mutation occurring in >90% of patients with PDAC, is likely to give rise to a more personalized therapeutic regimen. Nevertheless, Immunotherapeutic approaches such as PD-1/PD-L1 and CTLA-4 immune blockade are under investigation to overcome the immune suppressive microenvironment of pancreatic cancer. It also shown the GVAX and agnatical-L, both vaccine-based therapies, were designed to activate the immune response against Pancreatic Adenocarcinoma Cells (Neoptolemos et al., 2018). Such as Chemoresistance, Intertumoral Heterogeneity, and the Fibrotic stroma that obstructs Drug delivery. Novel combination strategies, biomarker-based patient selection, and multimodal integration are paving the way towards maximizing Therapeutic potency. The success of novel Adjuvant Therapies can lead to improved survival and enhanced quality of life in patients with Pancreatic Cancer (Klaiber et al., 2018).

Pancreatic Cancer persists to be among the aggressive and most mortal subtypes of malignancy, characterized as late-stage diagnosis, poor prognosis, and has limited clinical applications. The 5years survival rate of patients with Pancreatic Ductal Adeno Carcinoma (PDAC) remains less than 10% despite minor advances in Surgical resection, Chemotherapy, Radiotherapy, and Targeted therapies. Most of the mortality associated with Pancreatic Cancer results from the asymptomatic development, high metastatic potential, and intrinsic resistance to standard Cancer therapies (Cress et al., 2006). Adjuvant therapy is being applied post-surgical resection to eliminate microscopic residual disease, lower recurrence, and enhance overall survival is a critical part for improvement in treatment. Adjuvants in pancreatic cancer include Chemotherapy, Radiation, Immunotherapy, and new molecular targeted approaches (Farnell et al., 2005).

Adjuvant therapies primarily comprise chemotherapeutic agents like gemcitabine and fluoropyrimidine-based regimens (5-pruoroucil (5FU) and leucovorin) either alone or with the addition of oxaliplatin (e.g. FOLFIRINOX) or irinotecan. Radiation therapy is used in select patients to reduce local recurrence, particularly in patients with margin-positive resections. Therapeutic vaccines, dendritic cell-based therapies, and immune checkpoint inhibitors and adjuvants are used for their ability to modulate the tumour microenvironment and transform the Antitumor Immunity (Van Heek et al., 2005). The adjuvant-basedtherapieson targeted agents in the BRCA-Mutated Pancreatic Cancer (Type I) had been recently developed of molecular profiling, specific tyrosine kinase-inhibitor in some Molecular sub-types. Some advances had been made with nanoparticle-enabled drug delivery systems and new combination therapies that have the potential to overcome chemo resistance and improve drug bioavailability. They remain with optimizing adjuvant therapy to patient selection and treatment-related toxicities, and identifying reliable biomarkers associated with the Tumour Mediated Response. The precision of these Adjuvant therapies (Table 1) may be enhanced by analysis of multi-omics, including Genomics, Proteomics and Metabolomics (Lowenfels et al., 2001).

Table 1. Different Adjuvants and Their Efficacy in Treating Pancreatic Cancer

Adjuvant	Mechanism of Action	Key Clinical Trials	Efficacy Outcomes	Reference
Gemcitabine	Nucleoside analog; inhibits DNA synthesis, leading to apoptosis	CONKO-001	Median disease-free survival increased from 6.9 to 13.4 months compared to observation	Oettle et al. (2013)
5-Fluorouracil (5-FU) + Leucovorin	Antimetabolite; inhibits thymidylate synthase disrupting DNA synthesis	ESPAC-1	5-year survival improved to ~21% compared to 8% for surgery alone	Neoptolemos et al. (2001)
Gemcitabine + Capecitabine	Capecitabine is an oral prodrug of 5-FU, enhances cytotoxicity	ESPAC-4	Median overall survival improved to 28.0 months vs 25.5 months with gemcitabine alone	Neoptolemos et al. (2017)
Modified FOLFIRINOX	Combination of 5-FU, leucovorin, irinotecan, and oxaliplatin; multi-targeted cytotoxic effect	PRODIGE 24/CCTG PA.6	Median overall survival improved to 54.4 months vs 35.0 months with gemcitabine	Conroy et al. (2018)

2. PANCREATIC CANCER

The aggressive behavior and poor prognosis of pancreatic cancer well explains why extensive adjuvant therapy interventions after surgical resection are necessary to enhance survival and the advent of the chemotherapy use which is now part of the post surgical management, the CONKO-001 trial was the landmark trial that showed gemcitabine monotherapy as a standard treatment given a significant advancement in disease-free survival (Oettle et al., 2007) as supported by the ESPAC-4 trial which further showed increased survival advantage with gemcitabine: a low level of toxic The revolution in the treatment paradigm was also carried on by the PRODIGE 24 trial that associated a significant survival advantage of modified FOLFIRINOX (mFOLFIRINOX) over and above gemcitabine in terms of disease-free survival and overall survival, though with higher toxicity necessitating the selection of patients carefully (Conroy et al., 2018). Despite a decreased tendency to use adjuvant chemoradiation due to contradicting proofs of trial experiments, such as ESPAC-1 (Table 2) which did not demonstrate any advantage in survival when compared with chemotherapy agents alone (Neoptolemos et al., 2001), it can be used in cases of positive margins (R1 resection) or other high-risk features or capecitabine-based regimens with radiations. The emergence of targeted therapies in the has shown its potential in the context of adjuvant settings, especially in patients with molecular selection based on the POLO trial wherein a PARP inhibitor, in this case, olaparib, was demonstrated to enhance progression-free survival of germline BRCA-mutated pancreatic cancer after undergoing platinum-based chemotherapy, whereas, in immunotherapy, even though it exhibited only a limited efficacy in unselected pancreatic adenocarcinoma, the prototype of The growing adoption of neoadjuvant treatment of Locally advanced disease, with the aim of increasing resection rates using regimens such as FOLFIRINOX and gemcitabine/nab-paclitaxel must also have affected the adjuvant strategies, including the development of predictive biomarkers against personalized therapy as well as surgical margins, lymph node status, and molecular profiling to achieve better results in this difficult disease.

Table 2. The effect of CRT in the ESPAC-1 trial

Trial/ Analysis	Group	n	Median Survival (months)	2 years Survival (%)	5 years Survival (%)
ESPAC-1 (Interim analysis, 2001)	CRT	175	15.5	24.6	–
	No CRT	178	16.1	23.5	–
ESPAC-1 (2×2 factorial, final analysis, 2004)	CRT	145	15.9	29	10
	No CRT	144	17.9 ($p = 0.05$)	41	20
ESPAC-1 (Individual groups)	CRT	73	13.9	21.7	7.3
	Observation	69	16.9	38.7	10.7

3. TYPES OF PANCREATIC CANCER

3.1. Pancreatic Ductal Adenocarcinoma

Pancreatic ductal adenocarcinoma (PDAC) that constitutes approximately 90 percent of pancreatic cancer is considered one of the least survivable and most aggressive cancers whose adjuvant care plays a critical role in postoperative outcomes enhancement. There are three histological types of pancreatic cancer: the most common and fatal, PDAC, 1-2 percent of the rare and usually less far-reaching PNETs and cystic neoplasms, including IPMNs and MCNs, with a variable malignant potential. This amounted to 86.5 percent of the investments. The CONKO-001 study showed the observational efficacy of gemcitabine monotherapy in PDAC as an adjuvant drug and it was more effective in terms of median disease-free survival and favoured 5 years survival rates, than observation therapy. The introduction of the PRODIGE 24 trial also altered the treatment scene, as a disease-free and overall survival with additional toxicity left to be achieved by the selection of the patients

(Conroy et al., 2018). The adjuvant chemoradiation previously in common use has had its ESPAC-1 trial that proved no survival advantage over chemotherapy alone (Neoptolemos et al., 2001) reduce its usage, but can be utilised in accordance with the presence of other high-risk characteristics. The targeted treatments has ushered new approaches of precision medicine, among which is olaparib, a PARP inhibitor, that has shown better progression-free survival in cases of germline BRCA-mutated pancreatic cancer patients, as identified in the POLO trial. Although there has been only limited efficacy with immunotherapy in the PDAC (Figure 1), checkpoint inhibitors have been shown to exhibit activity in the rare mismatch repair-deficient (dMMR) or micro satellite instability-high (MSI-H) subtypes. Locally advanced disease is locally treated by neoadjuvant strategies with FOLFIRINOX or gemcitabine/nab-paclitaxel with the potential to promote resection. The current limitations involve maximizing exact patient selection, dealing with treatment toxicity, as well as development of predicting biomarkers, and promise to solve amongst ourselves the stromal-targeting agents and immunotherapies as well as novel treatments.

Figure 1. Vaccine Adjuvant for Immunotherapy

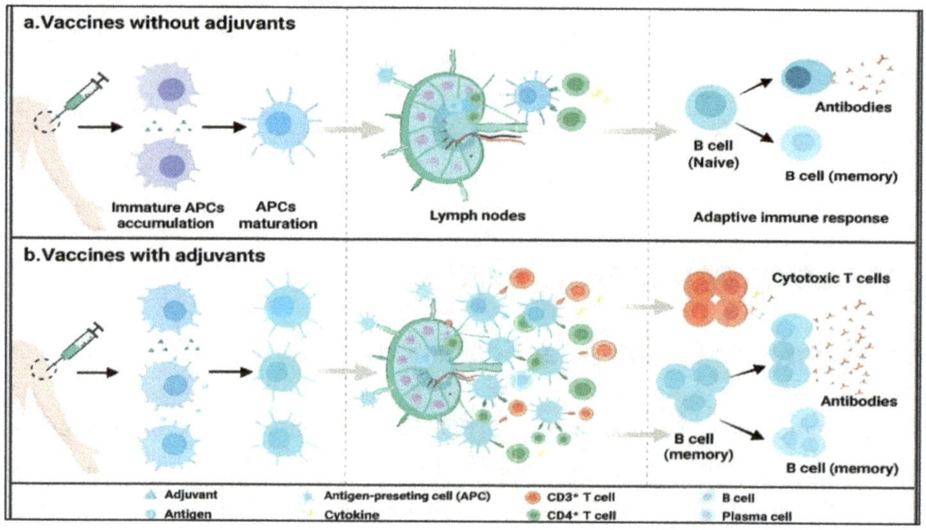

3.2. Pancreatic Neuroendocrine Tumours

Pancreatic neuroendocrine tumors (PNETs), also known as islet cell tumors, represent a distinct subset of pancreatic cancers, accounting for approximately 1-2% of all pancreatic malignancies, and are characterized by their origin from the hormone-producing cells of the pancreas, such as insulinomas, gastrinomas, and glucagonomas (Halfdanarson et al., 2008; Klimstra et al., 2010). Unlike pancreatic adenocarcinoma, PNETs often exhibit a more indolent course and better prognosis, with survival rates varying significantly based on tumor grade, stage, and functional status (Falconi et al., 2016). The treatment of PNETs typically involves a multimodal approach, including surgery, which remains the only curative option for localized disease, while systemic therapies, such as somatostatin analogs (e.g., octreotide and lanreotide), targeted agents (e.g., everolimus and sunitinib), and peptide receptor radionuclide therapy (PRRT), play critical roles in managing advanced or metastatic disease (Strosberg et al., 2017; Yao et al., 2016). Adjuvant therapy, although less established for PNETs compared to pancreatic adenocarcinoma, may be considered in high-risk cases, such as those with lymph node involvement or positive margins, with some evidence supporting the use of somatostatin analogs or targeted therapies to reduce recurrence (Pavel et al., 2020). The role of chemotherapy, particularly streptozocin-based regimens, remains controversial but may be employed in poorly differentiated or aggressive PNETs (Koumarianou et al., 2017). Recent advances in molecular profiling have identified potential biomarkers, such as MEN1, DAXX, and ATRX mutations, which may guide personalized adjuvant strategies (Scarpa et al., 2017). Despite these developments, clinical trials focusing specifically on adjuvant therapies for PNETs are limited, underscoring the need for further research to optimize treatment paradigms (Shah et al., 2021). In summary, while PNETs are relatively rare, their heterogeneous biology necessitates tailored adjuvant approaches, with ongoing studies aiming to refine the use of existing therapies and explore novel agents to improve outcomes for patients with this complex disease.

3.3. Acinar Cell Carcinoma

Acinar cell carcinoma (ACC) is a rare and aggressive subtype of pancreatic cancer, accounting for only 1 - 2% of all exocrine pancreatic malignancies, characterized by its distinct histological features and acinar cell differentiation, which often produces pancreatic enzymes such as trypsin, lipase, and amylase, leading to paraneoplastic syndromes like lipase hypersecretion syndrome in some patients (Wisnoski et al., 2008; La Rosa et al., 2016). Unlike Pancreatic ductal adenocarcinoma (PDAC), ACC typically presents with larger tumor sizes, a higher propensity for liver metastases, and a slightly better prognosis, with a median survival of approximately 36 months in resectable cases, though outcomes remain poor for advanced disease (Schmidt et al., 2007; Klimstra et al., 1992). Surgical resection remains the cornerstone of treatment for localized ACC, offering the only potential for cure, while adjuvant therapy though not as well-defined as in PDAC may include fluorouracil (5-FU)-based or gemcitabine-based chemotherapy regimens, with some evidence suggesting improved survival in patients receiving postoperative treatment (Lowery et al., 2011; Hester et al., 2020). For advanced or metastatic disease, systemic chemotherapy remains the primary approach, with regimens such as FOLFIRINOX (5-FU, leucovorin, irinotecan, and oxaliplatin) or gemcitabine plus nab-paclitaxel showing modest efficacy, though response rates are generally lower than in PDAC due to ACC's distinct biology (Hentic et al., 2012; Jiao et al., 2018). Targeted therapies and clinical trials exploring molecular alterations, such as alterations in the BRCA, PALB2, or DNA repair pathways, are under investigation, given the rarity of ACC and the lack of standardized treatment protocols (Agnihotri et al., 2021). Additionally, radiation therapy may play a palliative role in symptomatic control, though its use in the adjuvant setting is not well-established (Basturk et al., 2015). Given the rarity of ACC, most evidence derives from small retrospective studies or case series, highlighting the need for multicenter collaborations and prospective trials to refine adjuvant and systemic treatment strategies (Matthaei et al., 2012). Emerging research into the tumor's molecular profile, including recurrent APC/β-catenin pathway mutations and BRAF alterations, may pave the way for personalized therapies, such as EGFR or MEK inhibitors, though clinical validation is still pending (Abraham et al., 2002; Singhi et al., 2017). In summary, while ACC is a rare and poorly understood malignancy, aggressive surgical resection followed by adjuvant chemotherapy appears to offer survival benefits in select cases, with ongoing research needed to define optimal systemic therapies and explore targeted approaches for this unique pancreatic cancer subtype.

3.4. Colloid Carcinoma

Colloid carcinoma (CC), also known as mucinous non-cystic adenocarcinoma, is a rare variant of pancreatic cancer accounting for 1-3% of exocrine pancreatic malignancies, distinguished by its abundant extracellular mucin production comprising more than 50% of the tumor volume and frequent association with intestinal-type intraductal papillary mucinous neoplasms (IPMNs) (Adsay et al., 2001; Mino-Kenudson et al., 2010). This tumor type exhibits a markedly better prognosis compared to conventional pancreatic ductal adenocarcinoma (PDAC), with 5-year survival rates approaching 50 – 60% after resection, attributed to its indolent biological behavior and lower propensity for lymph node metastasis (Seidel et al., 2002). The molecular profile of CC is characterized by frequent GNAS mutations (seen in 40 – 60% of cases) and KRAS mutations (30 – 50%), while TP53 and SMAD4 alterations are less common than in PDAC, explaining its distinct clinical behavior (Wu et al., 2011; Furukawa et al., 2014). Surgical resection remains the mainstay of treatment for localized CC, with some studies suggesting that even node-positive cases may benefit from aggressive resection due to the tumor's favorable biology (Allen et al., 2006). The role of adjuvant therapy in CC is controversial due to its rarity, but current guidelines often recommend following PDAC protocols with gemcitabine or fluorouracil-based regimens for high-risk cases, particularly those with lymph node involvement or positive margins (Winter et al., 2013; Tempero et al., 2021). Notably, emerging evidence suggests CC may be less responsive to conventional chemotherapy than PDAC, prompting investigations into targeted approaches against mucin signaling pathways or *GNAS*-related mechanisms (Kaur et al., 2013). For advanced disease, combination regimens like FOLFIRINOX have shown some activity, though response rates appear lower than in PDAC, possibly due to the protective barrier created by abundant mucin. Recent studies highlight the potential of immunotherapy in CC, particularly in tumors with microsatellite instability (found in 5 – 10% of cases) or high tumor mutational burden, though clinical data remain limited (Hu et al., 2020). The tumor's unique extracellular matrix composition has also spurred interest in stroma-targeting agents and mucolytic therapies to enhance drug delivery (Provenzano et al., 2012). Diagnostic challenges persist, as preoperative differentiation from PDAC or mucinous cystic neoplasms can be difficult, often requiring immunohistochemical analysis (positive for MUC2 and CDX2, typically negative for MUC1) for definitive diagnosis (Yopp et al., 2011). Given CC's distinct molecular and clinical features, future clinical trials should consider stratifying pancreatic cancer subtypes rather than grouping all non-PDAC variants together, as current adjuvant protocols may not be optimal for this entity (Basturk et al., 2015). Ongoing research into the tumor's mucin biology and GNAS signaling may yield more tailored therapeutic strategies, potentially including MEK inhibitors or mucin-suppressing agents. In summary, while colloid carcinoma represents a more favorable pancreatic cancer subtype, optimal adjuvant approaches remain undefined, underscoring the need for subtype-specific studies to refine treatment paradigms for this rare mucin-producing malignancy.

4. NEOADJUVANT THERAPY

Neo-adjuvant therapy for pancreatic cancer that uses many patients are not candidates for adjuvant therapy because of postoperative complications. The incidence of postoperative incidence following major pancreatic resections remains in the range of 30 – 45% despite the substantially decreased postoperative mortality. Neo -adjuvant therapy with advanced loco - regional tumors are able to obtain a greater resection rates (Lowenfels et al., 1997). There have been large randomized controlled trials in neo-adjuvant therapy of Pancreatic Cancer. The number of patients actually had resection after neo-adjuvant therapy is quite small. Median survival rates typically range from 16 to 21 months is equivalent to both Adjuvant Systemic Chemotherapy and Regional Chemotherapy.

Table 3. Ongoing Adjuvant and Neoadjuvant studies in Pancreatic cancer

Study name	Study design	Treatment regimens	Primary outcome
NCT00058201: ESPAC-3	Randomised Phase III	5-FU bolus plus folinic acid (leucovorin) versus gemcitabine	Overall 2 years survival rate
NCT00064207: Gemcitabine and radiation therapy compared with gemcitabine alone after curative pancreatic oduodenectomy	Randomised Phase II/III	Adjuvant gemcitabine plus radiation versus gemcitabine alone	Feasibility and tolerability in Phase II; disease-free and overall survival in Phase III
NCT00068575: A trial of postoperative cisplatin, interferon, 5-FU with radiotherapy for patients with resected pancreatic adenocarcinoma	Open-label Phase II and open-label Phase III trials	Chemoradiation (5-FU, cisplatin, IFN-α plus concurrent radiotherapy) followed by chemotherapy (continuous infusion of 5-FU)	Overall survival
NCT00426738: A multi-institutional Phase II study of neoadjuvant gemcitabine and oxaliplatin with radiation therapy in patients with pancreatic cancer	Non-randomised, open-label Phase II	Neoadjuvant gemcitabine and oxaliplatin with concurrent radiation	2-year disease-free survival
NCT00335543: Preoperative chemoradiation in locally resectable adenocarcinoma of the pancreatic head without metastasis	Randomised, open-label Phase II	Neoadjuvant gemcitabine, cisplatin, and radiation followed by surgery versus surgery alone	Median survival
NCT00300950: Adjuvant trial of the efficacy, immunogenicity, and safety of GI-4000	Randomised, double-blind Phase II	Therapeutic vaccine GI-4000 plus gemcitabine versus gemcitabine plus placebo	Safety and efficacy
NCT00336648: A pilot study of preoperative gemcitabine and bevacizumab-based chemoradiation for patients with resectable adenocarcinoma of the pancreas	Non-randomised, open-label Phase II	Neoadjuvant gemcitabine and bevacizumab-based chemoradiation	Resectability rate
NCT00276744: A feasibility study for individualised treatment of patients with advanced pancreatic cancer	Open-label Phase II	Individualised adjuvant treatment with one of the following drugs: bortezomib, capecitabine, cetuximab, docetaxel, erlotinib, gemcitabine, irinotecan, mitomycin C, sirolimus or thalidomide	Feasibility

5. CHEMOTHERAPY

Pancreatic cancer is one of the most aggressive tumours with a poor prognosis, late diagnosis, early metastatic, and ineffective treatment. Adjuvant chemotherapy contributes significantly to improve survival after surgical resection remains that the only approach for localized pancreatic cancer (Wong et al., 2001). Adjuvant chemotherapy is given to eliminate microscopic residual disease, decrease the risk of recurrence, and improve overall survival. Gemcitabine and 5-fluorouracil (5-FU) have been the traditional bases for agents used in adjuvant settings, with gemcitabine showed advantages in survival advantage and tolerability. Combination regimens including modified FOLFIRINOX (5-FU, leucovorin, irinotecan and oxaliplatin) have demonstrated a marked benefit in disease-free survival and overall survival compared with Gemcitabine Immunotherapy. The high recurrence rates after complete surgical resection, the role of Adjuvant Chemotherapy is of particular importance. Micro metastases are not usually done during surgery and if not sufficiently treated (Breslin et al., 2001). The use of chemotherapy with immune inhibitors or targeted therapies is the impact of immune checkpoint inhibitors used with chemotherapy report positive outcomes, but clinical efficacy is still being investigated. New strategies such as algo rhythms for genomic profiling are being developed to customize adjuvant treatment to individual tumour biology as well as biomarker-based drugs.

The impact of adjuvant chemotherapy on the patient is a significant concern an 86% relative increase in survival is insufficient. Although targeted regimens, like Folfirinox, have a higher toxicity profile, they offer a better survival advantage, supportive care strategies. Adjuvant chemotherapy should be prescribed based on the status of the patients, comorbidities, and conditions at discharge (Regine, 2001). Even though research is still being done to determine the optimal Adjuvant therapy regimen in terms of duration, sequencing, and combinatorial approaches, the objective is always the same to maximize benefits that minimizing harm. Adjuvant chemotherapy represents an essential part of the overall treatment of pancreatic cancer, offering a survival benefit with surgical programmes. Recent innovations in combination regimens, personalized therapy, and novel therapeutic strategies will continue the evolution of adjuvant treatment strategies. More studies and clinical trials are needed to maximize treatment efficacy and minimize toxicity and to improve long-term patient outcomes in Pancreatic cancer management.

5.1. Advanced Pancreatic Cancer

Both single agents and combination regimens have been utilized. Currently, there is a no standard Chemotherapeutic agents for the treatment of Pancreatic cancer

(Mehta et al., 2001). The most potent and commonly used single Chemotherapy agent remains 5 - fluorouracil. 5-FU acts primarily through inhibition of enzymes like Thymidylate synthase and partially by the 5-FU metabolites into DNA and RNA (Haycox et al., 1998). In order to develop modulators had been the addition of folinic acid that shown to just marginally improve the on-treatment survival of patients on 5-FU at the cost of higher toxicity. Other potential modulators, such as Phosphonacetyl-L-aspartate (PALA), and interferon had not been associated either with significant improvements in survival. In randomized trials of 5-FU, there has been no advantage seen for a combined approach versus 5-FU alone (Haycox et al. 1998).

Gemcitabine had been compared with 5-FU in randomised multi-center Phase III clinical trial. Gemcitabine is a deoxycytidine analogue that is phosphorylated to an active form and competes with dCTP to be incorporated into the DNA. Averagely, 70% of patients had Stage IV disease 63 were randomized to receive gemcitabine and 63 to receive 5-FU. The gemcitabine group had median survival of 5.7 months and the 5-FU group 4.4 months but no patients survived beyond 19 months. Gemcitabine group also had significantly higher clinical benefit response (Moore et al., 1997). It had been evaluated the combination of Gemcitabine with 5-FU. It is well tolerated in general but unpredictable side effects like neutropoenia, liver function test abnormalities and nausea and vomiting can develop. In patients with previous radiotherapy to the mediastinum unpredictable reactions have been reported (Sauer-Heilborn et al., 1999).

Several randomized controlled trials have demonstrated that chemotherapy is beneficial and compared to no treatment in patients with advanced Pancreatic Cancer. Mallinson et al. (1980) reported a median survival of 11 months in patients treated for 5-FU, Cyclophosphamide, Methotrexate, Vincristine and Mitomycin C versus 2.2 months in the untreated control group. This regimen did not result in a significantly higher survival than 5-FU alone in a much larger randomized control trials. This regimen has a low overall survival benefit of 5-FU, doxorubicin and mitomycin C (FAM) produced median survival of 33 weeks compared with median survival of 15 weeks in untreated control patients.

5.2. Adjuvant Chemotherapy

Adjuvant Chemotherapy for Pancreatic Cancer have been done with ESPAC-1 trial, there had only been one randomized controlled trial comparing Surgery and Chemotherapy with Surgery. FAM regimen in 16 patients had undergone Pancreatoduodenectomy. Three-year survival was 24% versus three-year survival of 28%, in 36 patients had undergone surgery. Patients from two different eras were included in each group and there were only nine patients with pancreatic ductal adenocarcinoma in the adjuvant group and 18 in the surgery only group. Baumel et al. (1994) examined use of Adjuvant Chemotherapy in 43 of selected patients with a median survival of 12 months but no difference in median survival than those patients underwent surgery alone (12 months). Bakkevold et al. (1993) randomized 61 patients with previous Pancreatoduodenectomy for Pancreatic Cancer or Ampullary Cancer to six courses of FAM versus no Chemotherapy. The median survival between groups differed significantly: 23 months. The FAM regimen was also associated with quite a bit of toxicity. Of the 30 patients were randomized to treatment, only 24 patients started therapy.

6. RADIOTHERAPY

Pancreatic Cancer is a highly aggressive malignant tumour with a poor prognosis due to the failure of diagnosis, rapid metastasis, and low therapeutic activity. Surgical resection is the only potential therapy for localized neoplasm of the pancreas, adjuvant cycles of chemoradiation significantly extend survival post incision (Cullinan et al., 1990). Adjuvant chemotherapy is used to kill residual micro disease, decreases the risk of relapse and increases the overall survival. Adjuvant therapy is the most commonly used agents including gemcitabine and 5-fluorouracil (5-FU) that were the most favoured agents for hematologic stability. Combination regimens, including modified FOLFIRINOX (5-FU, leucovorin, irinotecan, oxaliplatin), have been shown to be significantly better than gemcitabine monotherapy in terms of disease-free survival and overall survival in the standard adjuvant regimen.

The primary role of adjuvant radiotherapy is to eradicate residual locoregional disease to lower local recurrence. The advent of IMRT, SBRT and other newer radiation technologies has improved its precision and targeting of delivery to the disease that sparing the adjacent soft tissue and Organ at Risk (OAR) safely. The role of adjuvant chemo radiotherapy in patients with resected Pancreatic Cancer and the impact on their survival outcomes. New treatment strategies, such as Immunotherapy and Targeted therapies, are being explored in the Adjuvants to enhance efficacy over Chemotherapy and Radiotherapy (Glimelius et al., 1996). The clinical applicability of combination therapies that include immune checkpoint inhibitors and the favourable preclinical centre indicated the use of immune checkpoint inhibitors in Conjunction with Chemotherapy. Other new approaches involve Personalized Medicine by using Genomic Profiling and modulation through Biomarkers to match Adjuvant Therapy with the characteristics of the tumour (Splinter et al., 1989).

Regimen combinations such as FOLFIRINOX that offer a significant survival benefit at the increased toxicity require appropriate patient selection and provision of supportive care. Radiotherapy can induce toxicity, including gastrointestinal and hematologic, as well to pursue this treatment modality. Active clinical trials are still in process for the optimal duration, sequencing, and combination of adjuvant therapies to maximize benefit and minimize harm. There is a strong adjuvant therapy-based treatment of Pancreatic Cancer as Surgical Resection of Pancreatic Cancer is gaining its survival due to the multicentre and aggressive nature of the cancer and that demonstrates that improved survival can be obtained Adjuvant Chemotherapy and Radio Therapy are applied post-resection with patients compared to patients with these types of therapies.

6.1. Advanced Pancreatic Cancer

EBRT (External Beam Radiation Therapy) is of use against advanced pancreatic cancer but it has never been examined in a randomized controlled trial against non-treated patients(non-EBRT). 5-Fluorouracil (5-FU), of the drugs available is the most common and effective radio-sensitizer used with EBRT for advanced Pancreatic Cancer (Gunderson et al., 1995). There has been no sustained improvement in overall survival time with the improved local control of disease afforded by EBRT, there have been numerous refinements and the efficacy of radiotherapy. Hepatic micro metastases have been treated with irradiation therapy. RTOG (Radiation Therapy Oncology Group) study involving 79 patients with irradiation of the pancreatic and hepatic regions was associated with a median survival of 8.4 months but a significant amount of toxicity. IORT (Intraoperative Radiation Therapy) aims to deliver higher doses of Radiotherapy more conformably away from Adjacent organs. This method is 2.5-5 times more effective than EBRT delivered at the same dose equivalent. The clinical use of IORT in Advanced Pancreatic Cancer (median survival 6 months) and its use has been primarily adjunctive to EBRT (Gunderson et al., 1987). A trial comparing EBRT + IORT + 5-FU vs. EBRT + 5-FU failed to demonstrate a significant difference in survival (12 and 13 months, respectively).

6.2. Adjuvant Radiotherapy

Adjuvant EBRT and IORT have been used as either single modalities or in combination in the adjuvant treatment of pancreatic cancer. EBRT with or without IORT has a substantial survival benefit in the IORT. The IORT had a 50% reduction in the local recurrence rate after surgery in a randomized trial, but no clinical survival benefit (I.E., 3-year survival with IORT = 7% vs no IORT 3%). In selected patients, three and 5years survival rates of 53% and 29% were achieved with IORT and resection. It also needs IORT-specialized facilities and may be associated with serious complications (Hiraoka, 1990).

EBRT (with concomitant chemotherapy) for resected disease is tolerable and the survival benefits. European Organization for Research and Treatment of Cancer (EORTC) that randomized patients to Chemoradiotherapy and Surgery with potentially curative resection for Pancreatic Cancer (Klinkenbijl et al., 1999). Between 1987 and 1995, 218 patients were randomly assigned to either Chemoradiotherapy or no Chemoradiotherapy following the resection of Pancreatic Cancer. There was also no difference in survival between the treatment and observation groups among patients with ampullary cancer. The Adjuvant Chemoradiotherapy for Pancreatic and Ampullary cancer is no more effective than no treatment (Klinkenbijl et al., 1999).

7. REGIONAL THERAPY

Adjuvant treatments, including Chemotherapy, Radiotherapy, and Immunotherapy, are therefore crucial for survival against these residual Malignant cells. Among these, regional therapy approaches that deliver therapeutic modalities directly to the tumour site or in its immediate Microenvironment have emerged as a strategy to enhance the activity of Systemic Therapies that limiting Systemic Toxicity. The regional therapies refer to different methods such as Intra-Arterial (IA) Chemotherapy, Intraperitoneal (IP) Chemotherapy and Localized Radiation that help to increase Drug concentrations at the tumour. Among the various forms of Regional Therapy in Pancreatic Cancer, Intra-Arterial Chemotherapy (IAC) is one of the more widely used techniques in Chemotherapeutic agents are infused directly into the pancreatic arterial supply (Willett & Warshaw, 1998). This method capitalizes on high intratumor drug concentration that overcomes the low vascularity and desmoplastic stroma of pancreatic tumours that would decrease penetration during conventional systemic therapy. Several IAC regimens evaluated agents such as gemcitabine and fluorouracil, demonstrating superior response rates with systemic delivery alone. Intra-arterial and isolated hepatic perfusion 10 has also been explored in the treatment of patients with pancreatic cancer with liver metastases and increases drug delivery to the hepatic lesions and normal hepatocytes.

Intraperitoneal (IP) Chemotherapy is an additional regional therapy of particular clinical relevance to peritoneal dissemination, an endemic pattern of spread in pancreatic cancer. Both biological and chemotherapy agents are instilled in the peritoneal cavity through a technique known as Hyperthermic Intraperitoneal Chemotherapy (HIPEC) in the chemotherapeutic agents, cisplatin or mitomycin, are given in the time of cytoreduction and under hyperthermic conditions. HIPEC allows drug penetration in normal anatomical, physiological and beneficial factors that also provides time dependent cytotoxic effect from hyperthermia (Jeekel et al., 2006). HIPEC is primarily utilized for peritoneal carcinomatosis from other gastrointestinal malignancies with the pancreatic cancer.

In addition to Chemotherapy, Regional Radiotherapy has been more widely used in patients with Pancreatic Cancer. Stereotactic Body Radiation Therapy (SBRT) is a technique that delivers high-dose, focused irradiation with the goal of preserving Adjacent normal tissue, allowing it to be utilized in advanced disease of the tumour (Bakkevold et al., 1993). SBRT affords local control, as well as possible tumour allowing for surgical resection. Intraoperative Radiation Therapy (IORT) has been also used to reduce local recurrence rate that directly irradiate to tumour bed during surgery.

Regional therapy development's other routes include new drug delivery systems such as nanoparticle-based nanocarriers that can target drug delivery into the tumor and promote better infiltration. These nanocarriers can be tagged with ligands or modified at the surface level to target Pancreatic Cancer cells selectively. Immunotherapeutic approaches are also here developed to promote Antitumor Immunity and minimize Systematic Immunosuppression (Takada et al., 2002). Nevertheless, many difficulties face Clinical Translation of Regional Therapies. Clinical trials with active Pancreatic Cancer treatments abound with emerging technologies seeking improvement of these strategies. Therefore, it is certain Regional Therapies will be integrated with Systemic Chemotherapy and Immunotherapy combinations to counter this deadly disease.

7.1. Advanced Pancreatic Cancer

Adjuvant combined therapy that combines several treatment modalities with the intention to increase therapeutic efficacy continues to both resectable and advanced pancreatic cancer. Adjuvant therapy (administered post-surgical resection) aims to eliminate undetectable residual disease, decrease recurrence risk and increase Overall Survival (OS). In the adjuvant pancreatic cancer had been shifted from single agent approaches with agents like Gemcitabine to Combination Therapy are Chemotherapy, Radiation Therapy, Targeted Therapy, and Immunotherapy (Kosuge et al., 2006). FOLFIRINOX (5-fluorouracil, leucovorin, irinotecan, and oxaliplatin), the most powerful agent, is the used Adjuvant Chemotherapy regimen based on multiagent Chemotherapeutics. PRODIGE 24/CCTG PA trial demonstrated that Adjuvant FOLFIRINOX improved Overall Survival (OS) compared with Gemcitabine (35.0 months *vs* 54.4 months). The toxic profile of FOLFIRINOX has evaluated the exploration of less toxic combinations, including the Gemcitabine plus that exhibited a survival difference in the ESPAC-4 trial. Chemotherapy-based combination involves Gemcitabine in combination with nab-paclitaxel, already widely used in the Metastatic phase and are being evaluated in Adjuvant clinical trials.

Chemoradiotherapy combinations beyond Chemotherapy-based Adjuvant approaches have been evaluated in Pancreatic Cancer. The utility of radiation therapy has been in the advanced radiation techniques that induce the higher radiation doses with less toxicity, including Stereotactic Body Radiation Therapy (SBRT) and Intensity-Modulated Radiation Therapy (IMRT), and as a result Radiotherapy can be done with the Combination Therapy. Radiotherapy with Chemotherapy has been used to reduce local recurrence in the patients. Radiation therapy to Chemotherapy will lead to improved survival with increased level of Pancreatic Cancer (Neoptolemos et al., 2001).

Besides Chemotherapy and Radiation Therapy, Targeted Therapies have become increasingly rational as Adjuvant combination strategies. Pancreatic cancer has a well-defined genomic landscape with around 5 – 7% of patients having functional mutations in BRCA1/2 that impair DNA damage repair pathways. These tumors are particularly sensitive to treatment with platinum-based chemotherapy agents (cisplatin, oxaliplatin) and PARP inhibitors (eg, olaparib, rucaparib). The POLO trial demonstrated that maintenance therapy with the PARP inhibitor Olaparib increased PFS in patients with Pancreatic Cancer and BRCA mutations, leading to the inclusion of PARP inhibitors in adjuvant combinations (Strobel et al., 2019). Some drugs targeting KRAS (sotorasib, adagrasib) and MEK inhibitors (trametinib) are under investigation based on the prevalence of KRAS mutations in >90% of Pancreatic Cancers. KRAS-driven pancreatic tumours present a tough target in the patients. Stroma Modulating Therapy in the form of Adjuvant combination with Anti-angiogenic agents.

Immune Checkpoint Inhibitors (ICIs) are responsive disease and the role of Adjuvant Therapy is still after Cytoreductive surgery has been suggested beneficial in Peritoneal Metastasis of Pancreatic Cancer. Nanotechnology-based drug delivery systems in a potential route for Adjuvant Combination Therapy that could help increase the efficiency of Chemotherapy, improve its Bioavailability, and reduce its Systemic Toxicity. Some agents include Liposomal irinotecan (nal-IRI) and Albumin-bound paclitaxel (nab-paclitaxel) that are associated with clinical applications, as well as new biodegradable Polymeric drug delivery formulations with the potential for sustained Intratumoral Drug Delivery (Oettle et al., 2007). Adjuvant therapy for Pancreatic Cancer should ideally be enhanced by incorporation of Gene Therapy, RNA-based Therapeutics, as well as Tumor-specific vaccine strategies to augment efficacy.

Despite these advances, optimizing Adjuvant Combination Therapy for PC has multiple challenges. Variations in Tumor Heterogeneity, Immune Evasion Mechanisms, and Stromal Resistance warrant a precision medicine-based approach for

Adjuvant treatment regimens to the Tumor Biology in individual patients. Liquid biopsy approaches (e.g., circulating tumor DNA, exosome-based diagnostics) are also under investigation to monitor treatment response and detect Early Resistance Mechanisms. There is a growing role of Artificial Intelligence (AI) and Machine Learning Algorithms in predictive modelling for treatment response, resulting in individualized Adjuvant combination therapy approaches (Neoptolemos et al., 2010). Adjuvant Combination Therapy, including Chemotherapy, Radiotherapy, Targeted Therapy, Immunotherapy, and Aided Drug Delivery Systems, is applied in Pancreatic Cancer to enhance the survival rate. In the Adjuvant Treatment of Pancreatic Cancer, a rational design of combination regimens will be crucial in overcoming divergent resistance mechanisms and enhancing Organ Therapeutic Efficacy.

7.2. Adjuvant Regional Therapy

Adjuvant regional therapy refers to localized post-surgical treatment strategies designed to target residual microscopic disease, reduce local recurrence, and enhance drug delivery to the tumour site while minimizing systemic toxicity. Given the anatomical complexity of the pancreas and the high rate of local recurrence even after surgical resection, regional therapies, including regional chemotherapy, intra-arterial therapy, loco-regional radiation, hyperthermia therapy, and novel drug delivery systems, have been explored as adjuncts to standard treatment (Valle et al., 2014). Intra-arterial or Regional Chemotherapy aims to deliver maximum concentrations of Cytotoxic agents directly to the Pancreatic tumor bed while minimizing side effects on the Systemic level. Systemic Chemotherapy agents, such as FOLFIRINOX and Gemcitabine-based regimens, often do not achieve satisfactory intratumor concentrations owing to the dense stroma hindering drug penetration into pancreatic tumors (Table 4).

Table 4. Survival Outcomes of Different Adjuvant Regimens in Pancreatic Cancer

Series	Patients	Regimen	Median survival (months)	3 years survival	5 years survival
GITSIG	21	5-FU/RT → 5-FU	20	–	14%
	22	Observation	11	–	4%
EORTC	104	5-FU/RT	17.1	–	20%
	103	Observation	12.6	–	10%
ESPAC-1	73	5-FU/RT	13.9	7%	
	75	5-FU/RT → 5-FU/ leucovorin	19.9	29%	

continued on following page

Table 4. Continued

Series	Patients	Regimen	Median survival (months)	3 years survival	5 years survival
	72	5-FU/leucovorin	21.6		13%
	69	Observation	16.9		11%
RTOG 97-04	221	Gem → 5-FU/RT → Gem	20.5	31%	–
	230	5-FU → 5-FU/RT → 5-FU	16.9	22%	–
CONKO-001	179	Gem	22.1	34%	–
	175	Observation	20.5	20.5%	–
ESPAC-3(v2)	537	Gem	23.6	–	–
		5-FU	23	–	–

Intra-arterial chemotherapy, or delivery of Chemotherapeutic agents such as Gemcitabine, Oxaliplatin, or Cisplatin into the Celiac axis or superior mesenteric arteries, has promising results to provide better local control of the tumor and lower recurrence rates. The enhanced local-regional response rates and survival times that may be achieved with intra-arterial drug delivery in LAPC (Locally Advanced Pancreatic Cancer) have been the subjects of several studies, although the roles in an Adjuvant setting need further confirmation through Randomized Controlled Trials (Neoptolemos et al., 2017). Besides intra-arterial chemotherapy, there are various regional perfusion modalities that have attempted to manage peritoneal and hepatic metastases of advanced pancreatic cancer, including isolated hepatic perfusion and Hyperthermia Intraperitoneal Chemotherapy (HIPEC). HIPEC employs heating agents and chemotherapy, which is administered in the abdominal cavity during surgery, and has been shown to impact peritoneal recurrence in Pancreaticoduodenectomy.

Hyperthermic chemotherapy may enhance certain drugs uptake and cytotoxicity; it may prolong survival for selected patients with peritoneal involvement. Locoregional radiation therapy is one integral element of adjuvant regional therapy that has been studied most concerning its effects on improving local control and recurrence of pancreatic cancer. Traditional External Beam Radiotherapy (EBRT) has produced generally mixed results. Some studies assume an impact on survival, such as the ESPAC-1 trial, which shows no significant beneficial effects (Conroy et al., 2018). New developments in radiotherapy techniques, such as Stereotactic Body Radiation Therapy (SBRT), Intensity-Modulated Radiation Therapy (IMRT), and Proton Beam Therapy (PBT), have enabled more precision in delivering radiation to tumors with decreased toxicity to surrounding normal tissue. High-dose radiation in a single treatment has made SBRT particularly popular and well-received in the management of locally advanced and borderline resectable Pancreatic Cancer.

Combining SBRT and sensitizers such as Gemcitabine or Paclitaxel has been promising for making Radiotherapy efficient by increasing DNA damage in Cancer cells. Hyperthermia will serve as another paradigm for Regional Adjuvant Therapy in Pancreatic Cancer, in the localized regions, which will lead to increased perfusion, improved drug delivery, and sensitization of Cancer cells to Radiation and Chemotherapy. Hyperthermia administered by Radiofrequency Ablation (RFA), High-Intensity Focused Ultrasound (HIFU), or Microwave Ablation (MWA) has shown synergy with Chemotherapeutic agents or Radiotherapy. Studies have also shown that hyperthermia can disrupt the dense desmoplastic stroma of Pancreatic Tumors and increase vascular permeability so that the drug can penetrate better, and the Immune Response can increase (Moutardier et al., 2004). Hyperthermia remains an investigational modality, but early clinical trials have reported promising improvement of local tumor control and survival in patients suffering from LAPC.

The use of regional drug delivery systems based on Nanotechnology has emerged as a promising approach toward improving the efficacy of Chemotherapy while reducing its Systemic Toxicities. Examples of Nanoparticle formulations, such as Liposomal irinotecan (nal-IRI) and Albumin-bound paclitaxel (nab-paclitaxel), have confirmed an increased bioavailability with prolonged circulation of the non-targeted delivery before being taken up into tumors. In the adjuvant setting, intratumoral administration of drug delivery through nanoparticles or biodegradable drug-eluting implants has been used for sustained Local Chemotherapy release in order to prevent Tumor recurrence (Evans et al., 1992). The approach uses implanted polymeric drug-eluting wafers containing Chemotherapeutic agents such as 5-fluorouracil or gemcitabine directly into the tumor bed after removing the tumor. Such Localized drug delivery systems may be able to sustain high Intratumoral drug concentrations while at the same time reducing systemic side effects, thus improving the tolerability and effectiveness of treatment.

Integrating gene therapy with Immunotherapy into regional Adjuvant Therapy fulfills an exciting frontier in research on Pancreatic Cancer. Concepts such as gene therapy with applications such as Oncolytic viruses, interference with RNA (RNAi), and CRISPR-based gene editing are being investigated to enhance chemosensitivity, inhibit oncogenic signalling pathways, and induce Tumor-specific immune responses (Hoffman et al., 1998). Oncolytic viral therapy targeting genetically engineered viruses to selectively infect and lyse Pancreatic Cancer cells showed very promising results in pre-clinical and early-phase clinical testing. Agents like T-VEC (talimogenela-herparepvec) and reolysin (pelareorep) can alter the tumor microenvironment and support immune-mediated tumor killing. On the other hand, dendritic cell vaccines and Tumor-Infiltrating Lymphocyte (TIL) therapy are also being evaluated as adjuvant regional immunotherapies to elicit a sustainable anti-tumor immune response. With all those encouraging developments, hurdles remain in the clinical translation of regional Adjuvant therapies for Pancreatic cancer. The extreme heterogeneity of Pancreatic tumors, with the accompaniment of an Immunosuppressive tumor microenvironment, is a roadblock to treatment efficacy.

The thick fibrotic stroma found in pancreatic cancer also poses challenges to drug delivery and, therefore, calls for novel strategies to increase the penetration of therapeutics into the tissue. Future research efforts will focus on integrating multi-omics technologies, high-throughput technologies that include genomics, transcriptomics, and proteomics, for the purpose of discovering new biomarkers for patient stratification and therapy selection (Ishikawa et al., 1989). In addition, the establishment of liquid biopsy methods, targeting Circulating tumor DNA (ctDNA) and exosome-based diagnostics, could allow real-time treatment response monitoring and early recurrence detection. The combination of regional adjuvant therapies in pancreatic cancer ultimately aims to develop multimodal approaches, integrating Regional Chemotherapy, Advanced Radiotherapy, Hyperthermia, Nanomedicine, and Immunotherapy in a synergistic way. Through these innovations, local tumor control may be enhanced, treatment tolerability improved, and ultimately, survival prolonged in this patient population. Regional adjuvant therapy should be the promise toward a cure for Pancreatic Cancer.

8. COMBINATION THERAPY

The high recurrence rates and resistance mechanisms that pancreatic tumors develop against Monotherapies have led to the emergence of combination Adjuvant Therapy as a cornerstone in improving survival outcomes. Adjuvant therapy refers to post-surgical interventions in the Microscopic disease, reducing local and distant recurrences, and enhancing overall treatment efficacy. Combination therapy refers to the strategic integration of multiple therapeutic modalities, including Chemotherapy, Radiation therapy, Immunotherapy, Targeted agents, and Novel delivery systems, to improve patient survival and reduce the risk of Disease progression (Jessup et al., 1993). The rationale behind Combination Therapy in Pancreatic Cancer lies in the tumor's intrinsic heterogeneity, its extensive desmoplastic stroma, and its highly Immunosuppressive microenvironment, all of which contribute to therapeutic resistance. Among the most established Adjuvant combinations, Chemotherapy-based regimens remain the standard of care, with FOLFIRINOX (a combination of 5-fluorouracil, leucovorin, irinotecan, and oxaliplatin) demonstrating superior efficacy over Gemcitabine Monotherapy.

The landmark PRODIGE 24/CCTG PA.6 trial showed that adjuvant FOLFIRINOX significantly improved median Overall Survival (OS) to 54.4 months compared to 35.0 months with gemcitabine alone, establishing it as the preferred regimen for fit patients. However, due to its high toxicity, alternative combinations such as Gemcitabine plus capecitabine have been explored, with the ESPAC-4 trial demonstrating improved survival over Gemcitabine (Kopelson, 1983). Beyond Chemotherapy, Chemoradiotherapy combinations have been extensively studied in the Adjuvant treatment of Pancreatic Cancer. Patients are combined with Chemotherapy, particularly 5-fluorouracil (5-FU) or Gemcitabine-based regimens, Radiation therapy has shown promise in improving local tumour control and reducing locoregional recurrence rates. The RTOG-0848 trial is currently evaluating whether the addition of Radiation Therapy to Chemotherapy confers a survival advantage in resected Pancreatic Cancer. Another rapidly evolving approach to Combination Therapy involves Targeted Therapies that exploit specific molecular vulnerabilities in Pancreatic tumours. The well-characterized Molecular target in Pancreatic Cancer is BRCA1/2 mutations that are present approximately in 5 – 7% of cases (Pilepich and Miller, 1980). These mutations impair DNA damage repair mechanisms, rendering tumors particularly sensitive to platinum-based chemotherapy (e.g., cisplatin, oxaliplatin) and PARP inhibitors (e.g., olaparib, rucaparib). The POLO trial demonstrated that maintenance therapy with the PARP inhibitor olaparib significantly prolonged progression-free survival in germline BRCA-mutated pancreatic cancer patients had responded to Platinum-based chemotherapy. While these findings are most relevant in the Metastatic setting, they underscore the potential role of PARP inhibitors in Adjuvant Combination regimens for BRCA-mutated Pancreatic Cancer patients. Other targeted agents under investigation include MEK inhibitors (trametinib), KRAS inhibitors (sotorasib, adagrasib), and anti-angiogenic agents (bevacizumab, aflibercept), though their efficacy in the adjuvant setting remains to be fully established. In addition to Chemotherapy and Targeted Agents, Immunotherapy-based combination strategies are being explored as Adjuvant treatments for Pancreatic Cancer (Breslin et al., 2001). Unlike melanoma or lung cancer, pancreatic cancer has demonstrated limited responsiveness to Immune Checkpoint Inhibitors (ICIs) due to its low Tumor Mutational Burden (TMB), lack of neo-antigen expression, and highly immunosuppressive tumor microenvironment.

Pancreatic tumors characterized by Microsatellite Instability-High (MSI-H) or Deficient Mismatch Repair (dMMR) status have exhibited significant responses to PD-1 inhibitors such as Pembrolizumab (KEYNOTE-158 trial). Given that MSI-H tumors represent less than 2% of Pancreatic cancers, ongoing research is focused on strategies to enhance Immune responsiveness through Combination

Immunotherapy approaches (Pisters et al., 1998). One promising approach is the combination of ICIs with Chemotherapy that has been shown to induce immunogenic cell death, thereby priming the immune system for a more robust anti-tumor response. Preclinical models suggest that pairing PD-1 inhibitors with agents like gemcitabine or nab-paclitaxel may promote immune infiltration into Pancreatic tumors. At the same time, translation into the clinical realm is an ongoing matter of concern. Furthermore, CD40 agonists, TGF-β inhibitors, and cancer vaccines are being experimented with in conjunction with ICIs to try to shift the immune landscape of pancreatic tumorseven more. Yet another pivotal combination therapy strategy would be blocking the stromal barriers of this pancreatic tumor stroma. The pancreatic tumor microenvironment comprises desmoplastic stroma loaded with cancer-associated fibroblasts, ECM components, and immunosuppressive cells such as regulatory T cells and myeloid-derived suppressor cells. This stroma serves as a physical barrier to drug penetration and facilitates immune evasion and tumor promotion. Concurrently, combination therapies introducing stroma-targeting agents have been explored, including the hyaluronidase inhibitor PEGPH20, the Vitamin D analog paricalcitol, and hedgehog pathway inhibitors such as Sarideg-iband Vismodegib. While early-phase trials have shown considerable promise, the complex Stromal interactions in Pancreatic Cancer have presented a challenge in developing any universally effective Stroma-Targeting Therapy (Ueno et al., 2009). Nanotechnology-based drug delivery systems also significantly improve the efficacy of Combination therapies. Nanoformulations such as nab-paclitaxel (nanoparticle albumin-bound paclitaxel) and liposomal irinotecan (nal-IRI) have already helped in clinical gains in Pancreatic Cancer, increasing Bioavailability and reducing Systemic Toxicity.

Novel theragnostic nanoparticles combining therapeutic and diagnostic functions are being explored to enable real-time drug distribution and tumor response monitoring. Future research is focused on developing biodegradable polymeric drug delivery systems that provide sustained intratumoral release of chemotherapeutic agents while minimizing systemic exposure. Despite these promising advances, challenges remain in optimizing combination therapy regimens for pancreatic cancer (Richter and Saif, 2010). The high degree of intertumoral and intratumoral heterogeneity necessitates a personalized medicine approach to tailor treatment combinations based on molecular, genetic, and immunological profiling. Additionally, real-time monitoring of treatment response using liquid biopsy approaches (circulating tumor DNA, exosomes, and CTCs) is being investigated to adjust combination therapies and prevent resistance dynamically. As research advances, integrating Artificial Intelligence (AI) and Machine Learning in clinical decision-making may enable precision-guided Combination Therapy strategies based on individual Tumor Biology. Ultimately, the future of Pancreatic Cancer treatment lies in rationally designed Combination therapies that integrate Chemotherapy, Radiotherapy, Targeted therapy, Immunotherapy, and Stromal-modulating agents in a synergistic and enhancing Therapeutic efficacy, combination Adjuvant therapies have the potential for the standard of care in Pancreatic Cancer for the patient survival and quality of life (Yamamoto et al., 2010).

8.1. Advanced Pancreatic Cancer

Adjuvant Therapy, which refers to post-surgical treatment aimed at eradicating residual microscopic disease and reducing recurrence, has played a crucial role in Pancreatic Cancer Management. In some advanced cases, Adjuvant Therapies have evolved to include Systemic Chemotherapy, Targeted Therapy, Immunotherapy, Radiotherapy, and novel loco-regional interventions to optimize treatment response and survival outcomes. The backbone of Adjuvant treatment in Pancreatic Cancer has traditionally been Chemotherapy, with Gemcitabine long considered the standard of care following Surgical Resection (Stocken et al., 2005). The introduction of multi-agent Chemotherapy regimens such as FOLFIRINOX (5-fluorouracil, leucovorin, irinotecan, and oxaliplatin) has significantly improved survival outcomes in adjuvant and advanced settings. The PRODIGE 24/CCTG PA.6 trial demonstrated that adjuvant FOLFIRINOX extended median Overall Survival (OS) to 54.4 months compared to 35.0 months with gemcitabine, highlighting its superior efficacy.

Due to toxicity concerns, the alternative gemcitabine-based combinations, such as gemcitabine plus capecitabine, have been explored, with the ESPAC-4 trial showing improved survival over Gemcitabine Monotherapy. In patients with Locally Advanced Pancreatic Cancer (LAPC), Induction Chemotherapy followed by Consolidative Chemoradiotherapy has been investigated as a strategy to enhance local tumor control and potentially downstage tumors to resectability (Boeck et al., 2007). The LAP07 trial assessed the benefit of adding Radiotherapy to Chemotherapy in LAPC, but found no significant improvement in survival, suggesting that Systemic Therapy remains the primary approach for Advanced disease. Another emerging Adjuvant Strategy in Advanced Pancreatic Cancer involves Targeted Therapies that exploit Molecular Vulnerabilities within Pancreatic Tumors. BRCA1/2 mutations, present in approximately 5 – 7% of Pancreatic Cancer cases, lead to defective DNA repair mechanisms, rendering tumors susceptible to Platinum-based Chemotherapy (Cisplatin, Oxaliplatin) and PARP inhibitors (Olaparib, Rucaparib). The POLO trial demonstrated that Maintenance Therapy with Olaparib significantly Prolonged Progression-Free Survival (PFS) in BRCA-Mutated Pancreatic Cancer patients who responded to Platinum-based chemotherapy. This marked a significant advancement in personalized treatment approaches.

In addition to Chemotherapy and Targeted agents, Immunotherapy-based approaches have gained attention in the treatment of advanced Pancreatic Cancer. However, unlike Cancers such as Melanoma or Lung cancer, Pancreatic Cancer has demonstrated limited responsiveness to Immune Checkpoint Inhibitors (ICIs) due to its low Tumor Mutational Burden (TMB), lack of neoantigen expression, and immunosuppressive Tumor Microenvironment (TME). The subset of patients with microsatellite instability-high (MSI-H) or deficient Mismatch Repair (dMMR) tumorshas shown remarkable responses to PD-1 inhibitors such as pembrolizumab (KEYNOTE-158 trial). Since MSI-H tumors account for less than 2% of pancreatic cancers, research efforts have focused on combining immunotherapy with chemotherapy, radiation therapy, and stroma-targeting agents to enhance immune infiltration and response rates (Butturini et al., 2008). Preclinical and early-phase clinical studies suggest that combining ICIs with gemcitabine, nab-paclitaxel, or CD40 agonists may modulate the Tumor Immune Microenvironment and enhance T-cell infiltration into Pancreatic Tumors. Another major challenge in advanced Pancreatic Cancer treatment is the presence of a dense Desmoplastic Stroma that acts as a physical and biochemical barrier to Drug Delivery and Immune Cell Infiltration. The use of Stromal-modulating agents such as hyaluronidase inhibitors like PEGPH20, Hedgehog pathway inhibitors, Saridegib, Vismodegib, and vitamin D analogs like Paricalcitol has been studied in Conjunction with Chemotherapy and Immunotherapy to increase drug access and efficacy.

In addition to Systemic Therapies, regional Adjuvant Therapies have been evaluated in treating locally advanced and Metastatic Pancreatic Cancer, including Stereotactic Body Radiation Therapy (SBRT), Intra-Arterial Chemotherapy, and Hyperthermic Intraperitoneal Chemotherapy (HIPEC). SBRT, which can deliver high doses of radiation while preserving surrounding normal tissue, is encouraging in achieving local control of the tumor and enabling conversion to surgical resectability in selected patients with LAPC. Intra-arterial chemotherapy was investigated to improve local drug concentration while reducing Systemic toxicity by giving Chemotherapeutic agents directly into the Pancreatic artery. In contrast, HIPEC, the process of introducing heated Chemotherapeutic agents into the peritoneal cavity, has been studied in Pancreatic cancer instances with Peritoneal metastasis; its use in the Adjuvant setting is still investigational (Farrell et al., 2009).

Nanotechnology-based drug delivery systems using Adjunct Therapy to improve Chemotherapy effectiveness in advanced Pancreatic Cancer, enhance the bioavailability of drugs, and reduce toxicity for the patient. Such Liposomal formulations have clinical efficacy; for example, Liposomal irinotecan (nal-IRI) and Albumin-bound paclitaxel (nab-paclitaxel) already show clinical merit. Specific mention can be made of new biodegradable polymeric carriers programmed to have an Intratumoral prolonged drug release (Haslam et al., 1973). For the future, Nanomedicine,

Gene therapy, and RNA-based therapeutics may herald a new paradigm in Adjuvant treatment of Pancreatic Cancer. However, these advances will not come without significant challenges for optimizing Adjuvant Therapy for advanced Pancreatic Cancer. High levels of Tumor heterogeneity combined with the Immune-evasive Pathophysiology of Pancreatic Cancer dictate a precision medicine approach that refines treatment regimens based on Molecular and Genetic profiling.

In addition, Monitoring Treatment Response and detecting early resistance mechanisms in real time is possible by adopting Liquid biopsy techniques such as ctDNA and exosome-based detection. Such predictive modelling for treatment response also incorporates advances offered by AI (Artificial Intelligence) and Machine Learning for personalized approaches to Adjuvant Therapy in Pancreatic Cancer. In the future, there will be more Adjuvant Treatment regimens that include a variety of Chemotherapy, Targeted Therapy, Immunotherapy, Radiotherapy, and new Drug delivery systems. These will be critical in addressing resistance mechanisms and enhancing survival outcomes in advanced Pancreatic Cancer (Moertel et al., 1969). These will further refine the strategies of Adjuvant therapy based on increasingly biomarker-directed treatment selection, multi-omics profiling, and innovative clinical trial designs. Finally, more efficient and individually tailored treatment approaches will be developed. With advances in research, Adjuvant Combination Therapy will soon change the standard of care for advanced Pancreatic Cancer. In this way, it promises to improve survival and reduce the cost of living for suffering patients.

8.2. Adjuvant Combination Therapy

Adjuvant combination therapy that comprises multiple treatment modalities to augment the therapeutic effect has been of great importance in the management of resectable and advanced pancreatic cancers. It aims to clear microscopic residual disease and tries to attain objectives such as reducing the risk of recurrences and increasing probabilistically Overall Survival (OS) in patients who have undergone Pancreatic Cancer Surgery. Shifted from pure approaches, like gemcitabine alone, to combinations involving all modalities, combinations in Adjuvant settings are mainly based on Chemotherapy, supported by Radiation, Targeted Therapy, and Immunotherapy. The most striking effects in terms of improved survival have been achieved through the implementation of Multiagent Chemotherapy Regimens, with FOLFIRINOX (5-fluorouracil, leucovorin, irinotecan, and oxaliplatin) established as the most effective Adjuvant Chemotherapy for fit patients (Fossati et al., 1995). The high toxicity seen in FOLFIRINOX has led to investigating combinations such as Gemcitabine plus Capecitabine that demonstrated a survival advantage in the ESPAC-4 trial. Other new exciting combinations that promise to outperform those based on Chemotherapy are Gemcitabine and nab-paclitaxel, a regimen widely used in the Metastatic setting.

It is an Adjuvant Therapy given post-surgery, geared towards the microscopic residual disease and the reduction of recurrences, in addition to improving Overall Survival (OS) in patients who have undergone surgery for Pancreatic cancer. These combinations in Adjuvant settings have shifted from Monotherapy approaches, such as Gemcitabine alone, to more effective Multimodal Chemotherapy, Radiation Therapy, Targeted Therapy, and Immunotherapy. The introduction of multi-agent Chemotherapy regimens has brought impressive gains in survival outcomes, with FOLFIRINOX (5-fluorouracil, leucovorin, irinotecan, and oxaliplatin) appearing to be the most effective Adjuvant Chemotherapy for the patients (Fossati et al., 1995). FOLFIRINOX does have a very high-causing Toxicity Profile and is therefore being studied for potentially better alternatives, such as Gemcitabine plus Capecitabine, which showed survival benefit in the ESPAC-4 trial. The combination of Chemotherapy that possibly has more efficacy alternatives is Gemcitabine and nab-paclitaxel, whichwas widely used in the Metastatic phase.

Adjuvant strategies that are mostly Chemotherapy-based have been examined using combinations, foremost with Radiation in Pancreatic Cancer. Advanced Radiation methodologies such as SBRTi and IMRT have delivered higher doses and provided less toxicity for Combination Therapy, thus qualifying Radiotherapy as one of the components (Zerbi et al., 1994). Chemotherapy and Radiotherapy have shown activity in reducing the local recurrence of diseases. The use of targeted agents in Adjuvant Combination strategies is also gaining interest. Pancreatic cancer has a well-characterized genomic landscape, with approximately 5-7% of patients harboring BRCA1/2 mutations that impair DNA damage repair mechanisms. These tumors exhibit increased sensitivity to Platinum-based chemotherapy (cisplatin, oxaliplatin) and PARP inhibitors (e.g., olaparib, rucaparib).

The POLO trial demonstrated that maintenance therapy with the PARP inhibitor Olaparib significantly Prolonged Progression-Free Survival (PFS) in BRCA-mutated Pancreatic Cancer patients, supporting the inclusion of PARP inhibitors in Adjuvant Combination regimens. KRAS-targeted therapies (Sotorasib, Adagrasib) and MEK inhibitors (Trametinib) are currently under investigation, as KRAS mutations are found in over 90% of Pancreatic Cancers. However, effective targeting of KRAS-driven pancreatic tumours remains a significant challenge. Another area of Adjuvant Combination Therapy research involves anti-angiogenic agents (e.g., Bevacizumab, Aflibercept) and stroma-modulating therapies that aim to overcome the dense desmoplastic Tumor Microenvironment (TME) that characterizes pancreatic cancer (Hiraoka et al., 1990).

Immunotherapy-based adjuvant strategies have also been explored, but Pancreatic Cancer has shown limited responsiveness to Immune Checkpoint Inhibitors

(ICIs) due to its Immunosuppressive TME, low Tumor Mutational Burden (TMB), and lack of Immunogenic Neo-antigens. However, a small subset of Microsatellite instability-high (MSI-H) or Deficient mismatch repair (dMMR) Pancreatic Tumors (~2% of cases) has shown significant responses to PD-1 inhibitors such as Pembrolizumab (as demonstrated in the KEYNOTE-158 trial). Given the low prevalence of MSI-H tumors, ongoing research is focused on enhancing Immune Response in Pancreatic Cancer through Combination Immunotherapy approaches (Coquard et al., 1997). Preclinical and early-phase clinical studies suggest that combining immune checkpoint inhibitors with Chemotherapy may increase Tumor Immunogenicity, as Chemotherapy can induce Immunogenic Cell Death, thereby priming the Immune system. Combination strategies involving CD_{40} agonists, ICIs, and Chemotherapy are currently under evaluation in clinical trials.

Another major challenge in adjuvant combination therapy for Pancreatic Cancer is the tumor's extensive desmoplastic stroma that acts as a physical and biochemical barrier to Drug penetration. Stroma-targeting agents have been investigated in combination with Chemotherapy and Immunotherapy. Other stroma-targeting approaches include Hedgehog pathway inhibitors (Saridegib, Vismodegib) and vitamin D analogs (paricalcitol), which have been explored in combination regimens to alter Fibroblast activity and improve Drug penetration (Reni et al., 2001). Regional adjuvant therapies, such as intra-arterial chemotherapy, Hyperthermic Intraperitoneal Chemotherapy (HIPEC), and Stereotactic Ablative Radiation Therapy (SABR), have been explored as Adjuncts to Systemic Therapy in locally advanced and Metastatic Pancreatic Cancer. Intra-arterial Chemotherapy that delivers High-Dose Chemotherapy directly into the pancreatic artery has been investigated to enhance local drug concentration while minimizing Systemic Toxicity.

The future of Adjuvant Therapy in Pancreatic Cancer may also be linked with Gene Therapy, RNA-based therapeutics, and Tumor-specific vaccine strategies to enhance further treatment efficacy (Sindelar and Kinsella, 1999). Several challenges remain in optimizing Adjuvant Combination Therapy for Pancreatic Cancer. The high degree of Tumor Heterogeneity, combined with Immune Evasion Mechanisms and Stromal Resistance, calls for a precision medicine approach to the Adjuvant Treatment regimens based on individual Tumor Biology (Kalser and Ellenberg, 1985). Artificial Intelligence (AI) and Machine Learning Algorithms are being integrated into predictive modelling for treatment response, paving the way for personalized Adjuvant Combination Therapy strategies. Adjuvant Combination Therapy in Pancreatic Cancer involves a multidimensional approach integrating Chemotherapy, Radiotherapy, Targeted Therapy, Immunotherapy, and Novel drug delivery mechanisms to improve survival rates.

Table 5. Some of the Agents Currently being Investigated in Clinical Trials in Advanced Pancreatic Cancer

S.No	Class of agents	Mode of action
1	Platinum analogues	This form adducts with DNA inhibiting transcription and replication causing cell death. Oxaliplatin is a third-generation platinum analogue (a diaminocyclohexane platinum derivative) that may have activity in tumours resistant to cisplatin or carboplatin and may have an additive/synergistic activity in doublet or triplet therapy. Trials are ongoing with cisplatin and oxaliplatin. Oxaliplatin may also have a role as second-line therapy with relapse on gemcitabine (Pelzer et al., 2002).
2	Proteasome inhibitors	PS-341 is a reversible and specific inhibitor of the proteasome with activity against Pancreatic Cancer. The 26S proteasome is a key part of the system that degrades regulatory proteins that govern cell trafficking, transcription factor activation, cell cycle regulation and apoptosis (Ryan et al., 2002).
3	Cyclo-oxygenase-2 inhibitors	Celecoxib has been found to be active against pancreatic cancer. Specific cyclo-oxygenase-2m (COX-2) inhibitors reduce proliferation, inhibit angiogenesis and promote apoptosis. First-generation COX-2 inhibitors include celecoxib and rofecoxib and second-generation agents include parecoxib, valdecoxib and etoricoxib (Xiong et al., 2002).
4	5-Lipoxygenase and thromboxane A2 inhibitor	CV6504 is a novel 5-lipoxygenase and thromboxane A2 synthase inhibitor shown in a phase II to produce stable disease in 32% of patients and a 1-year survival of ~25% (Ferry et al., 2000).
5	Histone deacetylase inhibitor	CI-994 (N-acetyl dinaline, PD 123654) is a novel orally active agent causing inhibition of both histone deacetylation and the G_1 to S transition phase of the cell cycle (Waterhouse et al., 2002).

9. FUTURE PERSPECTIVES

In Adjuvant Chemotherapy regimens and corresponding increases in postsurgical survival rates, a considerable minority of patients continue to have poor tumour responses to the Chemotherapy due to its adverse effects (Figure 2). One significant improvement in survival may be possible by stratifying patients into existing Chemotherapy regimens based on treatment-specific signatures that must be further developed and verified before being used in everyday practice within a clinically relevant time frame. Furthermore, direct functional response testing of personalized models of human pancreatic cancer, such as patient-derived tumour organoids, may be an effective method for predicting individual therapy responses. Specific prospective clinical trial designs are required to evaluate the potential oncological advantage of such personalized techniques compared to Traditional Therapy, even though response rates are dismal in most patients (Tiriac et al., 2018).

Tumour cell dissemination caused by Tumour manipulation during surgery may enhance the likelihood of early tumour recurrence and metastatic tumour spread in patients undergoing upfront resection. Intraoperative chemotherapy is plausible and is currently being studied in the prospective combiCaRe experiment (DRKS00015766). Furthermore, with the increased use of Neoadjuvant treatment techniques, particularly in patients with Borderline and Locally Advanced Pancreatic Cancer, the extent and value of Adjuvant treatment in these cases must be studied. The results of existing trials, such as the randomized ESPAC-5F feasibility trial (ISRCTN89500674), will serve as the foundation for future trials comparing the use of Neoadjuvant treatments to upfront surgery in patients with Borderline resectable Pancreatic Cancer (Marquart et al., 2018).

Figure 2. Future Perspectives of Adjuvants in Treating Pancreatic Cancer

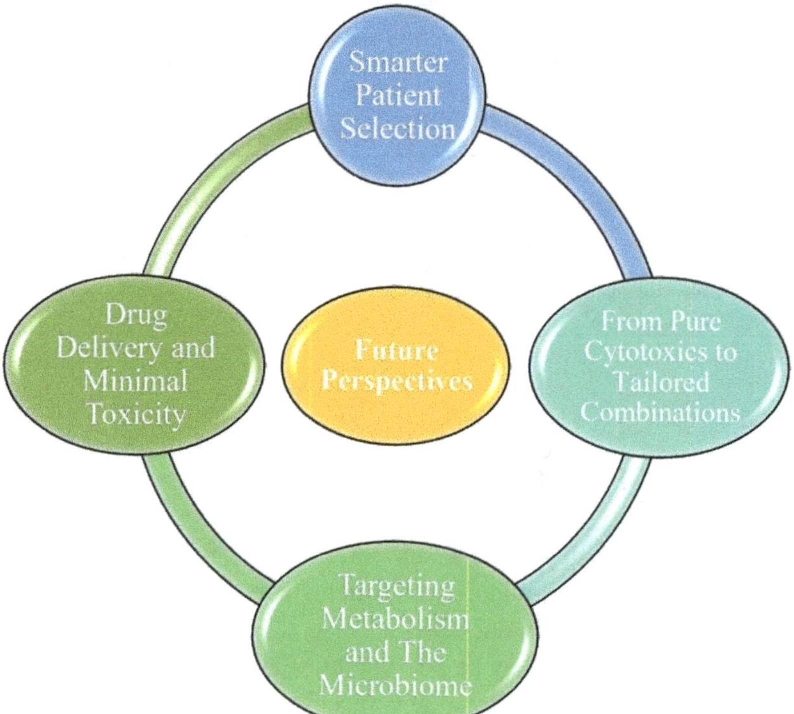

10. CONCLUSION

Neoadjuvant Therapy has emerged as a critical strategy in Pancreatic Cancer management, particularly for patients with advanced loco-regional tumors who face high postoperative complication rates (30 – 45%) that often preclude Adjuvant

Treatment. By enabling higher resection rates and addressing Micrometastatic disease preoperatively, Neoadjuvant approaches offer survival outcomes comparable to Adjuvant Therapies (median 16 – 21 months), though randomized trials remain limited by small patient cohorts undergoing resection post-neoadjuvant treatment. While studies highlight improved survival in borderline resectable cases, challenges persist in standardizing regimens and optimizing patient selection. Future research must focus on refining Neoadjuvant-adjuvant sequencing, integrating biomarkers for personalized therapy, and expanding clinical trials to validate its role in enhancing long-term outcomes, particularly in the context of evolving multimodal strategies and emerging technologies.

11. REFERENCES

Abraham, S. C., Wu, T. T., Klimstra, D. S., Finn, L. S., Lee, J.-H., Yeo, C. J., Cameron, J. L., & Hruban, R. H. (2002). Distinctive Molecular Genetic Alterations in Sporadic and Familial Adenomatous Polyposis-Associated Pancreatoblastomas. *American Journal of Pathology*, *160*(5), 1619–1627. DOI: 10.1016/S0002-9440(10)63008-8 PMID: 11696422

Adsay, N. V., Pierson, C., Sarkar, F., Abrams, J., Weaver, D., Conlon, K. C., Brennan, M. F., & Klimstra, D. S. (2001). Colloid (Mucinous Noncystic) Carcinoma of the Pancreas. *The American Journal of Surgical Pathology*, *25*(1), 26–42. DOI: 10.1097/00000478-200101000-00003 PMID: 11145249

Agnihotri, S., Kumar, N., & Coudière, P. (2021). Acinar Cell Carcinoma of the Pancreas: A Comprehensive Review. *The Oncologist*, *26*(7), e1122–e1132.

Allen, P. J., D'Angelica, M., Gonen, M., Jaques, D. P., Coit, D. G., Jarnagin, W. R., DeMatteo, R., Fong, Y., Blumgart, L. H., & Brennan, M. F. (2006). A selective approach to the resection of cystic lesions of the pancreas: Results from 539 consecutive patients. *Annals of Surgery*, *244*(4), 572–582. DOI: 10.1097/01.sla.0000237652.84466.54 PMID: 16998366

Bakkevold, K. E., Arnesjo, B., Dahl, O., & Kambestad, B. (1993). Adjuvant combination chemotherapy (AMF) following radical resection of carcinoma of the pancreas and papilla of Vater: Results of a controlled, prospective, randomised multicentre study. *European Journal of Cancer*, *29*(5), 698–703. DOI: 10.1016/S0959-8049(05)80349-1 PMID: 8471327

Basturk, O., Hong, S. M., Wood, L. D., Adsay, N. V., Albores-Saavedra, J., Biankin, A. V., Brosens, L. A. A., Fukushima, N., Goggins, M., Hruban, R. H., Kato, Y., Klimstra, D. S., Klöppel, G., Krasinskas, A., Longnecker, D. S., Matthaei, H., Offerhaus, G. J. A., Shimizu, M., Takaori, K., & Furukawa, T. (2015). A Revised Classification System and Recommendations from the Baltimore Consensus Meeting for Neoplastic Precursor Lesions in the Pancreas. *The American Journal of Surgical Pathology*, *39*(12), 1730–1741. DOI: 10.1097/PAS.0000000000000533 PMID: 26559377

Basturk, O., Tang, L., & Hruban, R. H. (2015). Poorly Differentiated Neuroendocrine Carcinomas of the Pancreas: A Clinicopathologic Analysis of 44 Cases. *The American Journal of Surgical Pathology*, *39*(5), 683–690. DOI: 10.1097/PAS.0000000000000408 PMID: 25723112

Baumel, H., Huguier, M., Manderscheid, J. C., Fabre, J. M., Houry, S., & Fagot, H. (1994). Results of resection for cancer of the exocrine pancreas: A study from the French Association of Surgery. *British Journal of Surgery*, *81*(1), 102–107. DOI: 10.1002/bjs.1800810138 PMID: 7906180

Boeck, S., Ankerst, D. P., & Heinemann, V. (2007). The role of adjuvant chemotherapy for patients with resected pancreatic cancer: Systematic review of randomized controlled trials and meta-analysis. *Oncology*, *72*(6), 314–321. DOI: 10.1159/000113054 PMID: 18187951

Bray, F., Ferlay, J., Soerjomataram, I., Siegel, R. L., Torre, L. A., & Jemal, A. (2018). Global cancer statistics 2018: GLOBOCAN estimates of incidence and mortality worldwide for 36 cancers in 185 countries. *CA: a Cancer Journal for Clinicians*, *68*(6), 394–424. DOI: 10.3322/caac.21492 PMID: 30207593

Breslin, T. M., Hess, K. R., Harbison, D. B., Jean, M. E., Cleary, K. R., Dackiw, A. P., Wolff, R. A., Abbruzzese, J. L., Janjan, N. A., Crane, C. H., Vauthey, J. N., Lee, J. E., Pisters, P. W. T., & Evans, D. B. (2001). Neoadjuvant chemoradiotherapy for adenocarcinoma of the pancreas: Treatment variables and survival duration. *Annals of Surgical Oncology*, *8*(2), 123–132. DOI: 10.1007/s10434-001-0123-4 PMID: 11258776

Butturini, G., Stocken, D. D., Wente, M. N., Jeekel, H., Klinkenbijl, J. H. G., Bakkevold, K. E., Takada, T., Amano, H., Dervenis, C., Bassi, C., Büchler, M. W., & Neoptolemos, J. P.Pancreatic Cancer Meta-Analysis Group. (2008). Influence of resection margins and treatment on survival in patients with pancreatic cancer: Meta-analysis of randomized controlled trials. *Archives of Surgery*, *143*(1), 75–83. DOI: 10.1001/archsurg.2007.17 PMID: 18209156

Conroy, T., Hammel, P., Hebbar, M., Abdelghani, M. B., Wei, A. C., & Raoul, J. L. (2018). FOLFIRINOX or gemcitabine as adjuvant therapy for pancreatic cancer. *The New England Journal of Medicine*, *379*(25), 2395–2406. DOI: 10.1056/NEJMoa1809775 PMID: 30575490

Coquard, R., Ayzac, L., Gilly, F. N., Romestaing, P., Ardiet, J. M., Sondaz, C., Sotton, M. P., Sentenac, I., Braillon, G., & Gerard, J. P. (1997). Intraoperative radiotherapy in resected pancreatic cancer: Feasibility and results. *Radiotherapy and Oncology : Journal of the European Society for Therapeutic Radiology and Oncology*, *44*(3), 271–275. DOI: 10.1016/S0167-8140(97)00107-2 PMID: 9380827

Cress, R. D., Yin, D., Clarke, L., Bold, R., & Holly, E. A. (2006). Survival among patients with adenocarcinoma of the pancreas: A population-based study (United States). *Cancer Causes & Control, 17*(4), 403–409. DOI: 10.1007/s10552-005-0539-4 PMID: 16596292

Cullinan, S., Moertel, C. G., Wieand, H. S., Schutt, A. J., Krook, J. E., Foley, J. F., Norris, B. D., Kardinal, C. G., Tschetter, L. K., & Barlow, J. F. (1990). A phase III trial on the therapy of advanced pancreatic carcinoma: Evaluations of the Mallinson regimen and combined 5-fluorouracil, doxorubicin, and cisplatin. *Cancer, 65*(10), 2207–2212. DOI: 10.1002/1097-0142(19900515)65:10<2207::AID-CNCR2820651007>3.0.CO;2-Y PMID: 2189551

Evans, D. B., Rich, T. A., Byrd, D. R., Ames, F. C., & Cleary, K. R. (1992). Preoperative chemoradiation and pancreaticoduodenectomy for adenocarcinoma of the pancreas. *Archives of Surgery, 127*(11), 1335–1339. DOI: 10.1001/archsurg.1992.01420110083017 PMID: 1359851

Falconi, M., Eriksson, B., Kaltsas, G., Bartsch, D. K., Capdevila, J., Caplin, M., Kos-Kudla, B., Kwekkeboom, D., Rindi, G., Klöppel, G., Reed, N., Kianmanesh, R., & Jensen, R. T. (2016). ENETS Consensus Guidelines Update for the Management of Patients with Functional Pancreatic Neuroendocrine Tumors and Non-Functional Pancreatic Neuroendocrine Tumors. *Neuroendocrinology, 103*(2), 153–171. DOI: 10.1159/000443171 PMID: 26742109

Farnell, M. B., Pearson, R. K., Sarr, M. G., DiMagno, E. P., Burgart, L. J., Dahl, T. R., Foster, N., & Sargent, D. J.the Pancreas Cancer Working Group. (2005). A prospective randomized trial comparing standard pancreatoduodenectomy with pancreatoduodenectomy with extended lymphadenectomy in resectable pancreatic head adenocarcinoma. *Surgery, 138*(4), 618–628. DOI: 10.1016/j.surg.2005.06.044 PMID: 16269290

Farrell, J. J., Elsaleh, H., Garcia, M., Lai, R., Ammar, A., Regine, W. F., Abrams, R., Benson, A. B., Macdonald, J., Cass, C. E., Dicker, A. P., & Mackey, J. R. (2009). Human equilibrative nucleoside transporter 1 levels predict response to gemcitabine in patients with pancreatic cancer. *Gastroenterology, 136*(1), 187–195. DOI: 10.1053/j.gastro.2008.09.067 PMID: 18992248

Ferry, D. R., Deakin, M., Babb, J., & Kerr, D. J. (2000). A Phase II study of the 5-lipoxygenase inhibitor, CV6504, in advanced pancreatic cancer: Correlation of clinical data with pharmacokinetic and pharmacodynamic endpoints. *Annals of Oncology : Official Journal of the European Society for Medical Oncology, 11*(10), 1165–1170. DOI: 10.1023/A:1008303715515 PMID: 11061613

Fossati, V., Cattaneo, G. M., & Clarke, L. (1995). The role of intraoperative therapy by electron beam and combination of Adjuvant Chemotherapy and External Radiotherapy in carcinoma of the Pancreas. *Tumori, 81*(1), 23–31. DOI: 10.1177/030089169508100106 PMID: 7754537

Furukawa, T., Hatori, T., Fujita, I., Yamamoto, M., Kobayashi, M., Ohike, N., Morohoshi, T., Egawa, S., Unno, M., Takao, S., Osako, M., Yonezawa, S., Mino-Kenudson, M., Lauwers, G. Y., Yamaguchi, H., Ban, S., & Shimizu, M. (2011). Prognostic relevance of morphological types of intraductal papillary mucinous neoplasms of the pancreas. *Gut, 60*(4), 509–516. DOI: 10.1136/gut.2010.210567 PMID: 21193453

Glimelius, B., Hoffman, K., Sjoden, P. O., Jacobsson, G., Sellstrom, H., Enander, L. K., Linne, T., & Svensson, C. (1996). Chemotherapy improves survival and quality of life in advanced pancreatic and biliary cancer. *Annals of Oncology : Official Journal of the European Society for Medical Oncology, 7*(6), 593–600. DOI: 10.1093/oxfordjournals.annonc.a010676 PMID: 8879373

Gunderson, L. L., Martin, J. K., Kvols, L. K., Nagorney, D. M., Fieck, J. M., Wieand, H. S., Martinez, A., O'Connell, M. J., Earle, J. D., & McIlrath, D. C. (1987). Intraoperative and external beam irradiation ± 5-FU for locally advanced Pancreatic Cancer. *International Journal of Radiation Oncology, Biology, Physics, 13*(3), 319–329. DOI: 10.1016/0360-3016(87)90005-8 PMID: 3104244

Gunderson, L. L., Nagorney, D. M., Martenson, J. A., Donohue, J. H., Garton, G. R., Nelson, H., & Fieck, J. (1995). External beam plus intraoperative irradiation for gastrointestinal cancers. *World Journal of Surgery, 19*(2), 191–197. DOI: 10.1007/BF00308625 PMID: 7754622

Halfdanarson, T. R., Rabe, K. G., Rubin, J., & Petersen, G. M. (2008). Pancreatic Neuroendocrine Tumors (PNETs): Incidence, Prognosis, and Recent Trend Toward Improved Survival. *Annals of Oncology : Official Journal of the European Society for Medical Oncology, 19*(10), 1727–1733. DOI: 10.1093/annonc/mdn351 PMID: 18515795

) Haslam, J. B., Cavanaugh, P. J., & Stroup, S. L. (1973). Radiation therapy in the treatment of unresectable adenocarcinoma of the pancreas. *Cancer: A Journal of the American Cancer Society, 32*, 1341–1345. doi:DOI: 10.1002/1097-0142(197312)32:6

Haycox, A., Lombard, M., Neoptolemos, J. P., & Walley, T. (1998). Review article: Current treatment and optimal patient management in pancreatic cancer. *Alimentary Pharmacology & Therapeutics, 12*(10), 949–964. DOI: 10.1046/j.1365-2036.1998.00390.x PMID: 9798799

Hentic, O., Hammel, P., & Couvelard, A. (2012). FOLFIRI Regimen in Metastatic Pancreatic Adenocarcinoma Resistant to Gemcitabine and Platinum-Salts. *World Journal of Gastroenterology*, *18*(33), 4533–4541. DOI: 10.3748/wjg.v18.i33.4533 PMID: 22969226

Hester, C. A., Augustine, M. M., & Choti, M. A. (2020). Comparative Outcomes of Acinar Cell Carcinoma and Pancreatic Adenocarcinoma: A Population-Based Analysis. *Journal of Surgical Oncology*, *121*(5), 821–829.

Hiraoka, T. (1990). Extended radical resection of cancer of the pancreas with intraoperative radiotherapy. *Bailliere's Clinical Gastroenterology*, *4*(4), 985–993. DOI: 10.1016/0950-3528(90)90031-B PMID: 2078795

Hiraoka, T., Uchino, R., Kanemitsu, K., Toyonaga, M., Saitoh, N., Nakamura, I., Tashiro, S., & Miyauchi, Y. (1990). Combination of intraoperative radiation with resection of cancer of the pancreas. *International Journal of Pancreatology*, *7*(3), 201–207. DOI: 10.1007/BF02924238 PMID: 1964472

Hoffman, J. P., Lipsitz, S., Pisansky, T., Weese, J. L., Solin, L., & Benson, A. B.III. (1998). Phase II trial of preoperative radiation therapy and chemotherapy for patients with localized, resectable adenocarcinoma of the pancreas: An Eastern Cooperative Oncology Group Study. *Journal of Clinical Oncology*, *16*(1), 317–323. DOI: 10.1200/JCO.1998.16.1.317 PMID: 9440759

Hu, Z. I., Shia, J., & Stadler, Z. K. (2020). Evaluating Mismatch Repair Deficiency in Pancreatic Adenocarcinoma: Challenges and Recommendations. *Clinical Cancer Research*, *26*(6), 1346–1354. DOI: 10.1158/1078-0432.CCR-17-3099 PMID: 29367431

Ishikawa, O., Ohhigashi, H., Teshima, T., Chatani, M., Inoue, T., Tanaka, S., Kitamura, T., Wada, A., Sasaki, Y., Imaoka, S., & Iwanaga, T. (1989). Clinical and histopathological appraisal of preoperative irradiation for adenocarcinoma of the pancreatoduodenal region. *Journal of Surgical Oncology*, *40*(3), 143–151. DOI: 10.1002/jso.2930400303 PMID: 2918720

Jeekel, J., Garofalo, M. C., Regine, W. F., & Tan, M. T. (2006). Upon statistical reanalysis, the EORTC trial was found to bepositive for Adjuvant Chemoradiation in Pancreatic Cancer. *Annals of Surgery*, *244*, 332–333. DOI: 10.1097/00000658-200608000-00036 PMID: 16858208

Jessup, J. M., Steele, G. J., & Mayer, R. J. (1993). Neoadjuvant therapy for unresectable Pancreatic Adenocarcinoma. *Archives of Surgery*, *128*(5), 559–564. DOI: 10.1001/archsurg.1993.01420170093014 PMID: 8098206

Jiao, Y., Yonescu, R., & Offerhaus, G. J. (2018). Whole-Exome Sequencing of Pancreatic Neoplasms with Acinar Differentiation. *The Journal of Pathology, 234*(4), 545–555. DOI: 10.1002/path.4310 PMID: 24293293

Kalser, M. H., & Ellenberg, S. S. (1985). Pancreatic cancer: Adjuvant combined radiation and chemotherapy following curative resection. *Archives of Surgery, 120*(8), 899–903. DOI: 10.1001/archsurg.1985.01390320023003 PMID: 4015380

Kaur, S., Kumar, S., Momi, N., Sasson, A. R., & Batra, S. K. (2013). Mucins in Pancreatic Cancer and Its Microenvironment. *Nature Reviews. Gastroenterology & Hepatology, 10*(10), 607–620. DOI: 10.1038/nrgastro.2013.120 PMID: 23856888

Klaiber, U., Leonhardt, C. S., Strobel, O., Tjaden, C., Hackert, T., & Neoptolemos, J. P. (2018). Neoadjuvant and adjuvant chemotherapy in pancreatic cancer. *Langenbeck's Archives of Surgery, 403*(8), 917–932. DOI: 10.1007/s00423-018-1724-8 PMID: 30397779

Klimstra, D. S., Heffess, C. S., Oertel, J. E., & Rosai, J. (1992). Acinar Cell Carcinoma of the Pancreas: A Clinicopathologic Study of 28 Cases. *The American Journal of Surgical Pathology, 16*(9), 815–837. DOI: 10.1097/00000478-199209000-00001 PMID: 1384374

Klimstra, D. S., Modlin, I. R., Coppola, D., Lloyd, R. V., & Suster, S. (2010). The Pathologic Classification of Neuroendocrine Tumors: A Review of Nomenclature, Grading, and Staging Systems. *Pancreas, 39*(6), 707–712. DOI: 10.1097/MPA.0b013e3181ec124e PMID: 20664470

Klinkenbijl, J. H., Jeekel, J., Sahmoud, T., van Pel, R., Couvreur, M. L., Veenhof, C. H., Arnaud, J. P., Gonzalez Gonzalez, D., de Wit, L. T., Hennipman, A., & Wils, J. (1999). Adjuvant radiotherapy and 5-fluorouracil after curative resection of cancer of the pancreas and periampullary region: Phase III trial of the EORTC gastrointestinal tract cancer cooperative group. *Annals of Surgery, 230*(6), 776–782. DOI: 10.1097/00000658-199912000-00006 PMID: 10615932

Kopelson, G. (1983). Curative surgery for adenocarcinoma of the pancreas/ampulla of Vater: The role of adjuvant pre- or postoperative radiation therapy. *International Journal of Radiation Oncology, Biology, Physics, 9*(6), 911–915. DOI: 10.1016/0360-3016(83)90018-4 PMID: 6408038

Kosuge, T., Kiuchi, T., Mukai, K., & Kakizoe, T. (2006). A multicenter randomized controlled trial to evaluate the effect of adjuvant cisplatin and 5-fluorouracil therapy after curative resection in cases of pancreatic cancer. *Japanese Journal of Clinical Oncology, 36*(3), 159–165. DOI: 10.1093/jjco/hyi234 PMID: 16490736

Koumarianou, A., Kaltsas, G., Kulke, M. H., Oberg, K., Strosberg, J. R., Spada, F., Galdy, S., Barberis, M., Fumagalli, C., Berruti, A., & Fazio, N. (2017). Temozolomide in Advanced Neuroendocrine Neoplasms: Pharmacological and Clinical Aspects. *Neuroendocrinology, 105*(3), 274–288. DOI: 10.1159/000430816 PMID: 25924937

La Rosa, S., Adsay, V., & Albarello, L. (2016). Clinicopathologic Study of 62 Acinar Cell Carcinomas of the Pancreas: Insights into the Morphology and Immunophenotype and Search for Prognostic Markers. *Modern Pathology, 25*(7), 1038–1052. DOI: 10.1097/PAS.0b013e318263209d PMID: 23026929

Lowenfels, A. B., Maisonneuve, P., DiMagno, E. P., Elitsur, Y., Gates, L. K., Perrault, J., & Whitcomb, D. C. (1997). Hereditary pancreatitis and the risk of pancreatic cancer. *Journal of the National Cancer Institute, 89*(6), 442–446. DOI: 10.1093/jnci/89.6.442 PMID: 9091646

Lowenfels, A. B., Maisonneuve, P., Whitcomb, D. C., Lerch, M. M., & DiMagno, E. P. (2001). Cigarette smoking as a risk factor for Pancreatic cancer in patients with hereditary pancreatitis. *Journal of the American Medical Association, 286*(2), 169–170. DOI: 10.1001/jama.286.2.169 PMID: 11448279

Lowery, M. A., Klimstra, D. S., Shia, J., Yu, K. H., Allen, P. J., Brennan, M. F., & O'Reilly, E. M. (2011). Acinar Cell Carcinoma of the Pancreas: New Genetic and Treatment Insights into a Rare Malignancy. *The Oncologist, 16*(12), 1714–1720. DOI: 10.1634/theoncologist.2011-0231 PMID: 22042785

Mallinson, C. N., Rake, M. D., Cocking, J. B., Fox, C. A., Cwynarski, M. T., Diffey, B. L., Jackson, G. A., & Wass, V. J. (1980). Chemotherapy in pancreatic cancer: Results of a controlled, prospective, randomised, multicentre trial. *British Medical Journal, 281*(6255), 1589–1591. DOI: 10.1136/bmj.281.6255.1589 PMID: 7004559

Marquart, J., Chen, E. Y., & Prasad, V. (2018). Estimation of the percentage of US patients with cancer who benefit from genome-driven oncology. *JAMA Oncology, 4*(8), 1093–1098. DOI: 10.1001/jamaoncol.2018.1660 PMID: 29710180

Matthaei, H., Norris, A. L., Tsiatis, A. C., Olino, K., Hong, S.-M., dal Molin, M., Goggins, M. G., Canto, M., Horton, K. M., Jackson, K. D., Capelli, P., Zamboni, G., Bortesi, L., Furukawa, T., Egawa, S., Ishida, M., Ottomo, S., Unno, M., Motoi, F., & Hruban, R. H. (2012). Clinicopathological Characteristics and Molecular Analyses of Multifocal Intraductal Papillary Mucinous Neoplasms of the Pancreas. *Annals of Surgery, 255*(2), 326–333. DOI: 10.1097/SLA.0b013e3182378a18 PMID: 22167000

Mehta, V. K., Fisher, G., Ford, J. A., Poen, J., Koong, A., & Bastidas, J. A. (2001). Preoperative chemoradiation for marginally resectable adenocarcinoma of the pancreas. *Journal of Gastrointestinal Surgery*, *5*(1), 27–35. DOI: 10.1016/S1091-255X(01)80010-X PMID: 11309645

Mino-Kenudson, M., Fernández-del Castillo, C., & Baba, Y. (2010). Prognosis of Invasive Intraductal Papillary Mucinous Neoplasm Depends on Histologic Subtype. *Human Pathology*, *41*(6), 810–819. DOI: 10.1136/gut.2010.232272 PMID: 21508421

Moertel, C. G., Childs, D. S., Reitemeier, R. J., Colby, M. Y., & Holbrook, M. A. (1969). Combined 5-fluorouracil and supervoltage radiation therapy of locally unresectable gastrointestinal cancer. *Lancet*, *294*(7626), 865–867. DOI: 10.1016/S0140-6736(69)92326-5 PMID: 4186452

Moore, M. J., Andersen, J. S., Burris, H. A., Tarassoff, P., Green, M. R., & Casper, E. S. (1997). A randomized trial of gemcitabine versus 5-FU as first-line therapy in advanced pancreatic cancer. *Journal of Clinical Oncology*, *15*(6), 2403–2410. DOI: 10.1200/JCO.1997.15.6.2403 PMID: 9196156

Moutardier, V., Magnin, V., Turrini, O., Viret, F., Hennekinne-Mucci, S., Gonçalves, A., Pesenti, C., Guiramand, J., Lelong, B., Giovannini, M., Monges, G., Houvenaeghel, G., & Delpero, J.-R. (2004). Assessment of pathologic response after Preoperative Chemoradiotherapy and Surgery in Pancreatic Adenocarcinoma. *International Journal of Radiation Oncology, Biology, Physics*, *60*(2), 437–443. DOI: 10.1016/j.ijrobp.2004.04.004 PMID: 15380577

Neoptolemos, J. P., Cunningham, D., & Friess, H. (2001). Adjuvant 5-fluorouracil plus folinic acid vs observation in resected pancreatic cancer: ESPAC-1 results. *Lancet*, *357*(9268), 1559–1565. DOI: 10.1016/S0140-6736(00)04639-6

Neoptolemos, J. P., Kleeff, J., Michl, P., Costello, E., Greenhalf, W., & Palmer, D. H. (2018). Therapeutic developments in pancreatic cancer: Current and future perspectives. *Nature Reviews. Gastroenterology & Hepatology*, *15*(6), 333–348. DOI: 10.1038/s41575-018-0005-x PMID: 29717230

Neoptolemos, J. P., Palmer, D. H., Ghaneh, P., Psarelli, E. E., Valle, J. W., Halloran, C. M., Faluyi, O., O'Reilly, D. A., Cunningham, D., Wadsley, J., Darby, S., Meyer, T., Gillmore, R., Anthoney, A., Lind, P., Glimelius, B., Falk, S., Izbicki, J. R., Middleton, G. W., & Büchler, M. W. (2017). Comparison of adjuvant gemcitabine and capecitabine with gemcitabine monotherapy in patients with resected pancreatic cancer (ESPAC-4): A multicentre, open-label, randomised, phase 3 trial. *Lancet*, *389*(10073), 1011–1024. DOI: 10.1016/S0140-6736(16)32409-6 PMID: 28129987

Neoptolemos, J. P., Palmer, D. H., Ghaneh, P., Psarelli, E. E., Valle, J. W., Halloran, C. M., Faluyi, O., O'Reilly, D. A., Cunningham, D., Wadsley, J., Darby, S., Meyer, T., Gillmore, R., Anthoney, A., Lind, P., Glimelius, B., Falk, S., Izbicki, J. R., Middleton, G. W., & Büchler, M. W. (2017). Comparison of adjuvant gemcitabine and capecitabine with gemcitabine monotherapy in resected pancreatic cancer (ESPAC-4): A multicentre, open-label, randomized, phase 3 trial. *Lancet*, *389*(10073), 1011–1024. DOI: 10.1016/S0140-6736(16)32409-6 PMID: 28129987

Neoptolemos, J. P., Stocken, D. D., Bassi, C., Ghaneh, P., Cunningham, D., Goldstein, D., Padbury, R., Moore, M. J., Gallinger, S., Mariette, C., Wente, M. N., Izbicki, J. R., Friess, H., Lerch, M. M., Dervenis, C., Oláh, A., Butturini, G., Doi, R., Lind, P. A., & European Study Group for Pancreatic Cancer, . (2010). Adjuvant chemotherapy with fluorouracil plus folinic acid vs gemcitabine following pancreatic cancer resection: A randomized controlled trial. *Journal of the American Medical Association*, *304*(10), 1073–1081. DOI: 10.1001/jama.2010.1275 PMID: 20823433

Neoptolemos, J. P., Stocken, D. D., Dunn, J., Almond, J., Beger, H. G., Pederzoli, P., Bassi, C., Dervenis, C., Fernandez-Cruz, L., Lacaine, F., Buckels, J., Deakin, M., Adab, F. A., Sutton, R., Imrie, C., Ihse, I., Tihanyi, T., Olah, A., Pedrazzoli, S., & Büchler, M. W. (2001). Influence of resection margins on survival for patients with pancreatic cancer treated by adjuvant chemoradiation and chemotherapy in the ESPAC-1 randomized controlled trial. *Annals of Surgery*, *234*(6), 758–768. DOI: 10.1097/00000658-200112000-00007 PMID: 11729382

Oettle, H., Neuhaus, P., Hochhaus, A., Hartmann, J. T., Gellert, K., Ridwelski, K., Niedergethmann, M., Zülke, C., Fahlke, J., Arning, M. B., Sinn, M., Hinke, A., & Riess, H. (2013). Adjuvant chemotherapy with gemcitabine and long-term outcomes among patients with resected pancreatic cancer: The CONKO-001 randomized trial. *Journal of the American Medical Association*, *310*(14), 1473–1481. DOI: 10.1001/jama.2013.279201 PMID: 24104372

Oettle, H., Post, S., Neuhaus, P., Gellert, K., Langrehr, J., Ridwelski, K., Schramm, H., Fahlke, J., Zuelke, C., Burkart, C., Gutberlet, K., Kettner, E., Schmalenberg, H., Weigang-Koehler, K., Bechstein, W.-O., Niedergethmann, M., Schmidt-Wolf, I., Roll, L., Doerken, B., & Riess, H. (2007). Adjuvant chemotherapy with gemcitabine vs observation in patients undergoing curative-intent resection of pancreatic cancer: A randomized controlled trial. *Journal of the American Medical Association*, *297*(3), 267–277. DOI: 10.1001/jama.297.3.267 PMID: 17227978

Pavel, M., Öberg, K., & Falconi, M. (2020). ENETS Consensus Guidelines Update for the Management of Distant Metastatic Disease of Intestinal, Pancreatic, and Bronchial Neuroendocrine Neoplasms. *Neuroendocrinology, 110*(9–10), 988–1008. DOI: 10.1159/000443167 PMID: 26731013

Pelzer, U., Hempel, C., Stieler, J., & Oettle, H. (2002). Oxaliplatin (OXA) in combination with high-dose 5-FU (24 h)/folinic acid (FA) as salvage therapy in patients with gemzar-refractory advanced pancreatic cancer. *Proceedings of the American Society of Clinical Oncology, 21*, 172–180.

Pilepich, M. V., & Miller, H. H. (1980). Preoperative irradiation in carcinoma of the pancreas. *Cancer, 46*(9), 1945–1949. DOI: 10.1002/1097-0142(19801101)46:9<1945::AID-CNCR2820460908>3.0.CO;2-X PMID: 7427900

Pisters, P. W., Abbruzzese, J. L., Janjan, N. A., Cleary, K. R., Charnsangavej, C., Goswitz, M. S., Rich, T. A., Raijman, I., Wolff, R. A., Lenzi, R., Lee, J. E., & Evans, D. B. (1998). Rapid-fractionation preoperative chemoradiation, pancreaticoduodenectomy, and intraoperative radiation therapy for resectable Pancreatic adenocarcinoma. *Journal of Clinical Oncology, 16*(12), 3843–3850. DOI: 10.1200/JCO.1998.16.12.3843 PMID: 9850029

Provenzano, P. P., Cuevas, C., Chang, A. E., Goel, V. K., Von Hoff, D. D., & Hingorani, S. R. (2012). Enzymatic Targeting of the Stroma Ablates Physical Barriers to Treatment of Pancreatic Ductal Adenocarcinoma. *Cancer Cell, 21*(3), 418–429. DOI: 10.1016/j.ccr.2012.01.007 PMID: 22439937

Regine, W. F. (2001). Postoperative adjuvant therapy: past, present, and future trial development. In Evans, D. B., Pisters, P. W. T., Abbruzzese, J. L., & Pollock, R. E. (Eds.), *MD Anderson Solid Tumor Oncology Series: Pancreatic Cancer* (pp. 235–242). Springer-Verlag., DOI: 10.1007/978-1-4613-0089-0_20

Reni, M., Panucci, M. G., Ferreri, A. J. M., Balzano, G., Passoni, P., Cattaneo, G. M., Cordio, S., Scaglietti, U., Zerbi, A., Ceresoli, G. L., Fiorino, C., Calandrino, R., Staudacher, C., Villa, E., & Di Carlo, V. (2001). Effect on local control and survival of electron beam intraoperative irradiation for resectable pancreatic adenocarcinoma. *International Journal of Radiation Oncology, Biology, Physics, 50*(3), 651–658. DOI: 10.1016/S0360-3016(01)01470-5 PMID: 11395232

Richter, J., & Saif, M. W. (2010). Updates in adjuvant therapy in pancreatic cancer: Gemcitabine and beyond. Highlights from the "2010 ASCO Gastrointestinal Cancers Symposium". Orlando, FL, USA. January 22–24, 2010. *Journal of the Pancreas, 11(2),* 144–147. doi:pubmed.ncbi.nlm.nih.gov/20208323/

Ryan, D. P., Eder, J. P., Winkelmann, J., & Clark, J. W. (2002). Pharmacokinetic and pharmacodynamic Phase I study of PS-341 and gemcitabine in patients with advanced solid tumors. *Proceedings of the American Society of Clinical Oncology, 21*, 95–102.

Sauer-Heilborn, A., Kath, R., Schneider, C. P., & Höffken, K. (1999). Severe non-haematological toxicity after treatment with gemcitabine. *Journal of Cancer Research and Clinical Oncology, 125*(11), 637–640. DOI: 10.1007/s004320050327 PMID: 10541971

Scarpa, A., Chang, D. K., Nones, K., Corbo, V., Patch, A.-M., Bailey, P., Lawlor, R. T., Johns, A. L., Miller, D. K., Mafficini, A., Rusev, B., Scardoni, M., Antonello, D., Barbi, S., Sikora, K. O., Cingarlini, S., Vicentini, C., McKay, S., Quinn, M. C. J., & Grimmond, S. M. (2017). Whole-Genome Landscape of Pancreatic Neuroendocrine Tumors. *Nature, 543*(7643), 65–71. DOI: 10.1038/nature21063 PMID: 28199314

Schmidt, C. M., Matos, J. M., & Bentrem, D. J. (2007). Acinar Cell Carcinoma of the Pancreas in the United States: Prognostic Factors and Comparison to Ductal Adenocarcinoma. *Journal of Gastrointestinal Surgery, 11*(7), 829–836. DOI: 10.1007/s11605-008-0705-6 PMID: 18836784

Seidel, G., Zahurak, M., Iacobuzio-Donahue, C., Sohn, T. A., Adsay, N. V., Yeo, C. J., Lillemoe, K. D., Cameron, J. L., Hruban, R. H., & Wilentz, R. E. (2002). Almost All Infiltrating Colloid Carcinomas of the Pancreas and Periampullary Region Arise from In Situ Papillary Neoplasms: A Study of 39 Cases. *The American Journal of Surgical Pathology, 26*(1), 56–63. DOI: 10.1097/00000478-200201000-00006 PMID: 11756769

Shah, M. H., Goldner, W. S., Benson, A. B., Bergsland, E., Blaszkowsky, L. S., Brock, P., Chan, J., Das, S., Dickson, P. V., Fanta, P., Giordano, T., Halfdanarson, T. R., Halperin, D., He, J., Heaney, A., Heslin, M. J., Kandeel, F., Kardan, A., Khan, S. A., & Hochstetler, C. (2021). Neuroendocrine and Adrenal Tumors, Version 2.2021, NCCN Clinical Practice Guidelines in Oncology. *Journal of the National Comprehensive Cancer Network : JNCCN, 19*(7), 839–868. DOI: 10.6004/jnccn.2021.0032 PMID: 34340212

Sindelar, W. F., & Kinsella, T. J. (1999). Studies of intraoperative radiotherapy in carcinoma of the pancreas. *Annals of Oncology : Official Journal of the European Society for Medical Oncology, 10*(4), 226–230. DOI: 10.1093/annonc/10.suppl_4.S226 PMID: 10436828

Singhi, A. D., Liu, T. C., Roncaioli, J. L., Cao, D., Zeh, H. J., Zureikat, A. H., Tsung, A., Marsh, J. W., Lee, K. K., Hogg, M. E., Bahary, N., Brand, R. E., McGrath, K. M., Slivka, A., Cressman, K. L., Fuhrer, K., & O'Sullivan, R. J. (2017). Alternative Lengthening of Telomeres and Loss of DAXX/ATRX Expression Predicts Metastatic Disease and Poor Survival in Patients with Pancreatic Neuroendocrine Tumors. *Clinical Cancer Research, 23*(2), 600–609. DOI: 10.1158/1078-0432.CCR-16-1113 PMID: 27407094

Splinter, T. A. W., Obertop, H., Kok, T. C., & Jeekel, J. (1989). Adjuvant Chemotherapy after resection of Adenocarcinoma of the periampullary region and the head of the pancreas: A non-randomised pilot study. *Journal of Cancer Research and Clinical Oncology, 115*(2), 200–202. DOI: 10.1007/BF00397924 PMID: 2715169

Stocken, D. D., Büchler, M. W., Dervenis, C., Bassi, C., Jeekel, H., Klinkenbijl, J. H., Bakkevold, K. E., Takada, T., Amano, H., & Neoptolemos, J. P. (2005). Meta-analysis of Randomised Adjuvant Therapy trials for Pancreatic Cancer. *British Journal of Cancer, 92*(8), 1372–1381. DOI: 10.1038/sj.bjc.6602513 PMID: 15812554

Strobel, O., Neoptolemos, J., Jager, D., & Buchler, M. W. (2019). Optimizing the outcomes of Pancreatic Cancer Surgery. *Nature Reviews. Clinical Oncology, 16*(1), 11–26. DOI: 10.1038/s41571-018-0112-1 PMID: 30341417

Strosberg, J. R., Halfdanarson, T. R., & Bellizzi, A. M. (2017). NANETS Consensus Guidelines for the Diagnosis and Management of Poorly Differentiated (High-Grade) Extrapulmonary Neuroendocrine Carcinomas. *Pancreas, 46*(1), 1–12. DOI: 10.1097/MPA.0b013e3181ebb56f PMID: 27977625

Takada, T., Amano, H., Yasuda, H., Nimura, Y., Matsushiro, T., Kato, H., Nagakawa, T., & Nakayama, T. (2002). Is postoperative adjuvant chemotherapy useful for gallbladder carcinoma? A Phase III multicenter prospective randomized controlled trial in patients with resected Pancreaticobiliary Carcinoma. *Cancer, 95*(8), 1685–1695. DOI: 10.1002/cncr.10831 PMID: 12365016

Tempero, M. A., Malafa, M. P., Al-Hawary, M., Behrman, S. W., Benson, A. B., Cardin, D. B., Chiorean, E. G., Chung, V., Czito, B., Del Chiaro, M., Dillhoff, M., Donahue, T. R., Dotan, E., Ferrone, C. R., Fountzilas, C., Hardacre, J., Hawkins, W. G., Klute, K., Ko, A. H., & George, G. V. (2021). Pancreatic Adenocarcinoma, Version 2.2021, NCCN Clinical Practice Guidelines in Oncology. *Journal of the National Comprehensive Cancer Network : JNCCN, 19*(4), 439–457. DOI: 10.6004/jnccn.2021.0017 PMID: 33845462

Tiriac, H., Belleau, P., Engle, D. D., Plenker, D., Deschênes, A., Somerville, T. D. D., Froeling, F. E. M., Burkhart, R. A., Denroche, R. E., Jang, G.-H., Miyabayashi, K., Young, C. M., Patel, H., Ma, M., LaComb, J. F., Palmaira, R. L. D., Javed, A. A., Huynh, J. C., Johnson, M., & Tuveson, D. A. (2018). Organoid profiling identifies common responders to Chemotherapy in Pancreatic Cancer. *Cancer Discovery*, *8*(9), 1112–1129. DOI: 10.1158/2159-8290.CD-18-0349 PMID: 29853643

Ueno, H., Kosuge, T., Matsuyama, Y., Yamamoto, J., Nakao, A., Egawa, S., Doi, R., Monden, M., Hatori, T., Tanaka, M., Shimada, M., & Kanemitsu, K. (2009). A randomised Phase III trial comparing gemcitabine with surgery-only in patients with resected Pancreatic Cancer: Japanese Study Group of Adjuvant Therapy for Pancreatic Cancer. *British Journal of Cancer*, *101*(6), 908–915. DOI: 10.1038/sj.bjc.6605256 PMID: 19690548

Valle, J. W., Palmer, D., Jackson, R., Cox, T., Neoptolemos, J. P., Ghaneh, P., Rawcliffe, C. L., Bassi, C., Stocken, D. D., Cunningham, D., O'Reilly, D., Goldstein, D., Robinson, B. A., Karapetis, C., Scarfe, A., Lacaine, F., Sand, J., Izbicki, J. R., Mayerle, J., & Büchler, M. W. (2014). Optimal duration and timing of Adjuvant Chemotherapy after definitive surgery for ductal adenocarcinoma of the pancreas: Ongoing lessons from the ESPAC-3 study. *Journal of Clinical Oncology*, *32*(6), 504–512. DOI: 10.1200/JCO.2013.50.7657 PMID: 24419109

van Heek, N. T., Kuhlmann, K. F. D., Scholten, R. J. P. M., de Castro, S. M. M., Busch, O. R. C., van Gulik, T. M., Obertop, H., & Gouma, D. J. (2005). Hospital volume and mortality after pancreatic resection: A systematic review and an evaluation of intervention in the Netherlands. *Annals of Surgery*, *242*(6), 781–788. DOI: 10.1097/01.sla.0000188462.00249.36 PMID: 16327488

Waterhouse, D. M., Richards, D., & Wagener, D. J. (2002). CA 19-9 levels in patients with Advanced Pancreatic Cancer (APC) treated in a randomized, Phase II trial with the histone deacetylase inhibitor CI-994 + gemcitabine (CI-994 + G) versus placebo + gemcitabine (P + G). *Proceedings of the American Society of Clinical Oncology*, *21*, 148–156.

Willett, C. G., & Warshaw, A. L. (1998). Intraoperative radiation therapy of pancreatic cancer. In Beger, H. G., Warshaw, A. L., Büchler, M. W., Carr-Locke, D. L., Neoptolemos, J. P., Russell, C., & Sarr, M. G. (Eds.), *The Pancreas: A Clinical.*, Textbook.

Winter, J. M., Jiang, W., & Basturk, O. (2013). Recurrence and Survival After Resection of Small Intraductal Papillary Mucinous Neoplasm-associated Carcinomas (≤20 mm Invasive Component). *Annals of Surgery*, *258*(2), 313–320. DOI: 10.1097/SLA.0000000000001319 PMID: 23360922

Wisnoski, N. C., Townsend, C. M.Jr, Nealon, W. H., Freeman, J. L., & Riall, T. S. (2008). 672 Patients with Acinar Cell Carcinoma of the Pancreas: A Population-Based Comparison to Pancreatic Adenocarcinoma. *Surgery*, *144*(2), 141–148. DOI: 10.1016/j.surg.2008.03.006 PMID: 18656619

Wong, T., Howes, N., Threadgold, J., Smart, H. L., Lombard, M. G., Gilmore, I., Sutton, R., Greenhalf, W., Ellis, I., & Neoptolemos, J. P. (2001). Molecular diagnosis of early pancreatic ductal adenocarcinoma in high-risk patients. *Pancreatology*, *1*(5), 486–509. DOI: 10.1159/000055852 PMID: 12120229

Wu, J., Matthaei, H., Maitra, A., Dal Molin, M., Wood, L. D., Eshleman, J. R., Goggins, M., Canto, M. I., Schulick, R. D., Edil, B. H., Wolfgang, C. L., Klein, A. P., Diaz, L. A.Jr, Allen, P. J., Schmidt, C. M., Kinzler, K. W., Papadopoulos, N., Hruban, R. H., & Vogelstein, B. (2011). Recurrent GNAS mutations define an unexpected pathway for pancreatic cyst development. *Science Translational Medicine*, *3*(92), 92ra66. Advance online publication. DOI: 10.1126/scitranslmed.3002543 PMID: 21775669

Xiong, H. Q., Du, M., Wolff, R. A., & Abbruzzese, J. L. (2002). Pharmacology study of celecoxib in combination with gemcitabine for advanced pancreatic cancer. *Proceedings of the American Society of Clinical Oncology*, *21*, 113–118.

Yamamoto, J., Saiura, A., Koga, R., Seki, M., Katori, M., Kato, Y., Sakamoto, Y., Kokudo, N., & Yamaguchi, T. (2010). Improved survival of left-sided pancreatic cancer after surgery. *Japanese Journal of Clinical Oncology*, *40*(6), 530–536. DOI: 10.1093/jjco/hyq015 PMID: 20363769

Yao, J. C., Fazio, N., Singh, S., Buzzoni, R., Carnaghi, C., Wolin, E., Tomasek, J., Raderer, M., Lahner, H., Voi, M., Pacaud, L. B., Rouyrre, N., Sachs, C., Valle, J. W., Fave, G. D., Van Cutsem, E., Tesselaar, M., Shimada, Y., Oh, D.-Y., & Pavel, M. E. (2016). Everolimus for the Treatment of Advanced, Non-Functional Neuroendocrine Tumours of the Lung or Gastrointestinal Tract (RADIANT-4): A Randomised, Placebo-Controlled, Phase 3 Study. *Lancet*, *387*(10022), 968–977. DOI: 10.1016/S0140-6736(15)00817-X PMID: 26703889

Yopp, A. C., Katabi, N., Janakos, M., Klimstra, D. S., D'Angelica, M. I., DeMatteo, R. P., Fong, Y., Brennan, M. F., Jarnagin, W. R., & Allen, P. J. (2011). Invasive carcinoma arising in intraductal papillary mucinous neoplasms of the pancreas: A matched control study with conventional pancreatic ductal adenocarcinoma. *Annals of Surgery*, *253*(5), 968–974. DOI: 10.1097/SLA.0b013e318214bcb4 PMID: 21422912

Zerbi, A., Fossati, V., Parolini, D., Carlucci, M., Balzano, G., Bordogna, G., Staudacher, C., & Di Carlo, V. (1994). Intraoperative radiation therapy adjuvant to resection in the treatment of Pancreatic Cancer. *Cancer*, *73*(12), 2930–2935. DOI: 10.1002/1097-0142(19940615)73:12<2930::AID-CNCR2820731209>3.0.CO;2-M PMID: 8199990

Chapter 9

Emerging Therapies: The Future of Pancreatic Cancer Treatment

Vinay Dwivedi
https://orcid.org/0000-0001-8294-0298
Amity University, Gwalior, India

Aarti Dwivedi
Amity University, Gwalior, India

Raghvendra Kumar Mishra
Amity University, Gwalior, India

Gayatri Abhay Kerkar
Amity University, Gwalior, India

Diksha Shrivastava
Amity University, Gwalior, India

Niharika Singh Tomar
Amity University, Gwalior, India

Ragini Singh
Amity University, Gwalior, India

ABSTRACT

Pancreatic cancer remains one of the deadliest malignancies due to aggressive progression, early metastasis, and lack of reliable early detection. Advances in chemotherapy, targeted therapy, immunotherapy, nanomedicine, and organoid-based precision medicine offer hope. Neoadjuvant therapies have improved outcomes in resectable and borderline cases. Emerging strategies, including KRAS-targeted agents, liposomal drug delivery, and checkpoint inhibitors, show clinical promise. A major barrier is the dense stromal matrix that impedes drug delivery. Nanotechnology, through advanced nanoparticle systems, enhances drug solubility, circulation, tumor targeting, and controlled release, reducing toxicity. Organoid technologies and biomarkers are advancing early diagnosis and personalized treatment. The dense stroma presents both a barrier and a target for innovation. Continued translational research is vital to overcome resistance and improve survival.

DOI: 10.4018/979-8-3373-1469-3.ch009

INTRODUCTION

Pancreatic cancer (PC) originating in the pancreas, having a terrible prognosis and is frequently hard to detect on its early stages arising from unchecked cell growth and tumour formation in the pancreas, a gland situated beneath the stomach (Pancreatic Cancer Treatment, 2024). PC are of two types: Pancreatic Ductal Adenocarcinoma (PDAC) which is the most common type originating in the calls that line the pancreatic ducts and Pancreatic Neuroendocrine Tumors (NETs) which is less common originating in the hormone-producing cells of the pancreas (Pancreatic Cancer Action Network, 2025). Although PDAC is the tenth most frequent disease, its poor survival results makes it the seventh greatest cause of cancer-related deaths worldwide. It is still a very dangerous gastrointestinal illness that is difficult to detect early and has a poor 5 year survival rate, even with the quick advancements in contemporary medical technology and the notable improvements in the survival rates of many cancers (Hu *et al.*, 2021). The development of PC is typically detected at a late stage with clinical signs because of the unique anatomical placement of the pancreas (Hu *et al.*, 2021). Knowing and recognising the risk factors for PC aids in its prevention and early detection (Chandana *et al.*, 2023). PDAC has several risk factors such as environmental, lifestyle, and genetic factors. Numerous medical disorders, including demographic and regional factors, age-related factors, and ethnicity, are also associated with PC development. Finding high-risks variables may offer chances for improved results and early PC detection and treatment (Sharma *et al.*, 2025). A comprehensive knowledge of these risks factors will be necessary for promoting the preventive screening and implementation of effective treatment plans to lower incidence and death rates, as well as for better PC management and improved results (Sharma *et al.*, 2025). The classification and metastatic pathways of pancreatic cancer have been illustrated in Figure 1. The destructive nature of PC and the dearth of efficient early detection techniques make early identification and therapy extremely difficult. Timely diagnosis is made more difficult by the lack of distinct symptoms and trustworthy biomarkers for early identification (Chen *et al.*, 2025). The low survival rate despite improvements in peri-operative care and surgical techniques highlights the need for better diagnostic and treatment approaches (Casà *et al.*, 2025). Although immunotherapy and targeted medicines are being developed, their use is constrained by the requirement for particular genetic abnormalities (Daamen *et al.*, 2023). The substantial shortcomings of the existing standard treatments for pancreatic cancer, which include surgery, chemotherapy, and radiation, make emerging medicines essential. The only possible cure is surgery, especially the Whipple method, however it is useful in 15% to 20% of cases because of the late detection and high metastatic rates. The number of patients who are eligible for surgery has not increased substantially despite improvements in imaging and surgical procedures (Banigallapati, 2024). Despite promising methods such as stereostatic body radiation therapy (SBRT) radiotherapy is rarely employed because of its poor efficacy in treating non-resectable tumours (Baker & Craft, 2023). Emerging Therapies include Immunotherapy, Neoadjuvant Therapy (NAT) and Novel Agents. Immunotherapies, including as immune checkpoint inhibitors and mRNA vaccines, are being investigated to improve recurrence-free survival and get past immune evasion mechanisms. In order to reduce tumours and boost surgical eligibility, NAT uses chemotherapy and radiation before to surgery. It has been shown to improve response rates and improve survival (Dallavalle *et al.*, 2024). Clinical trials examining Poly (ADP-ribose polymerase (PARP) inhibitors, new cytotoxic chemotherapies, and tumour microenvironment modifiers are examples of novel agents that may provide effectiveness with lower toxicity. Emerging treatments have potential, but they also confront obstacles such immune evasion and the requirement for individualised treatment plans. To get over these obstacles and enhance the prognosis of patients with pancreatic cancer, more study into molecular pathways and creative therapeutic approaches is necessary. This book chapter gives a brief overview of pancreatic cancer, the current Treatment Landscapes such as Immunotherapy, Targeted therapy and different Molecular Approaches, Tumour Microenvironment Targeting, Nanomedicine and Drug Deliver Innovations, Organoids, AI, and Precision Oncology. It also explores the clinical trials and ethical considerations needed to be followed in pancreatic cancer along with its future outlooks.

CURRENT TREATMENT LANDSCAPE

First-line treatment strategies

The best available possibly curative therapy at the moment is a multimodal strategy that involves surgical resection followed by adjuvant chemotherapy with FOLFIRINOX, which has a 3-year survival rate of above 60%. However because of its toxicity profile (the rate of grade 3-4 adverse events: 75.9%), this technique is only feasible in a small percentage of patients. Following the ESPAC-4 data, gemcitabine/capecitabine maty be an alternative for less fit people over 70 with an Eastern Cooperative Oncology Group (ECOG) performance status (PS) of 2 or patients who have any contraindication to the medications utilised in FOLFORINOX. Only pateints who are really weak should be treated with gemcitabine aalone, the first medication to show promise in the post-operative phase (De Dosso *et al.*, 2021). Tumours classified as 'borderline resectable' are those that respond well to neoadjuvant therapy, mostly because they have contact with the superior mesenteric vein or portal vein of $>180^{o}$ or with the superior mesenteric or coeliac artery of $\leq 180^{o}$

(Katz *et al.*, 2021). Randomised studies are being conducted in these situations as there is currently no clear standard procedure. Although chemotherapy or chemotherapy plus radiation therapy may be an option, the majority of recommendations are based on retrospective series, meta-analyses, and systematic reviews. However, new information points to FOLFORINOX as the most promising preoperative approach in this situation (Ghaneh *et al.*, 2020). Long-term survival rates are often low, with significant recurrence rates, despite the adjuvant and neoadjuvant approach being optimised For this reason, alternative therapeutic alternatives are urgently needed (McGuigan *et al.*, 2018). About half of the patients have distant metastases when they are diagnosed, according to this. The most common treatment method in this case is still systematic chemotherapy, which aims to reduce cancer-related symptoms and increase survival. The use if gemcitabine as a therapy for metastatic PC has long been established (Gemcitabin Labatec®, 2019).

It is crucial to base the selection of first-line therapy on the availability and overlap with possible second-line choices in order to optimise the continuum of care for patients with PC (De Dosso *et al.*, 2021). While gemcitabine plus nab-paclitaxel would enable second-line treatment with nanoliposomal irinotecan (nal-IRI) plus 5-fluorouracil (5FU), the only second-line therapy for metastatic PC that has demonstrated a survival advantage in a phase III study, following progression to gemcitabine-based regimen, FOLFIRINOX as a front-line treatment lacks clinically validated second-line options (Macuralla Mercadé *et al.*, 2020).

Second-line treatment strategies

Between 40-50% of patients with advanced PC eventually get second or later line chemotherapy. Treatment decision may be influenced by a number of factors, such as medication availability, patient characteristics, physician preference, and previous first-line therapy (Lambert *et al.*, 2019). Additionally, before selecting second-line treatment for patients with PC, the risk: benefit ratio should be examined. The choice of first-line treatment may be influenced by the changing situation in the second line. For example, folinic acid (leucovorin [LV] and nal-IRI with 5-FU is a novel second-line treatment that is only appropriate for patients who are making progress on gemcitabine-based therapy (Taieb *et al.*, 2020). Notably, this combination is also utilised as a third-line treatment in the clinical context if it hasn't been used before. However, despite the paucity of randomised clinical trials, the combination of gemcitabine and nab-paclitaxel may be a second-line therapeutic option when FOLFIRINOX therapy in the first-line fails. Small retrospective and cohort studies have demonstrated that this combination is more successful than gemcitabine monotherapy (de Jesus *et al.*, 2018). Strategies of treatment for first, second and third line therapy of patients with PDAC has been given in the form of flowchart (Figure 2).

Surgical options

Depending on where the tumour is located, different surgical options may be available. While tumours in the head and uncinate process necessitate a Pancreatic Duodenectomy (PD) for full resection, tumours distal to the pancreatic head are typically amenable to distal pancreatectomy. The Italian physician Dr. Codivilla introduced PD in1889, and Dr. Whipple used his two-step description to thoroughly define it in 1935 (Whipple *et al.*, 1935). The first laparoscopic PD (LPD) procedure for treating chronic pancreatis localised in the pancreatic head (pancreas divisum) was described by Gagner and Pomp in 1994. Since then, the approach has been more well-liked. New research has shown that patients with LPD have shorter hospital stays and comparable rates of complications, overall survival, and 5-year survival to those with PD (Hayat *et al.*, 2025). Nevertheless, there is a strong correlation between these surgical treatments and short-term morbidity and mortality. Pancreatic fistula (average frequency of 5-15%) and delayed stomach emptying (20%) are two of the most prevalent PD-related problems. Due to advances in surgical procedures, such as vascular resection and reconstruction, surgical results for PDAC have improved over the past few decades. A higher survival rate of 20-30% results from this. Nevertheless, surgical procedures continue to have greater recurrence rates, most likely because to the existence of micro metastases during the surgical procedure (Kolbeinsson *et al.*, 2023).

Chemotherapy – Adjuvant

The prognosis is still bad even for patients with localised, resectable tumours; the 5-year survival rate after surgery alone is only 20%, and with adjuvant treatment, it rises to 30% to 405. Gemcitabine and capecitabine or gemcitabine alone are commended for patients with poor functional level, while modifies FOLFIINOX is recommended for individuals with good functional status (Mizrahi *et al.*, 2020). In the six months after surgical resection, participants treated with gemcitabine has a slightly higher median overall survival (OS) (22.8 months) than those who were observed (20.2 months), according to the CONKO-001 trial. In an adjuvant scenario, gemcitabine's results were not improved by the addition of erlotinib. In a phase II trial with 22 patients, the adjuvant gemcitabine and cisplatin combination was assessed; where the median OS was 35.5 months. The combination was possible, despite the fact that a significant portion of patients (59%) had grade ¾ toxicity (Hayat *et al.*, 2025).

Chemotherapy – Neoadjuvant

Due to numerous studies demonstrating its efficacy in treating Locally Advanced pancreatic Cancer (LAPC) and Borderline Resectable Pancreatic Cancer (BRPC), neoadjuvant chemotherapy has grown in popularity throughout the past ten years. Patients using neoadjuvant treatment should have restaging scans before surgery if no signs of disease progression are seen. A multi-institutional trial showed that patients with BRPC undergoing neoadjuvant therapy had higher margin-negative resection rates. Its benefit in resectable PDAC is still being studies, though. One possible drawback of neoadjuvant therapy is that it may promote tumour growth when there is insufficient tumour response (Mokdad *et al.*, 2017).

Radiation Therapy

Radiation therapy's involvement in PDAC is debatable, and research is still being done to determine the best course of action. In patients with resectable PDAC, the PREOPANC trial discovered that neoadjuvant gemcitabine-based chemoradiography increased OS when compared to upfront surgery and adjuvant gemcitabine (Artinyan *et al.*, 2011). Its unclear how chemoradiation affects LAPC. Following R1 resection, it may be taken into consideration as an adjuvant; following a multidisciplinary evaluation, it may be considered as a neoadjuvant for certain patients. Retrospective analysis and data from small studies indicate that R0 resection rates are enhanced by chemoradiation in the neoadjuvant setting; nevertheless, further data from randomised clinical trials is required. However, it is not advised to utilise radiation with FOLFIRINOX in a neoadjuvant situation (Sohal *et al.*, 2021).

Emergent Therapies: Target Therapy, Immunotherapy and CAR-T

The field of pancreatic treatments is constantly evolving, and in recent years, new and developing treatments have gathered steam. Many targeted cancer medicines that can be utilised for any metastatic cancer with specific mutations for which first-line therapies have run out and been approved in recent years (Hayat *et al.*, 2025). Traditional targeted therapy is identifying germline or somatic alterations in cancer cells and developing a drug that selectively targets the impacted pathways. KRAS, which involves the G12 codon, is one of the genes with the highest mutation rates in pancreatic cancer. Clinical trials are now being conducted to examine how sotorasib may be used in conjunction with other treatments. Another targeted treatment for the G12C codon pathway under investigation is adagrasib. It is said to be well tolerated and has shown promising benefits (Bekaii-Saab *et al.*, 2023). Other pathways, like tyrosine kinase signalling, have proven advantageous in alternative cancer treatments in addition to KRAS signalling pathways. This route is being investigated as a promising cancer treatment option for pancreatic cancer. Patients with metastatic pancreatitis have been previously been treated with the EGFR inhibitor erlotinib, with evidence showing a longer survival time. Additional EGFR inibitors, including humanised nimotuzumab anitibodies are being researched at the moment. Focal adhesion kinases, which are non-receptor tyrosine kinase inhibitors that postpone tumour growth, have been employed in a variety of ways (Buckely & O'Reilly, 2024). The effectiveness of immunotherapy in treating PC has been disputed. For example, research examining the response to PC in combination with or without chemotherapy has gained some attention due to the assessment of CD40 agonists. Additionally, there is little proof that chimeric antigen receptor T-cell therapy is effective in treating PC, despite it having been examined. Numerous clinical trials are being conducted to further investigate the role of CAR-T (Buckely & O'Reilly, 2024). A flowchart of all the therapeutic options has been shown in the Figure 3. The above metioned Conventional treatment strategies, including surgical resection, chemotherapy, and radiotherapy, offer limited survival benefits. Gemcitabine, a standard chemotherapeutic agent, has demonstrated modest efficacy, extending overall survival by only 6 to 12 weeks. However, its effectiveness is hindered by a short half-life and low concentration in tumour tissues. Furthermore, a significant proportion of patients are ineligible for surgery due to late-stage diagnosis, early metastasis, and extensive local invasion. The absence of reliable biomarkers, high recurrence rates, and chemoresistance further exacerbate the poor prognosis associated with pancreatic cancer. These challenges underscore the urgent need for the development of more effective therapeutic approaches.

IMMUNOTHERAPY IN PANCREATIC CANCER

Immune checkpoint inhibitors

Anti- CTLA-4 and anti-PD-1/ anti PD-L1 drugs that block immunological checkpoints activate T cells and offer a successful tumour immunotherapy strategy. However, the majority of phase I and II clinical trials have not demonstrated any clinical efficacy in PAC although showing strong outcomes in certain malignancies. It is interesting to note that immune checkpoint inhibitor based treatment regimens combined with radiation and chemotherapy have shown positive outcomes.

Ipilimumab

Ipilimumab, a fully humanized anti- CTLA- 4 IgG1 monoclonal antibody (mAb), was approved for clinical use in the US and Europe in 2011; nevertheless, patients with locally progressed or metastatic PAC, the outcomes have been unsatisfactory. Furthermore, higher toxicity has been linked to the use of Ipilimumab in PAC patients. Remarkably, the combination with chemotherapy has yielded more encouraging outcomes. Gemcitabine, a popular treatment for advanced PAC, has actually been demonstrated to increase the immune response by increasing the activation of naïve T cells. Ipilimumab plus gemicitabine were used in phase Ib clinical trial (NCT01473940), with early findings showing a median OS of 8.5 months (95% CI 2.2 -10.3) and 2.5 months as the median progression- free survival (FPS) (95% CL 0.8-4.8) (Mohindra *et al.*, 2015). The most frequent toxicities were haematologic, with five patients having stable diseases (SD) and 2 in 11 examined patients experiencing (PR) Partial response. Ipilimumab and anti- PD- 1 drug Nivolumab are also being evaluated in another current clinical research NCT01928394; however, findings have not yet been released (Bristol-Myers Squibb, 2013) (Table 1)

Tremelimumab

Tremelimumab, another anti-CTLA-4 inhibitor and human IgG2 mAb, was evaluated as monotherapy in the phase II open label research (NCTO2527432). Eligible participants in the cohort of patients with metastatic PAC experienced tumour progression after receiving a 5- FU gemcitabine regimen. With the low median OS of 4 months (95% cl 2.83 – 5.42) and worsening illness in 18 out of 20 patients, tremelimumab yielded disappointing results . However, in phase I trial (Aglietta *et al).* assessed the effectiveness of gemcitabine and Tremelimumab together (NCT00556023) (Table 1 According to an efficacy research, durvalumab monotherapy had no effect on patients, but the combination had on objective response rate (ORR) of 3.1% (95% cl 0.08 – 16.22). The study was intended to be a randomized clinical trial based on the findings of part A, was not carried out as part A failed to achieve the intended threshold efficacy of 10% (Aglietta *et al.,* 2014)

Pembrolizumab

In PAC, immunohistochemical research has shown a correlation between poorer OS and PD-L1 expression. Immunomodulatory effects of gemcitabine and paclitaxel, a common first- line chemotherapeutic treatment for metastatic PAC, have been documented in the past (Nomi *et al.,* 2007). The safety and effectiveness of pembrolizumab, a PD-1 inhibitor, in conjunction with gemcitabine and nab- paclitaxel chemotherapy were assessed in the phase Ib /II research (NCT02331251). Evaluations of PFS and OS at 9.1 and 15.0 months respectively, revealed a significant positive association with OS and PFS (r = 0.777), whereas only 53% of patients experienced grade 3 incidents (Weiss *et al.,* 2019) (Table 1)

Atezolizumab

Atezolizumab is a designed IgG1 mAb that targets PD- L1, atezolizumab, demonstrated tolerability at dosages up to 20 mg/kg every three weeks in a phase I dose- escalating study. There is presently a phase I/II trial (NCT03829501) (Mizugaki et al.,2016) (Table 1)

Table 1. Immune Checkpoints inhibitor

Intervention	Cancer stage	Strategy	Clinical phase/ Identifier	Outcomes Median Overall Survival (months)	References
Ipilimumab, Gemcitabine	Locally advanced / unresectable(Stage III/ IV or metastatic pancreatic cancer.	CTLA-4 inhibitor, Cytotoxic drugs	Phase Ib, NCT01473940	8.5 (95% CI 2.2-10.3)	Mohindra *et al.,* 2015
Ipilimumab, Nivolumab	Advanced / metastatic pancreatic cancer	CTLA-4 inhibitor, PD-1 inhibitor	Phase I/II, NCT01928394	Ongoing	National Institute of health
Ipilimumab	Advanced / metastatic pancreatic cancer	CTLA- 4 Inhibitor	Phase II, NCT00112580	No improvement in survival rate.	Royal *et al.,* 2010
Tremelimumab, Durvalumab	Metastatic pancreatic ductal adenocarcinoma	CTLA-4 inhibitor, PD-1 inhibitor	Phase II, NCT02558894	3.1 (95%, 2.2- 6.1), Combination therapy 3.6(95%CI, 2.7-6.1), Durvalumab alone	O' Reilly *et al.,* 2019
Tremelimumab	Advanced / metastatic pancreatic cancer	CTLA-4 inhibitor	Phase II, NCT02527434	4 (95% CI, 2.83-5.42)	AstraZeneca, 2015
Atezolizumab	Advanced pancreatic cancer	PD-L1 inhibitor	Phase I/II, NCT03829501	Ongoing	Clinical Trials.gov.
Perbrolizumab, Gemcitabine, Nab-paclitaxel	Advanced / metastatic pancreatic cancer	PD-1 inhibitor cytotoxic drugs	Phase Ib/II, NCT02331251	15.0 (95%CI, 6.8- 22.6)	Weiss *et al.,* 2019

Nanomedicine and Drug Delivery Innovations

Nanomedicine is a rapidly growing field that applies principles and techniques from nanoscience to medical biology, focusing on disease prevention, diagnosis, and treatment. It involves the use of nano-sized materials—including nanorobots and nanosensors—for diagnostic and therapeutic functions, as well as actuating materials within living cells. One notable example is the development of nanoparticle-based platforms that integrate both therapeutic and imaging capabilities, offering a powerful tool for cancer diagnosis and treatment (Brigger *et al.*, 2012).

The first generation of nanoparticle-based therapies introduced lipid-based systems such as liposomes and micelles, many of which have received FDA approval (Allen & Cullis, 2013). These structures can encapsulate inorganic nanoparticles like gold or magnetic particles, enhancing their functionality in both therapeutic and diagnostic applications (Gupta & Gupta, 2005). As a result, the use of inorganic nanoparticles has expanded significantly, particularly in the areas of drug delivery, medical imaging, and targeted therapies.

Nanostructures offer several advantages in drug delivery. They help protect drugs from degradation in the gastrointestinal tract and improve the delivery of poorly water-soluble compounds to specific target sites. Additionally, nanostructures circulate in the bloodstream for extended periods, allowing for the controlled and sustained release of drugs, which minimizes plasma level fluctuations and reduces the risk of side effects. In fact, cellular absorption of nanoparticles is significantly higher than that of larger particles in the 1–10 μm range (Desai *et al.*, 1996).

The key advantages of nanoparticles in drug delivery stem from their unique surface properties, which allow for the attachment of various biomolecules and proteins to enhance functionality. For example, gold nanoparticles are commonly used as biomarkers and tumor labels in biomolecular detection assays due to their excellent biocompatibility and surface reactivity (Dreaden *et al.*, 2012). In designing nanoparticle-based drug delivery systems, the selection of nanoparticles is often guided by the physicochemical properties of the therapeutic agents involved. An emerging and promising strategy in this field is the integration of nanotechnology with bioactive natural compounds. This combination offers several therapeutic advantages, particularly in the treatment of cancer and infectious diseases. Natural compounds are gaining attention for their biological activities, including their ability to trigger tumor-suppressing autophagy—as demonstrated by agenLets like curcumin and caffeine—and their potent antimicrobial effects, shown by compounds such as cinnamaldehyde, carvacrol, curcumin, and eugenol (Huang *et al.*, 2018; Marchese *et al.*, 2017; Tyagi *et al.*, 2015).

Encapsulation of these natural compounds into nanocarriers significantly improves their pharmacological properties. It enhances bioavailability, ensures targeted delivery, and enables controlled release. For instance, thymoquinone, the active constituent of *Nigella sativa*, exhibited a sixfold increase in bioavailability when encapsulated in lipid-based nanocarriers compared to its free form. This formulation also provided better protection in the gastrointestinal tract and improved its pharmacokinetic profile, ultimately resulting in enhanced therapeutic efficacy (Ahmad *et al.*, 2020).

Both synthetic polymers—such as polyvinyl alcohol, poly-l-lactic acid, polyethylene glycol, and poly (lactic-co-glycolic acid)—and natural polymers like chitosan and alginate are frequently utilized in nanoparticle fabrication (Zhang *et al.*, 2022). The choice of an appropriate nanocarrier system is primarily determined by the physicochemical characteristics of the drug to be delivered (Wang *et al.*, 2021). However, despite their numerous advantages, the potential toxicity of nanoparticles remains a major concern. To address this, the integration of natural products with nanoparticles has emerged as a promising approach to mitigate toxicity. In particular, green synthesis methods—employing plant-based or biological materials in nanoparticle production—have gained considerable attention for their ability to reduce or eliminate the use of hazardous chemicals during fabrication, making the process more environmentally friendly and safer (Iravani, 2011).

Lipid nanoparticles (LNPs) have emerged as highly versatile delivery systems in the pharmaceutical industry, facilitating the transport of a broad range of therapeutic agents. In addition to their medical applications, LNPs have been explored in other fields, including medical imaging, cosmetics, nutrition, agriculture, and even nanoreactor design. Liposomes, the precursors to modern LNPs, are highly flexible nanocarriers capable of encapsulating both hydrophobic and hydrophilic substances, such as small molecules, proteins, and nucleic acids (Nsairat *et al.*, 2022). The next generation of lipid nanoparticles (LNPs), including solid lipid nanoparticles (SLNs) (Figure 4), nanostructured lipid carriers (NLCs), and cationic lipid–nucleic acid complexes, feature more sophisticated internal structures and offer enhanced physical stability compared to earlier formulations. These advanced systems enable precise control over the spatial and temporal release of drugs, making them highly effective for treating a wide range of diseases (Alavi & Nokhodchi, 2021; Zhong *et al.*, 2022). As biomedical research progresses, there is an increasing focus on therapies that target diseases at the genetic level, such as gene silencing and editing. In this regard, LNPs are particularly valuable due to their ability to safely and efficiently deliver nucleic acids and other complex therapeutic agents to targeted areas within the body (Hou *et al.*, 2021).

Liposomes typically range in diameter from 20 nm to several hundred micrometers, with those between 80 and 150 nm considered optimal for drug delivery (Figure 5). Particle size plays a crucial role in influencing pharmacokinetics, tissue distribution, hepatic clearance, renal elimination, and cellular uptake (Bozzuto & Molinari, 2015). Liposomal formulations have made significant strides in cancer treatment by enhancing drug delivery and reducing systemic toxicity. Doxil, the first PEGylated liposomal formulation of doxorubicin, boosts the drug's anticancer effects by inducing caspase-dependent apoptosis and oxidative DNA damage through topoisomerase II inhibition and free radical generation (Barenholz, 2012). Similarly, paclitaxel, which disrupts microtubule function to inhibit tumor cell division, has been reformulated to reduce its toxicity. Since paclitaxel is poorly water-soluble, liposomal formulations such as LEP-ETU, EndoTAG™, and Lipusu® have been developed to avoid toxic solvents like Cremophor EL. These liposomal versions improve bioavailability and more effectively target tumor vasculature (Wang *et al.*, 2015).

Targeted Therapies and Molecular Approaches

Targeted drug delivery systems often utilize various receptors to achieve enhanced specificity, and several biological ligands have been extensively studied for this purpose. (Table 2)

1. Antigens, particularly tumor-associated antigens like the carcinoembryonic antigen found in gastrointestinal, lung, and breast cancers, have been widely used for antibody-mediated targeting due to their overexpression in tumor tissues compared to normal.
2. Cadherins, a group of Ca^{2+}-dependent glycoproteins involved in cell-cell adhesion, have shown potential in inhibiting metastasis, particularly E-cadherin, whose dysfunction is associated with tumour progression (Takeichi, 1991).
3. Selectins, which bind to carbohydrate ligands on cell surfaces, contribute to tumor metastasis through multivalent interactions involving molecules like sialyl Lewis X and sialyl Lewis A (Borsig, 2018).
4. Integrins, composed of α and β subunits, are essential in cell adhesion and signaling and are promising targets in cancer therapy due to their role in tumor invasion and angiogenesis (Desgrosellier & Cheresh, 2010).
5. Vitamins such as folic acid and biotin can be used as ligands since their receptors are often overexpressed in cancer cells, enabling receptor-mediated endocytosis for targeted drug delivery (Sudimack & Lee, 2000).
6. Transferrin, which mediates iron transport, has also been explored as a carrier due to its receptor's high expression on tumor cells (Qian *et al.*, 2002).
7. Hormones and their receptors, overexpressed in cancers like ovarian, endometrial, and breast cancer, offer additional opportunities for targeted delivery of chemotherapeutic agents (Jiang *et al.*, 2014)

Table 2. Targeted Treatments in Pancreatic Ductal Adenocarcinoma (PDAC)

Gene Targeted Therapy	Targets of Gene	Mechanism	Details
KRAS Prohibitor	KRAS Gene mutations	The KRAS protein, a crucial component of cell signaling pathways that control cell division and proliferation, is the target of KRAS inhibitors. These medications try to stop the unchecked development of cancer cells by inhibiting KRAS activity.	KRAS mutations are commonly found in pancreatic ductal adenocarcinoma (PDAC), particularly G12C, G12D, G12V, and G12R. Clinical trials focusing on these mutations have demonstrated promising effects with KRAS inhibitors such sotorasib and adagrasib.
PARP Prohibitor	BRCA1/2 Gene Mutations	The PARP enzyme, which is necessary for fixing single-strand DNA breaks, is the target of PARP inhibitors. When PARP is blocked in cancer cells with BRCA mutations, DNA damage accumulates and eventually results in cell death.	Patients with PDAC who have BRCA1 or BRCA2 mutations are treated with olaparib, especially after platinum-based chemotherapy. The potential efficacy of other PARP inhibitors, like talazoparib, is also being studied.
Immune checkpoint blockers	PD-1/PD-L1 Gene Alterations	These inhibitors increase the immune system's capacity to identify and eliminate cancer cells by interfering with the interaction between PD-1 receptors on immune cells and PD-L1 proteins on cancer cells.	Pembrolizumab is allowed to treat PDAC that exhibits mismatch repair deficiency (dMMR) or high microsatellite instability (MSI-H). Immunotherapy may be more successful when combined with chemotherapy, vaccines, or other therapeutic treatments.
SMAD4-Targeted Therapy	SMAD4 Gene Alterations	SMAD4 is a specific part of the TGF-β signaling pathway, which controls cell growth and apoptosis. Targeting SMAD4 seeks to restore normal signaling and prevent tumor progression.	Metformin can assist to treat PDAC with SMAD4 deficiency by affecting the metabolism of cancer cells and inhibiting the emergence of tumors.
RET Prohibitors	RET Insertion	RET inhibitors block the activity of RET proteins, which can promote cancer cell growth when abnormally activated.	Selpercatinib targets RET gene fusions and has demonstrated durable responses in PDAC patients.
NTRK Prohibitors	NTRK Insertion	NTRK inhibitors block the action of TRK proteins, which, when abnormally activated in certain types of cancer, can result in uncontrolled proliferation of cells	Tumors with NTRK fusions, including PDAC, can be treated with larotrectinib and entrectinib.

Li & Vederas, (2009)

Tumour Microenvironment Targeting

Pancreatic stellate cells (PSCs), immune cells, and cancer-associated fibroblasts (CAFs) are among the cell types that make up the PDAC stroma. Recent studies have focused on reprogramming the stroma to produce a more advantageous milieu for therapy. Strategies for Stromal Reprogramming include FAK inhibition, Nanocarriers and Immunomodulators. A comparison of therapeutic strategies targeting the PDAC stroma has been given in Table 3. Meanwhile, various strategies for immunotherapy enhancement include: targeting CAFs, Inhibiting Regulatory T cells (Tregs) and Exogenous neoantigen vaccination.

Table 3. Comparison of therapeutic Strategies targeting the PDAC Stroma

Therapeutic Strategy	**Target/Mechanism**	**Key Effects**	**References**
Hyaluronidase (PEGPH20)	Degrades hyaluronan, remodels ECM, and reduces immunosuppression	Enhanced drug penetration, reduced HA levels, improved immune infiltration	(Zhou *et al.*, 2024) (Lee *et al.*, 2024).
Hedgehog Pathway Inhibitors	Inhibit Hh signalling in HPSCs, reduce ECM deposition, and mitigate desmoplasia	Improved drug delivery, reduced tumour growth, enhanced immunotherapy efficacy	(Hwang *et al.*, 2023) (Spivak-Kroizman *et al.*, 2023).
Nanocarriers and Immunomodulators	Deliver chemotherapeutic agents and immunomodulators, remodel stroma, and boose immunity	Synergistic anti tumour effects, enhanced immunogenic cell death, improved drug delivery	(Chattopadhyay *et al.*, 2023) (T *et al.*, 2023)
FAK Inhibition	Inhibits FAK, reduces ECM deposition, and enhances radiation therapy and immunotherapy	Improved tumour regression, enhanced T-cell priming, increased survival	(Shu & Wikison, 2022) (Liu *et al.*, 2024)

Li & Vedera (2009)

ORGANOIDS, AI, AND PRECISION ONCOLOGY

Patient- derived organoids

Patient-derived organoids provide the opportunity to study the behavior of individual cancers for both direct precision medicine and translational research. Another most recent and major breakthrough in the study of pancreatic cancer has been the development of pancreatic organoids. The Tuveson and Clevers labs used a 3D tissue culture method called pancreatic organoids to create human and animal models of the evolution of pancreatic ductal adenocarcinoma (PDAC) (Kim *et al.*, 2024). It has been shown that PDOs preserve the primary tumor's differentiation status, phenotypic heterogeneity, and histoarchitecture, making them representative of the particular patient. Additionally, PDOs preserve physiological changes unique to each patient, such as hypoxia, oxygen consumption, and epigenetic markers (Zhang *et al.*, 2024). PDOs could also be utilised for orthotopic transplantation into animal models and genetic modification. Beyond the various significant applications of mechanistic cancer research, it has been shown that PDOs can be used to test medication responsiveness in pancreatic cancer pre-clinical trials. As a result, PDOs are crucial for advancing cancer biology research and customizing pancreatic cancer treatment (Zhang *et al.*, 2024).

Personalized drug testing

PDOs, or patient-derived cancer organoids, have great potential to upgrade patient outcomes and tailor therapeutic choices. Scientists studying cancer are looking into similar strategies, gaining motivation from microbiology, where the Kirby-Bauer disk diffusion test allows for precise antibiotic selection by comparing several medicines against bacteria obtained from patients. Organoid models created from patient tumors are therefore a potential method. These organoids help screen a variety of therapeutic drugs to discover the best course of action for a person's cancer cells (Xu *et al.*, 2025). According to recent research, patient-derived organoids (PDOs) may indicate how well a patient would react to treatment. PDOs have the potential to be used in personalized cancer treatment since they can accurately preserve and replicate the genetic makeup and histological characteristics of the tumors from which they originate. PDOs and PDXs offer a unique balance between genetic fidelity and the potential of individualized medicine, setting them apart from other models such as 2D cell cultures, cancer-on-chip systems, spheroids, genetically engineered mouse models (GEMMs), and cell line-derived xenografts (CDX) (Xu *et al.*, 2025). These models have evident advantages over the more complex, but frequently resource-intensive, GEMMs and cancer-on-chip systems, as well as the simplicity of 2D cultures (Doe & Smith, 2023). One of the main uses of PDOs in PC research is dynamic chemotherapy sensitivity profiling, which evaluates how susceptible individual tumors are to different chemotherapeutic drugs and may reduce the need for animal models in drug screening. This method enables the customized assessment of each tumor's reaction to various chemotherapeutic drugs, that may help decide which treatment plans are best for a certain patient (Zhang *et al.*, 2024). The ethical implications of patient-centered medicine must be addressed, regardless of the vast potential of PDO technology. It is required to carefully handle issues including informed consent, genetic privacy, commercial organoid use, and biological material ownership (Choi *et al.*, 2024). Maintaining patient trust and handling unexpected genetic findings that could influence patients or their family members successfully depend on clearly established consent procedures and ethical standards (Xu *et al.*, 2025).

Clinical Trials

In oncology research, PDOs are playing a bigger role, especially in clinical trials. They can speed up medication development and personalize cancer treatment. Clinical trials are investigations into the effectiveness of novel therapies, processes, or equipment. They play a significant role in cancer prevention, treatment, and cure. Clinical trials were used to examine nearly all cancer treatments before being administered to patients. Researchers can verify if new medicines are helpful for patients by looking at the number of patients who respond to the tested therapy. There are numerous ongoing clinical trials, and participating in one could provide important data that would assist researchers in advancing treatment. Through trial participation, patients may occasionally have access to novel medicines that can improve their quality of life in ways that traditional therapy cannot. (Memorial Sloan Kettering Cancer Center, n.d.). New pancreatic cancer treatments are being tested by Memorial Sloan Kettering (MSK) Cancer Center. Drugs, drug combinations, technologies, and methods of performing operations, surgery, or radiation therapy are all tested in treatment studies. They are investigating the use of novel immunotherapy treatments for metastatic pancreatic cancer and pancreatic cancer following surgery. Immunotherapy is a promising treatment option for advanced pancreatic cancer, according to their clinical trials. Their experiment investigates the use of two immune-boosting medications as a substitute for chemotherapy. Immunotherapy is being investigated in another experiment for pancreatic tumors with KRAS or NRAS gene mutations that were surgically excised (Memorial Sloan Kettering Cancer Centre, n.d.).

Current clinical trial landscape

Clinical trials are the finest way to investigate the question of prospective remedies since they represent the most advanced stages in the development of new treatments. Here, experts profile the state of experimental treatments that are further along in the development pipeline by presenting the entire compilation of ongoing clinical trials in pancreatic cancer. The goal of this analysis is to arrange, evaluate, and compile the interventions that are currently being studied. Experts use this information to characterize the entire range of medicines in study and to calculate the number of current studies.

There were 430 ongoing therapeutic interventional studies assessing 590 treatments as of May 18, 2019. Phase III testing accounts for a very small percentage of studies (n = 37, 8.6%). Immunotherapies make up 189 (31%) of the interventions, followed by cell signaling pathways. (69; 11%), cell cycle or DNA biology (154; 26%), and metabolic pathways (35; 6%). Just 14 of the late phase trials are presently evaluating innovative therapies. Instead, 23 phase III trials look at novel approaches to provide currently approved FDA medications, treatments, or pain relief (Katayama *et al.*, 2020).

CONCLUSION

PC due to its aggressive progression, late detection, and resistance to standard treatments continues to pose significant oncology challenge. Although there is little chance of long-term survival with conventional treatments like radiation, chemotherapy, and surgery, new approaches offer hope. Improvements in precision medicine, including AI-assisted diagnostics and patient-derived organoids, targeted therapies immunotherapies, and nanomedicine are forming a more individualised and successful treatment strategy. While immunotherapies are gradually overcoming the immunosuppressive tumour microenvironment, drug delivery systems based on nanoparticles improve therapeutic efficacy and lower systemic toxicity. Notwithstanding setbacks, novel combinations and delivery systems are helping agents like immune checkpoint inhibitors and CAR-T cell therapies gain traction. Organoid technologies help to understand tumour biology in addition to enabling personalised drug screening. The lack of reliable biomarkers, low mutational burden, and desmoplastic stroma, however, continue to be major obstacles. Clinical trials and ongoing multidisciplinary research are essential to converting these advancements into better results. Navigating the complicated terrain of PC requires cooperation between researchers, clinicians, and the biotech sector. Ultimately, patients suffering from this terrible illness may experience a new era of hope if emerging therapies are combined with current standards.

Figure 1. Classification of Metastatic pathways of Pancreatic Cancer

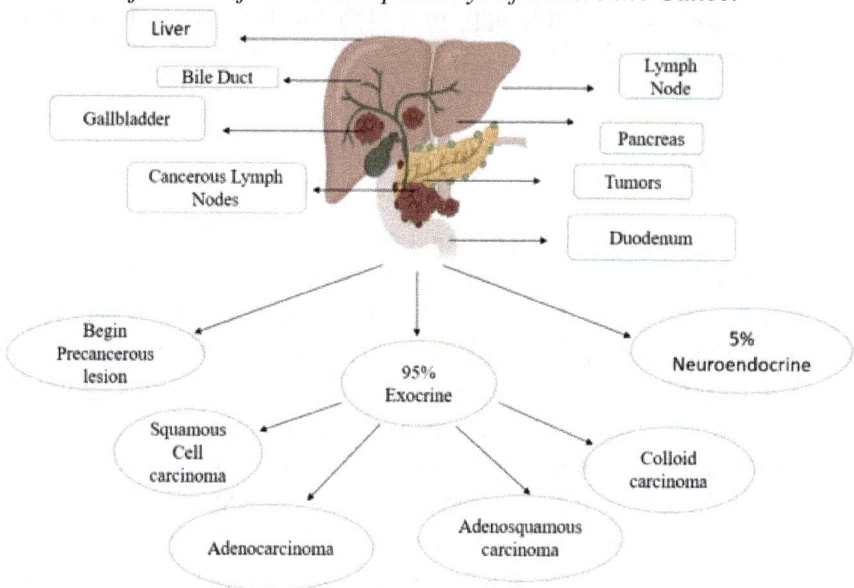

Figure 2. Strategies of treatment for first, second and third line therapy of patients with Pancreatic Ductal Adenocarcinoma Cancer (PDAC). PS, performance status

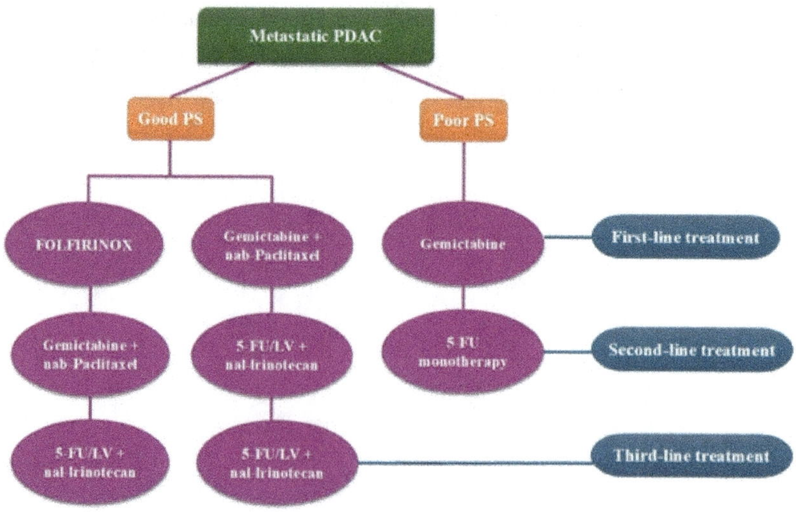

Figure 3. Flow chart of all available therapeutic options

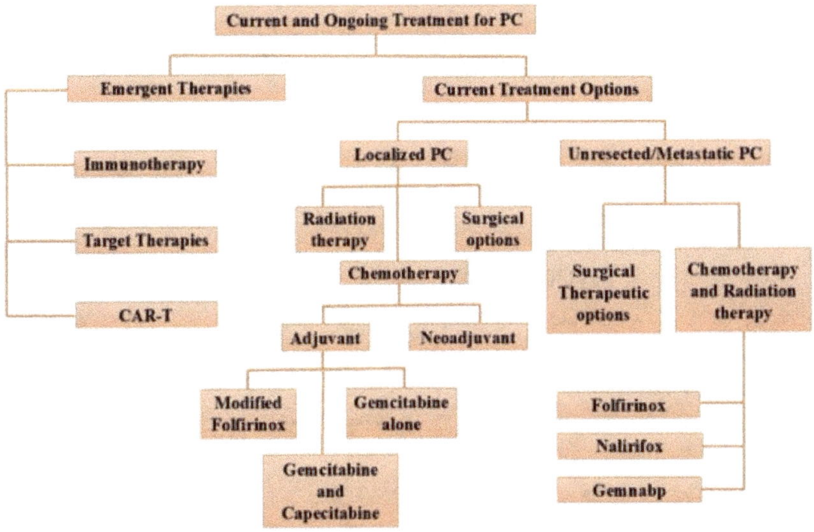

Figure 4. Schematic diagram of Solid Lipid Nanoparticles (SLNs)

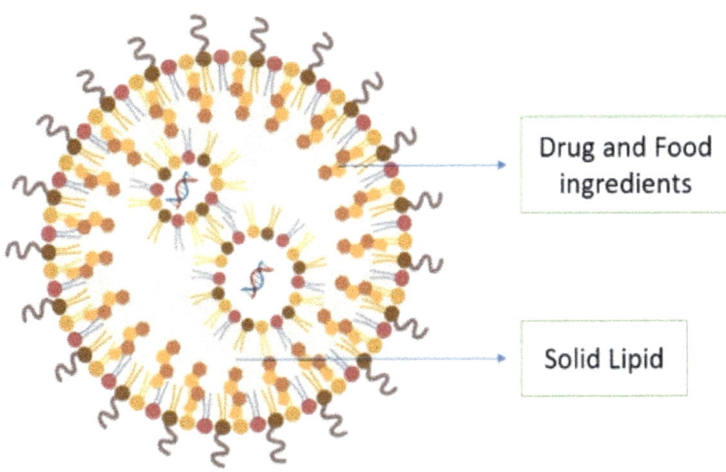

Figure 5. Diagram of a Liposome

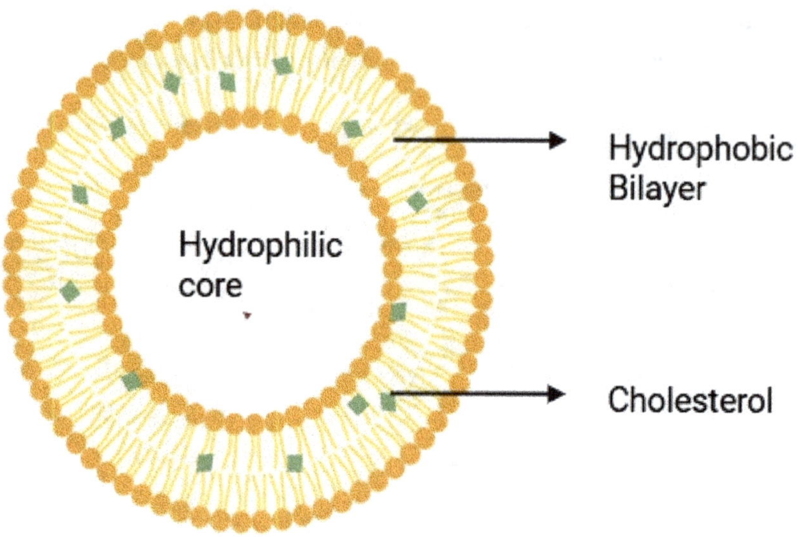

REFERENCES

Aglietta, M., Barone, C., Sawyer, M. B., Moore, M. J., Miller, W. H.Jr, Bagalà, C., Colombi, F., Cagnazzo, C., Gioeni, L., Wang, E., Huang, B., Fly, K. D., & Leone, F. (2014). A phase I dose escalation trial of tremelimumab (CP-675,206) in combination with gemcitabine in chemotherapy-naive patients with metastatic pancreatic cancer. *Annals of Oncology : Official Journal of the European Society for Medical Oncology*, *25*(9), 1750–1755. DOI: 10.1093/annonc/mdu205 PMID: 24907635

Ahmad, N., Ahmad, R., Naqvi, A. A., Alam, M. A., Ashafaq, M., Samim, M., & Ahmad, F. J. (2020). Thymoquinone lipid nanocarrier for the treatment of *Nigella sativa*-induced neurotoxicity in experimental epilepsy: Behavioral and biochemical evidences. *Journal of Drug Delivery Science and Technology*, *57*, 101696. DOI: 10.1016/j.jddst.2020.101696

Alavi, M., & Nokhodchi, A. (2021). Micro and nano liposomal carriers for lung cancer therapy: An updated review. *Advanced Drug Delivery Reviews*, *174*, 73–102. DOI: 10.1016/j.addr.2021.04.006

Allen, T. M., & Cullis, P. R. (2013). Liposomal drug delivery systems: From concept to clinical applications. *Advanced Drug Delivery Reviews*, *65*(1), 36–48. DOI: 10.1016/j.addr.2012.09.037 PMID: 23036225

Artinyan, A., Anaya, D. A., McKenzie, S., Ellenhorn, J. D., & Kim, J. (2011). Neoadjuvant therapy is associated with improved survival in resectable pancreatic adenocarcinoma. *Cancer*, *117*(10), 2044–2049. DOI: 10.1002/cncr.25763 PMID: 21523715

AstraZeneca. (2015). *Study of tremelimumab in patients with advanced solid tumors* (ClinicalTrials.gov Identifier No. NCT02527434). ClinicalTrials.gov. https://clinicaltrials.gov/show/NCT02527434

. Baker, E., & Craft, H. (2023). Pancreatic Ductal Adenocarcinoma: Current and Emerging Treatments. *Journal of Student Research*. https://doi.org/DOI: 10.47611/jsrhs.v12i3.4657

Banigallapati, S. (2024). *Current Treatment Methods in Pancreatic Cancer and the Need for Improvement*. https://doi.org/DOI: 10.20944/preprints202410.1569.v1

Barenholz, Y. (2012). Doxil®—the first FDA-approved nano-drug: Lessons learned. *Journal of Controlled Release*, *160*(2), 117–134. DOI: 10.1016/j.jconrel.2012.03.020 PMID: 22484195

Bekaii-Saab, T. S., Yaeger, R., Spira, A. I., Pelster, M. S., Sabari, J. K., Hafez, N., Barve, M., Velastegui, K., Yan, X., Shetty, A., Der-Torossian, H., & Pant, S. (2023). Adagrasib in advanced solid tumors harboring a KRASG12C mutation. *Journal of Clinical Oncology, 41*(20), 4097–4106. DOI: 10.1200/JCO.23.00434 PMID: 37099736

Borsig, L. (2018). Selectins in cancer immunity. *Glycobiology, 28*(9), 648–655. DOI: 10.1093/glycob/cwx105 PMID: 29272415

Bozzuto, G., & Molinari, A. (2015). Liposomes as nanomedical devices. *International Journal of Nanomedicine, 10*, 975–999. DOI: 10.2147/IJN.S68861 PMID: 25678787

Brigger, I., Dubernet, C., & Couvreur, P. (2012). Nanoparticles in cancer therapy and diagnosis. *Advanced Drug Delivery Reviews, 64*, 24–36. DOI: 10.1016/j.addr.2012.09.006 PMID: 12204596

Bristol-Myers Squibb. (2013). *A study of nivolumab by itself or nivolumab combined with ipilimumab in patients with advanced or metastatic solid tumors* (ClinicalTrials.gov Identifier: NCT01928394). ClinicalTrials.gov. https://clinicaltrials.gov/show/NCT01928394

Buckley, C. W., & O'Reilly, E. M. (2024). Next-generation therapies for pancreatic cancer. *Expert Review of Gastroenterology & Hepatology, 18*(1), 55–72. DOI: 10.1080/17474124.2024.2322648 PMID: 38415709

Casà, C., Portik, D., Abbasi, A. N., & Micciché, F. (2025). Radiomics in early detection of bilio-pancreatic lesions: A narrative review. *Best Practice & Research. Clinical Gastroenterology, 65*, 101997. DOI: 10.1016/j.bpg.2025.101997 PMID: 40210337

Chandana, S. R., Woods, L. M., Maxwell, F., Gandolfo, R., & Bekaii-Saab, T. (2023). Risk factors for early-onset pancreatic ductal adenocarcinoma: A systematic literature review. *European Journal of Cancer, 198*, 113471. DOI: 10.1016/j.ejca.2023.113471 PMID: 38154392

Chen, M., Liu, H., Xiao, Y., Liang, R., Xu, H., Hong, B., & Qian, Y. (2025). Predictive biomarkers of pancreatic cancer metastasis: A comprehensive review. *Clinica Chimica Acta, 550*, 120176. DOI: 10.1016/j.cca.2025.120176 PMID: 39914505

Choi, D., Gonzalez-Suarez, A. M., Dumbrava, M. G., Medlyn, M., de Hoyos-Vega, J. M., Cichocki, F., Miller, J. S., Ding, L., Zhu, M., Stybayeva, G., Gaspar-Maia, A., Billadeau, D. D., Ma, W. W., & Revzin, A. (2024). Microfluidic organoid cultures derived from pancreatic cancer biopsies for personalized testing of chemotherapy and immunotherapy. *Advancement of Science*, *11*(5), 2303088. Advance online publication. DOI: 10.1002/advs.202303088 PMID: 38018486

Daamen, L. A., Molenaar, I. Q., & Groot, V. P. (2023). Recent Advances and Future Challenges in Pancreatic Cancer Care: Early Detection, Liquid Biopsies, Precision Medicine and Artificial Intelligence. *Journal of Clinical Medicine*, *12*(23), 7485. Advance online publication. DOI: 10.3390/jcm12237485 PMID: 38068536

. Dallavalle, S., Campagnoli, G., Pastena, P., Martinino, A., Schilirò, D., & Giovinazzo, F. (2024). New Frontiers in Pancreatic Cancer Management: Current Treatment Options and the Emerging Role of Neoadjuvant Therapy. *Medicina-Lithuania, 60*(7), 1070. https://doi.org/DOI: 10.3390/medicina60071070

De Dosso, S., Siebenhüner, A. R., Winder, T., Meisel, A., Fritsch, R., Astaras, C., Szturz, P., & Borner, M. (2021). Treatment landscape of metastatic pancreatic cancer. *Cancer Treatment Reviews*, *96*, 102180. DOI: 10.1016/j.ctrv.2021.102180 PMID: 33812339

de Jesus, V. H. F., Camandaroba, M. P. G., Donadio, M. D. S., Cabral, A., Muniz, T. P., de Moura Leite, L., & Sant'Ana, L. F. (2018). Retrospective analysis of efficacy and safety of gemcitabine-based chemotherapy in patients with metastatic pancreatic adenocarcinoma experiencing disease progression on FOLFIRINOX. *Journal of Gastrointestinal Oncology*, *9*(5), 806–819. DOI: 10.21037/jgo.2018.06.08 PMID: 30505579

Desai, M. P., Labhasetwar, V., Amidon, G. L., & Levy, R. J. (1996). Gastrointestinal uptake of biodegradable microparticles: Effect of particle size. *Pharmaceutical Research*, *13*(12), 1838–1845. DOI: 10.1023/A:1016085108889 PMID: 8987081

Desgrosellier, J. S., & Cheresh, D. A. (2010). Integrins in cancer: Biological implications and therapeutic opportunities. *Nature Reviews. Cancer*, *10*(1), 9–22. DOI: 10.1038/nrc2748 PMID: 20029421

Doe, J., & Smith, A. (2023). Exploring new methodologies in data science. *Journal of Data Science : JDS*, *15*(2), 123–134. DOI: 10.1016/j.jds.2023.01.001

Dreaden, E. C., Alkilany, A. M., Huang, X., Murphy, C. J., & El-Sayed, M. A. (2012). The golden age: Gold nanoparticles for biomedicine. *Chemical Society Reviews*, *41*(7), 2740–2779. DOI: 10.1039/C1CS15237H PMID: 22109657

Ghaneh, P., Palmer, D. H., Cicconi, S., Halloran, C., Psarelli, E. E., Rawcliffe, C. L., Sripadam, R., Mukherjee, S., Wadsley, J., Al-Mukhtar, A., Jiao, L. R., Wasan, H. S., Carter, R., Graham, J. S., Ammad, F., Evans, J., Tjaden, C., Hackert, T., Buchler, M. W., & Neoptolemos, J. P. (2020). ESPAC-5F: Four-arm, prospective, multicenter, international randomized phase II trial of immediate surgery compared with neoadjuvant gemcitabine plus capecitabine (GEMCAP) or FOLFIRINOX or chemoradiotherapy (CRT) in patients with borderline resectable pancreatic cancer. *Journal of Clinical Oncology*, *38*(15, suppl), 4505. DOI: 10.1200/JCO.2020.38.15_suppl.4505

Gupta, A. K., & Gupta, M. (2005). Synthesis and surface engineering of iron oxide nanoparticles for biomedical applications. *Biomaterials*, *26*(18), 3995–4021. DOI: 10.1016/j.biomaterials.2004.10.012 PMID: 15626447

Hayat, U., Croce, P. S., Saadeh, A., Desai, K., Appiah, J., Khan, S., Khan, Y. I., Kumar, K., & Hanif, A. (2025). Current and emerging treatment options for pancreatic cancer: A comprehensive review. *Journal of Clinical Medicine*, *14*(4), 1129. DOI: 10.3390/jcm14041129 PMID: 40004658

Hou, X., Zaks, T., Langer, R., & Dong, Y. (2021). Lipid nanoparticles for mRNA delivery. *Nature Reviews. Materials*, *6*(12), 1078–1094. DOI: 10.1038/s41578-021-00358-0 PMID: 34394960

Hu, J., Zhao, C., Chen, W., Liu, Q., Li, Q., Lin, Y., & Gao, F. (2021). Pancreatic cancer: A review of epidemiology, trend, and risk factors. *World Journal of Gastroenterology*, *27*(27), 4298–4321. DOI: 10.3748/wjg.v27.i27.4298 PMID: 34366606

Huang, J., Zhan, J., Ye, B., Hu, W., Zhang, J., Wang, S., & Wang, L. (2018). Autophagy induced by curcumin and caffeine ameliorates oxidative stress-induced aging. *Cellular Physiology and Biochemistry*, *47*(3), 1241–1252. DOI: 10.1159/000490189

. Hwang, R. F., Moore, T. T., Hattersley, M. M., Scarpitti, M., Yang, B., Devereaux, E., Ramachandran, V., Arumugam, T., Ji, B., Logsdon, C. D., Brown, J. L., & Godin, R. (2023). *Data from Inhibition of the Hedgehog Pathway Targets the Tumor-Associated Stroma in Pancreatic Cancer*. https://doi.org/DOI: 10.1158/1541-7786.c.6541501.v1

Iravani, S. (2011). Green synthesis of metal nanoparticles using plants. *Green Chemistry*, *13*(10), 2638–2650. DOI: 10.1039/c1gc15386b

Jiang, W., Zhao, X., Wang, L., & Li, W. (2014). Hormone receptor-targeted nanoparticles for cancer imaging and therapy. *Journal of Controlled Release*, *193*, 139–153. DOI: 10.1016/j.jconrel.2014.05.032

Katayama, E. S., Hue, J. J., Bajor, D. L., Ocuin, L. M., Ammori, J. B., Hardacre, J. M., & Winter, J. M. (2020). A comprehensive analysis of clinical trials in pancreatic cancer: What is coming down the pike? *Oncotarget, 11*(38), 3489–3501. DOI: 10.18632/oncotarget.27727 PMID: 33014285

Katz, M. H. G., Shi, Q., Meyers, J. P., Herman, J. M., Choung, M., Wolpin, B. M., Ahmad, S., Marsh, R. W., Schwartz, L. H., Behr, S., Frankel, W. L., Collisson, E. A., Leenstra, J. L., Williams, T. M., Vaccaro, G. M., Venook, A. P., Meyerhardt, J. A., & O'Reilly, E. M. (2021). Alliance A021501: Preoperative mFOLFIRINOX or mFOLFIRINOX plus hypofractionated radiation therapy (RT) for borderline resectable (BR) adenocarcinoma of the pancreas. *Journal of Clinical Oncology, 39*(3, suppl), 377. DOI: 10.1200/JCO.2021.39.3_suppl.377

Kim, J. Y., Lim, Y., Cho, S., & Kim, J. (2024). Multiomics analysis identifies AQP1 as a prognostic marker and potential therapeutic target in pancreatic cancer. *Experimental & Molecular Medicine, 56*, 13. https://www.nature.com/articles/s12276-024-01378-w

Kolbeinsson, H. M., Chandana, S., Wright, G. P., & Chung, M. (2023). Pancreatic cancer: A review of current treatment and novel therapies. *Journal of Investigative Surgery, 36*(1), 2129884. DOI: 10.1080/08941939.2022.2129884 PMID: 36191926

Lambert, A., Schwarz, L., Borbath, I., Henry, A., Van Laethem, J.-L., Malka, D., Ducreux, M., & Conroy, T. (2019). An update on treatment options for pancreatic adenocarcinoma. *Therapeutic Advances in Medical Oncology, 11*, 1758835919875568. DOI: 10.1177/1758835919875568 PMID: 31598142

Lee, D. U., Han, B. S., Jung, K. H., & Hong, S.-S. (2024). Tumor Stroma as a Therapeutic Target for Pancreatic Ductal Adenocarcinoma. *Biomolecules & Therapeutics, 32*(3), 281–290. Advance online publication. DOI: 10.4062/biomolther.2024.029 PMID: 38590092

Li, J. W. H., & Vederas, J. C. (2009). Drug discovery and natural products: End of an era or an endless frontier? *Science, 325*(5937), 161–165. DOI: 10.1126/science.1168243 PMID: 19589993

Liu, X., Sun, L., & Zhang, W. (2020). The role of nanotechnology in pancreatic cancer treatment: A review of nanoparticle-based drug delivery systems. *Journal of Cancer Research and Clinical Oncology, 146*(9), 2165–2177. DOI: 10.1007/s00432-020-03288-x

Marchese, A., Orhan, I. E., Daglia, M., Barbieri, R., Di Lorenzo, A., Nabavi, S. F., Gortzi, O., Izadi, M., & Nabavi, S. M. (2017). Antibacterial and antifungal activities of thymol: A brief review of the literature. *Food Chemistry*, *210*, 402–414. DOI: 10.1016/j.foodchem.2016.04.111 PMID: 27211664

McGuigan, A., Kelly, P., Turkington, R. C., Jones, C., Coleman, H. G., & McCain, R. S. (2018). Pancreatic cancer: A review of clinical diagnosis, epidemiology, treatment and outcomes. *World Journal of Gastroenterology*, *24*(43), 4846–4861. DOI: 10.3748/wjg.v24.i43.4846 PMID: 30487695

Memorial Sloan Kettering Cancer Center. (n.d.). *Pancreatic cancer clinical trials & research*. https://www.mskcc.org/cancer-care/types/pancreatic/clinical-trials

Mizrahi, J. D., Surana, R., Valle, J. W., & Shroff, R. T. (2020). Pancreatic cancer. *Lancet*, *395*(10242), 2008–2020. DOI: 10.1016/S0140-6736(20)30974-0 PMID: 32593337

Mizugaki, H., Yamamoto, N., Murakami, H., Kenmotsu, H., Fujiwara, Y., Ishida, Y., Kawakami, T., & Takahashi, T. (2016). Phase I dose-finding study of monotherapy with atezolizumab, an engineered immunoglobulin monoclonal antibody targeting PD-L1, in Japanese patients with advanced solid tumors. *Investigational New Drugs*, *34*(4), 596–603. DOI: 10.1007/s10637-016-0371-6 PMID: 27363843

Mohindra, N. A., Kircher, S. M., Nimeiri, H. S., Benson, A. B., Rademaker, A., Alonso, E., Blatner, N., Khazaie, K., & Mulcahy, M. F. (2015). Results of the phase Ib study of ipilimumab and gemcitabine for advanced pancreas cancer. *Journal of Clinical Oncology*, *33*(15, suppl), e15281. DOI: 10.1200/jco.2015.33.15_suppl.e15281

Mokdad, A. A., Minter, R. M., Zhu, H., Augustine, M. M., Porembka, M. R., Wang, S. C., Yopp, A. C., Mansour, J. C., Choti, M. A., & Polanco, P. M. (2017). Neoadjuvant therapy followed by resection versus upfront resection for resectable pancreatic cancer: A propensity score matched analysis. *Journal of Clinical Oncology*, *35*(5), 515–522. DOI: 10.1200/JCO.2016.68.5081 PMID: 27621388

National Institutes of Health. (n.d.). *A study of nivolumab by itself or nivolumab combined with ipilimumab in patients with advanced or metastatic solid tumors* (ClinicalTrials.gov Identifier: NCT01928394). ClinicalTrials.gov. https://clinicaltrials.gov/show/NCT01928394

Nomi, T., Sho, M., Akahori, T., Hamada, K., Kubo, A., Kanehiro, H., Nakamura, S., Enomoto, K., Yagita, H., Azuma, M., & Nakajima, Y. (2007). Clinical significance and therapeutic potential of the programmed death-1 ligand/programmed death-1 pathway in human pancreatic cancer. *Clinical Cancer Research*, *13*(7), 2151–2157. DOI: 10.1158/1078-0432.CCR-06-2746 PMID: 17404099

Nsairat, H., Khater, D., Sayed, U., Odeh, F., Al Bawab, A., & Alshaer, W. (2022). Liposomes: Structure, Composition, Types, and Clinical Applications. *Heliyon*, *8*(9), e09394. DOI: 10.1016/j.heliyon.2022.e09394 PMID: 35600452

O'Reilly, E. M., Oh, D. Y., Dhani, N., Renouf, D. J., Lee, M. A., Sun, W., Fisher, G., Hezel, A., Chang, S.-C., Vlahovic, G., Takahashi, O., Yang, Y., Fitts, D., & Philip, P. A. (2019). Durvalumab with or without tremelimumab for patients with metastatic pancreatic ductal adenocarcinoma: A phase 2 randomized clinical trial. *JAMA Oncology*, *5*(10), 1431–1438. DOI: 10.1001/jamaoncol.2019.1588 PMID: 31318392

Pancreatic Cancer Action Network. (2025, January 16). *What is pancreatic cancer? – Pancreatic Cancer Action Network*. https://pancan.org/facing-pancreatic-cancer/about-pancreatic-cancer/what-is-pancreatic-cancer/

Pancreatic cancer treatment. (2024, August 28). Cancer.gov. https://www.cancer.gov/types/pancreatic/patient/pancreatic-treatment-pdq

Qian, Z. M., Li, H., Sun, H., & Ho, K. (2002). Targeted drug delivery via the transferrin receptor-mediated endocytosis pathway. *Pharmacological Reviews*, *54*(4), 561–587. DOI: 10.1124/pr.54.4.561 PMID: 12429868

Royal, R. E., Levy, C., Turner, K., Mathur, A., Hughes, M., Kammula, U. S., Sherry, R. M., Topalian, S. L., Yang, J. C., Lowy, I., & Rosenberg, S. A. (2010). Phase 2 trial of single agent ipilimumab (anti-CTLA-4) for locally advanced or metastatic pancreatic adenocarcinoma. *Journal of Immunotherapy*, *33*(8), 828–833. DOI: 10.1097/CJI.0b013e3181eec14c PMID: 20842054

Sharma, R., Ghosh, R., Kumar, S., Komal, K., & Kumar, M. (2025). Decoding pancreatic cancer: Key risk factors across genetics and lifestyle. *Expert Review of Molecular Diagnostics*, *25*(4), 95–99. Advance online publication. DOI: 10.1080/14737159.2025.2464563 PMID: 39918844

Sohal, D. P. S., Duong, M., Ahmad, S. A., Gandhi, N. S., Beg, M. S., Wang-Gillam, A., Wade, J. L.III, Chiorean, E. G., Guthrie, K. A., Lowy, A. M., Philip, P. A., & Hochster, H. S. (2021). Efficacy of perioperative chemotherapy for resectable pancreatic adenocarcinoma: A phase 2 randomized clinical trial. *JAMA Oncology*, *7*(3), 421–427. DOI: 10.1001/jamaoncol.2020.7328 PMID: 33475684

. Spivak-Kroizman, T. R., Hostetter, G., Posner, R. A., Aziz, M., Hu, C., Demeure, M. J., Von Hoff, D. D., Hingorani, S. R., Palculict, T. B., Izzo, J., Kiriakova, G., Abdelmelek, M., Bartholomeusz, G., James, B. P., & Powis, G. (2023). *Data from Hypoxia Triggers Hedgehog-Mediated Tumor–Stromal Interactions in Pancreatic Cancer*. https://doi.org/DOI: 10.1158/0008-5472.c.6504098

Sudimack, J., & Lee, R. J. (2000). Targeted drug delivery via the folate receptor. *Advanced Drug Delivery Reviews, 41*(2), 147–162. DOI: 10.1016/S0169-409X(99)00062-9 PMID: 10699311

Taieb, J., Prager, G. W., Melisi, D., Westphalen, C. B., D'Esquermes, N., Ferreras, A., Carrato, A., & Macarulla, T. (2020). First-line and second-line treatment of patients with metastatic pancreatic adenocarcinoma in routine clinical practice across Europe: A retrospective, observational chart review study. *ESMO Open, 5*(1), e000698. DOI: 10.1136/esmoopen-2019-000587 PMID: 31958291

Takeichi, M. (1991). Cadherin cell adhesion receptors as a morphogenetic regulator. *Science, 251*(5000), 1451–1455. DOI: 10.1126/science.2006419 PMID: 2006419

Tyagi, A. K., Prasad, S., Majeed, M., & Aggarwal, B. B. (2015). Curcumin, a component of turmeric: From farm to pharmacy. *BioFactors (Oxford, England), 41*(1), 1–9. DOI: 10.1002/biof.1214 PMID: 25545372

Wang, F., Li, L., Liu, B., Xin, H., & Cheng, L. (2015). Advances with liposomal carriers for paclitaxel: A review. *Journal of Nanoscience and Nanotechnology, 15*(1), 1–12. DOI: 10.1166/jnn.2015.10289 PMID: 26328301

Wang, J., Mao, W., Lock, L. L., & Tang, J. (2021). Targeted delivery strategies for precision medicines. *Nature Reviews. Materials, 6*(11), 924–939. DOI: 10.1038/s41578-021-00317-6 PMID: 34950512

Wang, L., Wang, H., Zhang, Q., & Zhang, H. (2021). Recent advances in nanomedicine for cancer therapy. *Biomaterials Science, 9*(4), 1137–1152. DOI: 10.1039/D0BM01928K

Wang, X., Zhang, Y., & Luo, Y. (2021). Toxicity concerns and stability of nanoparticles in pancreatic cancer therapy. *Cancer Nanotechnology, 8*(6), 289–296. DOI: 10.1002/cncr.33698

Weiss, G. J., Blaydorn, L., Beck, J., Bornemann-Kolatzki, K., Urnovitz, H., Schütz, E., & Khemka, V. (2019). Correction to: Phase Ib/II study of gemcitabine, nab-paclitaxel, and pembrolizumab in metastatic pancreatic adenocarcinoma. *Investigational New Drugs, 37*(4), 761. DOI: 10.1007/s10637-019-00763-x PMID: 31020607

Whipple, A. O., Parsons, W. B., & Mullins, C. R. (1935). Treatment of carcinoma of the ampulla of Vater. *Annals of Surgery*, *102*(4), 763–777. DOI: 10.1097/00000658-193510000-00023 PMID: 17856666

Xu, Q., Zhou, Y., Zhang, H., Li, H., Qin, H., & Wang, H. (2023). Bibliometric analysis of hotspots and frontiers of immunotherapy in pancreatic cancer. *Health Care*, *11*(3), 304. DOI: 10.3390/healthcare11030304 PMID: 36766879

Zhang, T., Liu, Q., & Zhou, S. (2020). Nanomedicine: An overview of nanotechnology in cancer treatment. *Journal of Nanoscience and Nanotechnology*, *20*(5), 2691–2704. DOI: 10.1166/jnn.2020.18113

Zhang, X., Zhang, T., Wang, S., Jiang, C., & Yu, X. (2022). Advances in polymeric nanoparticles for drug delivery: An updated review. *International Journal of Molecular Sciences*, *23*(4), 1906. DOI: 10.3390/ijms23041906

Zhang, Y., Liu, X., Wang, L., & Chen, H. (2024). Advanced nanomaterials for targeted cancer therapy: A comprehensive review. *International Journal of Pharmaceutics*, *635*, 122845. DOI: 10.1016/j.ijpharm.2024.122845

Zhong, G., Zhang, X., Zhao, R., Guo, Z., Wang, C., Yu, C., Liu, D., Hu, K., Gao, Y., Zhao, B., Liu, X., Shi, X., Chen, L., Li, Y., & Yu, L. (2025). The high efficacy of claudin18.2-targeted CAR-T cell therapy in advanced pancreatic cancer with an antibody-dependent safety strategy. *Molecular Therapy : the Journal of the American Society of Gene Therapy*, *33*(6), 2778–2788. Advance online publication. DOI: 10.1016/j.ymthe.2025.01.012 PMID: 39797399

Zhong, Y., Goltsche, K., Cheng, L., Xie, F., & Morsbach, S. (2022). Nanostructured lipid carriers in cancer therapy: Advances and challenges. *Journal of Controlled Release*, *351*, 370–389. DOI: 10.1016/j.jconrel.2022.09.019

Zhou, Y., Ma, Y., Sheng, J., Ma, Y., Ding, J., & Zhou, W. (2024). Breaking Down Barriers in Drug Delivery by Stromal Remodeling Approaches in Pancreatic Cancer. *Molecular Pharmaceutics*, *21*(8), 3764–3776. Advance online publication. DOI: 10.1021/acs.molpharmaceut.4c00329 PMID: 39049481

Chapter 10
Precision Treatment: The Promise of Targeted Therapies Against Pancreatic Cancer

Sangam Singh
https://orcid.org/0000-0002-1341-4451
Oxford College of Pharmacy, India

Punet Kumar
https://orcid.org/0000-0001-6047-6615
Shri Gopichand College of Pharmacy, India

Deepak Kumar
https://orcid.org/0009-0002-7598-5484
Shri Gopichand College of Pharmacy, India

Arun Kumar Mishra
SOS School of Pharmacy, Faculty of Pharmacy, IFTM University, Moradabad, India

ABSTRACT

Pancreatic cancer remains one of the deadliest malignancies due to late diagnosis, aggressive progression, and limited treatment options. This chapter highlights the promise of precision treatment approaches, focusing on targeted therapies guided by genetic and molecular profiles. Key oncogenic drivers such as KRAS mutations, EGFR/HER2 signaling, and Hedgehog pathways are critically evaluated for their therapeutic potential. Advances in tyrosine kinase inhibitors, PARP inhibitors, and anti-angiogenic agents are discussed with support from clinical trial outcomes and real-world applications. The chapter further explores mechanisms of resistance, the

DOI: 10.4018/979-8-3373-1469-3.ch010

role of biomarkers, and innovations such as liquid biopsies, AI-assisted treatment strategies, and personalized immunotherapy. Future perspectives emphasize combinatorial regimens, organoid-guided therapy, and spatial omics, underscoring a precision medicine roadmap for improving pancreatic cancer survival.

INTRODUCTION

Pancreatic cancer is an extremely aggressive malignancy derived from pancreas a key organ that carries out both (endocrine i.e. insulin secretion), and exocrine (digestive enzymes) functions. Closely dubbed the "silent killer" by many often shows no signs early on and thus is missed until it's too late to be diagnosed properly, resulting in dismal clinical outcomes (John, et al., 2024). Pancreatic cancer is one of the most lethal cancers because of silent metastasis, few therapeutic options and non-responding to treatment in most cases. Late-stage diagnosis and aggressive biology make it clear that there is an absolute need for new diagnostic modalities, systemic therapeutics and individual score-guided treatment to improve survival outcomes (Wood, et. al., 2022). Pancreatic cancer is the seventh leading cause of cancer-related deaths globally, an estimated more than 495,000 new cases and approximately 466,000 deaths each year. The condition is most commonly found in people over 60, with a slight male predilection. Significant geographic distribution differences were apparent with developed regions having among the highest incidence rates, presumably due to the mix of lifestyle behaviors, diagnostic access and exposure to environmental factors (Rawla, et. al., 2019).

Well known risk factors include tobacco use, chronic pancreatitis, diabetes mellitus and heavy alcohol use as well as genetic susceptibilities such as BRCA1/BRCA2 and Lynch syndrome. There have been enormous advances in medical research but pancreatic cancer five-year survival is virtually 10% and thus, the cry for building better preventive /cure interventions ensues (Capasso, et. al., 2018). The dismal outlook is primarily based on its aggressive biology: rapid metastatic spread, impediment to various drug penetration due desmoplastic stroma and immunosuppressive tumor microenvironment that attenuates chemotherapy or immunotherapy (Yu, et. al., 2024).

In the majority of patients at diagnosis, only 10–20% are potentially operable with curative intent as most present with locally advanced or metastatic disease. Even surgery fails at recurrence, so that adjuvant regimen has been of limited help to these patients. While efficacious, recent standard of care chemotherapy regimens (gemcitabine-based and FOLFIRINOX) have modest survival benefit in patients with very poor performance status (Pereira & Corrêa, 2018). Routine imaging such as CT, MRI and endoscopic ultrasound may not be able to detect early-stage disease

(Lee, et. al., 2018). Although biomarkers such as CA19-9 are commonly used, they do not provide sufficient sensitivity or specificity for population-based screening (especially in the asymptomatic setting. The molecular heterogeneity only adds to the difficultly in designing and moving forward with broadly effective targeted therapies, as the genes most commonly mutated- KRAS, TP53, CDKN2A and SMAD4 pancreatic their kinases are not druggable (Stefanoudakis, et. al., 2024).

Researchers are testing novel approaches to overcome these hurdles, from nanoparticle drug delivery to CAR-T cell therapy and combination of chemotherapy with checkpoint inhibitors (Garg, et. al., 2024). In addition, liquid biopsies, advanced imaging techniques and full-genome sequencing intended as a precision medicine model are aimed at identifying high-risk subjects and cancers well suited to therapies right from the time of diagnosis. However, these exciting strategies are confronted great scientific, operational and economical challenges, mostly in low-resource settings where healthcare disparities will bias the outcomes (Ma, L., et. al., 2024). This chapter takes a look at molecular pathways defining the progression of pancreatic cancer, analyzes the prospects and shortcomings of new targeted therapies in the clinic as well as provides clinical real-world applications whether with resistance issues and avenues for future research in precision oncology.

Key Molecular Pathways Driving Pancreatic Cancer

The network of molecular pathways that control cell proliferation, survival and differentiation drives pancreatic cancer pathogenesis. KRAS, EGFR and Hedgehog pathways are some of the most important for the initiation, progression and therapeutic resistance of pancreatic ductal adenocarcinoma (PDAC) which is the most common form of pancreatic cancer (Mustafa, et. al., 2024). Aberrant activation of these pathways, allows for tumour initiation, maintains the growth of cancer cells and establishes a pro-metastatic pro-immunoevasive milieu. Insight into these pathways is highly relevant to target compounds for therapeutic interventions (Biray Avci, et. al., 2024).

KRAS Pathway

KRAS mutations are the most frequent genetic alterations in pancreatic ductal adenocarcinoma (PDAC), occurring above 90% of all cases. Mutations occur mainly at codons 12,13 and 61 resulting in KRAS being constitutively active. KRAS is a small peptide (GTPase) wherein it functions as a molecular switch that modulates critical signaling pathways in the body (de Jesus, et. al., 2023). In the absence of ligands, normal KRAS is kept in check by upstream receptor tyrosine kinases (RTKs), for instance epidermal growth factor receptor (EGFR). RTKs autophosphorylate upon binding a ligand, then bring into complex adaptor proteins (e.g., GRB2, SOS) that subsequently exchange GDP for GTP on KRAS activating it transiently (Kim, et. al., 2021). Unfortunately, pancreatic cancer KRAS is constantly active in the GTP-bound state by oncogenic mutations in a GOF manner and not dependent on extracellular signals to keep downstream pathways constitutively activated. Two of the main cascades downstream of oncogenic-activated KRAS are the RAF-MEK-ERK and next level PI3K-AKT-mTOR pathway. In the RAF-MEK-ERK axis, K-Ras co localizes and phosphorylates RAF kinases which in turn phosphorylate MEK1/2, thus activating ERK1/2 (Yang & Wu, 2024). ERK is transported into nucleus region, stimulating gene expression to support cell proliferation and survival. When KRAS signals PI3K, the PI3K-AKT-mTOR pathway is then activated to generate PIP3 and subsequently activating AKT. AKT promotes cell survival by counteracting apoptotic proteins and mTOR, an upstream kinase that governs protein synthesis as well as metabolism reprogramming (Klomp, et. al., 2021). Moreover, RalGDS is an upstream activator of RalA and RalB being small GTPases known to participate in cytoskeleton organization vesicle trafficking and tumor metastasis. These pathways collectively scaffold a tumor enabling milieu of uncontrolled growth, escape from apoptosis/ differentiation, metabolic rewiring and immune evasion. KRAS although central to pancreatic cancer, has been called forlornly "undruggable" due to its extremely high affinity for GTP and lack of putative ligand pockets (Zhou, et. al., 2024). This has changed recently though as mutant-specific inhibitors, mostly focused on the G12C KRAS mutant have entered clinical development. These drugs, including sotorasib and adagrasib, covalently bind to the mutant cysteine and irreversibly tether KRAS in a GDP-bound inactive state (Alturki, et. al., 2025).

EGFR Pathway

Epidermal Growth Factor Receptor (EGFR) is a central signaling hub that contributes to the rational and pathophysiology of pancreatic cancer. EGFR is a transmembrane (tyrosine kinase) receptor subclass. The binding of certain ligands, e.g., epidermal growth factor (EGF) to the cell surface-targeted receptor called EGFR, results in dimerization and autophosphorylation of specific cell surface receptors (Murphrey, et. al., 2023). This priming leads to activation of downstream signaling cascades, which are two among the most famously known; RAS-RAF-MEK/ERK pathway and PI3K-AKT. They all play critical roles in basic cellular functionality such as proliferation, survival, migration and angiogenesis (Guo, et. al., 2020). EGFR is overexpressed or aberrantly activated in most pancreatic cancer samples which contribute to the uncontrolled growth and progression of tumor cells. It also promotes angiogenesis (new blood vessel formation), providing nutrients to the tumor an aspect that makes EGFR an attractive target for drug development (Chinnadurai, et al., 2023).

Pancreatic Tumors: Despite Overexpression of EGFR, EGFR-targeted therapies have failed to give any significant clinical benefit. This failure comes in part from multiple downstream KRAS mutations that are often co-selected with each other to maintain constitutive signaling downstream of proliferative pathways independently of EGFR blockades. This molecular back-up scheme completely makes any EGFR inhibition in most PDAC patients futile (Halder, et. al., 2023). Notably, the responses of these NSCLC patients (who lack KRAS mutations and harbor a specific EGFR activating mutation) such as to gefitinib/osimertinib etc. are profound. That shows just how critical the mutation type and driver dependency of an oncogene is in targeted therapy success. Hence, the poor results of EGFR inhibitors in pancreatic cancer reflect the lack a biomarker-driven approach and highlight the necessity of determining molecular fingerprints (Harrison, et. al., 2020).

Hedgehog Pathway

The Hedgehog (Hh) signaling pathway is involved in embryo growth and tissue homeostasis as well as keeping both adult cells young Systemic and repair. Though in pancreatic cancer this pathway is overly stimulated particularly in the stroma of the tumor, this like helps cancer grow (Dosch, et. al., 2010). In the absence of Hedgehog proteins PTCH1 will "cover" another protein called Smoothened (SMO) that would normally function. However, if a Hedgehog protein binds to PTCH1 this block is unblocked, SMO is activated, and the process of Hedgehog signal inside the cell begins. It is this activation that causes the activation of the GLI transcription factors, which then translocate to the nucleus and induce target gene expression (Klieser, et. al., 2016). These genes make an important contribution to many of the hallmarks that are essential for cancer evolution. The importance of Hedgehog pathway in pancreatic cancer is not by its effect in cancer cells directly., but by effects on tumor microenvironment. It contributes to the formation of a large fibrous stroma the desmoplasia that physically filters chemotherapy drugs out of working range to cancer cells. It also contributes to immune suppression, so the body can't get at the cancer as much (Jing, et. al., 2023).

Since Hedgehog pathway is requisite for the growth of cancer, it became a candidate that can be targeted eventually. Vismodegib and sonidegib, two good examples of SMO protein blockers in vitro/ in vivo experiments. It highlights that, if not to the hedgehog pathway, then definitely with other treatments e.g. chemotherapy or immunotherapy together could block it better. Right now, scientists are working on better strategies to block this pathway so that this path of treatment can be improved for patients with pancreatic cancer (Miyashita, et. al., 2024). Figure

1 illustrates the key molecular pathways involved in the progression of pancreatic cancer, highlighting critical targets such as KRAS mutations, EGFR/HER2 signaling, and Hedgehog pathways.

Figure 1. Key Molecular Pathways Driving Pancreatic Cancer

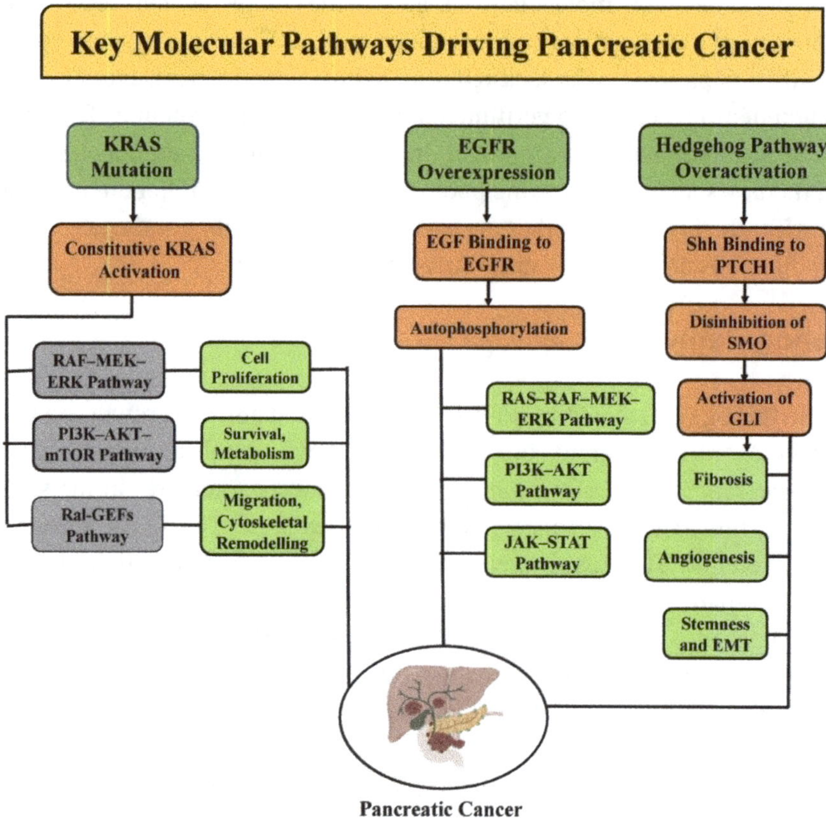

Table 1. Comparative Analysis of Key Molecular Pathways in Pancreatic Cancer

Pathway	Key Role in Pancreatic Cancer	Clinical Significance	Therapeutic Targeting & Limitations
KRAS	>90% mutation rate; drives proliferation, survival, immune evasion	Central driver mutation; hallmark of PDAC	Recently druggable (KRAS G12C inhibitors) but resistance emerges rapidly (Chunxiao Zhu, at al, 2022)
EGFR	Overexpressed in PDAC; activates MAPK & PI3K-AKT pathways	Promotes proliferation & angiogenesis	EGFR inhibitors (erlotinib) approved with gemcitabine; limited efficacy due to KRAS co-mutations (Fagman JB et al, 2019)
Hedgehog	Activates stromal desmoplasia & immune evasion	Contributes to drug resistance & tumor microenvironment (TME) remodelling	SMO inhibitors (vismodegib, sonidegib) under study; best in combination therapies (Amakye D, at al., 2013)

Among the three pathways, the KRAS pathway is the most significant in pancreatic cancer. Over 90% of pancreatic ductal adenocarcinoma (PDAC) cases harbor activating KRAS mutations, mainly at codons 12, 13, and 61. This leads to constitutive activation of downstream RAF-MEK-ERK and PI3K-AKT signaling cascades, promoting uncontrolled proliferation, metabolic rewiring, and resistance to therapy. Unlike EGFR or Hedgehog signaling, KRAS mutations occur early in tumorigenesis and are considered the "founding event" in PDAC. Although long deemed "undruggable," novel KRAS G12C inhibitors (e.g., sotorasib, adagrasib) show promising results in early trials, making KRAS the most critical therapeutic target in precision treatment of pancreatic cancer. A comparative overview of the KRAS, EGFR, and Hedgehog pathways is presented in Table 1, highlighting their relative roles, clinical significance, and therapeutic implications in pancreatic cancer.

Therapeutic Implications

The focus on targeting KRAS, EGFR and Hedgehog regulatory pathways in the search for additional treatments of pancreatic cancer continues. Research into improved inhibitors continues with a deeper understanding of these signaling networks to interfere at the level of the tumor and microenvironment in general. Ongoing clinical development of combination treatment strategies with therapies based on KRAS/EGFR inhibitors in combination with chemotherapy, immunotherapy or Hedgehog pathway modulators are aimed at improving response and overcoming resistance (Lyman, and Moses, 2016). But equally important at the time, we are finding biomarker discovery and patient selection underway that will be key to ensure these therapies are used in those with best chance of benefit. This highly targeted treatment gives us the best chance at success and also preserves less toxicities for the patients that are highly unlikely to do better. Taken together, the elaborate nature of these molecular pathways underscores the importance of novel and integrative medicines. Coordinated disruption of these cores signaling pathways offers a rational basis for improving outcomes in a disease that has proven unyielding to standard therapies (Bhat, et. al., 2024).

Targeted Therapies Reshaping Treatment Landscape

The recent progress of targeted therapies in a deadly pancreatic cancer is bringing new hope to patients with this aggressive disease. These have focused treatments to molecular hallmarks of growth/survival/metasis in cancer, with the hope of improving treatment efficacy. Designed to target the very basis of the tumor growth itself, these formulations are formulated to have superior efficacy and fewer side effects as compared to standard care. Much research also still needs to be done, in order to find novel approaches which might change the paradigm of pancreatic cancer management (Li et. al., 2024).

1. Tyrosine Kinase Inhibitors (TKIs)

The tyrosine kinase inhibitors (TKIs) have emerged as a potential targeted therapeutic group for pancreatic cancer. Tyrosine kinases are enzymes that are involved to the basic cellular process of growth, differentiation and survival, by which they add phosphate groups to specific proteins. The abnormal over-expressing or mutations of tyrosine kinases that play a central role in activating pancreatic cancer since these are considered as drugs worthy of targeting (Long, et. al., 2021). TKIs have had tremendous success in a variety of cancers, but their activity against pancreatic cancer has been curtailed by the intricacies of the disease and resistance mechanisms. TKIs inhibit the ATP-binding site of tyrosine kinases, halting the activation of signaling pathways required for tumor growth, angiogenesis, metastasis and cell survival (Bahar ME, et. al., 2023). The TKIs in pancreatic cancer target the activated signalling cascades of the Epidermal Growth Factor Receptor (EGFR), Vascular Endothelial Growth Factor Receptor (VEGFR) and in some cases the Platelet-Derived Growth Factor Receptor (PDGFR). All are essential for progression of tumor which function through similar mechanism. In pancreatic cancer there are multiple TKIs being studied. Erlotinib that was the most investigated first generation of EGFR inhibitors in this setting (He, et. al., 2021). It is only approved in combination with gemcitabine, modest survival benefits have been demonstrated from clinical trials. But its efficacy is only profound in patients with wild-type KRAS, as mutations in KRAS confer resistance by skipping the activated EGFR. Frequency of side effects e.g. rash and diarrhea is expected because the results reflect its normal epithelial tissue inhibition (Yang X, and Wu H, 2024). TKIs have completely changed the treatment paradigm for cancers such as CML, renal cell carcinoma and NSCLC but were an underdog in pancreatic cancer. One possible explanation is the characteristic of tumor microenvironment in PDAC: dense stroma, low vascularity and limited drug perfusion. Pancreatic cancer lacks frequent actionable mutations like ALK or EGFR seen in NSCLC, limiting the effectiveness of single-agent TKIs. As a result, combination therapies are preferred, and agents like sunitinib have shown potential in targeting tumor vasculature and preventing PNET metastasis (Kelley & Ko, 2008).

2. PARP Inhibitors

The biggest strides in pancreatic cancer treatment have come using PARP inhibitors, particularly in those patients with BRCA1/BRCA2 gene mutations. The PARP enzymes act to repair damaged DNA through, basically, base excision repair (BER). When tumors have other issues: with a different repair process (e.g. homologous recombination repair, as is the case for BRCA mutations, blocking PARP results in more of what Hecht calls "synthetic lethality". The cancer cells are literally unable to fix their DNA and therefore die. All of that said, this treatment is a potential option for a handful of pancreatic cancer patients with particular genetic mutations (Rose, et. al., 2020). This simply means that PARP inhibitors inhibit the PARP enzymes that cleave single strand breaks of DNA. No repair leads to the formation of double-strand breaks when these chromosomes will be replicated in the next cell cycle. Healthy cells normally can fix the break itself but some cancer cells harboring defective BRACA (del Rivero & Kohn, 2017).

PARP inhibitors have made a big step forward in treating pancreatic cancer, especially for people with certain gene changes like BRCA1 or BRCA2. PARP enzymes normally help fix damaged DNA through a repair process called base excision repair (BER). But when tumors already have problems in another repair system called homologous recombination repair (HRR), like in BRCA-mutated cancer, blocking PARP becomes very effective (Chi, et. al., 2021). PARP inhibitors exploit synthetic lethality by blocking DNA repair in BRCA-mutated pancreatic cancer cells, leading to accumulated damage and cell death offering a promising option for a small subset of hard-to-treat cases (Cortesi, et. al., 2021).

There are a bunch of PARP inhibitors being researched for pancreatic cancer. Olaparib, the first PARP inhibitor to come down this road in this setting with well-established clinical benefit for BRCA-mutated patients. Olaparib is the maintenance treatment in the POLO trial of metastatic pancreatic cancer patients with BRCA mutations who progressed after initial platinum-based chemotherapy. However, the effect on overall survival from this treatment appears to be modest at best. Rucaparib has also had success in Phase I trials, be it as a single agent or in combination with other treatments (Dibitetto, et. al., 2024). Niraparib and Talazoparib are being investigated in clinical studies in hopes of better understanding whether this could provide unique advantages or increased potency in a wider array of cancer types with

DNA repair deficiencies. The maintenance regimen is used mostly post chemo for disease control. There is ongoing work to potentially use PARP inhibitors in other tumor sites harboring a homologous recombination deficiency, such as those with PALB2/ RAD51/RAD51L3/ATM mutations (Annese, et. al., 2019). As shown in Figure 2, the mechanism of PARP inhibition leverages synthetic lethality by targeting cancer cells with defective DNA repair pathways, such as those harboring BRCA mutations.

Figure 2. Mechanism of PARP Inhibition (Synthetic lethality)

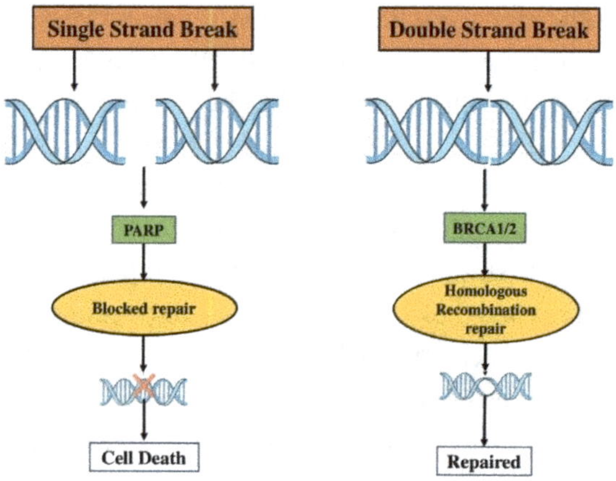

3. Anti-Angiogenic Agents

Anti-angiogenic agents are special cancer treatments that work by stopping the growth of new blood vessels. Tumors need these blood vessels to get oxygen and nutrients to grow and spread. In pancreatic cancer especially the common and aggressive type called pancreatic ductal adenocarcinoma (PDAC) the tumor often has low oxygen levels, which triggers the body to make more blood vessels (Liu, et. al., 2023). These drugs try to block that process, starving the tumor and helping other treatments like chemotherapy and radiation work better. In pancreatic cancer, the growth of blood vessels is mainly controlled by a protein called VEGF (vascular endothelial growth factor) and its receptors, along with other signals like PDGF (platelet-derived growth factor), FGF (fibroblast growth factor), and angiopoietins (Matuszewska, et. al., 2021). Anti-angiogenic drugs work by either blocking VEGF or stopping its receptor from working. Some drugs also target several of these pathways at once to stop blood vessel growth more effectively. Another way these agents help is by making the tumor's blood vessels more normal and less leaky. This can improve how well drugs reach the tumor and reduce the low-oxygen environment inside it, making the treatment more successful (Gerriets & Katz, 2025). Sunitinib, FDA-approved for pancreatic neuroendocrine tumors (PNETs), targets multiple angiogenic receptors and has shown significant survival benefits in advanced PNET patients. Other agents like sorafenib and ramucirumab (a VEGFR-2 antibody) have shown limited success alone but are being studied in combination therapies for pancreatic cancer (Clarke & Hurwitz, 2013). As shown in Table 2, several drug classes with defined targets have emerged-some FDA-approved, others still under clinical evaluation.

Table 2. Targeted Therapies in Pancreatic Cancer – Drug Classes, Targets, and FDA Status

Drug Class	Examples	Primary Target	FDA Status	Notes
EGFR Inhibitors	Erlotinib	EGFR	Approved (with gemcitabine)	Limited efficacy; KRAS mutation reduces benefit
TKIs (multi-targeted)	Sunitinib, Sorafenib	VEGFR, PDGFR, KIT	Approved (PNETs) / Not for PDAC	Modest benefit in neuroendocrine tumors
PARP Inhibitors	Olaparib, Rucaparib	PARP enzymes (DNA repair)	Approved (BRCA-mutated PDAC)	For maintenance therapy
Anti-VEGF Antibodies	Bevacizumab	VEGF-A	Not approved	Studied in combo; limited efficacy
KRAS G12C Inhibitors	Adagrasib, Sotorasib	KRAS G12C	Investigational	Active trials; early promising data

Case Studies and Clinical Trials: Successful Applications and Real-World Outcomes in Pancreatic Cancer

Case studies and clinical trials reveal important information for the performance of next generation therapies against pancreatic cancer to be at best well evidence and at worst what is translating poorly in to real-world outcomes. Despite being relatively resistant to many drugs, pancreatic ductal adenocarcinoma (PDAC), targeted therapies, and even immunotherapy. combination regimens have shown some successes in select patient populations. Several innovative therapies have demonstrated significant improvements in patient outcomes, particularly when tailored to individual genetic profiles. As shown in Table 3, "Case Studies and

Clinical Trials: Successful Applications and Real-World Outcomes in Pancreatic Cancer," these approaches have led to increased survival rates and better quality of life in select patient populations.

Table 3. Precision Medicine in Pancreatic Cancer: Case Studies, Clinical Trials, and Real-World Outcomes

S. No.	Case Study / Focus	Clinical Trial (If applicable)	Trial Number (NCT No.)	Key Findings	Real-World Impact
1	BRCA-mutated PDAC treated with Olaparib	POLO Trial	NCT02184195	Olaparib maintenance therapy doubled PFS compared to placebo (7.4 vs 3.8 months).	First FDA approval for a PARP inhibitor in pancreatic cancer (Golan T, et. al., 2019).
2	dMMR PDAC treated with Pembrolizumab	KEYNOTE-158	NCT02628067	~29% objective response rate in PDAC patients with dMMR/ MSI-H tumors.	Checkpoint inhibitors now used for dMMR pancreatic cancers (Marabelle A, et. al., 2020).
3	KRAS G12C mutation targeted with Adagrasib	KRYSTAL-1 Study	NCT04104672	Tumor size reduction observed; disease control achieved in KRAS G12C mutated PDAC.	First promising approach for previously 'undruggable' KRAS mutations (Hallin J, et. al., 2020).
4	mRNA vaccine (Autogene Cevumeran) in early PDAC	Personalized Tumor Vaccine Trial	NCT05968326	Half of vaccinated patients cancer-free at 3 years.	Opened new frontier of mRNA-based immunotherapy (Rojas LA, et. al., 2023).
5	Nanoliposomal Irinotecan after gemcitabine failure	NAPOLI-1 Trial	NCT01494506	Improved median OS (6.1 months vs 4.2 months).	Second-line therapy option post-gemcitabine failure (Wang-Gillam A, et. al., 2016).
6	Standard chemotherapy FOLFIRINOX efficacy	-	-	Median OS extended to 11.1 months vs 6.8 months with gemcitabine.	FOLFIRINOX became standard for fit patients (Conroy T, et. al., 2018).
7	Gene therapy (CAN-2409) with valacyclovir	CAN-2409 Gene Therapy Trial	NCT03224117	71.4% 2-year survival vs 16.7% in control; median OS 28.8 months.	Fast-tracked by FDA for pancreatic cancer (He J, et. al., 2021).

continued on following page

Table 3. Continued

S. No.	Case Study / Focus	Clinical Trial (If applicable)	Trial Number (NCT No.)	Key Findings	Real-World Impact
8	Tumor Treating Fields (TTFields) + chemo	PANOVA-3 Trial	NCT03377491	13% increase in survival (16.2 vs 14.16 months).	Non-invasive device addition to standard therapy (Motzer RJ, et. al., 2023).
9	Olaparib for PALB2-mutated PDAC	PARP Inhibitor Trial	NCT06078787	Study ongoing; expanding PARP use beyond BRCA.	Potential new biomarker-driven therapy option(National Library of Medicine (US); 2023).
10	Chemotherapy + Statin combination	Statin Trial	NCT06241352	Study ongoing; evaluating statins' synergistic effects.	Possible low-cost adjunct therapy for PDAC (ClinicalTrials.gov 2024).
11	Real-world precision medicine outcomes: 'Know Your Tumor'	Observational Study	-	Matched therapies → OS 2.58 years vs 1.51 years.	Validates molecular profiling approach in real-world setting (Pishvaian MJ, et. al., 2020).
12	XCELSIOR Real-world Study: Trametinib + Hydroxychloroquine	Observational Study	-	Median OS 7.4 months; some partial responses/ stable disease.	Encouraging results for late-line targeted therapies (ClinicalTrials.gov, 2019).
13	Early detection with PAC-MANN Blood Test	Diagnostic Study	-	85% accuracy in early PDAC detection; improved with CA 19-9 combination.	Potential to detect pancreatic cancer earlier, improving outcomes (Montoya Mira J, et. al., 2023).

Table 4. Resistance Mechanisms in Pancreatic Cancer and Potential Solutions

Resistance Mechanism	Example	Therapeutic Implication	Proposed Solutions
KRAS Secondary Mutations	KRAS Y96C mutation after G12C inhibition	Loss of inhibitor binding	Next-gen KRAS inhibitors; combo with MEK inhibitors (Awad, et. al., 2021).
Stromal Barrier (Desmoplasia)	Dense fibrotic matrix	Impaired drug delivery	Stromal-depleting agents; TGF-β inhibitors (Kopecka, et. al., 2021).
Efflux Pump Overexpression	P-glycoprotein (P-gp)	Reduced intracellular drug levels	Inhibitors of efflux transporters (Karamitopoulou, 2020)
EMT & Phenotypic Plasticity	Transition to mesenchymal state	Increased invasiveness and drug resistance	EMT blockers; epigenetic modulators (Nunes-Xavier & Pulido, 2020).
Alternative Pathway Activation	HGF/MET activation after EGFR blockade	EGFR-independent proliferation	Dual inhibition or pathway combination (Tolstonog, & Krupitza, 2019).
Immunosuppressive TME	Tregs, MDSCs, PD-L1 upregulation	Limited immunotherapy success	Checkpoint inhibitors + TME-modifying agents (Tariq, & Badar, 2019)

Challenges in Precision Treatment

One of the hardest cancers to treat, pancreatic cancer is a very biologically and molecularly complex, as well as aggressive disease. Precision medicine strives to match the right therapies with individual genetic and molecular profiles albeit presents many challenges to translate into practice successfully. A major obstacle is resistance mechanisms that decrease the durability of targeted therapies. The heterogeneous tumor and dense stromal microenvironment also blur the treatment approach. Targeting / overcoming the resistance pathways will play a pivotal role to improve patient outcomes

Resistance Mechanisms in Pancreatic Cancer

Precision medicine has revolutionized the care of patient with pancreatic cancer by delivering therapies based on precise genetic, molecular, and environmental profiles of an individual patient. The main obstruction is the emergence resistance, which reduces target efficacity and typically disease progresses. Resistance can be categorized into intrinsic (present before therapy) and acquired (developed during or after treatment) (Perello-Reus, et. al., 2022).

Intrinsic Resistance Mechanisms

Pancreatic tumors are characterized by extensive both inter- and intra-tumor heterogeneity. Tumor can harbinger multiple molecular subtypes, which leads to an intertwined nature of response to therapy. In some subpopulations, the targeted pathway is non-essential so that treatments for a specific pathway do not work more broadly on the tumour (Mengistu, et. al., 2024). The pancreatic tumors are shrouded by high dense fibrotic tissue that serves as a physical barrier to drug delivery and cancer cell shelter. The Tumor microenvironment (TME) also releases growth factors, cytokines such as TGF-β and interleukins that tumors can use to increase resistance against therapies. When a cancer cell hits the road to survival the other exit becomes activated when one pathway is blocked. If for example the inhibitor hits a cell expressing EGFR it may then transition to growing by using the HGF/MET signaling pathway (Herbst & Zheng, 2019).

Acquired Resistance Mechanisms

Cancer cells may eventually acquire secondary mutations within the target protein that are resistant to drug binding overtime. Such as the KRAS mutations within oncogenes like KRAS Y96C for example have been suggested as possible resistance drivers for drug targeting KRAS G12C. These mutations restore pathway activation and tumorigenesis. Epigenetic changes that relaunch tumor cells can create resistance for example histone modifications or DNA methylation could hyperactivate survival paths or efflux pump of the cells making PARP inhibitors and/or chemo backend less effective (Fan, et. al., 2025). Phenotypic plasticity is high in pancreatic cancer cells, allowing them to go through epithelial-mesenchymal transition (EMT). The mesenchymal state is linked to resistance, increased invasiveness and immune suppression making treatment difficult (Myo Min, et. al., 2023). Overexpression of efflux transporters like P-glycoprotein (P-gp) are known to occur in some cancer cells and this facilitates the active extrusion of drugs out of the cell, resulting in sub micromolar drug concentrations inside of cancer cells. Furthermore, metabolic reprogramming (glycolysis and glutamine metabolism among others) often makes existing therapies less potent (Chour A, et. al., 2024). Tumor microenvironment is known to be immunosuppressive that explains why immune checkpoint inhibitors have not shown much success in pancreatic cancer. Mechanisms including PD-L1 up-regulation, regulatory T cells (Tregs) and myeloid-derived suppressor cells (MDSCs) that generate an immune-mediated tumor eradication (Philipp, et. al., 2024).

Overcoming Resistance: Strategies and Innovations

Administering targeted agents along with those that target compensatory pathways or resistance mechanisms together seems most effective. KRAS inhibitors plus MEK inhibitors prevent pathway reactivation e.g. other examples of pairing PARP inhibitors with immune checkpoint inhibitors to take advantage of the DNA damage-driven immune response (Karthika, et. al., 2022). However, identification and monitoring predictive biomarkers (e.g. circulating tumor DNA and exosomal proteins) may allow early detection of emerging resistance, allowing for prompt treatment interventions (Li, et. al., 2021). Strategies to alter the TME stomal-depleting agents, and TGF-β signaling targeted therapies and so on, are designed to improve drug delivery off suppression of tumor support systems (Li, Q, et. al., 2024). Identified strategies to overcome resistance include targeting epigenetic regulators (histone deacetylase inhibitors, Bromodomain inhibitors for reversal of epigenetic reprogramming caused resistance. In basket and umbrella trials treatment strategy can be dynamically adjusted as per next generation molecular profiles, paving the way for individualized approaches to treatment resistance (Cheng, et. al., 2016). Table 4 presents key resistance mechanisms and potential strategies to overcome them, offering insights into improving therapeutic outcomes.

Biomarker Discovery and Validation in Pancreatic Cancer

Early steps towards precision medicine for pancreatic cancer involve biomarker discovery and validation. Biomarkers are important to understand tumor biology and to predict the response to treatment, as well to single-out patient subsets that may derive benefit from certain therapies. But this complexity makes it hard to identify and validate biomarkers that can be used in the clinic, when translated out of the laboratory to cancer patients (Dai, et. al., 2024).

Challenges in Biomarker Discovery

A big hurdle is tumor heterogeneity. Pancreatic cancers are so heterogeneous that a biomarker identified on one patient will likely not translate into the next. Circulating biomarker such as ctDNA and tumor-derived exosomes are extensively present in nano-molar level which make them low quantity required to track or measure with high accuracy (Menis, et. al., 2014). A second limitation is the lack of standard procedures for sample collection, storage and subsequently analysis. There is also significant lack of standard operating procedures to ensure that a biomarker will act in the same way across different labs/clinics in non-consistent processes (Lowery & O'Reilly, 2011). In addition, biomarker need to cross-validated across real world populations because genetic backgrounds environmental impact and other health problems can influence how well a biomarker can translate. But this is hard to do without significant access to big pools of high-quality patient groups, samples. At last, most of the highly promising biomarkers need specialized tests that not yet provide and available everyday clinical contexts making it hard to bring them into routine care (Zhou, et. al., 2024).

Strategies for Effective Biomarker Validation

Now so that biomarkers can be more robust, researchers conduct large multicenter studies that include a broad and heterogeneous patient set. This also maintains to ensure that results are generalisable across populations and healthcare systems. One more step is to standardize how samples are collected, stored and analyzed. This eliminates variability and thus, increases accuracy of the results (O'Connor, et. al., 2017). Approaches using "omics" technologies for example proteomics, genomics and metabolomics etc are also becoming important. They leverage these methods to identify new biomarkers based on what is happening to proteins, genes and metabolic changes that are specific to pancreatic cancer. The era of real-time monitoring cytokine data with liquid biopsies using ctDNA/circulating tumor cells/ exosomes to explore disease evolution and treatment responses is now. Collaboration is important as well. Academic-university and biotech-company-partnerships with regulatory bodies can help accelerate the identification and verification of novel biomarkers. Organizations like PanCAN are engaged in supporting these efforts (Ahmad A, et. al., 2023).

Promising Biomarkers in Pancreatic Cancer

Circulating Tumor DNA (ctDNA)

Non-invasive detection of mutations, such as KRAS, and the monitoring of minimal residual disease (MRD) have shown significant promise in advancing pancreatic cancer diagnosis and treatment. KRAS mutations are prevalent in pancreatic cancer, and their detection can aid in early identification and personalized therapeutic strategies. MRD monitoring, which tracks remaining cancer cells after treatment, offers valuable insights into the likelihood of recurrence, helping to tailor subsequent treatment plans (Kerr KM, et. al., 2021, and Uesato, et. al., 2020). However, challenges persist, particularly in the sensitivity of these techniques for detecting early-stage pancreatic cancer. Despite advancements, the ability to detect subtle mutations or low levels of residual disease in the early stages remains limited, which hinders the early diagnosis and effective management of the disease (Guan, et. al., 2022).

Exosomal Biomarkers

Glypican-1 (GPC1) on exosomes has emerged as a potential diagnostic marker for pancreatic cancer, offering a promising tool for distinguishing this aggressive cancer from benign conditions. Exosomes, small vesicles released by cells, carry proteins like GPC1 that are specific to cancer cells, making them an attractive biomarker for non-invasive detection (Bunduc, et. al., 2022). The use of GPC1 as a diagnostic marker can help differentiate pancreatic cancer from other conditions, improving the accuracy of diagnosis. However, challenges remain in the clinical application of this marker, primarily due to the lack of standardization in the methods used for exosome isolation and quantification. Variability in these processes can lead to inconsistencies in results, hindering the widespread adoption of GPC1 as a reliable diagnostic tool (Wu, et al, 2020).

Metabolic Biomarkers

Elevated serum levels of metabolites such as sarcosine or branched-chain amino acids have gained attention as potential biomarkers for the early detection and prognosis prediction of various cancers, including pancreatic cancer. These metabolites are involved in metabolic pathways that are often altered in cancer cells, and their presence at elevated levels in the serum can signal the onset of malignancy. Early detection using these biomarkers could enable timely intervention, improving patient outcomes (Mehta, et. al., 2017). Additionally, monitoring changes in their levels may offer valuable insights into disease progression and the patient's prognosis. However, challenges persist, including the need for more extensive validation studies and the development of standardized assays to ensure consistency and accuracy in metabolite measurement (Perazzoli, et. al., 2023).

Immunological Biomarkers

Tumor mutational burden (TMB) and immune cell infiltration profiles are emerging as key indicators for predicting a patient's response to immunotherapies. TMB refers to the total number of mutations within a tumor's genome, with higher mutational burdens often correlating with better responses to immune checkpoint inhibitors. Additionally, the infiltration of immune cells into the tumor microenvironment can provide valuable insights into the immune landscape of the tumor, helping to assess its potential for immune recognition and response (van der Sijde, et. al., 2021). Together,

TMB and immune cell infiltration profiles can guide clinicians in selecting the most appropriate immunotherapy for a patient, optimizing treatment outcomes. However, challenges remain, such as variability in the methods for calculating TMB and the complexity of interpreting immune cell profiles, which can complicate their routine clinical use (Khomiak A, et. al., 2020). Figure 3 demonstrates how biomarker-based therapy is applied in pancreatic cancer, enabling personalized treatment strategies based on molecular profiling and predictive markers.

Figure 3. Biomarker-Based Therapy for Pancreatic Cancer

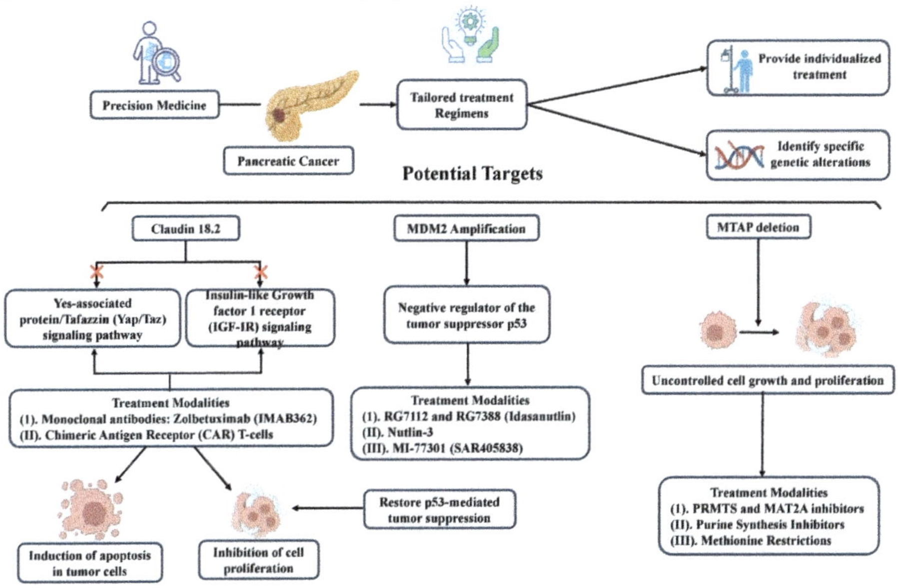

Future Perspectives in Precision Treatment of Pancreatic Cancer

Precision medicine for pancreatic cancer will be defined by advanced technologies and expanding tumor biology. Surveillance strategies are emerging to dispel these inadequacies, which comprise tumor heterogeneity, non-specific drug delivery and drug resistance. Artificial Intelligence (AI) is increasingly influential in oncological decision-making. Platform companies such like Tempus, Foundation Medicine, and PathAI are in the business of using machine learning to digest massive genomic as well transcriptomic data from hundreds of hospitals in radiological datasets (Imtiaz, et. al., 2025). These approaches are designed to predict response to therapy, identify actionable mutations and support real time treatment adaptation. AI-powered models are further applied to patient-stratification in clinical trials and to improve drug repurposing. The success of mRNA vaccines for COVID-19 has accelerated interest in applying mRNA-based therapies to oncology. Driven by the successes of COVID-19 vaccines, personal mRNA cancer vaccines (like Moderna's mRNA-4157) are being tested as it allows to encode neoantigens specific for each patient thus potentially generating an immune response (Dhudum, et. al., 2024).

CAR-T cell therapy, traditionally effective in hematologic malignancies, is evolving for pancreatic cancer through innovative engineering. Armored CAR-T cells, dual-antigen targeting CARs, and oncolytic virus-armed CAR-T constructs are being tested to overcome the immunosuppressive tumor microenvironment (Ali, and DiPersio, 2024). Clinical trials combining CAR-T with checkpoint inhibitors (e.g., anti-PD-1) and stromal-targeting agents are underway (e.g., NCT03323944), aiming to improve intratumoral penetration and persistence. Patient-derived organoids (PDOs) are transforming ex vivo drug screening (Grosser, et. al., 2019). These 3D models retain the genetic and phenotypic traits of the parent tumor and are now being used in real-time clinical settings. A new method, 'organoid-guided therapy' was recently tested on pancreatic cancer patients (PDAC) publicly in a recent study published in Nature Medicine in the year of 2022. The answers were promising, as they corresponded to what one recorded in actual patient response to therapy by matching treatment chosen using organoids (mini-tumors) grown from the sample (Gong, et. al., 2023). This approach is indeed being tested further in clinical trials through NCT04296944. This approach may help identify effective treatments and mechanisms of drug resistance. Spatial omics (complementary to single omics data generated) is another recent tool rapidly used by researchers they allow to analyze the tumor microenvironment in high fidelity (spatial omics include spatial transcriptomics and proteomics). They are giving scientists a view of where all the cell types reside within the tumor, how immune cell behavior is playing out and what signals are coming from specific areas. Visium platform, recently launched by 10x Genomics for pancreatic cancer research allows to map tumors in more detail and potentially plan effective combination treatment toward different subdomains within the tumor (Du, et. al., 2023).

Together, these new advances offer hope for overcoming the tough challenges of treating pancreatic cancer. They aim to turn it from a disease that's hard to treat into one that can be managed using personalized, data-driven approaches. The combination of artificial intelligence, custom-made immunotherapy, organoid testing, and spatial biology is opening the door to a new kind of cancer care, one that adapts to each patient. As more clinical studies confirm their benefits, these technologies are expected to help patients live longer and improve their quality of life.

CONCLUSION

Pancreatic cancer continues to pose major therapeutic challenges due to its late detection, molecular heterogeneity, and drug resistance. Precision oncology is transforming the treatment paradigm by targeting key molecular drivers such as KRAS, EGFR, and Hedgehog pathways, and by integrating novel therapies including PARP inhibitors, TKIs, and anti-angiogenic agents. Recent advances in biomarkers, liquid biopsies, and next-generation sequencing are enabling more personalized approaches. Innovative technologies such as organoid-guided therapy, artificial intelligence, and spatial omics are further enhancing drug discovery and patient stratification. Although significant barriers remain, particularly resistance mechanisms and the immunosuppressive tumor microenvironment, the future of pancreatic cancer therapy lies in rationally designed combination regimens and biomarker-driven strategies. With continued clinical innovation and cross-disciplinary collaboration, precision treatment offers a realistic path toward improving survival and quality of life for pancreatic cancer patients.

REFERENCES

Ahmad, A., Imran, M., & Ahsan, H. (2023). Biomarkers as biomedical bioindicators: Approaches and techniques for the detection, analysis, and validation of novel biomarkers of diseases. *Pharmaceutics, 15*(6), 1630. DOI: 10.3390/pharmaceutics15061630 PMID: 37376078

Ali, A., & DiPersio, J. F. (2024). ReCARving the future: Bridging CAR T-cell therapy gaps with synthetic biology, engineering, and economic insights. *Frontiers in Immunology, 15*, 1432799. DOI: 10.3389/fimmu.2024.1432799 PMID: 39301026

Alturki, M. S., Tawfeeq, N., Alissa, A., Ahbail, Z., Gomaa, M. S., Al Khzem, A. H., & Alshehri, A. A. (2025). Targeting KRAS G12C and G12S mutations in lung cancer: In silico drug repurposing and antiproliferative assessment on A549 cells. *Informatics in Medicine Unlocked, 52*, 101612. DOI: 10.1016/j.imu.2024.101612

Amakye, D., Jagani, Z., & Dorsch, M. (2013). Unraveling the therapeutic potential of the Hedgehog pathway in cancer. *Nature Medicine, 19*(11), 1410–1422. DOI: 10.1038/nm.3389 PMID: 24202394

Annese, T., Tamma, R., Ruggieri, S., & Ribatti, D. (2019). Angiogenesis in Pancreatic Cancer: Pre-Clinical and Clinical Studies. *Cancers (Basel), 11*(3), 381. DOI: 10.3390/cancers11030381 PMID: 30889903

Awad, M. M., Liu, S., Rybkin, I. I., Arbour, K. C., Dilly, J., Zhu, V. W., & Riely, G. J. (2021). Acquired resistance to KRAS G12C inhibition in cancer. *The New England Journal of Medicine, 384*(25), 2382–2393. DOI: 10.1056/NEJMoa2105281 PMID: 34161704

Bahar, M. E., Kim, H. J., & Kim, D. R. (2023). Targeting the RAS/RAF/MAPK pathway for cancer therapy: From mechanism to clinical studies. *Signal Transduction and Targeted Therapy, 455*(1), 455. DOI: 10.1038/s41392-023-01705-z PMID: 38105263

Bhat, G. R., Sethi, I., Sadida, H. Q., Rah, B., Mir, R., Algehainy, N., Albalawi, I. A., Masoodi, T., Subbaraj, G. K., Jamal, F., Singh, M., Kumar, R., Macha, M. A., Uddin, S., Akil, A. S. A., Haris, M., & Bhat, A. A. (2024). Cancer cell plasticity: From cellular, molecular, and genetic mechanisms to tumor heterogeneity and drug resistance. *Cancer and Metastasis Reviews, 43*(1), 197–228. DOI: 10.1007/s10555-024-10172-z PMID: 38329598

Biray Avci, C., Goker Bagca, B., Nikanfar, M., Takanlou, L. S., Takanlou, M. S., & Nourazarian, A. (2024). Tumor microenvironment and cancer metastasis: Molecular mechanisms and therapeutic implications. *Frontiers in Pharmacology, 15*, 1442888. DOI: 10.3389/fphar.2024.1442888 PMID: 39600368

Bunduc, S., Gede, N., Vancsa, S., Lillik, V., Kiss, S., Juhász, M. F., Erőss, B., Szakács, Z., Gheorghe, C., Mikó, A., & Hegyi, P. (2022). Exosomes as prognostic biomarkers in pancreatic ductal adenocarcinoma—A systematic review and meta-analysis. *Translational Research; the Journal of Laboratory and Clinical Medicine, 244*, 126–136. DOI: 10.1016/j.trsl.2022.01.001 PMID: 35066189

Capasso, M., Franceschi, M., Rodriguez-Castro, K. I., Crafa, P., Cambiè, G., Miraglia, C., Barchi, A., Nouvenne, A., Leandro, G., & Meschi, T., De' Angelis, G. L., & Di Mario, F. (2018). Epidemiology and risk factors of pancreatic cancer. *Acta Biomedica, 89*(9-S), 141–146. DOI: 10.23750/abm.v89i9-S.7923 PMID: 30561407

Cheng, F., Su, L., & Qian, C. (2016). Circulating tumor DNA: A promising biomarker in the liquid biopsy of cancer. *Oncotarget, 7*(30), 48832–48841. DOI: 10.18632/oncotarget.9453 PMID: 27223063

Chi, J., Chung, S. Y., Parakrama, R., Fayyaz, F., Jose, J., & Saif, M. W. (2021). The role of PARP inhibitors in *BRCA* mutated pancreatic cancer. *Therapeutic Advances in Gastroenterology, 14*, 17562848211014818. DOI: 10.1177/17562848211014818 PMID: 34025781

Chinnadurai, R. K., Khan, N., Meghwanshi, G. K., Ponne, S., Althobiti, M., & Kumar, R. (2023). Current research status of anti-cancer peptides: Mechanism of action, production, and clinical applications. *Biomedicine and Pharmacotherapy, 164*, 114996. DOI: 10.1016/j.biopha.2023.114996 PMID: 37311281

Chour, A., Toffart, A. C., Berton, E., & Duruisseaux, M. (2024). Mechanisms of resistance to KRASG12C inhibitors in KRASG12C-mutated non-small cell lung cancer. *Frontiers in Oncology, 14*, 1328728. DOI: 10.3389/fonc.2024.1328728 PMID: 39301544

Clarke, J. M., & Hurwitz, H. I. (2013). Targeted inhibition of VEGF receptor 2: An update on ramucirumab. *Expert Opinion on Biological Therapy, 13*(8), 1187–1196. DOI: 10.1517/14712598.2013.810717 PMID: 23803182

ClinicalTrials.gov. [Internet]. Bethesda (MD): National Library of Medicine (US). Identifier NCT06241352, A Study of Modified FOLFIRINOX With Simvastatin in Metastatic Pancreatic Adenocarcinoma; 2024 [cited 2025 Apr 29]. Available from: https://clinicaltrials.gov/ct2/show/NCT06241352

Conroy, T., Hammel, P., Hebbar, M., Ben Abdelghani, M., Wei, A. C., Raoul, J. L., Chone, L., Francois, E., Artru, P., Biagi, J. J., Lecomte, T., Assenat, E., Faroux, R., Ychou, M., Volet, J., Sauvanet, A., Breysacher, G., Di Fiore, F., Cripps, C., & Bachet, J.-B. (2018). FOLFIRINOX or gemcitabine as adjuvant therapy for pancreatic cancer. *The New England Journal of Medicine*, *379*(25), 2395–2406. DOI: 10.1056/NEJMoa1809775 PMID: 30575490

Cortesi, L., Rugo, H. S., & Jackisch, C. (2021). An overview of PARP inhibitors for the treatment of breast cancer. *Targeted Oncology*, *16*(3), 255–282. DOI: 10.1007/s11523-021-00796-4 PMID: 33710534

Dai, W., Qiao, X., Fang, Y., Guo, R., Bai, P., Liu, S., Li, T., Jiang, Y., Wei, S., Na, Z., Xiao, X., & Li, D. (2024). Epigenetics-targeted drugs: Current paradigms and future challenges. *Signal Transduction and Targeted Therapy*, *9*(1), 332. DOI: 10.1038/s41392-024-02039-0 PMID: 39592582

de Jesus, V. H. F., Mathias-Machado, M. C., de Farias, J. P. F., Aruquipa, M. P. S., Jácome, A. A., & Peixoto, R. D. (2023). Targeting KRAS in Pancreatic Ductal Adenocarcinoma: The Long Road to Cure. *Cancers (Basel)*, *15*(20), 5015. DOI: 10.3390/cancers15205015 PMID: 37894382

del Rivero, J., & Kohn, E. C. (2017). PARP Inhibitors: The Cornerstone of DNA Repair-Targeted Therapies. *Oncology (Williston Park, N.Y.)*, *31*(4), 265–273. PMID: 28412778

Dhudum, R., Ganeshpurkar, A., & Pawar, A. (2024). Revolutionizing Drug Discovery: A Comprehensive Review of AI Applications. *Drugs and Drug Candidates*, *3*(1), 148–171. DOI: 10.3390/ddc3010009

Dibitetto, D., Widmer, C. A., & Rottenberg, S. (2024). PARPi, BRCA, and gaps: Controversies and future research. *Trends in Cancer*, *10*(9), 857–869. DOI: 10.1016/j.trecan.2024.06.008 PMID: 39004561

Dosch, J. S., Pasca di Magliano, M., & Simeone, D. M. (2010). Pancreatic cancer and hedgehog pathway signaling: new insights. *Pancreatology: official journal of the International Association of Pancreatology (IAP) ... [et al.]*, *10*(2-3), 151–157. DOI: 10.1159/000225923

Du, J., An, Z. J., Huang, Z. F., Yang, Y. C., Zhang, M. H., Fu, X. H., Shi, W.-Y., & Hou, J. (2023). Novel insights from spatial transcriptome analysis in solid tumors. *International Journal of Biological Sciences*, *19*(15), 4778–4792. DOI: 10.7150/ijbs.83098 PMID: 37781515

Fagman, J. B., Ljungman, D., Falk, P., Iresjö, B. M., Engström, C., Naredi, P., & Lundholm, K. (2019, June). EGFR, but not COX-2, protein in resected pancreatic ductal adenocarcinoma is associated with poor survival. *Oncology Letters*, *17*(6), 5361–5368. DOI: 10.3892/ol.2019.10224 PMID: 31186753

Fan, Z., Xiao, Y., Du, Y., Zhang, Y., & Zhou, W. (2025). Pancreatic cancer subtyping - the keystone of precision treatment. *Frontiers in Immunology*, *16*, 1563725. DOI: 10.3389/fimmu.2025.1563725 PMID: 40264765

Feng, Z., Prentice, R., & Srivastava, S. (2004). Research issues and strategies for genomic and proteomic biomarker discovery and validation: A statistical perspective. *Pharmacogenomics*, *5*(6), 709–719. DOI: 10.1517/14622416.5.6.709 PMID: 15335291

Garg, P., Pareek, S., Kulkarni, P., Horne, D., Salgia, R., & Singhal, S. S. (2024). Next-Generation Immunotherapy: Advancing Clinical Applications in Cancer Treatment. *Journal of Clinical Medicine*, *13*(21), 6537. DOI: 10.3390/jcm13216537 PMID: 39518676

Gerriets, V., & Kasi, A. (2025 Jan). Bevacizumab. [Updated 2023 Aug 28] In *StatPearls* [Internet]. StatPearls Publishing., Available from https://www.ncbi.nlm.nih.gov/books/NBK482126/

Golan, T., Hammel, P., Reni, M., Van Cutsem, E., Macarulla, T., Hall, M. J., Park, J. O., Hochhauser, D., Arnold, D., Oh, D. Y., Reinacher-Schick, A., Tortora, G., Algül, H., O'Reilly, E. M., McGuinness, D., Cui, K. Y., Schlienger, K., Locker, G. Y., & Kindler, H. L. (2019). Maintenance olaparib for germline BRCA-mutated metastatic pancreatic cancer. *The New England Journal of Medicine*, *381*(4), 317–327. DOI: 10.1056/NEJMoa1903387 PMID: 31157963

Gong, M., Meng, H., Tan, D., Li, P., Qin, J., An, Q., Shi, C., & An, J. (2023). Establishment of organoid models for pancreatic ductal adenocarcinoma and screening of individualized therapy strategy. *Animal Models and Experimental Medicine*, *6*(5), 409–418. DOI: 10.1002/ame2.12352 PMID: 37890865

Grosser, R., Cherkassky, L., Chintala, N., & Adusumilli, P. S. (2019). Combination Immunotherapy with CAR T Cells and Checkpoint Blockade for the Treatment of Solid Tumors. *Cancer Cell*, *36*(5), 471–482. DOI: 10.1016/j.ccell.2019.09.006 PMID: 31715131

Guan, S., Deng, G., Sun, J., Han, Q., Lv, Y., Xue, T., Ding, L., Yang, T., Qian, N., & Dai, G. (2022). Evaluation of circulating tumor DNA as a prognostic biomarker for metastatic pancreatic adenocarcinoma. *Frontiers in Oncology*, *12*, 926260. DOI: 10.3389/fonc.2022.926260 PMID: 36081557

Guo, Y. J., Pan, W. W., Liu, S. B., Shen, Z. F., Xu, Y., & Hu, L. L. (2020). ERK/MAPK signalling pathway and tumorigenesis. *Experimental and Therapeutic Medicine, 19*(3), 1997–2007. PMID: 32104259

Halder, S., Basu, S., Lall, S. P., Ganti, A. K., Batra, S. K., & Seshacharyulu, P. (2023). Targeting the EGFR signaling pathway in cancer therapy: What's new in 2023? *Expert Opinion on Therapeutic Targets, 27*(4-5), 305–324. DOI: 10.1080/14728222.2023.2218613 PMID: 37243489

Hallin, J., Engstrom, L. D., Hargis, L., Calinisan, A., Aranda, R., Briere, D. M., Sudhakar, N., Bowcut, V., Baer, B. R., Ballard, J. A., Burkard, M. R., Fell, J. B., Fischer, J. P., Vigers, G. P., Xue, Y., Gatto, S., Fernandez-Banet, J., Pavlicek, A., Velastagui, K., & Christensen, J. G. (2020). The KRASG12C inhibitor MRTX849 provides insight toward therapeutic susceptibility of KRAS-mutant cancers in mouse models and patients. *Cancer Discovery, 10*(1), 54–71. DOI: 10.1158/2159-8290.CD-19-1167 PMID: 31658955

Harrison, P. T., Vyse, S., & Huang, P. H. (2020). Rare epidermal growth factor receptor (EGFR) mutations in non-small cell lung cancer. *Seminars in Cancer Biology, 61*, 167–179. DOI: 10.1016/j.semcancer.2019.09.015 PMID: 31562956

He, J., Mo, Z., Mai, Q., & Chen, X. (2021). Serum neutrophil/lymphocyte ratio as a potential predictor of treatment response for immune checkpoint inhibitors in patients with advanced hepatocellular carcinoma. *Journal of Clinical Oncology, 39*(15, suppl), e16156. Advance online publication. DOI: 10.1200/JCO.2021.39.15_suppl.e16156

He, Y., Sun, M. M., Zhang, G. G., Yang, J., Chen, K. S., Xu, W. W., & Li, B. (2021). Targeting PI3K/Akt signal transduction for cancer therapy. *Signal Transduction and Targeted Therapy, 6*(1), 425. DOI: 10.1038/s41392-021-00828-5 PMID: 34916492

Herbst, B., & Zheng, L. (2019). Precision medicine in pancreatic cancer: treating every patient as an exception. *The lancet. Gastroenterology & hepatology, 4*(10), 805–810. doi:.1016/S2468-1253(19)30175-X

Imtiaz, S., Ferdous, U. T., Nizela, A., Hasan, A., Shakoor, A., Zia, A. W., & Uddin, S. (2025). Mechanistic study of cancer drug delivery: Current techniques, limitations, and future prospects. *European Journal of Medicinal Chemistry, 290*, 117535. DOI: 10.1016/j.ejmech.2025.117535 PMID: 40132495

Jing, J., Wu, Z., Wang, J., Luo, G., Lin, H., Fan, Y., & Zhou, C. (2023). Hedgehog signaling in tissue homeostasis, cancers and targeted therapies. *Signal Transduction and Targeted Therapy, 8*(1), 315. DOI: 10.1038/s41392-023-01559-5 PMID: 37596267

John, K. M., Tenner, J., Franco, Y., Croocks, R., Perez, M., McEvoy, T., Zavadsky, T., Beyer, K., Mercieca, R., Nadella, S., Carvino, A., Barish, M., & King, D. A. (2024). Abstract PR01: Implementation of a real-time AI-guided navigation service for pancreas cancer. *Cancer Research*, *84*(2, Supplement), PR01–PR01. DOI: 10.1158/1538-7445.PANCA2023-PR01

Karamitopoulou, E. (2020). Pancreatic ductal adenocarcinoma: Almost a century of attempting to solve the mystery of its early dissemination. *Cancers (Basel)*, *12*(4), 1021. DOI: 10.3390/cancers12041021 PMID: 32326377

Karthika, C., Sureshkumar, R., Zehravi, M., Akter, R., Ali, F., Ramproshad, S., Mondal, B., Tagde, P., Ahmed, Z., Khan, F. S., Rahman, M. H., & Cavalu, S. (2022). Multidrug Resistance of Cancer Cells and the Vital Role of P-Glycoprotein. *Life (Basel, Switzerland)*, *12*(6), 897. doi:3390/life12060897

Kelley, R. K., & Ko, A. H. (2008). Erlotinib in the treatment of advanced pancreatic cancer. *Biologics*, *2*(1), 83–95. DOI: 10.2147/BTT.S1832 PMID: 19707431

Kerr, K. M., Bibeau, F., Thunnissen, E., Botling, J., Ryska, A., Wolf, J., Öhrling, K., Burdon, P., Malapelle, U., & Büttner, R. (2021). The evolving landscape of biomarker testing for non-small cell lung cancer in Europe. *Lung Cancer (Amsterdam, Netherlands)*, *154*, 161–175. DOI: 10.1016/j.lungcan.2021.02.026 PMID: 33690091

Khomiak, A., Brunner, M., Kordes, M., Lindblad, S., Miksch, R. C., Öhlund, D., & Regel, I. (2020). Recent discoveries of diagnostic, prognostic and predictive biomarkers for pancreatic cancer. *Cancers (Basel)*, *12*(11), 3234. DOI: 10.3390/cancers12113234 PMID: 33147766

Kim, H. J., Lee, H. N., Jeong, M. S., & Jang, S. B. (2021). Oncogenic KRAS: Signaling and Drug Resistance. *Cancers (Basel)*, *13*(22), 5599. DOI: 10.3390/cancers13225599 PMID: 34830757

Klieser, E., Swierczynski, S., Mayr, C., Jäger, T., Schmidt, J., Neureiter, D., Kiesslich, T., & Illig, R. (2016). Differential role of Hedgehog signaling in human pancreatic (patho-) physiology: An up-to-date review. *World Journal of Gastrointestinal Pathophysiology*, *7*(2), 199–210. DOI: 10.4291/wjgp.v7.i2.199 PMID: 27190692

Klomp, J. E., Klomp, J. A., & Der, C. J. (2021). The ERK mitogen-activated protein kinase signaling network: The final frontier in RAS signal transduction. *Biochemical Society Transactions*, *49*(1), 253–267. DOI: 10.1042/BST20200507 PMID: 33544118

Kopecka, J., Campia, I., & Riganti, C. (2021). Pharmacologically targeting the tumor microenvironment to overcome resistance in pancreatic cancer. *Molecular Pharmaceutics*, *18*(6), 2094–2108. DOI: 10.1021/acs.molpharmaceut.4c00329

Lee, T., Teng, T. Z. J., & Shelat, V. G. (2020). Carbohydrate antigen 19-9 - tumor marker: Past, present, and future. *World Journal of Gastrointestinal Surgery*, *12*(12), 468–490. DOI: 10.4240/wjgs.v12.i12.468 PMID: 33437400

Li, B., Zhang, Q., Castaneda, C., & Cook, S. (2024). Targeted Therapies in Pancreatic Cancer: A New Era of Precision Medicine. *Biomedicines*, *12*(10), 2175. DOI: 10.3390/biomedicines12102175 PMID: 39457488

Li, K., Shi, H., Zhang, B., Ou, X., Ma, Q., Chen, Y., Shu, P., Li, D., & Wang, Y. (2021). Myeloid-derived suppressor cells as immunosuppressive regulators and therapeutic targets in cancer. *Signal Transduction and Targeted Therapy*, *6*(1), 362. DOI: 10.1038/s41392-021-00670-9 PMID: 34620838

Li, Q., Geng, S., Luo, H., Wang, W., Mo, Y. Q., Luo, Q., Wang, L., Song, G.-B., Sheng, J.-P., & Xu, B. (2024). Signaling pathways involved in colorectal cancer: Pathogenesis and targeted therapy. *Signal Transduction and Targeted Therapy*, *9*(1), 266. DOI: 10.1038/s41392-024-01953-7 PMID: 39370455

Liu, Z. L., Chen, H. H., Zheng, L. L., Sun, L. P., & Shi, L. (2023). Angiogenic signaling pathways and anti-angiogenic therapy for cancer. *Signal Transduction and Targeted Therapy*, *8*(1), 198. DOI: 10.1038/s41392-023-01460-1 PMID: 37169756

Long, J., Zhang, Y., Yu, X., Yang, J., LeBrun, D. G., Chen, C., Yao, Q., & Li, M. (2011). Overcoming drug resistance in pancreatic cancer. *Expert Opinion on Therapeutic Targets*, *15*(7), 817–828. DOI: 10.1517/14728222.2011.566216 PMID: 21391891

Lowery, M. A., & O'Reilly, E. M. (2011). Pancreatic cancer: The role of molecular markers in diagnosis and management. *Clinical Advances in Hematology & Oncology*, *9*(12), 900–908. PMID: 22252658

Lyman, G. H., & Moses, H. L. (2016). Biomarker tests for molecularly targeted therapies-the key to unlocking precision medicine. *The New England Journal of Medicine*, *375*(1), 4–6. DOI: 10.1056/NEJMp1604033 PMID: 27353537

Ma, L., Guo, H., Zhao, Y., Liu, Z., Wang, C., Bu, J., Sun, T., & Wei, J. (2024). Liquid biopsy in cancer current: Status, challenges and future prospects. *Signal Transduction and Targeted Therapy*, *9*(1), 336. DOI: 10.1038/s41392-024-02021-w PMID: 39617822

Marabelle, A., Le, D. T., Ascierto, P. A., Di Giacomo, A. M., De Jesus-Acosta, A., Delord, J. P., Geva, R., Gottfried, M., Penel, N., Hansen, A. R., Piha-Paul, S. A., Doi, T., Gao, B., Chung, H. C., Lopez-Martin, J., Bang, Y.-J., Frommer, R. S., Shah, M., Ghori, R., & Diaz, L. A.Jr. (2020). Efficacy of pembrolizumab in patients with noncolorectal high microsatellite instability/mismatch repair–deficient cancer: Results from the phase II KEYNOTE-158 study. *Journal of Clinical Oncology*, *38*(1), 1–0. DOI: 10.1200/JCO.19.02105 PMID: 31682550

Matuszewska, K., Pereira, M., Petrik, D., Lawler, J., & Petrik, J. (2021). Normalizing Tumor Vasculature to Reduce Hypoxia, Enhance Perfusion, and Optimize Therapy Uptake. *Cancers (Basel)*, *13*(17), 4444. DOI: 10.3390/cancers13174444 PMID: 34503254

Mehta, K. Y., Wu, H. J., Menon, S. S., Fallah, Y., Zhong, X., Rizk, N., Unger, K., Mapstone, M., Fiandaca, M. S., Federoff, H. J., & Cheema, A. K. (2017). Metabolomic biomarkers of pancreatic cancer: A meta-analysis study. *Oncotarget*, *8*(40), 68899–68915. DOI: 10.18632/oncotarget.20324 PMID: 28978166

Mengistu, B. A., Tsegaw, T., Demessie, Y., Getnet, K., Bitew, A. B., Kinde, M. Z., Beirhun, A. M., Mebratu, A. S., Mekasha, Y. T., Feleke, M. G., & Fenta, M. D. (2024). Comprehensive review of drug resistance in mammalian cancer stem cells: Implications for cancer therapy. *Cancer Cell International*, *24*(1), 406. DOI: 10.1186/s12935-024-03558-0 PMID: 39695669

Menis, J., Hasan, B., & Besse, B. (2014). New clinical research strategies in thoracic oncology: Clinical trial design, adaptive, basket and umbrella trials, new end-points and new evaluations of response. *European Respiratory Review : an Official Journal of the European Respiratory Society*, *23*(133), 367–378. DOI: 10.1183/09059180.00004214 PMID: 25176973

Miyashita, H., Kato, S., & Hong, D. S. (2024). KRAS G12C inhibitor combination therapies: Current evidence and challenge. *Frontiers in Oncology*, *14*, 1380584. DOI: 10.3389/fonc.2024.1380584 PMID: 38756650

Montoya Mira, J., Bayani, N., Kesavan, M., Zhu, Y., Chen, L., & Housman, G.. (2023, April 5). A multimodal blood test for early detection of pancreatic cancer. *Science Translational Medicine*, *15*(693), eabq5734. Advance online publication. DOI: 10.1126/scitranslmed.abq5734

Motzer, R. J., Porta, C., Eto, M., Powles, T., Grünwald, V., Hutson, T. E., Alekseev, B., Rha, S. Y., Merchan, J. R., Goh, J. C., Kapoor, A., De Giorgi, U., Melichar, B., Hong, S.-H., Gurney, H., Rodriguez-Lopez, K., He, C. S., Okpara, C., McKenzie, J., & Choueiri, T. K. (2023). Final prespecified overall survival (OS) analysis of CLEAR: 4-year follow-up of lenvatinib plus pembrolizumab (L+ P) vs sunitinib (S) in patients (pts) with advanced renal cell carcinoma (aRCC). *Journal of Clinical Oncology*, *41*(16, suppl), 4502. Advance online publication. DOI: 10.1200/JCO.2023.41.16_suppl.4502

Murphrey, M. B., Quaim, L., Rahimi, N., & Varacallo, M. (2023). Biochemistry, epidermal growth factor receptor. In *StatPearls* [Internet]. StatPearls Publishing.

Mustafa, M., Abbas, K., Alam, M., Habib, S., Zulfareen, , Hasan, G. M., Islam, S., Shamsi, A., & Hassan, I. (2024). Investigating underlying molecular mechanisms, signaling pathways, emerging therapeutic approaches in pancreatic cancer. *Frontiers in Oncology*, *14*, 1427802. DOI: 10.3389/fonc.2024.1427802 PMID: 39087024

Myo Min, K. K., Ffrench, C. B., Jessup, C. F., Shepherdson, M., Barreto, S. G., & Bonder, C. S. (2023). Overcoming the Fibrotic Fortress in Pancreatic Ductal Adenocarcinoma: Challenges and Opportunities. *Cancers (Basel)*, *15*(8), 2354. DOI: 10.3390/cancers15082354 PMID: 37190281

Nunes-Xavier, C. E., & Pulido, R. (2020). Targeting EMT in pancreatic cancer. *Cancers (Basel)*, *12*(6), 1374. DOI: 10.3390/cancers12061374 PMID: 32471123

O'connor, J. P., Aboagye, E. O., Adams, J. E., Aerts, H. J., Barrington, S. F., Beer, A. J., Boellaard, R., Bohndiek, S. E., Brady, M., Brown, G., Buckley, D. L., Chenevert, T. L., Clarke, L. P., Collette, S., Cook, G. J., deSouza, N. M., Dickson, J. C., Dive, C., Evelhoch, J. L., & Waterton, J. C. (2017). Imaging biomarker roadmap for cancer studies. *Nature Reviews. Clinical Oncology*, *14*(3), 169–186. DOI: 10.1038/nrclinonc.2016.162 PMID: 27725679

Perazzoli, G., García-Valdeavero, O. M., Pena, M., Prados, J., Melguizo, C., & Jimenez-Luna, C. (2023). Evaluating metabolite-based biomarkers for early diagnosis of pancreatic cancer: A systematic review. *Metabolites*, *13*(7), 872. DOI: 10.3390/metabo13070872 PMID: 37512579

Pereira, N. P., & Corrêa, J. R. (2018). Pancreatic cancer: Treatment approaches and trends. [N-A.]. *Journal of Cancer Metastasis and Treatment*, •••, 4.

Perello-Reus, C. M., Rubio-Tomás, T., Cisneros-Barroso, E., Ibargüen-González, L., Segura-Sampedro, J. J., Morales-Soriano, R., & Barceló, C. (2022). Challenges in precision medicine in pancreatic cancer: A focus in cancer stem cells and microbiota. *Frontiers in oncology, 12*, 995357. doi:.3389/fonc.2022.995357

Philipp, L. M., Yesilyurt, U. U., Surrow, A., Künstner, A., Mehdorn, A. S., Hauser, C., Gundlach, J. P., Will, O., Hoffmann, P., Stahmer, L., Franzenburg, S., Knaack, H., Schumacher, U., Busch, H., & Sebens, S. (2024). Epithelial and Mesenchymal-like Pancreatic Cancer Cells Exhibit Different Stem Cell Phenotypes Associated with Different Metastatic Propensities. *Cancers (Basel)*, *16*(4), 686. DOI: 10.3390/cancers16040686 PMID: 38398077

Pishvaian, M. J., Blais, E. M., Brody, J. R., Lyons, E., DeArbeloa, P., Hendifar, A., Mikhail, S., Chung, V., Sahai, V., Sohal, D. P. S., Bellakbira, S., Thach, D., Rahib, L., Madhavan, S., Matrisian, L. M., & Petricoin, E. F.III. (2020). Overall survival in patients with pancreatic cancer receiving matched therapies following molecular profiling: A retrospective analysis of the Know Your Tumor registry trial. *The Lancet. Oncology*, *21*(4), 508–518. DOI: 10.1016/S1470-2045(20)30074-7 PMID: 32135080

Rawla, P., Sunkara, T., & Gaduputi, V. (2019). Epidemiology of Pancreatic Cancer: Global Trends, Etiology and Risk Factors. *World Journal of Oncology*, *10*(1), 10–27. DOI: 10.14740/wjon1166 PMID: 30834048

Rojas, L. A., Sethna, Z., Soares, K. C., Olcese, C., Pang, N., Patterson, E., Lihm, J., Ceglia, N., Guasp, P., Chu, A., Yu, R., Chandra, A. K., Waters, T., Ruan, J., Amisaki, M., Zebboudj, A., Odgerel, Z., Payne, G., Derhovanessian, E., & Balachandran, V. P. (2023). Personalized RNA neoantigen vaccines stimulate T cells in pancreatic cancer. *Nature*, *618*(7963), 144–150. DOI: 10.1038/s41586-023-06063-y PMID: 37165196

Rose, M., Burgess, J. T., O'Byrne, K., Richard, D. J., & Bolderson, E. (2020). PARP Inhibitors: Clinical Relevance, Mechanisms of Action and Tumor Resistance. *Frontiers in Cell and Developmental Biology*, *8*, 564601. DOI: 10.3389/fcell.2020.564601 PMID: 33015058

Stefanoudakis, D., Frountzas, M., Schizas, D., Michalopoulos, N. V., Drakaki, A., & Toutouzas, K. G. (2024). Significance of TP53, CDKN2A, SMAD4 and KRAS in Pancreatic Cancer. *Current Issues in Molecular Biology*, *46*(4), 2827–2844. DOI: 10.3390/cimb46040177 PMID: 38666907

Tariq, S., & Badar, A. (2019). Immune evasion strategies of pancreatic cancer and the emerging role of immunotherapy. *Journal of Experimental & Clinical Cancer Research : CR*, *38*, 162. DOI: 10.1186/s13046-019-1153-8

Tolstonog, G. V., & Krupitza, G. (2019). HGF/c-MET as a therapeutic target in pancreatic cancer: Past achievements and future perspectives. *Frontiers in Oncology*, *9*, 1227. DOI: 10.3389/fonc.2019.01227

Uesato, Y., Sasahira, N., Ozaka, M., Sasaki, T., Takatsuki, M., & Zembutsu, H. (2020). Evaluation of circulating tumor DNA as a biomarker in pancreatic cancer with liver metastasis. *PLoS One*, *15*(7), e0235623. DOI: 10.1371/journal.pone.0235623 PMID: 32614932

van der Sijde, F., Mustafa, D. A., Vietsch, E. E., Katsikis, P. D., & van Eijck, C. H. (2021). Circulating immunological biomarkers: Prognosis of pancreatic cancer patients reflected by the immune system. *Pancreas*, *50*(7), 933–941. DOI: 10.1097/MPA.0000000000001862 PMID: 34643608

Wang-Gillam, A., Li, C. P., Bodoky, G., Dean, A., Shan, Y. S., Jameson, G., Macarulla, T., Lee, K. H., Cunningham, D., Blanc, J. F., Hubner, R. A., Chiu, C.-F., Schwartsmann, G., Siveke, J. T., Braiteh, F., Moyo, V., Belanger, B., Dhindsa, N., Bayever, E., & Wong, M. (2016). Nanoliposomal irinotecan with fluorouracil and folinic acid in metastatic pancreatic cancer after previous gemcitabine-based therapy (NAPOLI-1): A global, randomised, open-label, phase 3 trial. *Lancet*, *387*(10018), 545–557. DOI: 10.1016/S0140-6736(15)00986-1 PMID: 26615328

Wood, L. D., Canto, M. I., Jaffee, E. M., & Simeone, D. M. (2022). Pancreatic Cancer: Pathogenesis, Screening, Diagnosis, and Treatment. *Gastroenterology*, *163*(2), 386–402.e1. DOI: 10.1053/j.gastro.2022.03.056 PMID: 35398344

Wu, L., Zhou, W. B., Zhou, J., Wei, Y., Wang, H. M., Liu, X. D., Chen, X.-C., Wang, W., Ye, L., Yao, L., Chen, Q.-H., & Tang, Z. G. (2020). Circulating exosomal microRNAs as novel potential detection biomarkers in pancreatic cancer. *Oncology Letters*, *20*(2), 1432–1440. DOI: 10.3892/ol.2020.11691 PMID: 32724386

Yang, X., & Wu, H. (2024, November 9). RAS signaling in carcinogenesis, cancer therapy and resistance mechanisms. *Journal of Hematology & Oncology*, *17*(1), 108. DOI: 10.1186/s13045-024-01631-9 PMID: 39522047

Yang, X., & Wu, H. (2024). RAS signaling in carcinogenesis, cancer therapy and resistance mechanisms. *Journal of Hematology & Oncology*, *17*(1), 108. DOI: 10.1186/s13045-024-01631-9 PMID: 39522047

Yu, B., Shao, S., & Ma, W. (2024). Frontiers in pancreatic cancer on biomarkers, microenvironment, and immunotherapy. *Cancer Letters*, •••, 217350. PMID: 39581219

Zhou, Y., Kuang, Y., Wang, C., Yu, Y., Pan, L., & Hu, X. (2024). Impact of KRAS mutation on the tumor microenvironment in colorectal cancer. *International Journal of Biological Sciences*, *20*(5), 1947–1964. DOI: 10.7150/ijbs.88779 PMID: 38481800

Zhou, Y., Tao, L., Qiu, J., Xu, J., Yang, X., Zhang, Y., Tian, X., Guan, X., Cen, X., & Zhao, Y. (2024). Tumor biomarkers for diagnosis, prognosis and targeted therapy. *Signal Transduction and Targeted Therapy*, *9*(1), 132. DOI: 10.1038/s41392-024-01823-2 PMID: 38763973

Zhu, C., Guan, X., Zhang, X., Luan, X., Song, Z., Cheng, X., Zhang, W., & Qin, J.-J. (2022). Targeting KRAS mutant cancers: From druggable therapy to drug resistance. *Molecular Cancer*, *21*(1), 159. DOI: 10.1186/s12943-022-01629-2 PMID: 35922812

Chapter 11
Role of Artificial Intelligence in the Future of Pancreatic Cancer

K. Gayathri
https://orcid.org/0009-0007-3786-2009
Department of Microbiology, Sacred Heart College, Tirupattur, India

K. Kesavardhini
Department of Microbiology, Sacred Heart College, Tirupattur, India

E. Tharani
Department of Microbiology, Sacred Heart College, Tirupattur, India

ABSTRACT

Pancreatic cancer is still one of the deadliest cancers, with a survival rate of less than 10% at five years. Artificial Intelligence (AI) has become a potential key in transforming the treatment of pancreatic cancer by improving early detection, treatment planning, and prognostic prediction. AI-based diagnostic software has the potential to identify pancreatic tumours from imaging scans, even at the early stage when symptoms cannot be detected. They are capable of markedly enhancing diagnostic specificity, minimizing the influence of human bias, and facilitating the detection of pancreatic lesions with increased ease. AI has the ability to support the formation of personalized therapeutic strategies in analysing genetic data and anticipating therapy responses. It can help to reduce needless side effects, enable more ideal treatment modalities to be chosen, and increase general survival in the outcomes. The AI models are becoming more skilled at tracking treatment and recurrence prediction through the analysis of change in medical imaging and bio-markers. AI tool may be able to predict the incipient pancreatic cancer three years

DOI: 10.4018/979-8-3373-1469-3.ch011

ahead of diagnosis by analyzing medical patient results to a large extent. Overall, the future of pancreatic cancer treatment is most likely to be dramatically influenced by AI technologies that optimize early detection, enhance diagnostic precision, and enable individualized treatment modalities to transform early detection, diagnosis, treatment, and patient monitoring, artificial intelligence in pancreatic cancer.

1. INTRODUCTION

Pancreatic Cancer (PC) is the leading cause of cancer. With a mere 11%, PC boasts the lowest five-year relative survival rate of all cancers (Ryan et al., 2014). PC was the cause of 466003 deaths and 495773 new cases in 2022 worldwide, making up 2.6% of all new cancers and 4.7% of all cancer-related deaths (Zheng et al., 2022). The frequency and mortality rate of PC among Chinese tumors are 2.47% and 3.64%, respectively (Kenner et al., 2021). The primary cause of poor pancreatic cancer prognosis is that just 20% of patients undergo an early diagnosis (Aier et al., 2019). The majority of patients present with symptoms such as fatigue, indigestion, jaundice, and bowel habit changes difficult to differentiate from non-cancerous diseases (Klein, 2021). Primarily, Chemotherapy, Targeted Therapy, and Immunotherapy are futile as the majority of patients are already in an advanced stage with local invasion and distant metastases (Heinemann et al., 2013). PC patients identified by screening had a median survival time of 9.8 years and a 5 years survival rate of 73.3%, but non-screening found had a median survival time of 1.5 years (Tripathi, 2021).

AI is being used in the field of medicine that includes healthcare, oncology, and cardiology (Chen et al., 2022). AI may be applied in a wide range of tasks since it is more adaptable and scalable than normal biometric information techniques (Topol, 2019). It also possessed the capacity regarding bring together a broad variety of data kinds and sophisticated variable interactions in a flexible approach (Ngiam and Khor, 2019). As the volume of health-related data continues to grow and computer processing capacity continues to expand, Artificial Intelligence (AI) is exhibiting significant benefits in dealing with massive data (Bhinder et al., 2021). In practice, AI is able to execute multi-tasking applications well and leverages the doctor's time to tackle more sophisticated clinical issues of pancreatic cancer (Laranjo et al., 2018).

AI-enhanced PC diagnostic procedures are on the rise (Schuurmans et al., 2022). AI and Early Detection during Pancreatic Breast cancer Virtual Summit, the AI potential for early PC surveillance was discussed alongside highlighted (Kenner et al., 2021). Pancreas is highly vascularized milieu that encourages cancer spread and causes the disease extremely aggressive in character (Ryan et al., 2014). The challenges notwithstanding, there are and have been developments in imaging technology for better accuracy in pancreatic cancer detection and therapy (Young et al., 2020). Computed Tomography (CT), Magnetic Resonance Imaging (MRI), Endoscopic Ultrasound (EUS), and 18-fluoro-2-deoxy-d-glucose Positron Emission Tomography/Computed Tomography (18FDG PET/CT) are some of these technologies (Chen et al., 2020). Biopsies are still widely utilized to diagnose pancreatic cancer (Ryan et al., 2014). Histological assessment is extremely difficult owing to the high morphological heterogeneity in tumors and the limited tissue that can be obtained (Juiz et al., 2019). Histologic assessment of treatment response remains imprecise, similar to imaging features (Kenner et al., 2021).

The medical industry is changing and Artificial Intelligence (AI) offers innovative answers to challenging situations (Topol, 2019). Designed to make decisions, sort through and make sense of a lot of data, and learn from experience, artificial intelligence algorithms are Medical use of artificial intelligence is improving diagnosis, therapy, and patient care (Chen et al., 2022). Its capacity to improve diagnostic accuracy, Young et al. (2020) makes it most beneficial to medicine. With great accuracy in reading medical pictures such CT, MRI, and X-ray scans, doctors can identify ailments early enough to AI systems (Schuurmans et al., 2022). Quick processing AI-based diagnosis systems can show doctors their exact diagnosis (Kumar et al., 2022). Artificial intelligence (AI) tools could examine large data sets including genetic features, clinical history, and therapy response to identify patterns and associations that can be used to individualise treatment plans for unique patients (Bhinder et al., 2021). This helps medical personnel to provide customised treatment, predict the course of diseases, and reduce side effects (Kenner et al., 2021). AI is also improving operational efficiency and automating administrative task in hospitals (Laranjo et al., 2018).

Medical coding activities that alleviate medical practitioners from some of their burden and lower errors by Natural Language Processing (NLP) methods help Artificial intelligence (AI) chatbots are helping patients around-the-clock, respond to questions, arrange appointments, and even offer them simple medical advice (Laranjo et al., 2018). Machine learning is a practical application of artificial intelligence that uses a range of applications like Bayesian methods, logistic regression, support vector machines, decision trees, random forests, artificial neural networks and K-nearest neighbours (Tripathi, 2021). Among such techniques is deep learning classified under artificial neural networks and with remarkable image processing ability, particularly when used with convolutional neural networks (Ngiam and Khor, 2019). Deep learning can explore statistical dependencies between these values and corresponding outcomes in pancreatic cancer (Si et al., 2021). To enable early screening and assist in the management of complications following pancreatic cancer surgery, deep learning is able to build early high-risk prediction models for the disease as well as postoperative recurrence risk prediction models (Lee et al.,

2021). AI-based radiomics can diagnose pancreatic cancer accurately (Mukherjee et al., 2022).

2. ARTIFICIAL INTELLIGENCE (AI) IN EARLY SCREENING AND PREDICTION OF PANCREATIC CANCER

Pancreatic cancer is among the most malignant tumors, with a poor prognosis and high fatality rate owing to its early asymptomatic stages and late detection (Ryan et al., 2014). The dearth of strong biomarkers and the fact that the disease is hard to diagnose before it becomes advanced make early management extremely tough (Singhi and Wood, 2021). Nonetheless, Artificial Intelligence (AI) is now a fast-emerging methodology for the boosting of pancreatic cancer early screening, diagnosis, and prediction founded on sophisticated. The Machine Learning (ML) algorithms and Deep Learning (DL) methodology (Ngiam and Khor, 2019). The AI-based tools process huge relational databases of imaging scans, genetic material, clinical information, and biomarker profiles in order to pick up on minor patterns suggestive of early-stage pancreatic cancer (Young et al., 2020).

Machine Learning algorithms, particularly supervised along with unsupervised learning models, have demonstrated to be exceptionally competent at distinguishing between malignant and benign the pancreatic lesions (Kumar et al., 2022). Supervised learning models that are actually trained from labeled data in Computed Tomography (CT), Magnetic Resonance Imaging (MRI), and Endoscopic Ultrasound (EUS) scans can discover early Pancreatic Cancers with greater accuracy compared to standard diagnosis approaches (Schuurmans et al., 2022). Convolutional Neural Networks (CNNs), being a sort of deep learning, have done remarkably well in image detection and therefore are the appropriate tool for the diagnosis of pancreatic cancers from radiological images (Ma et al., 2020). Studies have indicated that AI-based imaging analysis boosts the sensitivity and specificity of tumor diagnosis, with less false-negative and fewer false-positive outcomes compared to detection by Human Radiologists (Si et al., 2021).

Apart from imaging, artificial intelligence is revolutionising research on Molecular and Genetic markers of Pancreatic cancer (Xiao et al., 2021). Particularly relevant in the carcinogenesis of pancreatic cancer is genomic data comprising mutations in KRAS, TP53, CDKN2A, and SMAD4 genes (Yang et al., 2016). Linking genetic changes with clinical indicators, AI-based predictive models evaluate individual risk variables and project disease development (Cheerla and Gevaert, 2019). Apart from that, transcriptome and proteome data can also be investigated using artificial intelligence techniques to identify fresh biomarkers capable of acting as previous markers of pancreatic cancer (Xiao et al., 2021). By means of artificial intelligence analysis in liquid biopsies, researchers have identified Circulating Tumour DNA (ctDNA) and microRNA fingerprints unique to pancreatic cancer, therefore enabling non-invasive early diagnosis (Radon et al., 2015).

Artificial Intelligence (AI) Natural Language Processing (NLP) has also been used to extract significant information from literature and Electronic Health Records (EHRs). Analysing unstructured clinical notes, pathology data, and patient histories, NLP tools find trends implying early pancreatic cancer (Laranjo et al., 2018). Based on patient demographics, lifestyle choices, and comorbidities, risk stratification algorithms based on artificial intelligence aim to deliver individualised risk scores that enable doctors to prioritise high-risk patients for extra screening (Sharma et al., 2018). Predictive models of pancreatic cancer outcomes have also been produced in great relevance by artificial intelligence (Lee et al., 2021).

Predicting disease onset, danger of recurrence, and response to therapy, the machine learning models grounded in past and present data generate Reinforcement learning methods and survival analysis let the AI models learn from patient data as iterations, thereby improving their forecasting capacity with time (Kumar et al., 2022). By means of predictive analysis of this kind, oncologists can make evidence-based judgements in treatment planning, therefore optimising treatment regimens, and hence increasing patient outcomes (Kenner et al., 2021).

Though promising, AI for pancreatic cancer screening and prognosis has some difficulties to be cleared (Yin et al., 2021). Among the major obstacles are the heterogeneity of pancreatic cancer, dearth of large-quality databases, and need for outside validation of AI algorithms (Mikdadi et al., 2022). To have AI generally accepted clinically, ethical issues including patient confidentiality, algorithmic bias, and explainability of AI-driven judgements must be resolved (Choudhury and Asan, 2020).

To solve these challenges and improve artificial intelligence models for practical use, cooperative data science, clinical, and research projects are absolutely essential (Kenner et al., 2021). Early pancreatic cancer (Ngiam and Khor, 2019) prognosis and diagnosis are quite promising for artificial intelligence. Integrating AI-driven imaging evaluation, biomarker discovery, and predictive modelling (Young et al., 2020) will help clinicians improve prediction accuracy, early diagnosis, and personalised treatment methods. Coupled with interdisciplinarity approaches, future innovations in artificial intelligence technology will be crucial in helping to reduce the load of pancreatic cancer and raise patient survival (Kenner et al., 2021). Future studies should concentrate on improving AI models, broadening datasets, and addressing ethicality issues to successfully translate AI innovation into clinical applications (Yin et al., 2021).

Predictive models created by Artificial Intelligence (AI) could let early intervention and diagnosis possible as well as assess the risk of pancreatic cancer development

(Sharma et al., 2018). Pancreatic cancer arises from a tumour known as Intraductal Papillary Mucinous Neoplasm (IPMN) (Kuwahara et al., 2019). Angulated 3,970 Endoscopic Ultrasonic Scanning (EUS) from patients, IPMN was histologically confirmed. Images then were loaded into sophisticated deep learning models. In malignant IPMN, mean artificial intelligence values were much more than in benign ones (0.808 vs. 0.104, P 0.01). AI diagnosis exceeded the 56.0% diagnosis effectiveness of clinicians (Kuwahara et al., 2019). Model predictive especially for identifying high-risk subgroups of diabetic individuals susceptible to Pancreatic Cancer (Sharma et al., 2018). It also integrated the key variables such as body mass index, glucose fluctuations and diabetes onset age at the onset of diabetes. In a period not more than three years, this complex prediction ratings were able to predict the premature progression of pancreatic tumors. Nearly, 80% sensitivity and specificity in Pancreatic Carcinoma Diagnosis (AUC=0.87), the presence of a score of 3 or higher, a 4.4 fold increase in incidence of Pancreatic Cancer over their Diabetic peers was noted in (Sharma et al., 2018). Patients with Type 2 Diabetes through logistic regression and artificial neural network methods. Application of anti-diabetic drugs as risk indicators of Pancreatic Cancer (Sharma et al., 2018). Likewise, they created a novel urine biomarker-based pancreatic cancer patient risk scoring system (PancRisk) (Blyuss et al., 2020). They also evaluated three urine biomarkers (LYVE1, REC1B, and TFF1) in 199 patients with Pancreatic Ductal Adenocarcinoma and 180 healthy controls. The logistic regression model was excellent at diagnostics with AUC = 0.94 and are identified tumor marker CA19-9 in sensitivity and diagnostic specificity were 96% (Blyuss et al., 2020).

3. ARTIFICIAL INTELLIGENCE (AI) IN THE DIAGNOSIS OF PANCREATIC CANCER

Diagnosis of Pancreatic cancer is a multi-step process that generally involves imaging methods like Endoscopic Ultra Sound (EUS), serum tumor markers, high-risk factors, and clinical presentation in pancreatic cancer (Ryan et al., 2014). Imaging assessment is still the most important method of clinical diagnosis of pancreatic cancer (Chen et al., 2020). CT and MRI are the most frequent methods in the diagnosis of pancreatic cancer (Young et al., 2020). Deep learning models have been a highly promising diagnostic tool for pancreatic cancer in recent years (Si et al., 2021). Averagely, 319 patient's abdominal contrast-enhanced CT scans were employed to train a deep learning model proposed by Zhejiang University. Pancreatic tumors can be identified directly from the original abdominal CT scans with the help of this model. The model obtained an AUC value of 0.871 and F1 value of 88.5%, with overall average diagnostic performance of 82.7% in all tumor cell types (Si et al., 2021). In addition, with accuracy levels of 87.6% and 100%, respectively, the model showed outstanding capacity to differentiate between pancreatic ductal adenocarcinoma and IPM (Si et al., 2021). Besides, 7245 CT scans of 222 pathologically diagnosed pancreatic cancer and 190 normal pancreas individuals were used to construct a convolutional neural network. network model in Chinese research (Ma et al., 2020). The diagnostic accuracy (95.47%) with high sensitivity (91.58%) and specificity (98.27%) for the light exposure of the Pancreatic Cancer (Ma et al., 2020). It was employed to classify the three sets of no cancer, tumor in body or tail of pancreas, as well as tumor in the neck or completely of pancreas and two classes to or without the pancreatic cancer. Three-category approach performed remarkably well in the diagnosis of pancreatic head/neck tumors with the assistance of arterial the time period of the pancreatic cancer (Ma et al., 2020). Endoscopic Ultra Sonography (EUS) is very significant diagnostic modalitiy of Chronic Pancreatitis and Pancreatic Carcinoma (Marya et al., 2021).

With the introduction of AI, EUS images have been found to be very helpful in diagnosis (Marya et al., 2021). The challenge of diagnosing Autoimmune Pancreatitis (AIP) from pancreatic ductal cancer, chronic pancreatitis, and normal pancreas (Marya et al., 2021). The model was trained them on static images and videos of EUS patient examinations (Marya et al., 2021). AIP from the normal digestive tract (99% and 98%, respectively), chronic pancreatitis (94% and 71%, respectively), and the pancreatic ductal cancer (90% and 93%, respectively), the model showed high sensitivity and specificity rates (Marya et al., 2021). AI-based on tissue pathology sections and the tumor biology markers has also achieved significant breakthroughs (Xiao et al., 2021). It is particularly noteworthy that the unsupervised learning models were able to identify a number of tumor markers for pancreatic cancer, and this provides a new the procedure through which to find potential indicators whose values can change into therapeutic (Xiao et al., 2021). One of the areas in the area of medical research with immense potential towards improving pancreatic cancer screening methods and therapy strategies is one such advanced model, which can effectively identify pancreatic cancers (Mukherjee et al., 2022). Such AI tools have the potential to revolutionize clinical practice and on pancreatic cancer (Kenner et al., 2021).

4. ARTIFICIAL INTELLIGENCE (AI) IN THE PROGNOSIS OF PANCREATIC CANCER

Artificial intelligence (AI) has become a leading tool in pancreatic cancer prediction, a disease that is notoriously well known for its late detection and poor survival rates (Ryan et al., 2014). Pancreatic cancer remains one of the deadliest diseases, with a five-year remaining alive rate of less than 10% owing to thus aggressive behavior and lack of sensitivity to conventional therapy (Ryan et al., 2014). AI, emphasizing Machine Learning (ML) and Deep Learning (DL) Techniques, has been found to possess great potential in enabling early diagnosis, predictions prediction, and individualized therapy regimens (Kumar et al., 2022). Leaning on large data sets like medical image processing, genomic data, and patient history, AI-based frameworks can identify subtle signals that might be hard to discern for human doctors (Young et al., 2020). This ability significantly enhanced disease progression, recurrence, and patient the outcome prediction, allowing physicians to make better-informed decisions (Lee et al., 2021). The most promising use of AI in pancreatic cancer prognosis may be for medical image analysis (Schuurmans et al., 2022). Conventional imaging methods like Computed Tomography (CT), Magnetic Resonance Imaging (MRI), and Endoscopic Ultrasound (EUS) are of central importance in staging and pancreatic cancer diagnosis (Chen et al., 2020).

Despite this, differentiation between malignant and benign tumors or accurate evaluation of the aggressiveness of a tumor is still challenging (Marya et al., 2021). Artificial Intelligence Systems that have been trained on massive annotated imaging datasets can accurately quantify radiographic features, automatically segment tumors, predict stages, and estimate survival (Mukherjee et al., 2022). Radiomics, one of the fields of imaging analysis through AI, draws quantitative data from medical images linked to tumor biology, allowing for the identification of high-risk patients that can be in need of more intensive treatment protocols (Mukherjee et al., 2022). Other than imaging, AI has revolutionized biomarker discovery and genetic examination of pancreatic cancer prognosis (Xiao et al., 2021). Genomic profiling of cancers provides vital information regarding mutations, levels of gene expression, and molecular subtypes that drive infections progression (Singhi and Wood, 2021).

AI-based bioinformatics tools can analyze vast genomic data to identify prognostic biomarkers and forecast therapy outcomes (Cheerla and Gevaert, 2019).

Transcriptomistically derived AI models, for instance, can predict patients depending on molecular subtypes including classical or basal-like pancreatic cancer, which have differing treatment and prognosis consequences (Cheerla and Gevaert, 2019). Furthermore, artificial intelligence may use multi-omics data including genomics, proteomics, and metabolomics to create sophisticated prognostic models in an aim to enhance risk stratification and inform precision medicine approaches (Xiao et al., 2021). Another urgent contribution of artificial intelligence in the prognosis of pancreatic cancer is therapeutic outcome predictive modelling and recurrence risk prediction (Lee et al., 2021). Conventional statistical models can understate the survival probabilities since they make general predictions based on few inputs (Tong et al., 2020). Predictive analytics using artificial intelligence, however, contain varied patient-specific data including demographics, history, treatment outcomes, and real-world experience from past instances (Kumar et al., 2022). By means of Machine Learning approaches including neural networks and support vector machines, these models can create tailored survival estimates, pinpoint high-risk individuals for recurrence, and suggest better treatment plans (Lee et al., 2021).

Furthermore, by use of specific patient variables, Artificial Intelligence can assist doctors in analysing the efficacy of Chemotherapy, Immunotherapy, and newly Targeted Medications so raising the success rate of treatment (Kenner et al., 2021). Although effective, the use of Artificial Intelligence in Pancreatic Cancer Prediction is prone to restrictions under the cover of data heterogeneity, model interpretability, and regulatory difficulties (Yin et al., 2021). AI cannot be therapeutically applied without the strongness, fairness, and openness of AI models (Choudhury and Asan, 2020). Standardised, morally appropriate AI tools necessitate multidisciplinary co-operation among data scientists, oncologists, and legislators (Kenner et al., 2021). Future developments in artificial intelligence could change the prognosis of Pancreatic Cancer, therefore offering hope for Earlier Diagnosis, better risk stratification, and increased patient survival in one of the most lethal tumours (Ngiam and Khor, 2019).

5. APPLICATIONS OF ARTIFICIAL INTELLIGENCE (AI) IN PANCREATIC CANCER

One of the most fatal diseases with notable death rates, pancreatic cancer diagnosis, treatment, and care is being revolutionised by Artificial Intelligence (AI) (Ryan et al., 2014). Early diagnosis, predictive modelling, personalised therapy, and drug discovery (Kumar et al., 2022) are much enabled by technologies connected to artificial intelligence like Machine Learning (ML) and Deep Learning (DL). Usually identified in their late stage, pancreatic cancer lacks early symptoms or reliable biomarkers (Singhi and Wood, 2021). By spotting minor patterns in CT, MRI, and Endoscopic Ultrasound (EUS) images that might be missed by Human Radiologists, Artificial Intelligence (AI)-driven imaging techniques including Convolutional Neural Networks (CNNs) are improving the accuracy of radiological diagnosis. Faster and more accurate diagnosis follows from these technologically based equipment's ability to distinguish cancerous from benign pancreatic tumours (Si et al., 2021).

Furthermore able to screen high-risk individuals based on genetic profiles, live biomarkers, and clinical history and enable better screening methods are artificial intelligence models using large datasets (Sharma et al., 2018).

Along with patient response to various therapeutic regimens, artificial intelligence is supporting accuracy oncology in treatment (Kenner et al., 2021). Running on multi-omics data including Genomes, Transcriptomics, and Proteomics, Artificial Intelligence systems deliver patient-specific treatment alternatives (Xiao et al.,

2021). For example, Artificial Intelligence Decision Support Systems assist doctors in determining, based on Tumour Genetic Markers, the most suitable Chemotherapy, Immunotherapy, and Tailored treatment (Bhinder et al., 2021). By simplifying Tumour Classification and Treatment Planning and reducing radiation exposure to surrounding healthy tissue, Artificial Intelligence also maximises Radiation Therapy (Kenner et al., 2021). By increasing accuracy and minimising human error, Artificial Intelligence supports robotic surgery in Surgical Cancer (Kenner et al., 2021).

By means of virtual screening paired with molecular docking simulation, AI is also expediting drug discovery and repurposing by discovering possible therapeutic molecules, hence drastically lowering drug development time and cost (Bhinder et al., 2021). By extracting significant data from Digital Electronic Health Records (EHRs) and real-world evidence (Choudhury and Asan, 2020), Natural Language Processing (NLP) technology enabled by AI is also improving clinical documentation, patients monitoring, and predictive modelling.

Around-the-clock patient care offered by virtual assistants and AI-powered chatbots enhances communication between patients and healthcare professionals (Laranjo et al., 2018). Moreover, by including several traits including tumour stage, genetic mutation, and response to therapy, which enables enhanced-informed clinical decision-making, AI-driven predictive models improve survival estimates (Lee et al., 2021). With problems such data privacy, model interpretability, and the necessity of meticulous validation still present, it nevertheless offers great promise (Yin et al., 2021). AI models must be trained on high-quality, varied datasets if one hopes to lower bias and maximise generalisability (Mikdadi et al., 2022). To adapt the developments of Artificial Intelligence to Clinical Practice, Oncologists, Radiologists, Bioinformaticians, and in addition to AI researchers must work across disciplines (Kenner et al., 2021). Furthermore, developed should be ethical rules and regulatory clearance to enable safe and efficient application of artificial intelligence for the treatment of Pancreatic cancer (Choudhury and Asan, 2020). With continuous developments in Artificial Intelligence technology, its use in cancer is projected to transform pancreatic cancer treatment, thereby improving early detection, therapy success, and patient survival (Ngiam and Khor, 2019).

5.1. Early Detection

Early identification of pancreatic cancer is critical for improving patient survival rates, as this illness is commonly diagnosed in its advanced stage when the treatment options are restricted (Ryan et al., 2014). The pancreas is recessed deep into the abdomen, and therefore, early malignancies are difficult to approach by the standard physical examination (Kenner et al., 2021). Moreover, pancreatic cancer displays few or vague indications in the early stages, which leads to diagnostic delays (Singhi and Wood, 2021). Newer diagnostic technologies and Artificial Intelligence (AI) are leading the way in advancing early detection forward through biomarker detection, enhanced image analysis, and risk stratification optimization (Young et al., 2020). Traditional diagnostic procedures such as CT, MRI, and EUS are based on the intelligence of radiologists and thereby entail the fallibility of human interpretation (Schuurmans et al., 2022). Imaging algorithms based on artificial intelligence, specifically Deep Learning-based Convolutional Neural Networks (CNNs), have been found superior to the correct identification of pancreatic lesions that would indicate precancerous stages of cancer (Si et al., 2021).

These models of Machine Learning browse vast amounts of imaging data, picking up patterns not evident to human observers (Mukherjee et al., 2022). With reduced diagnostic errors and real-time image interpretation, AI enhances early and accurate pancreatic cancer diagnosis (Ma et al., 2020). Concurrently with imaging technology advancements, blood-based biomarkers increase as a minimally invasive approach to early detection (Xiao et al., 2021). Carbohydrate Antigen 19-9 (CA 19-9) is the most prevalent Biomarker for Pancreatic Cancer, but because of its poor specificity and sensitivity, researchers are looking for alternative Biomarker panels (Radon et al., 2015). AI-based computational models integrate multi-omics data, like genomes, proteomics, and metabolomics, to uncover possible biomarker signatures that assist early detection (Xiao et al., 2021). Liquid biopsy, which identifies Circulating Tumor DNA (ctDNA) and extracellular vesicles in the blood, is yet another promising tool that AI is making more efficient by enabling the interpretation of complicated molecular data (Radon et al., 2015).

AI is changing risk assessment by integrating patient data from Electronic Health Records (EHRs), genetic predisposition, and lifestyle factors to forecast an individual's vulnerability to pancreatic cancer (Sharma et al., 2018). Machine Learning algorithms employ big data to identify high-risk individuals and hence enable early screening in asymptomatic patients (Sharma et al., 2018). AI can recognize modest abnormalities of laboratory test results, like variations in glucose metabolism or inflammatory markers, as earliest warning indications of pancreatic cancer (Sharma et al., 2018). In addition, AI-based Natural Language Processing (NLP) software also pulls useful information from clinical notes, radiological reports, and pathology reports to offer a more thorough assessment of illness development (Choudhury and Asan, 2020).

Although these technologies are promising, challenges must still be addressed before AI-based early detection methods can become widely adopted and accepted clinically (Yin et al., 2021). Properly high-quality and diverse data sets are needed to train generalizable AI models that can operate well on different populations (Mikdadi et al., 2022). Regulatory sign-offs, ethical approval, and doctor buy-in are all crucial to implement AI into daily clinical practice (Choudhury and Asan, 2020).

Advances in AI, with inter-specialty coordination among oncologists, radiologists, bioinformaticians, and data scientists, in the future will potentially revolutionize early detection strategies (Kenner et al., 2021). AI has the potential to improve the efficacy of treatments, improve survival, and ultimately reduce the burden of pancreatic cancer on individuals and health care systems worldwide by improving early diagnosis (Ngiam and Khor, 2019).

5.2. Diagnosis and Classification

Effective treatment methods and patient outcomes depend on a diagnosis and classification of Pancreatic Cancer (Ryan et al., 2014). Diagnosis of Pancreatic Cancer remains difficult since this malignancy is anatomically deeply seated, lacks early signs, and is mistakenly identified with benign pancreatic diseases (Kenner et al., 2021). Common but relying on Radiologists and Pathologists experience for diagnosis are Computed Tomography (CT), Magnetic Resonance Imaging (MRI), Endoscopic Ultrasonic (EUS), and Biopsy (Chen et al., 2020). Advancements in Artificial Intelligence (AI) and Machine Learning (ML) during the past few years have revolutionised Pancreatic Cancer detection by means of augmentation, automation of classification, and improvement of diagnostic performance (Si et al., 2021). Driven by Convolutional Neural Networks (CNNs), Artificial Intelligence (AI) Deep Learning Computer Systems can screen millions of imaging data sets to discover small pancreatic lesions, differentiate benign from malignant tumours, and forecast aggressiveness of tumours (Ma et al., 2020). Artificial Intelligence improves early and accurate detection by spotting minute radiological imaging patterns that human observers could miss, hence reducing misdiagnosis and treatment delay (Mukherjee et al., 2022).

Using multi-omics data integrating Genomic, Proteomic, and Metabolomic Information, AI-powered predictive models also help to better identify Pancreatic Cancer (Xiao et al., 2021). For the molecular subtype-based Pancreatic Cancer Categorisation, Transcriptomics and Whole-Genome Sequencing provide evidence of heterogeneity in the tumour (Cheerla and Gevaert, 2019). Most widely used classification scheme for Pancreatic Cancer is four basic sub-types: Squamous, Pancreatic progenitor, Aberrantly Differentiated Endocrine Exocrine (ADEX), and Immunogenic (Cheerla and Gevaert, 2019). Correct classification is therefore crucial for focussed therapy since every subtype has unique genetic changes and reactions to drugs (Cheerla and Gevaert, 2019). Often found in PDAC, Artificial Intelligence-based methods classify Tumours depending on Genetic Alterations including KRAS, TP53, SMAD4, and CDKN2A by processing large amounts of Molecular data (Yang et al., 2016). Artificial Intelligence-based algorithms can predict patient prognosis in addition to assist Oncologists in selecting the optimum course of treatment (Lee et al., 2021).

Pathogenic typing of Pancreatic cancer is another area Artificial Intelligence is fundamentally altering. Still the gold standard for Pancreatic Cancer Diagnosis is Histological Evaluation of Tissue Biopsies (Singhi and Wood, 2021). But, microscopic investigation takes time and is prone to interobserver variance (Juiz et al., 2019). AI-facilitated digital pathology tools utilize deep learning models to analyze Histopathological slides, where cancer cells are identified automatically by computer vision, tumor severity graded, and histological subtypes recognized correctly (Xiao et al., 2021). These tools assist pathologists in providing improved accuracy and reproducibility of diagnoses with reduced workload and turnaround time (Xiao et al., 2021). Additionally, NLP technology powered by AI retrieves key diagnostic information from Electronic Health Records (EHRs), pathology reports, and radiology reports, and facilitate whole and data-driven decision-making (Choudhury and Asan, 2020).

Liquid biopsy is emerging as a promising, non-invasive diagnosis that detects circulating tumor DNA (ctDNA) and extracellular vesicles in the blood (Radon et al., 2015). AI-powered computational models enhance liquid biopsy data interpretation, identifying genetic mutations and epigenetic changes associated with pancreatic cancer (Xiao et al., 2021). They allow real-time tracking of disease progression and response to treatment (Radon et al., 2015). Though AI holds great promise in pancreatic cancer diagnosis and classification, model validation, data standardization, and clinical implementation remain challenging (Yin et al., 2021). There is a need for regulatory clearance and collaboration among AI researchers, Oncologists, and Pathologists to close the gap between AI-driven innovations and clinical use (Kenner et al., 2021). With continued developments in AI, it is expected to revolutionize pancreatic cancer diagnosis and classification, leading to improved detection at an earlier stage, prognosis, and individualized treatment approaches that ultimately enhance patient survival rates (Ngiam and Khor, 2019).

5.3. Biomarker Discovery

The discovery of biomarkers plays a critical role in improving early detection, diagnosis, prognosis, and treatment of pancreatic cancer (Xiao et al., 2021). Because PDAC is so virulent and often diagnosed at advanced stages, it becomes crucial to set reliable biomarkers that can detect the disease in the most curable initial stages (Singhi and Wood, 2021). Traditional diagnostic biomarkers such as carbohydrate antigen 19-9 (CA 19-9) are widely used in clinical practice but are hampered by specificity and sensitivity because they can be elevated in benign conditions such as pancreatitis (Radon et al., 2015). Advances in Multi-omics and Artificial Intelligence

(AI) are presently accelerating biomarker discovery by identifying new molecular signatures associated with pancreatic cancer, improving diagnostic sensitivity, and enabling precision medicine approaches (Xiao et al., 2021).

AI computational models leverage enormous compute-ready data, including genomic, transcriptomic, proteomic, and metabolomic data, to detect potential biomarkers with greater specificity and sensitivity (Xiao et al., 2021). Machine learning algorithms analyze current complex biological data, identifying genetic mutations, epigenetic changes, and protein expression signatures of pancreatic cancer (Xiao et al., 2021). For instance, Next-Generation Sequencing (NGS) and Whole-Genome Sequencing have detected primary mutations in genes like KRAS, TP53, SMAD4, and CDKN2A that are frequently mutated in PDAC (Yang et al., 2016). AI-driven bioinformatics software integrates these genomic alterations with RNA sequencing data to identify dysregulated pathways and predictive biomarkers that distinguish cancerous from normal pancreatic tissues (Cheerla and Gevaert, 2019).

Artificial Intelligence is revolutionising the finding of proteome and metabolomic biomarkers (Xiao et al., 2021). Liquid biopsy, a non-invasive method, is being promoted as a promising instrument for the identification of Circulating tumour DNA (ctDNA), Circulating tumour cells (CTCs), and Exosomal RNA in blood specimens (Radon et al., 2015). Algorithms based on Artificial Intelligence improve the processing of liquid biopsy data to detect tumor-specific alterations, including DNA methylation signatures, microRNA (miRNA) profiles, and extracellular vesicle profiles (Xiao et al., 2021). Studies have established that miRNA panels such as miR-21, miR-155, and miR-196a play a role in Pancreatic Cancer development and can serve as useful Biomarkers for Early Detection and Prognosis (Radon et al., 2015). Metabolomic profiling is a hopeful tool as well, which identified an altered lipid and amino acid metabolism in Pancreatic Cancer, AI models merging metabolically changed profiles to enhance on biomarker panels for early-diagnosis.

The application of biomarker discovery and AI is also transforming precision oncology, where AI will predict patient response to therapy (Bhinder et al., 2021). Immunotherapy has proven of little value for pancreatic cancer since the tumor has an immunosuppressive microenvironment, but AI algorithms are helping determine predictive biomarkers of immune checkpoint inhibitor chimeric antigen receptor T-cell therapy, and cancer vaccines. Artificial intelligence-based predictive models will direct personalized immunotherapy strategies (Xiao et al., 2021). Robotic-assisted surgery and minimally invasive methods will enhance pancreatic cancer treatment by enhancing accuracy, lowering complications, and facilitating patient recovery. Personalized radiation therapy, such as proton beam therapy and adaptive radiotherapy, will enhance tumor targeting while reducing injury to healthy tissues.

6. CONCLUSION

Pancreatic cancer, notorious for its late detection and dismal prognosis, is being transformed by Artificial Intelligence (AI), which offers unprecedented potential in early screening and prediction. By leveraging Machine Learning (ML) and Deep Learning (DL) Algorithms, AI analyzes complex datasets including Radiological Imaging (CT, MRI, EUS), Genomic Profiles, and Liquid Biopsies to detect subtle patterns indicative of early-stage malignancies, outperforming traditional diagnostic methods in sensitivity and specificity. AI-driven tools, such as Convolutional Neural Networks (CNNs), excel in distinguishing malignant lesions and identifying molecular Biomarkers like Circulating tumor DNA (ctDNA), enabling non-invasive risk stratification and personalized intervention. Despite challenges such as data heterogeneity, ethical concerns, and the need for robust validation, interdisciplinary collaboration and advancements in AI models promise to enhance early diagnosis, refine prognostic accuracy, and optimize therapeutic strategies. Addressing these barriers through standardized datasets, ethical frameworks, and clinical integration will be pivotal in translating AI innovations into tangible improvements in patient survival and reducing the global burden of this lethal disease.

7. REFERENCES

Aier, I., Semwal, R., Sharma, A., & Varadwaj, P. K. (2019). A systematic assessment of statistics, risk factors, and underlying features involved in pancreatic cancer. *Cancer Epidemiology*, *58*, 104–110. DOI: 10.1016/j.canep.2018.12.001 PMID: 30537645

Bhinder, B., Gilvary, C., Madhukar, N. S., & Elemento, O. (2021). Artificial intelligence in cancer research and precision medicine. *Cancer Discovery*, *11*(4), 900–915. DOI: 10.1158/2159-8290.CD-21-0090 PMID: 33811123

Blyuss, O., Zaikin, A., Cherepanova, V., Munblit, D., Kiseleva, E. M., Prytomanova, O. M., Duffy, S. W., & Crnogorac-Jurcevic, T. (2020). Development of PancRISK, a urine biomarker-based risk score for stratified screening of pancreatic cancer patients. *British Journal of Cancer*, *122*(5), 692–696. DOI: 10.1038/s41416-019-0694-0 PMID: 31857725

Cheerla, A., & Gevaert, O. (2019). Deep learning with multimodal representation for pancancer prognosis prediction. *Bioinformatics (Oxford, England)*, *35*(14), 446–454. DOI: 10.1093/bioinformatics/btz342 PMID: 31510656

Chen, T., Carter, J., Mahmud, M., & Khuman, A. S. (2022). *Artificial intelligence in healthcare: Recent applications and developments*. Springer Nature., DOI: 10.1007/978-981-19-5272-2

Chen, W., Butler, R. K., Zhou, Y., Parker, R. A., Jeon, C. Y., & Wu, B. U. (2020). Prediction of pancreatic cancer based on imaging features in patients with duct abnormalities. *Pancreas*, *49*(4), 413–419. DOI: 10.1097/MPA.0000000000001499 PMID: 32132511

Choudhury, A., & Asan, O. (2020). Role of artificial intelligence in patient safety outcomes: Systematic literature review. *JMIR Medical Informatics*, *8*(7), 18599. DOI: 10.2196/18599 PMID: 32706688

Heinemann, V., Haas, M., & Boeck, S. (2013). Neoadjuvant treatment of borderline resectable and non-resectable pancreatic cancer. *Annals of Oncology : Official Journal of the European Society for Medical Oncology*, *24*(10), 2484–2492. DOI: 10.1093/annonc/mdt239 PMID: 23852311

Juiz, N. A., Iovanna, J., & Dusetti, N. (2019). Pancreatic cancer heterogeneity can be explained beyond the genome. *Frontiers in Oncology*, *9*, 246. DOI: 10.3389/fonc.2019.00246 PMID: 31024848

Kenner, B., Chari, S. T., Kelsen, D., Klimstra, D. S., Pandol, S. J., Rosenthal, M., Rustgi, A. K., Taylor, J. A., Yala, A., Abul-Husn, N., Andersen, D. K., Bernstein, D., Brunak, S., Canto, M. I., Eldar, Y. C., Fishman, E. K., Fleshman, J., Go, V. L. W., Holt, J. M., & Wolpin, B. (2021). Artificial intelligence and early detection of pancreatic cancer: 2020 summative review. *Pancreas*, *50*(3), 251–279. DOI: 10.1097/MPA.0000000000001762 PMID: 33835956

Klein, A. P. (2021). Pancreatic cancer epidemiology: Understanding the role of lifestyle and inherited risk factors. *Nature Reviews. Gastroenterology & Hepatology*, *18*(7), 493–502. DOI: 10.1038/s41575-021-00457-x PMID: 34002083

Kumar, Y., Gupta, S., Singla, R., & Hu, Y.-C. (2022). A systematic review of artificial intelligence techniques in cancer prediction and diagnosis. *Archives of Computational Methods in Engineering*, *29*(4), 2043–2070. DOI: 10.1007/s11831-021-09648-w PMID: 34602811

Kuwahara, T., Hara, K., Mizuno, N., Okuno, N., Matsumoto, S., Obata, M., Kurita, Y., Koda, H., Toriyama, K., Onishi, S., Ishihara, M., Tanaka, T., Tajika, M., & Niwa, Y. (2019). Usefulness of deep learning analysis for the diagnosis of malignancy in intraductal papillary mucinous neoplasms of the pancreas. *Clinical and Translational Gastroenterology*, *10*(5), 1–8. DOI: 10.14309/ctg.0000000000000045 PMID: 31117111

Laranjo, L., Dunn, A. G., Tong, H. L., Kocaballi, A. B., Chen, J., Bashir, R., Surian, D., Gallego, B., Magrabi, F., Lau, A. Y. S., & Coiera, E. (2018). Conversational agents in healthcare: A systematic review. *Journal of the American Medical Informatics Association : JAMIA*, *25*(9), 1248–1258. DOI: 10.1093/jamia/ocy072 PMID: 30010941

Lee, K. S., Jang, J. Y., Yu, Y. D., Heo, J. S., Han, H. S., Yoon, Y. S., Kang, C. M., Hwang, H. K., & Kang, S. (2021). Usefulness of artificial intelligence for predicting recurrence following surgery for pancreatic cancer: Retrospective cohort study. *International Journal of Surgery*, *93*, 106050. DOI: 10.1016/j.ijsu.2021.106050 PMID: 34388677

Ma, H., Liu, Z. X., Zhang, J., Wu, F. T., Xu, C. F., Shen, Z., Yu, C.-H., & Li, Y.-M. (2020). Construction of a convolutional neural network classifier developed by computed tomography images for pancreatic cancer diagnosis. *World Journal of Gastroenterology*, *26*(34), 5156–5168. DOI: 10.3748/wjg.v26.i34.5156 PMID: 32982116

Marya, N. B., Powers, P. D., Chari, S. T., Gleeson, F. C., Leggett, C. L., Abu Dayyeh, B. K., Chandrasekhara, V., Iyer, P. G., Majumder, S., Pearson, R. K., Petersen, B. T., Rajan, E., Sawas, T., Storm, A. C., Vege, S. S., Chen, S., Long, Z., Hough, D. M., Mara, K., & Levy, M. J. (2021). Utilisation of artificial intelligence for the development of an EUS-convolutional neural network model trained to enhance the diagnosis of autoimmune pancreatitis. *Gut*, *70*(7), 1335–1344. DOI: 10.1136/gutjnl-2020-322821 PMID: 33028668

Mikdadi, D., O'Connell, K. A., Meacham, P. J., Dugan, M. A., Ojiere, M. O., Carlson, T. B., & Klenk, J. A. (2022). Applications of artificial intelligence (AI) in ovarian cancer, pancreatic cancer, and image biomarker discovery. *Cancer Biomarkers*, *33*(2), 173–184. DOI: 10.3233/CBM-210301 PMID: 35213360

Mukherjee, S., Patra, A., Khasawneh, H., Korfiatis, P., Rajamohan, N., Suman, G., Majumder, S., Panda, A., Johnson, M. P., Larson, N. B., Wright, D. E., Kline, T. L., Fletcher, J. G., Chari, S. T., & Goenka, A. H. (2022). Radiomics-based machine-learning models can detect pancreatic cancer on prediagnostic computed tomography scans at a substantial lead time before clinical diagnosis. *Gastroenterology*, *163*(5), 1435–1446.e3. DOI: 10.1053/j.gastro.2022.06.066 PMID: 35788343

Ngiam, K. Y., & Khor, I. W. (2019). Big data and machine learning algorithms for health-care delivery. *The Lancet. Oncology*, *20*(5), e262–e273. DOI: 10.1016/S1470-2045(19)30149-4 PMID: 31044724

Radon, T. P., Massat, N. J., Jones, R., Alrawashdeh, W., Dumartin, L., & Ennis, D. (2015). Identification of a three-biomarker panel in urine for early detection of pancreatic adenocarcinoma. *Clinical Cancer Research*, *21*(15), 3512–3521. DOI: 10.1158/1078-0432.CCR-14-2467 PMID: 26240291

Ryan, D. P., Hong, T. S., & Bardeesy, N. (2014). Pancreatic adenocarcinoma. *The New England Journal of Medicine*, *371*(11), 1039–1049. DOI: 10.1056/NEJMra1404198 PMID: 25207767

Schuurmans, M., Alves, N., Vendittelli, P., Huisman, H., & Hermans, J. (2022). Setting the research agenda for clinical artificial intelligence in pancreatic adenocarcinoma imaging. *Cancers (Basel)*, *14*(14), 3498. DOI: 10.3390/cancers14143498 PMID: 35884559

Sharma, A., Kandlakunta, H., Nagpal, S., Feng, Z., Hoos, W., Petersen, G. M., & Chari, S. T. (2018). Model to determine risk of pancreatic cancer in patients with new-onset diabetes. *Gastroenterology*, *155*(3), 730–739. DOI: 10.1053/j.gastro.2018.05.023 PMID: 29775599

Si, K., Xue, Y., Yu, X., Zhu, X., Li, Q., Gong, W., Liang, T., & Duan, S. (2021). Fully end-to-end deep learning-based diagnosis of pancreatic tumors. *Theranostics*, *11*(4), 1982–1990. DOI: 10.7150/thno.52508 PMID: 33408793

Singhi, A. D., & Wood, L. D. (2021). Early detection of pancreatic cancer using DNA-based molecular approaches. *Nature Reviews. Gastroenterology & Hepatology*, *18*(7), 457–468. DOI: 10.1038/s41575-021-00470-0 PMID: 34099908

Tong, Z., Liu, Y., Ma, H., Zhang, J., Lin, B., Bao, X., Xu, X., Gu, C., Zheng, Y., Liu, L., Fang, W., Deng, S., & Zhao, P. (2020). Development, validation and comparison of artificial neural network models and logistic regression models predicting survival of unresectable pancreatic cancer. *Frontiers in Bioengineering and Biotechnology*, *8*, 196. DOI: 10.3389/fbioe.2020.00196 PMID: 32232040

Topol, E. J. (2019). High-performance medicine: The convergence of human and artificial intelligence. *Nature Medicine*, *25*(1), 44–56. DOI: 10.1038/s41591-018-0300-7 PMID: 30617339

Tripathi, S. (2021). Artificial intelligence: A brief review. In *Analyzing future applications of AI, sensors, and robotics in society* (pp. 1–22). IGI Global., DOI: 10.4018/978-1-7998-3499-1.ch001

Xiao, Q., Zhang, F., Xu, L., Yue, L., Kon, O. L., Zhu, Y., & Guo, T. (2021). High-throughput proteomics and AI for cancer biomarker discovery. *Advanced Drug Delivery Reviews*, *176*, 113844. DOI: 10.1016/j.addr.2021.113844 PMID: 34182017

Yang, J., Li, S., Li, J., Wang, F., Chen, K., Zheng, Y., Wang, J., Lu, W., Zhou, Y., Yin, Q., Zhang, H., & Guo, C. (2016). A meta-analysis of the diagnostic value of detecting K-ras mutation in pancreatic juice as a molecular marker for pancreatic cancer. *Pancreatology*, *16*(4), 605–614. DOI: 10.1016/j.pan.2016.04.033 PMID: 27237100

Yin, J., Ngiam, K. Y., & Teo, H. H. (2021). Role of artificial intelligence applications in real-life clinical practice: Systematic review. *Journal of Medical Internet Research*, *23*(4), e25759. DOI: 10.2196/25759 PMID: 33885365

Young, M. R., Abrams, N., Ghosh, S., Rinaudo, J. A. S., Marquez, G., & Srivastava, S. (2020). Pre-diagnostic image data, artificial intelligence, and pancreatic cancer: A tell-tale sign to early detection. *Pancreas*, *49*(7), 882–886. DOI: 10.1097/MPA.0000000000001603 PMID: 32675784

Zheng, R., Zhang, S., Zeng, H., Wang, S., Sun, K., Chen, R., Li, L., Wei, W., & He, J. (2022). Cancer incidence and mortality in China, 2016. *Journal of the National Cancer Center*, *2*(1), 1–9. DOI: 10.1016/j.jncc.2022.02.002 PMID: 39035212

Chapter 12
Case Studies Highlighting Promising Therapies and Their Effectiveness in Pancreatic Cancer

Sayan Acharyya
https://orcid.org/0009-0004-0602-3980
Maulana Abul Kalam Azad University of Technology, West Bengal, India

Bikram Sarkar
https://orcid.org/0009-0007-7725-6687
Maulana Abul Kalam Azad University of Technology, West Bengal, India

Hridoy Ranjan Bairagya
https://orcid.org/0009-0001-7966-5755
Maulana Abul Kalam Azad University of Technology, West Bengal, India

ABSTRACT

Pancreatic cancer (PC) will soon become a leading cause of cancer death. Combined strategies for patients with unrespectable, non-metastatic disease, which include chemotherapy and radiation, show promise. Proper application of these treatments can also increase the rate of radical resections in respectable. Alternative treatments have been shown to enhance survival and quality of life in fit patients suffering from metastatic disease. New locoregional treatment approaches are emerging as vital options in the multimodal strategy for patients. As of now, when compared to other cancer, targeted therapies have not demonstrated significant efficacy, either alone or in combination with chemotherapy and are therefore not incorporated into current clinical practice. Despite the promising outcomes of such studies in various

DOI: 10.4018/979-8-3373-1469-3.ch012

tumors, immunotherapy is not yet included in the current therapeutic options for PC. We provide a review on (i) early detection, (ii) treatments, (iii) various biomarkers, (iv) focused treatments, and (v) future developments in PC to guide clinicians in managing PC.

INTRODUCTION

Due to the high mortality rate, pancreatic cancer is considered the most dreadful of all gastrointestinal cancers. The prognosis for pancreatic adenocarcinoma is poor, and it remains a significant source of cancer morbidity and mortality despite all efforts to establish an effective treatment (Moss & Lee, 2010). The number of deaths from pancreatic cancer (PC) has been increasing annually. There are still a number of barriers to pancreatic cancer treatment, despite the fact that India's 5-year survival rate has risen to 9–12%. Pancreatic cancer is estimated to have killed close to 470,000 people in 2022, accounting for over 500,000 new cases and ranking as the sixth most common cause of cancer-related fatalities (Garrido-Laguna & Hidalgo, 2015).

Pancreatic cancer responds poorly to chemotherapy and radiation, spreads rapidly, and metastasizes early. Nevertheless, the prognosis for PC patients has improved due to surgery and rigorous therapy. However, the effectiveness of immunotherapy and targeted therapy for pancreatic tumors is not anticipated, indicating considerable room for advancement. Utilizing multi-omics technology to identify and develop novel antigens and tumor vaccines for PC, as well as to screen patients for potential candidates for immunotherapy and targeted therapy, is one of the most promising approaches to improving treatment (Kolbeinsson et al., 2023). This bleak outlook is primarily due to the reality that early pancreatic cancer is asymptomatic; as a result, most individuals are diagnosed at an advanced stage, often associated with vague symptoms (those that are difficult to describe or pinpoint, often general like fatigue or pain, and can make diagnosis challenging). For these patients, surgery remains the only treatment that provides a chance for long-term survival with pancreatic disease. Although scientific understanding of the pancreatic disease is still limited and the overall prognosis poor, the quality of surgical therapy has improved with the help of AI, and survival rates have recently increased (Ma et al., 2024). In addition to surgery, researchers have increasingly focused on the use of potential biomarkers since they assist in the early detection of the disease, enhancing the prognosis and forecasting the tumor's response to specific therapies. Because the substances in this collection are directly produced by the tumor and circulate throughout the body, enabling communication between the tumor and its microenvironment, the secretome has been extensively utilized to examine these indicators. A liquid biopsy looks for tumor biomarkers in the blood, allowing for the procedure to be performed on this same group.

Currently, radiation therapy, chemotherapy, and surgery are the recommended treatments for pancreatic cancer disease. However, these traditional therapies often provide limited benefits, particularly in advanced stages of the illness. The chemotherapy agent's folfrinox (consists of oxaliplatin, leucovorin, irinotecanand fluorouracil) and gemcitabine with nab-paclitaxel are two well-established treatment regimens that have become essential components of the therapeutic arsenal. The folfrinoxhas proven effective in certain patient populations. Similarly, patients with advanced pancreatic cancer may find that gemcitabine with ab-paclitaxel is an effective treatment option. However, these regimens fail to achieve significant long-term survival benefits. Amidst these challenges, precision medicine has shown considerable promise and may provide a new strategy for the treatment of pancreatic cancer. Precision medicine has the potential to offer individualized treatments based on each patient's unique genetic profile by comprehending the complex molecular landscape of the disease. Thus, Gaining a deeper understanding of the molecular classification of pancreatic cancer is the aim of individualized treatment and utilize next-generation sequencing (NGS) to identify distinct genetic alterations for treatment that may be highly advantageous for a subset of patients. Exploring key DDR (DNA damage response and repair genes) genes such as BRCA (Breast CAncer gene)-1, BRCA-2 and KRAS, significantly linked to the development of pancreatic cancer, may present valuable targets for improving survival rates, particularly in cases of metastatic pancreatic cancer, thus opening new therapeutic avenues (Cortiana et al., 2024).

DIFFERENT STAGES OF PANCREATIC CANCER

Various staging classifications for pancreatic cancer are based on the tumor's size. For pancreatic cancer staging, the TNM staging approach [Fig.1], which stands for Tumor, Node, and Metastasis, is commonly utilized. In its eighth edition, the T-category was added to the TNM system by the American Joint Committee on Cancer (AJCC). The tumour's size and depth are described by this T-category; because the pancreas does not have a capsule-like structure, it is challenging to tell whether there is extra-pancreatic extension when inflammation or desmoplasia is present. Regional lymph node involvement is indicated by the N-category, but the prognosis is influenced by the quantity of metastatic lymph nodes (LNs). The *M-category* describes the presence or absence of distant metastases. Additionally, there is a number staging system that includes four stages.

Figure 1. Three stages of pancreatic cancer. TNM staging system stands for Tumour, Node, and Metastasis.

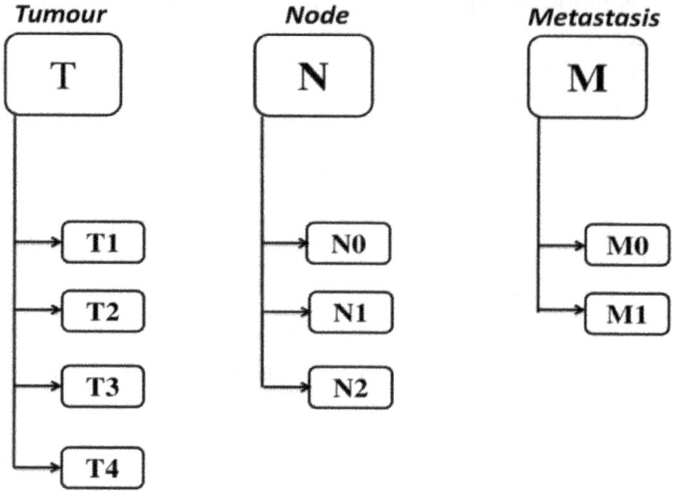

T (carcinoma in situ) represents a very early stage of pancreatic cancer (**Fig.2**). It hasn't spread to the deeper levels of pancreatic tissue. Such early diagnoses of pancreatic cancer are rare. T1 indicates that the malignancy is confined to the pancreas and is no more than 2 cm in any direction (**Fig. 2a**). T2 indicates that the malignancy remains within the pancreas and measures between 2cm and 4 cm in any direction (**Fig. 2b**). T3 signifies that the malignancy is present in the pancreas and exceeds 4 cm in any direction (**Fig. 2c**). T4 indicates that the malignancy has extended beyond the pancreas and into nearby large blood vessels (**Fig. 2d**).

Figure 2. Panel (a) indicates T1 stage of the Tumour (pancreas size no more than 2 cm). The panel (b) indicates T2 stage of pancreatic tumour measures between 2cm and 4 cm). The panel (c) indicates T3 stage of pancreatic tumour (exceeds 4 cm). The panel (d) indicates T4 stage of the malignancy (extended beyond the pancreas and into nearby large blood vessels).

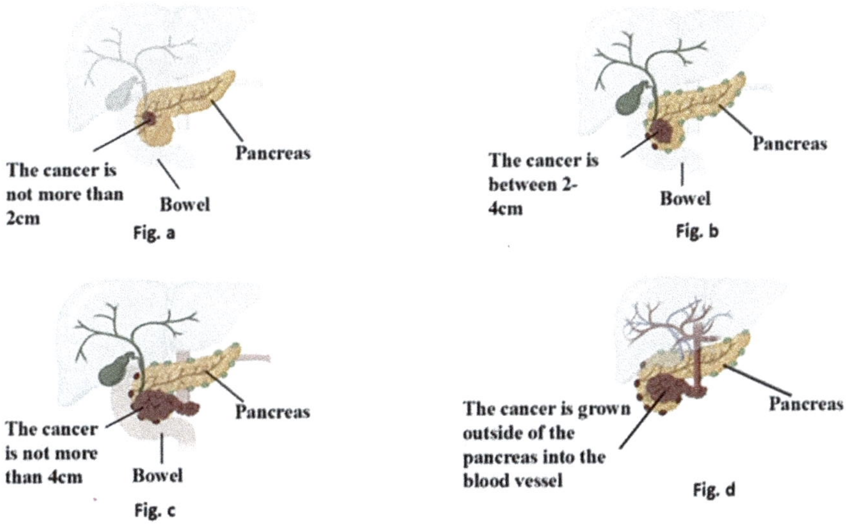

The N-category describes both the number of metastatic lymph nodes and the involvement of regional lymph nodes. The likelihood that cancer cells have spread outside of the pancreas is higher if the cancer has impacted the nearby lymph nodes. N0 indicates that no cancer cells are present in nearby lymph nodes. The N1 indicates that 1 to 3 lymph nodes contain cancer cells (**Fig. 3**). The N2 indicates that 4 or more lymph nodes contain cancer cells. (**Fig. 3**) he M-category describes the presence or absence of cancer in different parts of the body. M0 indicates that cancer has not spread to other organs, such as the liver. M1 indicates that cancer has spread to other organs (**Fig. 4**).

Figure 3. Panel A (left side) indicates N1 stage of the pancreatic node (1 to 3 lymph nodes contain cancer cells). The panel B (right side) indicates N2 stage of pancreatic node (4 or more lymph nodes contain cancer cells).

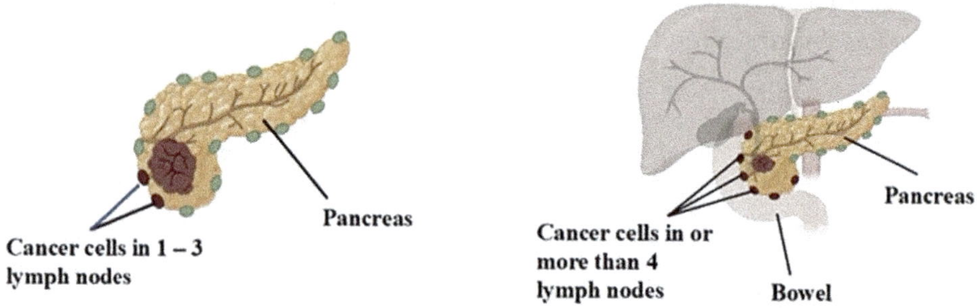

Figure 4. It indicates M1 stage of the pancreatic Metastasis (cancer has spread to other organs).

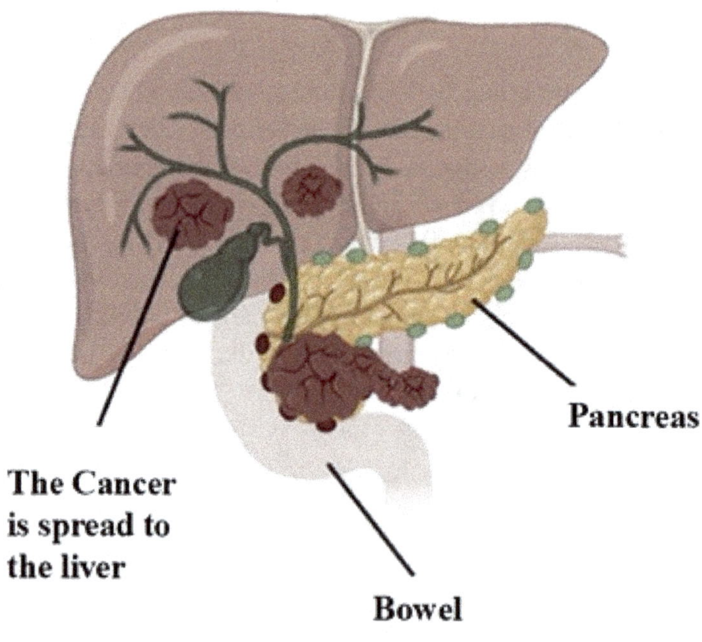

EARLY DETECTION OF PANCREATIC CANCER

Pancreatic cancer has a poor prognosis, and early detection is quite challenging because the disease is usually asymptomatic in its initial stages. Most diagnoses occur at later stages when the disease has progressed, often presenting symptoms such as vomiting, pain in the upper and middle abdomen, unexplained weight loss, and fatigue. Conventional methods for detecting pancreatic cancer, including imaging techniques like MRI (Magnetic Resonance Imaging) and CT (Computed Tomography) scans, often have limitations. These methods may lack the sensitivity needed to detect pancreatic cancer in its early stages or to identify small tumors. By the time these imaging techniques can identify a tumor, it is often already metastasized or has significantly increased in size. Another diagnostic approach is the tumor marker test, which measures the levels of specific chemicals produced by organs, tissues, or tumor cells in the body. Common markers include CA19-9 (Carbohydrate Antigen 19-9) and arcinoembryonic antigen (CEA), which can be detected in blood, urine, or tissue samples. Elevated levels of these compounds can be associated with particular types of cancer.

Using Biomarkers for Early Pancreatic Cancer Detection: A Case Study Perspective

The various types of biomarkers for the early detection of pancreatic cancer are shown in **Fig. 5**.

Figure 5. Different type of biomarkers used for identification of pancreatic cancer.

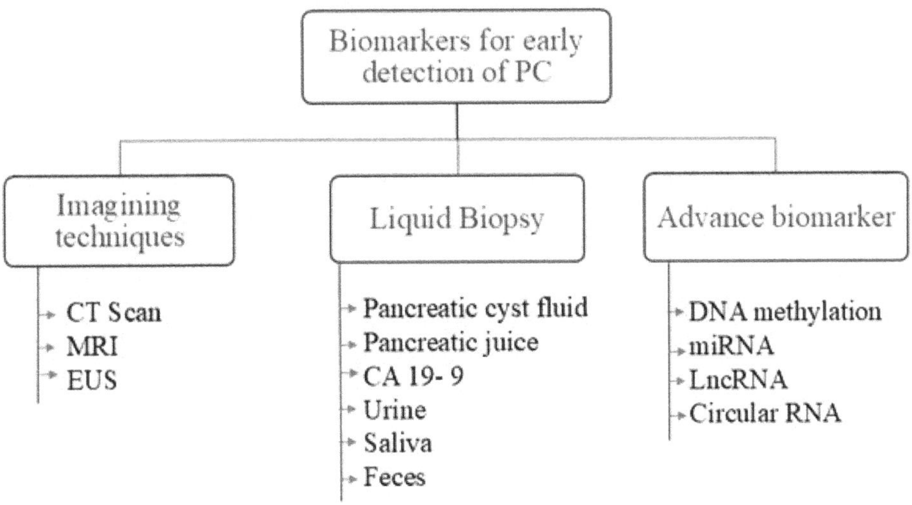

Imagining techniques for detection of pancreatic cancer

Medical imaging is important for pancreatic cancer screening and early detection, follow-up, differential diagnosis, proper evaluation and staging, and therapeutic evaluation. However, a standardized imaging screening process is not currently in place. According to the USPSTF (United State Preventive Services Task Force), there has been research into screening methods for high-risk populations with inherited genetic abnormalities or a family history of pancreatic cancer using imaging techniques such as CT (Computed Tomography), MRI (Magnetic resonance imaging), and EUS (endoscopic ultrasonography) (Vitale et al., 2024). EUS is particularly effective for screening high-risk individuals.

To elucidate the imaging features of 200 PDAC stage 0 and I cases (pancreatic ductal adenocarcinomas), of which 20% were symptomatic, a multicenter retrospective study was conducted in Japan. Transabdominal ultrasonography (TAUS), CT, MRI, and EUS (endoscopic ultrasonography) showed relative diagnostic accuracy rates of 67.5%, 98.0%, 86.5%, and 86.5%, respectively. Unlike thin-section triple-phase helical CT, which has low sensitivity for PDAC with a diameter of less than 2 cm, EUS can detect smaller solid lesions and has the extra advantage of not requiring contrast agents or ionizing radiation. Additionally, it might produce cytopathological consequences in a sequential manner (Yang et al., 2021).

Liquid Biopsy for detection of pancreatic cancer

Figure 6. Different type of biomarkers used for identification of pancreatic cancer.

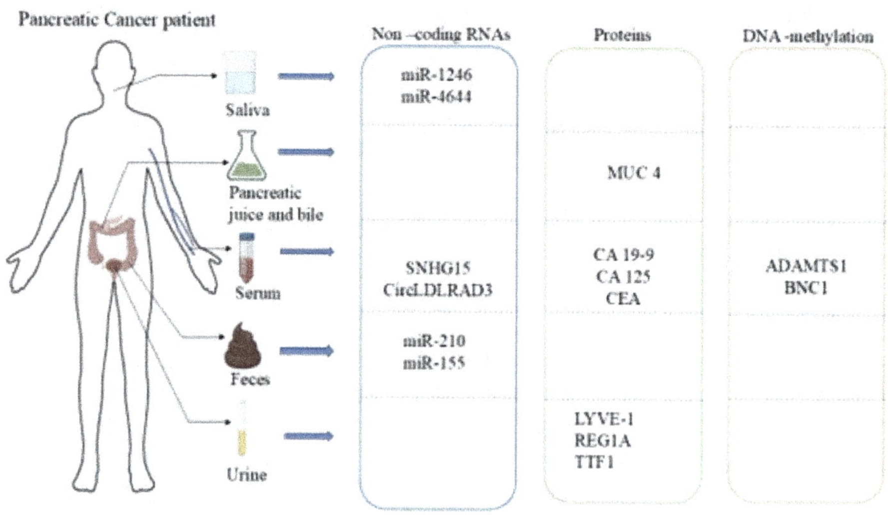

Small non-coding RNA molecules called miRNAs, which have between 18 and 22 nucleotides, control posttranscriptional gene expression and are crucial for oncogenesis and tumor metastasis. Diagnostic biomarkers of pancreatic cancer obviously need that the expression of miRNAs varies between normal tissues and pancreatic cancer or between phases of the disease. MiR-103 and miR-107 overexpression and miR-155 low expression were found to be able to differentiate pancreatic cancer from healthy controls. Blood miRNAs may be useful as biomarkers for the diagnosis of pancreatic cancer, according to a growing body of recent studies. Due to their high stability in blood, miRNAs can be detected by a number of methods, including miRNA microarray, in situ hybridization, next-generation sequencing, and reverse transcription-quantitative PCR (RT-qPCR) (Heredia-Soto et al., 2021).

Blood, other body fluids, or tissues includes biological molecules that show either normal or abnormal activity, or a condition or disease like cancer, is called a biomarker (NCI). Typically, biomarkers differentiate a patient with the illness from one who does not. The range of biomarkers is vast and includes proteins, peptides, antibodies, and nucleic acids (such as microRNA or other non-coding RNA). A biomarker can also encompass a group of changes, including metabolomic, proteomic, and gene expression profiles. Biomarkers can be found in secretions or excretions (stool, urine, sputum, or nipple discharge) or in circulation (whole blood, serum, or plasma) (**Fig. 6**).

Role of Urine Biomarker for pancreatic cancer detection

There are currently no reliable serum tumor biomarkers available for the early detection of pancreatic cancer. The Food and Drug Administration states that the only blood biomarker for PDAC (pancreatic ductal adenocarcinomas) is CA19-9 (Carbohydrate Antigen 19-9); however, the presence of benign tumors, inflammatory masses, or diabetes may cause CA19-9 levels to rise. Due to these limitations, its low sensitivity and specificity for early diagnosis of pancreatic cancer limit its usefulness. However, in patients with advanced pancreatic cancer, CA19-9 is frequently employed as a critical prognostic biomarker for assessing treatment outcomes, tracking metastases, and forecasting survival. Additionally, along with CA19-9, other tumor bio-markers like CEA (Carcinoembryonic antigen) and CA125 (Carbohydrate Antigen 125) are also employed to detect pancreatic cancer. Its diagnostic and prognostic performance for pancreatic tumors has been elucidated by clear evidence. According to reports, CA19-9 has a 70% to 95% sensitivity and a 72% to 90% specificity for pancreatic cancer. Additionally, several studies have shown that CA19-9 has a high potential for early detection of pancreatic cancer, with a median sensitivity of 76.1% and a median specificity of 82%. The sensitivity rose to 80.1% when all stages of pancreatic cancer were taken into account. The combined sensitivity and specificity of blood CA19-9, CEA, CA125, and CA242 (Carbohydrate Antigen 242) were 90.4% and 93.8%, respectively, which were noticeably greater than those of any one marker alone (Vitale et al., 2024). Using Sanger sequencing, a team from Fudan University's Shanghai Cancer Center separated the participants into three genotypes: Lewis-negative, mixed, and secretor-negative. They then determined the optimal cut-off value for each group and applied it to the detection of pancreatic cancer. From 76.1% to 87.2%, CA19-9's sensitivity for detecting pancreatic cancer in stages I and II increased.

Role of Urine Biomarker for pancreatic cancer detection

Another simple method for identifying potential pancreatic cancer biomarkers is urine collection. However, limited scientific information are available about the urine proteome. Using AUC (area under the curve) values of 0.89 and 0.92 in the training and validation datasets, respectively, investigated a biomarker panel composed of thyroid transcription factor 1, hyaluronan receptor 1, REG1A, and lymphatic vascular endothelial 1 (LYVE-1). They found that this panel may be able to detect pancreatic cancer (Vitale et al., 2024).

Role of Salivary Biomarkers for pancreatic cancer detection:

Saliva collection is easy, non-invasive, and cost-effective compared to blood draws. Additionally, it proves more practical for large-scale screenings than imaging methods. Over the last ten years, salivary diagnostics have expanded to cover a broader range of systemic disorders, including pancreatic cancer, alongside oral diseases. This highlights the exciting potential of salivary biomarkers to enhance PDAC (pancreatic ductal adenocarcinomas) outcomes by enabling early disease detection. With an AUC (Area under curve) of 0.993, analysis of saliva from 215 patients with various neoplasms identified 48 metabolites as potential biomarkers for distinguishing pancreatic cancer (Sugimoto et al., 2010). Salivary miRNAs have been shown to be stable, indicating their potential as diagnostic indicators. For example- miR-1246 and miR- 4644 (Al Balushi et al., 2024).

Role of Pancreatic Juice for pancreatic cancer detection:

Pancreatic juice is often acquired during ERCP (Endoscopic Retrograde Cholangiopancreatography), an invasive technique that involves risks of morbidity and mortality, and is frequently used as a screening approach. As an alternative, after secretin injection, pancreatic juice can be removed from the duodenum during an endoscopy; however, this method carries the risk of inducing pancreatitis due to secretin and contaminating the sample with gastric and duodenal juice. In the pancreatic juice of pancreatic cancer (PC) patients, the expression of numerous proteins particularly mucins have been thoroughly investigated. KL-6 (Krebs von den Lungen-6, a high-molecular-weight glycoprotein, has been investigated as a potential biomarker for pancreatic cancer) mucin expression in the pancreatic juice of pancreatic cancer patients was found to be superior to that in inflammatory lesions and IPMN (Intraductal Papillary Mucinous Neoplasm, a type of pancreatic cyst that has the potential to become cancerous) (Pflüger et al., 2023).

Role of Pancreatic cyst fluid for pancreatic cancer detection:

Pancreatic cysts (PCy) have immense potential in the area of specimen collecting for biomarker identification. IPMN, mucinous cystic neoplasms (MCN), serous cystic neoplasms, and pseudocysts are the most common forms of PCy, and their frequency increases with age. The examination of pancreatic cystic fluid (EUS-FNA) is done through aspiration during EUS. The CEA (Carcinoembryonic antigen), VEGF-A (Vascular Endothelial Growth Factor A), and mucins are the most significant isolated proteins from the PCy that have demonstrated potential effectiveness in differentiating benign lesions from premalignant and malignant ones. Since MUC4 (mucin 4) may contribute to early carcinogenesis, it is used for the early detection of pancreatic cancer (O'Neill & Stoita, 2021).

Role of Fecal Biomarkers for pancreatic cancer detection:

Since the pancreas is a digestive organ, pancreatic cancer (PC) may influence the fecal microbiota and stool composition. Therefore, only a limited number of studies have focused on using this medium to identify biomarkers or metabolic signals among the various non-invasive techniques aimed at detecting new biomarkers of disease. Fecal samples exhibited high consistency in miRNA detection. The feces of pancreatic cancer patients displayed lower levels of miR-216a, miR-196a, miR-143, and miR-155 compared to those of the control group (O'Neill & Stoita, 2021; Tarasiuk et al., 2021).

Role of advanced biomarker for detecting Pancreatic Cancer

13.3.1.3.1 miRNAs

MicroRNAs (miRNAs) are small RNA molecules that range from 19 to 25 nucleotides in length. They are created through a process that transforms them into mature miRNAs (Huang et al., 2016). While miRNAs do not directly make proteins, they play a vital role in regulating about half of the genes that do. These molecules influence many important processes in the body, such as blood vessel formation, cell differentiation, programmed cell death, and cell division.

In pancreatic cancer, the epithelial-mesenchymal transition (EMT) is critical for metastasis, and miRNAs are involved in this process. For instance, the overproduction of certain miRNAs, such as ex-miR-21 and ex-miR-155, is linked to increased invasion, growth, and resistance to the chemotherapy drug gemcitabine in pancreatic cancer cells. These miRNAs are found at much higher levels in the pancreatic juice of patients with pancreatic ductal adenocarcinoma (PDAC) compared to healthy individuals. MiR-21 is known as an oncogene, and other miRNAs like miR-155, miR-106a, miR-27a, and miR-221/222 are also found in higher amounts in cancer tissues (16-17).

DNA Methylation

By regulating tumor suppressor genes and proto-oncogenes, DNA methylation is believed to significantly contribute to the development and spread of pancreatic cancer. DNA methylation in peripheral blood is frequently detected for the diagnosis of PC. A study indicated a notable correlation between PC and the promoter DNA methylation of ADAMTS1 (A Disintegrin and Metalloproteinase with Thrombospondin type 1 motif, member 13) and BNC1 (basonuclin zinc finger protein 1). Moreover, DNA methylation of ADAMTS1 and BNC1 emerged as the most reliable biomarkers for assessing the TNM stage of pancreatic cancer. The percentages of BNC1 and ADAMTS1 DNA methylation in stage I PC patients were 62.5% and 87.5%, respectively (Yang et al., 2017).

LncRNAs (Long non-coding RNA)

Long noncoding RNAs have the potential to serve as useful biomarkers for early-stage prostate cancer (PC) identification, alongside microRNAs. For instance, pancreatic cancer patients exhibit higher levels of SNHG15 (small nucleolar RNA host gene 15) compared to healthy controls, which facilitates cell proliferation via enhancer of zeste homolog 2 (EZH2), an enzyme that is encoded by the EZH2 gene and functions as a histone-lysine N-methyltransferase mediated H3K27me3 (histone H3 lysine 27 trimethylation). Moreover, the expression of SNHG15 in serum demonstrates moderate diagnostic value, revealing an 89.6% specificity and a 68.3% sensitivity (Yang et al., 2017).

CircRNAs (Circular RNAs)

CircRNAs are stable enough to be used as molecules for cancer diagnosis due to their continuous closed circular shapes. Circ-LDLRAD3 (low-density lipoprotein receptor class A domain) contain was significantly elevated in pancreatic cancer tissues and plasma and showed a strong association with metastasis, venous invasion, and lymphatic invasion. Although it is not a perfect independent biomarker, circLDLRAD3 improved its AUC (area under curve) from 0.67 to 0.87 when merged with CA19-9, with sensitivity and specificity at 80.33% and 93.55%, respectively (Duan et al., 2023).

PANCREATIC CANCER THERAPIES/TREATMENTS

Pancreatic cancer has a bad prognosis and is difficult to identify early since it is frequently asymptomatic in its early stages. As a result, the disease is usually discovered later. Diabetes and obesity have been found to be risk factors for pancreatic cancer, a form of tumor in the digestive tract, and pancreatic ductal adenocarcinoma (PDAC) may be indicated by newly developed or worsening diabetes. The major treatment for pancreatic cancer at the moment is still surgery. For individuals with pancreatic cancer who are not candidates for surgical resection, chemotherapy, radiation, and immunotherapy may be considered as alternate therapeutic options (Springfeld et al., 2019).

Surgery

Due in significant part to growing surgical expertise at higher volume institutions, surgical results have improved over the last 20 years. Aggressive surgical procedures, such as vascular resection and reconstruction, have led to a greater number of patients being considered for resection. According to recent statistics, the median 5-year survival following surgery is about 20%. However, the overall recurrence rate of 70–80% is still high. The liver is the most frequent site of distant metastases following surgery, which are the primary means of disease recurrence. Micro-metastases that existed at the time of surgery are usually to blame for this. Regardless of resectability, this is what motivates current practice to treat patients with neoadjuvant chemotherapy prior to surgery.

Chemotherapy

One important component of the multimodal treatment of pancreatic cancer is chemotherapy. Adjuvant chemotherapy for pancreatic cancer can greatly increase overall survival and disease-free survival following curative resection. According to the European Study Group for Pancreatic Cancer (ESPAC) study, chemotherapy for six months is the usual course of treatment for pancreatic cancer. This treatment includes modified folinic acid, 5-fluorouracil, irinotecan, and oxaliplatin (known as mFOLFIRINOX) for patients who can handle it. If patients are not suitable for this treatment, they will receive six months of gemcitabine and capecitabine instead. Chemoradiation has long been used to treat pancreatic cancer that has spread locally (Malla et al., 2023).

Radiation

Particularly for borderline and locally advanced pancreatic cancer, radiation therapy has a demonstrated function in controlling the disease and may increase the resectability rate of a particular neoadjuvant treatment. Radiation therapy is frequently used to treat positive margins following pancreatic cancer surgery, however its relevance in resected pancreatic cancer is debatable. With improvements in delivery methods, combination strategies, and treatment modalities, radiation therapy paradigms are still changing. The significance of radiation therapy in treating this illness is still up for debate, despite the advancements (Salman et al., 2013).

Cancer vaccines and Targeted Treatments: A Case Study on Innovative Strategies for Pancreatic Tumor Management

Anticancer vaccinations for pancreatic cancer can be administered in a number of ways. Genetic and epigenetic alterations cause cancer cells to differ from healthy cells. Utilizing the immune system's natural capacity to identify and react to new antigens, especially TAAs, is the goal of vaccine-based anticancer immunotherapy. A successful anticancer vaccine must overcome the barriers that cancer cells erect to prevent immune activation and deliver potent immune stimulatory signals.

Antigen specific vaccines

Tumor indicators include carcinoembryonic antigen (CEA), mucin 1 (MUC1), and proteins that play a crucial role in the early onset of pancreatic ductal adenocarcinoma (PDA), serving as the ideal starting point for vaccinations against PDA. The first anti-PDA immunizations studied were peptide and protein-based vaccines, which aimed to utilize immuno-dominant tumor epitopes to elicit antitumor T-cell responses (Murray & López, 1994).

KRAS-targeting vaccines

KRAS (Kirsten rat sarcoma viral oncogene homolog gene), mutated in over 90% of pancreatic ductal adenocarcinoma (PDA) patients, was the first peptide-based vaccine's target, which was investigated in clinical trials with patients suffering from pancreatic cancer, proving the immunotherapeutic approach's safety. When patients with incurable pancreatic cancer received synthetic KRAS-derived peptides in a Phase I/II research, 2 out of 5 individuals showed an immune response (Kaufman et al., 2007).

Whole cancer cell-based vaccines

Targeting a particular tumor-associated antigen (TAA) is not necessary because whole cancer cell-based vaccines use irradiated tumor cells, which naturally express a wide variety of TAAs. Moreover, whole cell-based vaccinations offer a neutral method of vaccinating lymphocytes and sera against TAAs, potentially producing a reagent that can be used to find immunologically relevant TAAs to guide the development of vaccination plans that are specific to particular antigens. Two allogeneic whole cell-based anticancer vaccines are presently being researched for their safety and antitumor efficacy in patients with pancreatic ductal adenocarcinoma (PDA) (Principe et al., 2021).

Phase 1 Trial Reveals Persistent Immune Response Induced by mRNA Vaccine in Pancreatic Cancer Patients

The mRNA vaccines deliver neoantigens to PC patients, stimulating both immune system-mediated antibody responses and targeted cellular anti-tumor reactions. These vaccines are custom-made, safe, easy to produce, and do not integrate into the host's DNA, positioning them as a promising treatment option being explored for pancreatic ductal adenocarcinoma (PDAC). A significant phase I trial evaluated the capability of autogenecevumeran, an established mRNA neoantigen vaccine, to enhance T-cell activity in cases with surgically resected PDAC (Wandmacher et al., 2021). The study enrolled 32 patients, of whom 16 underwent surgery and proceeded with treatment using at ezolizumab (anti PD-L1 antibody), autogenecevumeran, and the chemotherapy regimen mFOLFIRINOX (which includes 5-fluorouracil, folinic acid, oxaliplatin, and irinotecan) (Torphy et al., 2018). Eight out of the sixteen patients receiving autogenecevumeran exhibited increased T-cell activity targeting at least one neoantigen. Further research is necessary to optimize neoantigen targeting and enhance the efficacy of mRNA vaccines.

Compared to other vaccination platforms, mRNA vaccines offer a number of noteworthy safety advantages, and safety is still of utmost importance. Because mRNA vaccines are made and administered without the use of hazardous chemicals, fewer PC patients and manufacturing employees are harmed. Because mRNA vaccines are produced quickly, there is less chance of contamination during manufacture. The host genome cannot incorporate mRNA, in contrast to other therapeutic approaches.

Furthermore, the exact regulation of the length and degree of protein expression is made possible by the mRNA's changeable half-life. Through the regulation of immune responses and any adverse effects, this skill improves safety (McCarthy, 2006).

Nonetheless, some issues with mRNA vaccines are brought out. It is essential to carefully choose and optimize suitable mRNA formulations (such as liposomes, polyplexes, and lipoplexes) and administration methods in order to enhance the effective transport of mRNA to antigen-presenting cells. Since several factors affect the pharmacologic and pharmacokinetic properties of mRNA-based therapeutics, controlling the in vivo half-life of the produced mRNA is crucial after successful mRNA delivery (Uehata & Takeuchi, 2020). Furthermore, the effectiveness of cancer mRNA vaccines can be increased by augmenting the immunostimulatory qualities of mRNA through the use of adjuvants like TriMix, which contains mRNA encoding for CD70, CD40L, and TLR4 (Lorentzen et al., 2022). The tetravalent vaccine mRNA-5671, which targets KRAS G12D, G12V, G13D, and G12C, was the subject of a clinical trial that was eventually terminated in 2022 due to its failure to fulfil efficacy standards. As a result, there have been no further advances or revelations about this vaccination. (Wadhwa et al., 2020).

Case Study: Engineered T Cells Shrank Pancreatic Cancer Tumors

Mesothelin is a protein found on the surface of cells and is often overproduced in pancreatic cancer and other solid tumors (Diken et al., 2011). This makes it a promising target for cancer immunotherapy. After surgery for pancreatic cancer, patients usually receive low-dose chemotherapy and radiation, but these treatments only extend survival by less than a year and have limited effectiveness. Research has shown that T cells targeting mesothelin, known as meso-CART cells, can reduce or eliminate tumors (Diken et al., 2011). These meso-CART cells are a type of engineered T cell therapy that uses specific mechanisms to enhance their effectiveness and are derived from human blood cells that have been modified in the lab.

Figure 7. Preparation of engineered T cells for Pancreatic Cancer Tumors.

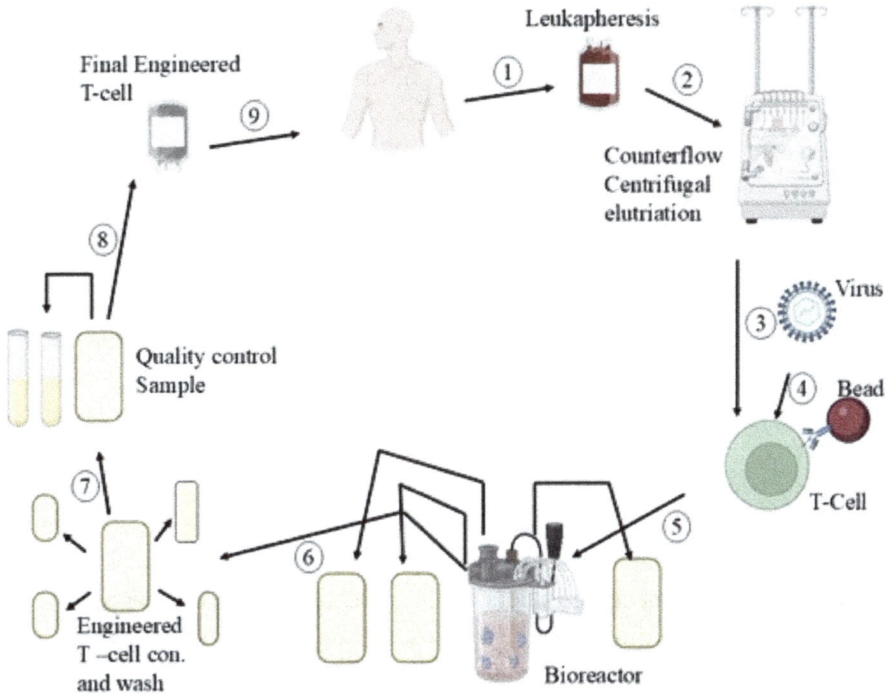

Other T cell therapies targeting different proteins like EGFRvIII and IL13Rα2 have also shown promise. EGFRvIII-CAR T cells have been effective against glioblastoma in early studies, and trials are currently testing their safety. Preparation of engineered T cells for pancreatic cancer tumors are schematically mentioned in (Fig7). To get to tumours, these T cells can also pass across the blood-brain barrier. Similarly, IL13Rα2-CAR T cells, which are given directly into the brain, have been safe in glioblastoma patients, and their effectiveness is still being evaluated. In addition to mesothelin, it's important to focus on minimizing harmful side effects when developing CAR T cell therapies. Reducing off-tumor effects is crucial because these can be dangerous and limit how these therapies are used. Targeting cancer stem cells (CSCs), found in many cancers like pancreatic cancer, may provide long-term benefits. Some studies and a clinical trial have suggested that specific CAR T cells can target and eliminate these CSCs. Creating strategies to focus on these cells could improve treatment results while reducing off-tumor effects.

Exploring Immunotherapy in Pancreatic Cancer: A Case Study on Advancing Treatment Strategies

A significant number of cancer patients have experienced positive outcomes from innovative immunotherapeutic strategies, particularly immune checkpoint inhibitors. Nevertheless, the lack of benefit from these and other immunotherapeutic advancements for patients with pancreatic ductal adenocarcinoma (PDAC) suggests significant immunosuppressive and immune evasion mechanisms. Tumors can modify immunological checkpoints to avoid the immune response, but they also help maintain self-tolerance (Jackson et al., 2016). Restoring T cell activation by therapies that target checkpoints like PD-1/PD-L1 and CTLA-4 improves the body's capacity to fight tumors (Table 1). Additionally, activating CD40 boosts the function of antigen-presenting cells and T cell responses, thereby improving tumor suppression.

Palliative chemotherapy using FOLFIRINOX (5-FU, Irinotecan, Leucovorin, and Oxaliplatin) or Gemcitabine/Nab-Paclitaxel is currently the main treatment choice for this sizable patient population. With respective durations of 11.1 and 8.5 months, these treatments provide a slight increase in overall survival. T cells are essential for immunological defense in immune checkpoint-based therapies because they can recognize and eliminate tumor cells thanks to costimulatory and inhibitory signals. Recent developments in checkpoint agonists and inhibitors have broadened anti-tumor treatment approaches and opened up new avenues for cancer immunotherapy. (Sun et al., 2018).

Table 1. Clinical trials for immunotherapy-related regimens in pancreatic cancer

Target	Name	Isotype/Type	Combination	Phase	Identifier
PD-1	Pembrolizumab	IgG4	Trametinib (a MEK inhibitor), SBRT, chemotherapy	I	NCT01295827
PD-1	Pembrolizumab	IgG4	Pelareorep (an oncolytic reovirus), chemotherapy	Ib	NCT03723915
PD-1	Pembrolizumab	IgG4	AMG 820 (an anti-CSF1R IgG2 monoclonal antibody)	I/Ib	NCT02713529
PD-1	Pembrolizumab	IgG4	BL-8040 (a CXCR4 antagonist)	I	NCT02826486
PD-1	Pembrolizumab	IgG4	NOX-A12 (a CXCL12 inhibitor)	I/II	NCT03168139
PD-1	Pembrolizumab	IgG4	Gemcitabine, Defactinib (a FAK inhibitor)	I	NCT02546531
PD-1	Nivolumab	IgG4	Ipilimumab	I	CA209-538
PD-1	Nivolumab	IgG4	Ipilimumab, Radiation therapy	I	NCT03104439

continued on following page

Table 1. Continued

Target	Name	Isotype/Type	Combination	Phase	Identifier
PD-1	Nivolumab	IgG4	Nivolumab, SBRT, with or without Ipilimumab	II	NCT02866383
PD-1	Nivolumab	IgG4	Nivolumab, SBRT, Ipilimumab, Tocilizumab (an anti-IL-6 receptor monoclonal antibody)	II	NCT04258150
PD-1	Nivolumab	IgG4	mFOLRINOX	I	JapicCTI-184230
PD-1	Nivolumab	IgG4	APPGC	I	NCT02754726
PD-1	Nivolumab	IgG4	Evofosfamide (an investigational hypoxia-activated prodrug)	I	NCT03098160
PD-1	Nivolumab	IgG4	IRE	I	NCT03080974
PD-1	Camrelizumab	IgG4	AG	I	NCT05061017
PD-1	Toripalimab	IgG4	AG	/	/
PD-L1	BMS-936559	IgG4	/	/	NCT00729664
PD-L1	Atezolizumab	IgG1	Binimetinib	I	JapicCTI-132208
PD-L1	Durvalumab	IgG1	Bevacizumab (an anti-VEGF IgG1 monoclonal antibody)	I	NCT03634791
PD-L1	Durvalumab	IgG1	Tremelimumab	I	NCT03074513
CTLA-4	Tremelimumab	IgG2	Tremelimumab, AG	II	NCT02558894
CTLA-4	Tremelimumab	IgG2	Galunisertib (a TGF-β type I receptor kinase inhibitor)	Ib	NCT02734160
CTLA-4	Ipilimumab	IgG1	Durvalumab	II	NCT02558894
CD40	Selicrelumab	IgG2	Gemcitabine	I	NCT01436585
CD40	Sotigalimab	IgG1	AG	I	NCT02588463
CCR4	Mogamulizumab	IgG1	Durvalumab or Tremelimumab	I	NCT02302130
EGFR	Cetuximab	IgG1	Gemcitabine, IMRT	II	ISCRTN 56652283

Immunocheckpoint inhibitors (ICIs), either alone or in combination, have not generally shown much promise in treating pancreatic ductal adenocarcinoma (PDAC), although they have shown promise in treating individuals with microsatellite instability-high (MSI-H) or DNA mismatch repair-deficient (dMMR) tumors. The pancreatic tumor microenvironment (TME) may be significantly altered by neoadjuvant chemotherapy, which also has the potential to increase the intra-tumoral concentrations of CD4, CD8, and T-cells in PDAC patients. Combinations of these therapies have been explored in PDAC (Sun et al., 2018). Several pancreatic cancer antigens, including carcinoembryonic antigen (CEA), mucin-1 (MUC-1), and the mutated product of KRAS, are commonly found across most pancreatic tumors.

These antigens can be utilized in vaccines targeting pancreatic cancer. According to the results of a phase II clinical trial, patients with surgically removable PDAC who received GVAX alone or in combination with oral or intravenous cyclophosphamide around the time of surgery (the first dose being a neoadjuvant treatment and subsequent doses being an adjuvant) showed immune responses, with GVAX activating a variety of immune cell types. Algenpantucel-L, sometimes referred to as the HAPa cancer vaccine, is the vaccine strategy for treating PDAC. It consists of two allogeneic pancreatic cancer cell lines that have been altered to express the murine α (1,3) GT gene. Mechanistically, Algenpantucel-L stimulates a strong immune response against PDAC peptides by using hyperacute rejection of mouse proteins. In a phase III clinical trial with 303 participants, this drug was clinically evaluated as part of a neoadjuvant strategy to complement the usual neoadjuvant chemotherapy and chemoradiation for patients with locally advanced unresectable PDAC or borderline resectable PDAC. (Lanitis et al., 2012).

Advancements in Systemic Therapy for Pancreatic Cancer

For patients with advanced pancreatic cancer, systemic therapy has historically advanced slowly. These developments have been based on the continuous development of cytotoxic chemotherapy combinations, such as gemcitabine plus nab-paclitaxel (2013), fluorouracil (FU)/nano liposomal irinotecan (2016), oxaliplatin, irinotecan, fluorouracil, and leucovorin (FOLFIRINOX; 2011), and NALIRIFOX (2023) (Chmielewski et al., 2011). The steady rise in targeted medicines for patients with pancreatic cancer has been another noteworthy development. The continued discovery of KRAS inhibit ors raises hopes that other research organisations may soon offer precision medicines to a wider percentage of patients, even though the number of patients eligible for focused treatment is still small (Casucci et al., 2013). According to results from the PRODIGE-4/ACCORD-111 trial and the MPACT trial, respectively, the majority of patients with metastatic pancreatic adenocarcinoma are currently treated with continuous cytotoxic chemotherapy using either FOLFIRINOX or gemcitabine in combination with nanoparticle albumin-bound (nab-) paclitaxel (Gill et al., 2014). FOLFIRINOX and gemcitabine-nab-paclitaxel have not been directly compared in a prospective clinical study, despite the fact that both treatment plans have improved patient outcomes when compared to the previous standard of gemcitabine monotherapy as the first-line treatment. However, gemcitabine-nab-paclitaxel is recommended for second-line therapy or as a first-line option for patients with other medical conditions, while FOLFIRINOX is typically preferred as the first-line therapy for advanced pancreatic cancer in patients deemed capable of handling it and is supported by the ASCO guidelines (Disis, 2010). This treatment strategy is further supported by indirect evidence from the recently released NAPOLI-3 trials, which compare NALIRIFOX to gemcitabine-nab-paclitaxel. These findings will be covered in more detail in later sections of this review (Furnari et al., 2015).

FOCUSED TREATMENTS IN PANCREATIC CANCER: A NEW ERA OF TAILORED MEDICINE

Fluoropyrimidines and the antimetabolite drug gemcitabine have been the standard chemotherapies for pancreatic cancer for the past thirty years. Randomised clinical trials have shown that these two drugs are generally equivalent (Jarboe et al., 2007). Chemoradiotherapy's role in treating locally advanced pancreatic adenocarcinomas (LAPC) and resectable ones is still up for dispute. Up to 30% of patients die from local progression of pancreatic cancer, despite the fact that it is evident that the disease is really systemic. Two randomised European trials (EORTC 61 and ESPAC 112) conducted over the last 20 years have concluded that radiation therapy is not beneficial after pancreatic cancer surgery.The RTOG 0848 trial (NCT01013649) is now examining the efficacy of adjuvant radiation therapy in conjunction with gemcitabine as opposed to gemcitabine alone after resection (O'Rourke et al., 2016). The inclusion of radiotherapy following a four-month chemotherapy induction phase did not improve survival for LAPC in the LAP-07 study (gemcitabine with or without capecitabine-based chemoradiotherapy and with or without erlotinib). The malignancy potential of cancer cells and the host microenvironment, which is made up of fibroblasts, myofibroblasts, pancreatic stellate cells, vascular cells, immune cells, and the extracellular matrix, as well as associated cytokines, affect how pancreatic cancer tumors behave (Rump et al., 2004).

Despite conflicting data about its efficacy, adjuvant radiation treatment (RT) is frequently used. The first randomised experiment to assess adjuvant chemoradiation against observation in 43 patients with negative margins following PDAC resection was the GITSG study, which was carried out in 1985. Even though the experiment was ended early because of poor enrolment (it was intended to recruit 100 patients), its results showed an overall survival advantage with CRT (median 20 months vs to 11 months). Consequently, CRT emerged as the new adjuvant therapy standard. Like chemotherapy, neoadjuvant radiation has potential benefits (Beatty, 2015). The neoadjuvant approach to radiation therapy may prove more effective, as expected, considering the significant morbidity after PDAC surgery and the possibility of an early systemic recurrence. Researchers have only found a slight benefit of neoadjuvant radiation since the 1980s. Stronger evidence for neoadjuvant chemoradiation in individuals with borderline resectable cancer was presented in 2018 by the PREOPANC-1 research (Tanyi, 2015). 246 patients with borderline resectable PDAC were randomised to either upfront surgery or neoadjuvant gemcitabine plus 36 Gy of radiation administered in between two gemcitabine cycles. Adjuvant chemotherapy was administered to both groups. There is moderate evidence to support the use of conventionally fractionated RT or SBRT for borderline or locally progressed PDAC, according to the 2019 American Society for Radiation Oncology guidelines. However, there is little evidence to suggest RT for unresectable or high-risk patients in the adjuvant situation (Zhao et al., 2015).

FUTURE DEVELOPMENTS IN PANCREATIC CANCER TREATMENTS

The accumulation of different gene deletions, mutations, and amplifications is a characteristic of pancreatic adenocarcinoma; the most common changes are deletions of tumour suppressor genes. The current targeted medicines assessed in phase III trials, with the exception of erlotinib and gemcitabine, have not been able to increase the survival rates of patients with pancreatic cancer (Yuan et al., 2004a). This finding emphasises how important it is to learn more about the molecular processes behind pancreatic carcinogenesis. The creation of targeted agents was predicated on their capacity to inhibit particular elements (an enzyme, a growth factor, or a cell receptor) of pathways thought to be involved in the development of pancreatic cancer. Because the biology of pancreatic cancer is complicated, concentrating on just one component of a pathway is insufficient. Future clinical studies may benefit from the use of multitargeted medicines or combinations of targeted drugs that can simultaneously inhibit various pathways by identifying numerous proteins (Yuan et al., 2004a). The impacted genes and pathways, however, differed for every individual case, indicating that a customised treatment strategy would be required. The many study groups of pancreatic cancer cells showed that the Hedgehog developmental signalling system was activated, that they could self-renew, and that they could create children that could differentiate. These findings are consistent with past research showing the presence of cancer stem cells (Yuan et al., 2004b). One of the most important recent developments in our knowledge of pancreatic cancer biology is the identification of pancreatic cancer stem cells, which could result in the creation of novel therapeutic approaches that employ substances that interfere with developmental pathways. These pathways have been identified to be overexpressed in pancreatic cancer samples, where they are believed to promote tumour growth and contribute to chemotherapy resistance. Normally, these pathways are inactive in the normal pancreas and active during tissue development (Yuan et al., 2004b).

CONCLUSION

An on-going concern in the field of oncology is the rising incidence of pancreatic cancer (PC) in recent years. While India has made advancements in the five-year survival rate, now reported at 9–12%, the treatment landscape still faces several hurdles. Traditional therapies such as chemotherapy and radiation have shown limited effectiveness, and the aggressive nature of pancreatic cancer often results in rapid spread and early metastasis. At present, targeted therapies have not demonstrated substantial efficacy in comparison to other cancer forms, either as standalone treatments or in combination with chemotherapy regimens like FOLFIRINOX. As such, these options have yet to find a comprehensive place within standard clinical practice. Importantly, while the results from various studies on immunotherapy have been promising in different cancer types, this approach has not yet been integrated into the treatment protocols for pancreatic cancer. This book chapter will give a comprehensive summary of the most recent developments in (i) early detection, (ii) therapies and treatments, (iii) various biomarkers, (iv) focused approaches to treatment in PC, and (v) future directions in pancreatic cancer research. Our goal is to equip clinicians with the most relevant insights for effective management of this challenging disease.

Consent for Publications

All the authors give consent for the publication of this book chapter.

Conflict of Interest

The authors declare no conflict of interest.

ACKNOWLEDGEMENT

The authors would like to convey their special thanks to the Department of Bioinformatics, Maulana Abul kalam Azad University of Technology, W.B. for providing the computational facility and other institutional facility to contribute to this work.

Authors' Note: Hridoy Ranjan Bairagya is the corresponding author. Sayan Acharyya and Bikram Sarkar contribute equally and share joint first authorship.

REFERENCES

Al Balushi, H., Chowdhury, P., Babu, H. M., Rehman, A., Bokhari, S. F. H., Al-Tarawneh, L. M., Al-Adwan, A. J., Cheran, M., Chilla, S. P., Addula, A. R., & Amir, M. (2024). The Potential of Salivary Biomarkers in Early Detection of Pancreatic Ductal Adenocarcinoma: A Systematic Review. *Cureus, 16*(2). Advance online publication. DOI: 10.7759/cureus.55003 PMID: 38550499

Beatty, G. L. Safety and antitumor activity of chimeric antigen receptor modified T cells in patients with chemotherapy refractory metastatic pancreatic cancer. ASCO Annu. Meet. Proc. 33, 3007 (2015). DOI: 10.1200/jco.2015.33.15_suppl.3007

Casucci, M., Nicolis di Robilant, B., Falcone, L., Camisa, B., Norelli, M., Genovese, P., Gentner, B., Gullotta, F., Ponzoni, M., Bernardi, M., Marcatti, M., Saudemont, A., Bordignon, C., Savoldo, B., Ciceri, F., Naldini, L., Dotti, G., Bonini, C., & Bondanza, A. (2013). CD44v6-targeted T cells mediate potent antitumor effects against acute myeloid leukemia and multiple myeloma. *Blood, 122*(20), 3461–3472. DOI: 10.1182/blood-2013-04-493361 PMID: 24016461

Chmielewski, M., Kopecky, C., Hombach, A. A., & Abken, H. (2011). IL-12 release by engineered T cells expressing chimeric antigen receptors can effectively Muster an antigen-independent macrophage response on tumor cells that have shut down tumor antigen expression. *Cancer Research, 71*(17), 5697–5706. DOI: 10.1158/0008-5472.CAN-11-0103 PMID: 21742772

Cortiana, V., Abbas, R. H., Chorya, H., Gambill, J., Mahendru, D., Park, C. H., & Leyfman, Y. (2024). Personalized medicine in pancreatic cancer: The promise of biomarkers and molecular targeting with dr. *Michael J. Pishvaian. Cancers, 16*(13), 2329. PMID: 39001391

Diken, M., Kreiter, S., Selmi, A., Britten, C. M., Huber, C., Türeci, Ö., & Sahin, U. (2011). Selective uptake of naked vaccine RNA by dendritic cells is driven by macropinocytosis and abrogated upon DC maturation. *Gene Therapy*, *18*(7), 702–708. DOI: 10.1038/gt.2011.17 PMID: 21368901

Disis, M. L. (2010). Immune regulation of cancer. *Journal of Clinical Oncology*, *28*(29), 4531–4538. DOI: 10.1200/JCO.2009.27.2146 PMID: 20516428

Duan, H., Li, L., & He, S. (2023). Advances and prospects in the treatment of pancreatic cancer. *International Journal of Nanomedicine*, *18*, 3973–3988. DOI: 10.2147/IJN.S413496 PMID: 37489138

Furnari, F. B., Cloughesy, T. F., Cavenee, W. K., & Mischel, P. S. (2015). Heterogeneity of epidermal growth factor receptor signalling networks in glioblastoma. *Nature Reviews. Cancer*, *15*(5), 302–310. DOI: 10.1038/nrc3918 PMID: 25855404

Garrido-Laguna, I., & Hidalgo, M. (2015). Pancreatic cancer: From state-of-the-art treatments to promising novel therapies. *Nature Reviews. Clinical Oncology*, *12*(6), 319–334. DOI: 10.1038/nrclinonc.2015.53 PMID: 25824606

Gill, S., Tasian, S. K., Ruella, M., Shestova, O., Li, Y., Porter, D. L., Carroll, M., Danet-Desnoyers, G., Scholler, J., Grupp, S. A., June, C. H., & Kalos, M. (2014). Preclinical targeting of human acute myeloid leukemia and myeloablation using chimeric antigen receptor–modified T cells. *Blood*, *123*(15), 2343–2354. DOI: 10.1182/blood-2013-09-529537 PMID: 24596416

Heredia-Soto, V., Rodríguez-Salas, N., & Feliu, J. (2021). Liquid biopsy in pancreatic cancer: Are we ready to apply it in the clinical practice? *Cancers (Basel)*, *13*(8), 1986. DOI: 10.3390/cancers13081986 PMID: 33924143

Huang, J., Liu, J., Chen-Xiao, K., Zhang, X., Lee, W. P., Go, V. L. W., & Xiao, G. G. (2016). Advance in microRNA as a potential biomarker for early detection of pancreatic cancer. *Biomarker Research*, *4*(1), 1–5. DOI: 10.1186/s40364-016-0074-3 PMID: 27795830

Jackson, H. J., Rafiq, S., & Brentjens, R. J. (2016). Driving CAR T-cells forward. *Nature Reviews. Clinical Oncology*, *13*(6), 370–383. DOI: 10.1038/nrclinonc.2016.36 PMID: 27000958

Jarboe, J. S., Johnson, K. R., Choi, Y., Lonser, R. R., & Park, J. K. (2007). Expression of interleukin-13 receptor α2 in glioblastoma multiforme: Implications for targeted therapies. *Cancer Research*, *67*(17), 7983–7986. DOI: 10.1158/0008-5472.CAN-07-1493 PMID: 17804706

Kaufman, H. L., Kim-Schulze, S., Manson, K., DeRaffele, G., Mitcham, J., Seo, K. S., Kim, D. W., & Marshall, J. (2007). Poxvirus-based vaccine therapy for patients with advanced pancreatic cancer. *Journal of Translational Medicine*, *5*(1), 1–10. DOI: 10.1186/1479-5876-5-60 PMID: 18039393

Kolbeinsson, H. M., Chandana, S., Wright, G. P., & Chung, M. (2023). Pancreatic cancer: A review of current treatment and novel therapies. *Journal of Investigative Surgery*, *36*(1), 2129884. DOI: 10.1080/08941939.2022.2129884 PMID: 36191926

Lanitis, E., Poussin, M., Hagemann, I. S., Coukos, G., Sandaltzopoulos, R., Scholler, N., & Powell, D. J.Jr. (2012). Redirected antitumor activity of primary human lymphocytes transduced with a fully human anti-mesothelin chimeric receptor. *Molecular Therapy : the Journal of the American Society of Gene Therapy*, *20*(3), 633–643. DOI: 10.1038/mt.2011.256 PMID: 22127019

Lorentzen, C. L., Haanen, J. B., Met, Ö., & Svane, I. M. (2022). Clinical advances and ongoing trials of mRNA vaccines for cancer treatment. *The Lancet. Oncology*, *23*(10), e450–e458. DOI: 10.1016/S1470-2045(22)00372-2 PMID: 36174631

Ma, Y., Zhang, F., & Yang, Y. (2024). Recent advances in the treatment of pancreatic cancer. *Holistic Integrative Oncology.*, *3*(1), 34. DOI: 10.1007/s44178-024-00089-6

Malla, M., Fekrmandi, F., Malik, N., Hatoum, H., George, S., Goldberg, R. M., & Mukherjee, S. (2023). The evolving role of radiation in pancreatic cancer. *Frontiers in Oncology*, *12*, 1060885. DOI: 10.3389/fonc.2022.1060885 PMID: 36713520

McCarthy, E. F. (2006). The toxins of William B. Coley and the treatment of bone and soft-tissue sarcomas. *The Iowa Orthopaedic Journal*, *26*, 154. PMID: 16789469

Moss, R. A., & Lee, C. (2010). Current and emerging therapies for the treatment of pancreatic cancer. *OncoTargets and Therapy*, •••, 111–127. DOI: 10.2147/OTT.S7203 PMID: 20856847

Murray, C. J., & López, A. D. (1994). Global and regional cause-of-death patterns in 1990. *Bulletin of the World Health Organization*, *72*(3), 447. PMID: 8062402

O'Neill, R. S., & Stoita, A. (2021). Biomarkers in the diagnosis of pancreatic cancer: Are we closer to finding the golden ticket? *World Journal of Gastroenterology*, *27*(26), 4045–4087. DOI: 10.3748/wjg.v27.i26.4045 PMID: 34326612

. O'Rourke, D. M., Nasrallah, M., Morrissette, J. J., Melenhorst, J. J., Lacey, S. F., Mansfield, K., ... & Maus, M. V. (2016). Pilot study of T cells redirected to EGFRvIII with a chimeric antigen receptor in patients with EGFRvIII+ glioblastoma.

Pflüger, M. J., Jamouss, K. T., Afghani, E., Lim, S. J., Franco, S. R., Mayo, H., & Wood, L. D. (2023). Predictive ability of pancreatic cyst fluid biomarkers: A systematic review and meta-analysis. *Pancreatology*, *23*(7), 868–877. DOI: 10.1016/j.pan.2023.05.005 PMID: 37230894

Principe, D. R., Underwood, P. W., Korc, M., Trevino, J. G., Munshi, H. G., & Rana, A. (2021). The current treatment paradigm for pancreatic ductal adenocarcinoma and barriers to therapeutic efficacy. *Frontiers in Oncology*, *11*, 688377. DOI: 10.3389/fonc.2021.688377 PMID: 34336673

Rump, A., Morikawa, Y., Tanaka, M., Minami, S., Umesaki, N., Takeuchi, M., & Miyajima, A. (2004). Binding of ovarian cancer antigen CA125/MUC16 to mesothelin mediates cell adhesion. *The Journal of Biological Chemistry*, *279*(10), 9190–9198. DOI: 10.1074/jbc.M312372200 PMID: 14676194

Salman, B., Zhou, D., Jaffee, E. M., Edil, B. H., & Zheng, L. (2013). Vaccine therapy for pancreatic cancer. *OncoImmunology*, *2*(12), e26662. DOI: 10.4161/onci.26662 PMID: 24498551

Springfeld, C., Jäger, D., Büchler, M. W., Strobel, O., Hackert, T., Palmer, D. H., & Neoptolemos, J. P. (2019). Chemotherapy for pancreatic cancer. *La Presse Medicale*, *48*(3), e159–e174. DOI: 10.1016/j.lpm.2019.02.025 PMID: 30879894

Sugimoto, M., Wong, D. T., Hirayama, A., Soga, T., & Tomita, M. (2010). Capillary electrophoresis mass spectrometry-based saliva metabolomics identified oral, breast and pancreatic cancer-specific profiles. *Metabolomics*, *6*(1), 78–95. DOI: 10.1007/s11306-009-0178-y PMID: 20300169

Sun, Q., Zhou, S., Zhao, J., Deng, C., Teng, R., Zhao, Y., Chen, J., Dong, J., Yin, M., Bai, Y., Deng, H., & Wen, J. (2018). Engineered T lymphocytes eliminate lung metastases in models of pancreatic cancer. *Oncotarget*, *9*(17), 13694–13705. DOI: 10.18632/oncotarget.24122 PMID: 29568387

. Tanyi, J. L.. Safety and feasibility of chimeric antigen receptor modified T cells directed against mesothelin (CART-meso) in patients with mesothelin expressing cancers. Cancer Res. 75, Abstr. CT105 (2015).

Tarasiuk, A., Mackiewicz, T., Małecka-Panas, E., & Fichna, J. (2021). Biomarkers for early detection of pancreatic cancer–miRNAs as a potential diagnostic and therapeutic tool? *Cancer Biology & Therapy*, *22*(5-6), 347–356. DOI: 10.1080/15384047.2021.1941584 PMID: 34224317

Torphy, R. J., Zhu, Y., & Schulick, R. D. (2018). Immunotherapy for pancreatic cancer: Barriers and breakthroughs. *Annals of Gastroenterological Surgery*, *2*(4), 274–281. DOI: 10.1002/ags3.12176 PMID: 30003190

Uehata, T., & Takeuchi, O. (2020). RNA recognition and immunity—Innate immune sensing and its posttranscriptional regulation mechanisms. *Cells*, *9*(7), 1701. DOI: 10.3390/cells9071701 PMID: 32708595

Vitale, F., Dal Verme, L. Z., Paratore, M., Negri, M., Nista, E. C., Ainora, M. E., & Nicoletti, A. (2024). The Past, Present, and Future of Biomarkers for the Early Diagnosis of Pancreatic Cancer. *Biomedicines*, *12*(12), 2840. DOI: 10.3390/biomedicines12122840 PMID: 39767746

Wadhwa, A., Aljabbari, A., Lokras, A., Foged, C., & Thakur, A. (2020). Opportunities and challenges in the delivery of mRNA-based vaccines. *Pharmaceutics*, *12*(2), 102. DOI: 10.3390/pharmaceutics12020102 PMID: 32013049

Wandmacher, A. M., Letsch, A., & Sebens, S. (2021). Challenges and future perspectives of immunotherapy in pancreatic cancer. *Cancers (Basel)*, *13*(16), 4235. DOI: 10.3390/cancers13164235 PMID: 34439389

Yang, F., Liu, D. Y., Guo, J. T., Ge, N., Zhu, P., Liu, X., Wang, S., Wang, G.-X., & Sun, S. Y. (2017). Circular RNA circ-LDLRAD3 as a biomarker in diagnosis of pancreatic cancer. *World Journal of Gastroenterology*, *23*(47), 8345–8354. DOI: 10.3748/wjg.v23.i47.8345 PMID: 29307994

Yang, J., Xu, R., Wang, C., Qiu, J., Ren, B., & You, L. (2021). Early screening and diagnosis strategies of pancreatic cancer: A comprehensive review. *Cancer Communications*, *41*(12), 1257–1274. DOI: 10.1002/cac2.12204 PMID: 34331845

Yuan, X., Curtin, J., Xiong, Y., Liu, G., Waschsmann-Hogiu, S., Farkas, D. L., Black, K. L., & Yu, J. S. (2004). Isolation of cancer stem cells from adult glioblastoma multiforme. *Oncogene*, *23*(58), 9392–9400. DOI: 10.1038/sj.onc.1208311 PMID: 15558011

Yuan, X., Curtin, J., Xiong, Y., Liu, G., Waschsmann-Hogiu, S., Farkas, D. L., Black, K. L., & Yu, J. S. (2004). Isolation of cancer stem cells from adult glioblastoma multiforme. *Oncogene*, *23*(58), 9392–9400. DOI: 10.1038/sj.onc.1208311 PMID: 15558011

Zhao, Q., Ahmed, M., Tassev, D. V., Hasan, A., Kuo, T. Y., Guo, H. F., O'Reilly, R. J., & Cheung, N. K. (2015). Affinity maturation of T-cell receptor-like antibodies for Wilms tumor 1 peptide greatly enhances therapeutic potential. *Leukemia*, *29*(11), 2238–2247. DOI: 10.1038/leu.2015.125 PMID: 25987253

Chapter 13

Hope on the Horizon: The Future of Pancreatic Cancer Treatment

Lovleen Marwaha
https://orcid.org/0009-0007-0196-4919
Lovely Professional University, India

ABSTRACT

Pancreatic cancer is considered one of the most deadly because often it diagnosed only in the late stage, while the early symptoms are not very pronounced. They remain undiagnosed most of the time when they are already widespread and treatment is complicated, admission and survival rare. This is because new technologies for diagnosis and cure have enhanced prospects. Cancer DNA or proteins from tissues are found in blood to diagnose them early through liquid biopsies. AI helps in imaging and in identification of early signs of cancer. For example, there is precision medicine which aims at genetic mutation for example BRCA and treats them with PARP inhibitors. Immuno is a therapy that enhances the body's immune system, whereas, Nano means the scaling down of devices and machinery to the nanometer range that aids in delivering drugs without generating side effects. Telemedicine intervention and hospice support allow patients to physically benefit from care and provided services. This advancement are enhancing survival and care of pancreatic cancer hence making it a manageable disease.

1. INTRODUCTION

Approximately, pancreatic cancer is regarded as a silent killer (Olajubutu *et al.*, 2023), and one of the most aggressive and hard to detect and treat types of cancer. This has been termed to be silent in that, most patients present with the symptoms

DOI: 10.4018/979-8-3373-1469-3.ch013

when the disease is already at the advanced stage. Such late diagnosis, coupled with the lack of effective screening, leads to very poor survival rates as more than 80 percent of patients survive less than five years after being diagnosed (Tang *et al.,* 2018). The other issue is desmoplasia, i.e. the surrounding tumor tissue is a dense layer of tissue that prevents treatments. In spite of these challenges, new studies are bringing in some hope. Radiological scans and blood tests are known to be inefficient in identifying the disease at an early stage, and the liquid blood biopsies will now be able to identify the cancer DNA and biomarkers in blood samples. Artificial intelligence (AI) enhances the accuracy of imaging because it can notice the patterns that cannot be identified by the human eye. The personalized medicine approach personalizes therapy based on genes of a patient such as BRCA mutation carriers have the opportunity to be treated with PARP inhibitors (Cortesi *et al.,* 2021). Nanoparticle drugs have increased tumor delivery of drugs and reduced toxicity by half and may synergize with immunotherapy to release more immune cells. Immunotherapy is a kind of cancer fighting utilizing the immune system. In spite of the stroma barrier that makes this treatment method less effective in the past, new strategies, including immune checkpoint inhibitors and CAR T-cell therapy are proving to be promising, particularly when used with chemotherapy or radiation (Rossi *et al.,* 2020; Malik *et al.,* 2023). Others are CRISPR-Cas9 gene editing to repair mutations that result in the development of cancer and cultured patient-made organoids to screen drugs in the laboratory before employing them in patients. This is shown in the title Hope on the Horizon which signifies this new dawn of innovation where there are enhanced diagnostics and more focused treatments that may lead to earlier diagnosis, improved survival and quality of life. Also, medical innovations cannot be considered separately without supportive care, pain management, nutrition, and psychological support. Innovation and holistic patient care continue to change pancreatic cancer into a disease with actual hope in mind about the future.

1.1 What Pancreatic Cancer Is?

Pancreatic cancer is an especially malignant and deadly disease which arises in the pancreas-a small but very important gland which is located in the abdominal cavity behind the stomach. The pancreas has two main jobs in the body: it aids in digestion and; there are indications that it is also good in managing diabetes. The first function which is called its exocrine function is secretion of specific enzymes that would otherwise be able to metabolise foods in the intestines in order to be transported in the blood stream or body fluids. Its second function, known as the endocrine function, is to secrete such hormones as insulin – which regulates high levels of sugar in the blood- and glucagon which raises the level of sugar in the blood (Qaid & Abdelrahman, 2016). Since such activity performs such important functions, contamination with the identified pathogen significantly impairs the ability of birds to survive. any disruption caused by cancer in the pancreas can lead to serious problems throughout the body. Pancreatic adenocarcinoma is the most prevalent and lethal type of pancreatic cancer that begins in the ducts that supply enzymes. It makes up over 90% of pancreatic cancers and is known to metastasize quickly to organs like the liver, stomach, lungs, and bones, among others. This accounts for the reason why many patients present symptoms of abdominal pain at very advanced stages (Nersesyan & Slavin, 2007). Some of the visible signs of cancer including fatigue, weight loss and stomach upsets are usually ignored thus patients present themselves to the hospital at the last stage and this reduces the survival rates. PDAC is inherently chemoresistant and it exhibits several properties such as dense stroma which hinders the delivery of chemotherapy and its potential to recover and withstand treatments. Currently, only about 10% of the patients reach the five-year survival level and therefore enhancing the early diagnosis is paramount. Some of the key measures that can improve treatment outcome and the survival rate of the patients comprise of the screening and diagnosis developments. (Table 1)

Table 1. Symptoms of Pancreatic Cancer by Disease Stage

Stage	Common Symptoms	Clinical Implications
Early Stage	Mild abdominal pain, indigestion, fatigue.	Often mistaken for less serious conditions.
Intermediate	Jaundice, unexplained weight loss, loss of appetite.	The progression indicator asks for diagnostic imaging tests.
Advanced Stage	Severe pain, ascites, bowel obstruction.	The patient needs comprehensive palliative care along with symptom control.

Types of Pancreatic Cancer

There are two broad categories of pancreatic cancer depending on the type of cell in the pancreas in which it originates. Two of these types are: exocrine and endocrine cancers which differ in their function and how they affect the body.

1. Exocrine Tumors

Exocrine advertisement is the most prevalent type of cancerous cells that are observed in the pancreatic region. Of all the exocrine carcinomas, pancreatic ductal adenocarcinoma (PDAC) is the most aggressive and common (Luchini *et al.*, 2020). The cells that form the walls of pancreatic ducts transform into PDAC tumors since these cells produce enzymes released into the small intestine. Many of these enzymes are integral within the process of the digestion of the presented food substances into forms that can be assimilated by the rest of the body as nutrients. Exocrine tumors may grow at a slow pace but most of them are aggressive and they infiltrate surrounding tissue early. They tend to obstruct the bile duct which leads to jaundice and may then metastasize to other distant organs before symptoms are visible. The establishment of location and spread of pancreas, ducts, and tumor site can be visualized through high quality imaging (Figure 1). Exocrine cancer is invasive, quick to metastasize in the liver, stomach skeleton, lungs and intestines. It is common in these cancers to spread early and silently, resulting to late stages' diagnosis and less favorable prognosis. This comes out clearly to demonstrate that there is need to come up with better ways of screening and treatment methods for the early stage patients to be given in order to increase there chances of survival and gain a better prognosis.

2. Endocrine Tumors

Much like the exocrine tumors, neuroendocrine tumors also known as pancreatic neuroendocrine tumors (PNETs) are relatively rare (Cives & Strosberg, 2018). They occur from the hormone secreting cells in pancreas. These cells are of the endocrine system and synthesize important hormones include insulin which lowers blood sugar levels and glucagon which raises them. Since these tumours may disturb hormonal regulation, they may result in serious disruptions in the blood sugar levels, including hypoglycemica or hyperglycaemia.

Whether or not the tumor is functional (produces hormones) behaviorally varies in endocrine tumors. Tumors may lead to early symptoms of hormone manifesstion as being functional or not functional ones going on silently many years. The figure 2 shows pancreatic cells of endocrine and the examples of hormone-producing tumors. PNETs are less malignant as compared to exocrine tumors and grow slowly with a favorable prognosis. While functional PNETs release hormones that result in symptoms such as diarrhea or ulcers, non-functional ones do not have symptoms at early stages and cause symptoms only in the late stages. The moderate cases require stringent control since they cause a lot of harm to one's health.

1.2 Problems in Identification and Therapy

Early identification challenges

Personalized cancer vaccines that prompt the immune system to be trained to recognize specific proteins on the tumor of individual patients are being studied in recent research. Reducing the resistance of pancreatic cancer to immunotherapy is promising with PecCell new combinations that also contain checkpoint inhibitors and drugs that alter the tumor microenvironment. A primary limitation in the treatment of pancreatic cancer is that in most cases, the disease is diagnosed at a later stage. It is located in the deep internal cavity behind the stomach, liver and intestine; thus, palpation or visualization by normal physical examination procedures or conventional imaging cannot readily reveal its condition. Therefore, their manifestation is not typically recognisable until the disease stage is relatively far progressed (Stathis & Moore, 2010). Also very subtle signs might include vomiting, loss of appetite or back pains and many a time are considered to be flu like symptoms and cannot be easily diagnosed until the cancer has advanced to higher levels. Other established diagnostic methods have their own restrictions in practice that one needs to recognize. Essential ordinary investigations like CT scan and MRI are not sensitive to diagnosing early stage and small tumours. This implies that by the time that such a tumor shows up on these scans, it may have expanded in size or metastasized to other organs. Anthropometrics are another frequently used ways of checking on the state of pancreatic cancer; a blood test called CA19-9 is typical in this regard. These tests are not informative for early detection as CA19-9 levels may be rise due the presence of other disorders such as pancreatitis or gallstones (Liu *et al.*, 2018). Such limitations call for the development of better and reliable techniques for early diagnosis desperately.

Conventional diagnostic tools have significant limitations:

Imaging Techniques

The practical use of newer technologies, such as Endoscopic Ultrasound (EUS), enables the patient to have an up-close view of the interior of the digestive system by penetrating the mucous lining, which enhances small tumor diagnosis in pancreatic cancer. PET scans may trace the intake of radioactive glucose to demonstrate activity of cancer as well as point out tumors that a regular CT or MRI could not discover. A flowchart of the steps of the diagnostic process between initial symptoms and advanced imaging may be depicted in Figure 3. Pancreatic cancer is usually diagnosed using CT and MRI scans, however, small tumors without rich blood supply are difficult to detect on these scans in the early stages. In addition to that, the pancreas is located in the deep abdominal cavity and it is surrounded by other organs making identification of its position even more complex. Unnhappily, most of the patients are the diagnosed when the tumor is developed or has spread and therefore the treatment yields low outcomes. New ways of endoscopic investigation such as EUS and PET are more accurate than simple CT-scans. These innovations enhance early diagnoses since they reach parts inaccessible to the conventional imaging, thus improving chances for early diagnosis (Kasban et al., 2015).

Biomarker Tests

Some proteins, fragments of mutated DNA, and alteration of methylation patterns of DNA are studied as biomarkers. An example is KRAS mutant, present in more than 90 percent of pancreatic malignancies, and it may be observed in blood tests. A diagram (Figure 4) may indicate the process of biomarkers transiting tumor cells consequently into the bloodstream and being identified in testing laboratories. Tumor markers such as CA 19–9 and CEA help in the diagnosis of pancreatic cancer as well as assessment of its progression. It involves cytokine CA 19-9 produced in pancreatic cancer, which increases in the blood but is not very specific because its level increases in pancreatitis and gallstones. Though can be useful in disease progression, it is not very useful in diagnosing the disease at its early stage. Further biomarkers are then being investigated and CA19-9 is being used together with other tests in a bid to increase specificity in order to widespread use a blood test for the early diagnosis of pancreatic cancer (Chen et al., 2015).

Issues with Current Therapies

Treatment for pancreatic cancer is further complicated by the unique biology of the disease:

Dense Stromal Barrier: Pancreatic cancer remains challenging to treat for the simple fact that it is encased in a thick connective tissue called stroma. This kind of matrix of tissues and proteins was a barrier of membranes and cells, preventing chemo drugs and immune cells from reaching the tumor site inside the body. It also limits the oxygen supply and thus discourages the treatment of cancer cells. Although the stroma is a part of the body's defense system, in the case of pancreatic cancer it actually helps to prevent the therapy. Scientists are trying to overcome this barrier for a better drug delivery and improving the immunological reactions (Borst, 2012).

Chemoresistance: Chemoresistance is a significant issue in pancreatic cancer since the tumor mass develops ways of defending itself after administration of drugs such as gemcitabine. This hampers the efficacy of the drug, enabling the cancer to continue to-progress and even metastasize. Scientists are still in the process of engineering new drugs and identifying better use of nanoparticles for treatment of chemotherapy and overcoming resistance (Borst, 2012).

Pancreatic cancer tends to have high rates of recurrences with the inability of the condition returning after a successful operation within 1-2 years, necessitating effective long-term follow-ups.

Heterogeneity of Tumor: In a tumor, not all cancer cells act in a similar manner in response to treatment which makes treatment less effective.

Inadequate Screening Services: There exists no common method of screening the general populations with pancreatic cancer, in comparison to breast cancer or cancer of the colon since comparatively few patients are diagnosed early.

Limited Surgical Options: Surgery is often used to manage pancreatic cancer but is possible only in 10–20% of the patients. It is estimated that most of the diagnosis takes place when it is already too late, surgery cannot be performed. If done, it may be done in conjunction with the removal of parts of the pancreas, stomach or intestines. They indicate that for non-eligible patients, treatment aims at providing comfort through controlling the diseases via chemotherapy, radiation, or some experimental treatments (Griffin *et al.,* 2015).

1.3 How New Ideas Are Helping to Increase Hope

Early Detection Innovations

It is now well understood that this type of cancer is often diagnosed late, when the efficiency of the treatment thereof is comparatively low; however, new technologies are being introduced frequently allowing for early detection of pancreatic cancer and thus, enhancing the efficacies of the tumor treatment rates. Pancreatic cancer is typically diagnosed at an advanced stage, at which time the prognosis is poor; detection therefore must be made as soon as possible. Some of the recent innovations of value in this area are liquid biopsies and artificial intelligence that brings about a change in the diagnosis and treatment of this disease (Kenner et al., 2021).

Circulating tumor DNA is one of the important biomarkers in liquid biopsy that is a newly approved diagnostic test from a blood sample (Tang et al., 2024). This method used in diagnosis is done from circulating tumor DNA and does not require surgery or any typical biopsy results. Liquid biopsies even better compared to traditional diagnosis reveal present carcinogenic changes, track tumor growth, and evaluate treatment outcomes. This makes a significant change in the diagnosis and treatment of pancreatic cancer.AI integrates CT and MRI data and thus, detects the patterns that patients with pancreatic cancer do not show. It makes comparisons, reminds the radiologists about suspicious regions, enhances the diagnosis, and shortens the diagnosis time, helping start the treatment at an early stage and ultimately positively influencing the survival rate (Hunter et al., 2022). Recent advancements in liquid biopsy, artificial intelligence for diagnosis and treatment provide more chances of success in treatment for patients. Pancreatic cancer research is vigorous and consequently, there have been new developments in the care of this disease.

Breakthroughs in Treatment

New treatments are unfolding the defects of former therapies and became the hope for the patients:

Precision Medicine: They are the specific treatment as well as diagnosis of diseases based on specific genetic profile of a certain person (Duffy, 2016). In pancreatic cancer, PARP inhibitors are used to treat the BRCA mutated patients because they prevent DNA repair pathway in cancer cells. It increases the efficiency of the treatment and thus has minimal side effects on the normal cells (Perkhofer et al., 2021). Precision medicine refers to the use of a tailored approach to treatment and is ideal in dealing since it aligns with the general goals of enhancing quantity and quality of life of the patients as well as minimizing the side effects of some treatments.

Immunotherapy: Immunotherapy refers to the use of the patient's immune system to fight cancer. Some of the promising strategies with respect to pancreatic cancer consist of checkpoint inhibitors, which revitalise immune cells to address the malignant tissues, and CAR-T cell therapy that modifies the immune cells to attack cancerous cells. However some obstacles, such as the possibility of having a dense stroma can be a downfall. New findings show that immunotherapy can better enhance the chemotherapy setting than overcoming barriers and patient success rates (Madorsky Rowdo et al., 2015).

Nanotechnology: Nanotechnology in delivering drugs for pancreatic cancer has undergone significant changes in the past. The sites of drug delivery through nanoparticles can also include the dense stromal barrier wherein the anti-cancer agents get delivered at the tumor site. This makes chemotherapy to be more effective with a less harm on the healthy cells; this increases the efficiency of the treatment besides reducing on side effects (Bahrami et al., 2017).

Comprehensive Patient Care

Consequently, besides the progression in diagnosing and managing this disease, supportive care is becoming an essential and valuable intervention for the patients. Unlike previous techniques that were only concerned with eradicating the tumor these procedures aim at helping patients and families live better lives. The supportive care includes tele health, palliative care, and psychosocial and nutritional support tailored to the needs of patient's with pancreatic cancer.

Telehealth Services: It is hard to overestimate the significance of telehealth in the process of increasing alone access to healthcare for a variety of populations, including but not limited to people in rural areas. This helps the patients avoid physical distress caused by traveling to access the services through teletriage, teleconsultation, and telemonitoring equipment. Telehealth also offers timely consultation, reviews patients' treatment progress and keeps up the patient-physician relationship (Lin et al., 2018).

Palliative Care: This chapter aims to determine satisfaction with and attitudes towards palliative care of pancreatic cancer patients, asserting that effective palliative care can lead to both increase in quantity and quality of life of such patients through controlling of pains and other symptoms. This is most essential in terminal phase where curative care can no longer be applied. Measures such as nerve blocks, antiemetics, and respiratory support make them less uncomfortable and respect the dignity of a person (Agarwal & Epstein, 2017).

Emotional and Nutritional Support: Pancreatic cancer impacts one's quality of life in areas of the body such as the physical, mental, and nutrition states. These references establish that support groups help in mitigaging depression, anxiety, and social isolation. Children may face some digestion issues as well as appetite loss as an effect of the disease and its treatment. Nurses give prescription of meals for enhancing energy, general health, and living standards (Lin et al., 2015).

2. NEW WAYS TO DETECT PANCREATIC CANCER

2.1 Problems with Traditional Tests

Diagnostic procedures used for pancreatic cancer have drawbacks, and they rarely diagnose the disease at a curable stage. One of the largest concerns is that the organ is located internally deep in the body, thus, cannot be observed easily throughout physical check-up. Cancer diagnosis can be made using CT and MRI but large carcinoma may not detect small-sized carcinomas in early stages. Still, these imaging tools have certain drawbacks, the major of which may result in missing a malignant lesion or invading a benign one.

The second common diagnostic procedure is blood test – CA19-9, which indicates signs of increased protein in pancreatic cancer cases. This test is not prone to early detection even though it is applicable in observing the advancement of the disease. However, CA19-9 is raised in other diseases such as pancreatitis or gallstones, which give false-third, DES-γ can also be upregulated in conditions other than PDAC, and thus give false positives. On the other hand, some patient with pancreatic cancer might present with normal CA19-9, which makes it give an outlook of negative results. These limitations however escalate the need for better and early detection methods.

Diagnostic Journey for Pancreatic Cancer

Figure 1.

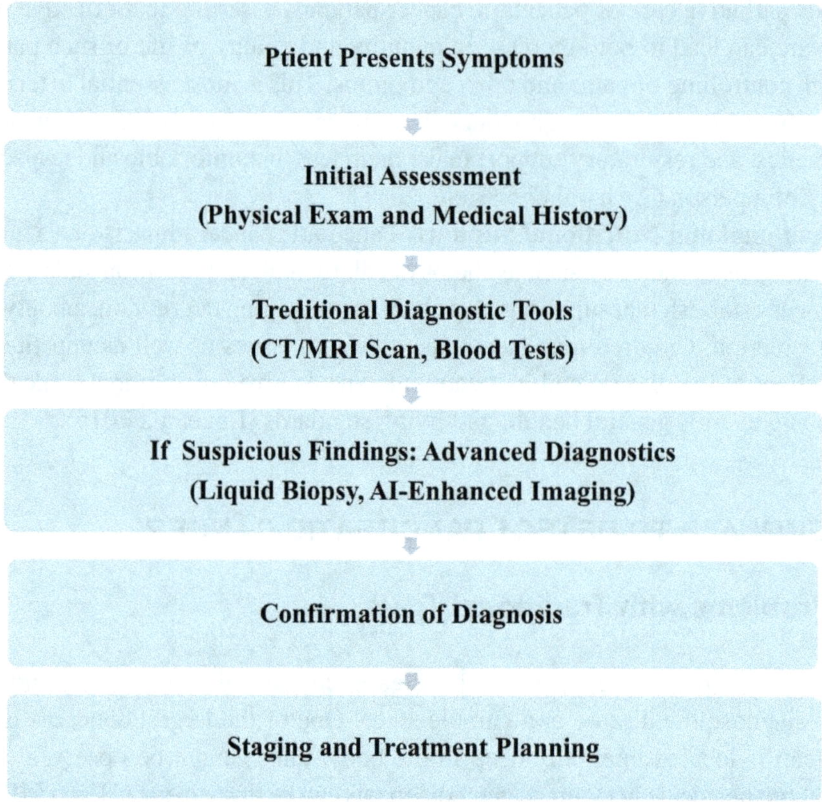

2.2 Liquid Biopsy: A Blood Test for Early Diagnosis

It is now clear that liquid biopsy is revolutionizing the diagnostic and therapeutic profiles of pancreatic cancer through offering a noninvasive approach to biopsy. Specifically, the conventional biopsies involve invasive means of obtaining tissue samples from the tumor, usually through surgery that may prove challenging and dangerous in overall system-threatening situations to the patient, including being in a frail physical condition. On the other hand, liquid biopsies are a blood test for nucleic acids and proteins released by cancer cells into the stream of blood plasma. This make such process safer, quicker, and comfortable for patients compared to other traditional procedures. Out of all the promising features of liquid biopsy, the greatest value is its early detection capabilities of pancreatic cancer compared with traditional approaches. Given that doctors can detect the presence of ctDNA and other biomarkers of early-stage disease well before symptoms develop, a greatly increased likelihood of successful treatment of the disease can be achieved. Pancreatic cancer is more often diagnosed at an advanced stage and hence early diagnosis is very important to increase the effectiveness of the treatment. Besides, the value of liquid biopsy consists in its ability to dynamically monitor pancreatic cancer progression and response to therapy (Santarpia *et al.,* 2018). Since ctDNA concentrations can change with time, the dynamics of the tumor and the efficiency of therapy can be determined. This has the advantage of enabling a doctor modifies a separate treatment if one particular technique turns out to be ineffectual. Liquid biopsy also includes genetic and molecular tumor characteristics for treatment choice of the cancer's vulnerable points, reducing toxicity and improving efficiency. This patient-oriented approach privatizes the treatment of pancreatic cancer into a flexible and accurate plan, improving the lives of patients with such a deadly illness.

Table 2. Types of Biomarkers for Pancreatic Cancer Detection

Biomarker Type	Example	Clinical Use
Protein Biomarkers	CA19-9, CEA	Monitors disease progression and treatment response.
Genetic Biomarkers	KRAS mutations	Identifies high-risk individuals; aids in targeted therapies.
Epigenetic Biomarkers	DNA methylation patterns	Early detection and risk assessment.
Immune Biomarkers	Cytokine levels	Evaluates immune response to therapies.

2.3 The Roles of Artificial Intelligence in Reducing Error Rates with Traditional Tests

AI is now transforming the field of pancreatic cancer diagnosis due to many drawbacks linked to conventional diagnosing processes. AI relies on the analysis of large doses of imaging losses; studies the CT or MRI images which can reveal the emerging signs of pancreatic cancer. These patterns can get very fine and highly multilayered, and, as a rule, it is very difficult to enhance and make obvious for everyone, including experienced radiologists. Introducing some level of artificial intelligence into the diagnostic situations allows the doctors to reveal patterns that are not discernable usually, making the diagnosis attempts much more accurate (Hameed & Krishnan, 2022). When implemented in the diagnosis of pancreatic cancer AI technology is hence highly significant in the reduction of diagnostic errors. In particular, they can identify cancer accurately and thereby minimising the false positive rates that indicate cancer is present but actually is not, and the false negative rates that deny a cancer is present although it is. But this level of precision is important to guarantee that the patients get the right treatment at the right time. In addition, with the help of AI, diagnostic activities are optimized due to the high-speed analysis of imaging data and possible areas of malignancy. This makes it possible for those healthcare providers to provide attention to patients who are critical and make faster decisions on other patients' treatment. AI technology performs superior disease diagnosis when supported with liquid biopsy tools. As far as liquid biopsy data is integrated with imaging, a detailed picture of the state of the disease is possible using an artificial neural network and the results can be personalized for each user. These aspects point to speed, accuracy and crucially personalisation which accentuates the role of AI in conquering pancreatic cancer (Ginghina *et al.*, 2022).

2.4 Real Stories: Where These Methods Are Helpful to the Patients

It is evident that the results of these new diagnostic approaches are best illustrated by patient's success stories of early and accurate diagnosis (Talley & O'Connor, 2010). For instance, a patient complaining of mere fatigue and random stomach aches was given a liquid biopsy after normal tests proved inconclusive. This study found ctDNA of pancreatic cancer by biopsy and received a early diagnose and early treatment. Early intertvention enhanced the patient's outcome and lifestyle. For instance, AI imaging systems detected a tiny tumor that was not seen in another scan. This approach was very productive because for the first time doctors were able to start treatment of the disease when it was still early, when the disease had not fully developed and killed the patient. Such stories are the vivid example that liquid biopsies and AI are not only equipment but the means that influence the fight for the defeat of PCa.

Table 3. Comparison of Traditional and Innovative Pancreatic Cancer Detection Methods

Methods	Description	Advantages	Limitations
CT/MRI Scans	Diverse methods exist to observe tumors through images.	Widely available; non-invasive.	It struggles to find small malignant growths before they become advanced.
Liquid Biopsy	Blood test to detect tumor DNA/proteins.	The method tests without affecting the body to find issues before they become severe.	Not yet universally standardized.
Artificial Intelligence	Studies medical visual images and patient data for recognizable patterns.	High accuracy; reduces diagnostic errors.	It demands sophisticated computing systems.

3. THE PRESENT MANAGEMENT AND CONVENTIONAL CHEMOTHERAPEUTIC APPROACHES TO PANCREATIC CANCER

Pancreatic cancer is one of the most difficult cancers to manage because of its aggressiveness and, in most cases, when diagnosed. Today's management plans involve surgery, chemotherapy, radiation, and supportive care to increase patients' lifespan and the quality of that lifespan. However, the initial treatment using conventional chemotherapy based on gemcitabine typically proves ineffective because the tumor establishes multiple defensive strategies along with dense stromal development. For that reason, new approaches that are beginning to emerge include precision medicine as well as Immunotherapy.

3.1 Precision Medicine: Personalized Gene-Based Cancer Treatment

According to clinical trials, patients with tumor-specific therapy have response rates and a reduction in side effects. This has been shown in e.g. the POLO trial that showed that BRCA-mutant patients with pancreatic cancer survived significantly longer without their disease progressing when they got a PARP inhibitor rather than usual chemotherapy. During personalized medicine physicians adapt medical treatments specifically for tumor genetics. That is why genetics and biomarkers allow for pinpointing practices that might work for a particular case and avoiding using treatments proven being ineffective in other cases. This in pancreatic cancer involves isolating them to mutations in other genes that include KRAS, TP53, CDKN2A,

SMAD4 genes. The practice of precision medicine includes targeted therapy as one example as demonstrated with PARP inhibitors for individuals with BRCA-mutant cancers. These therapies; not only make the treatment effective and efficient, but they also reduce side effects as compared to normal chemotherapy. Today, gene-based cancer treatment has become an undeniable part of the modern approach to treating pancreatic cancer because of the introduction of the next-generation sequencing and bioinformatics tools (Sisodiya, 2021).

3.2 Immunotherapy: Aiding the Immune System against Cancer

Cancer can be treated with the assistance of a patients own immune system through immunotherapy. In pancreatic cancer, however, this is especially difficult because the environment surrounding the tumor inhibits the activity of the immune system to detect the cancer. The drugs that treat cancer through immune checkpoint inhibitors, such as PD-1/PD-L1, and CTLA-4 have been effective in some forms of cancers but have not been equally helpful in pancreatic cancer, which tends to be immunosuppressive. These are issues that applicable to older immunotherapy approaches but newer immunotherapy approaches are being entertained. Novel cancer vaccines are designed to prompt immune response specific to particular types of tumour cells. CAR T cell therapy is actually a method of reprogramming a patient's immune system for it to focus on cancer. Immunotherapy can also be used together with other treatments, including chemotherapy or radiation, to get around the tumor's shield. These strategies lay the prospect for garnering a more hopeful immunotherapy method in the treatment of pancreatic cancer (Koury *et al.*, 2018).

3.3 Aiding Together: Complementary Treatment for a Better Outcome

It can be supposed that integrating conventional and NBM techniques alongside embedded innovative methodologies such as precision medicine and immunotherapy will have an additive effect on the efficiency of the treatments. For example, it has been known that combining chemotherapeutic drugs with immune checkpoint inhibitors or targets both improves the efficacy. Also, supportive care has a central role in treatment of the condition as well moving forward. As for possible treatments, nutritional support, psychological counselling, pain relieving are the key factors in the enhancement of quality of life of the pancreatic cancer patients. The employment of interdisciplinary care in that it pulls together professionals from a number of different backgrounds guarantees that all the needs of a patient are met. There is therefore a strong possibility that by combining traditional and innovative treatment with supportive care, physicians can offer improved clinical results as well as give a much more favorable care experience for pancreatic cancer patients (Kolbeinsson *et al.*, 2023).

4. NANOTECHNOLOGY: A SMARTER WAY TO DELIVER MEDICINE

Conventional systems of treatment of pancreatic cancer have low efficiency, but use of nanotechnology is a new concept on this field. Since it is targeted to kill cancerous cells, the drugs also impact the normal cells hence causing side effects such as nausea and fatigue. Nanoparticles are used in drug delivery to get to the tumor directly thus minimizing side effects and increasing the effectiveness of the treatment. They also invade the compact stromal layer that hinders other treatments, enhancing administration of medication in later stages. In the same way, the use of nanoparticles can transport one or several drugs or imaging agents, thus ensuring the accuracy in treatment of the disease. It, however, shows that nanotechnology opens new horizons in treating pancreatic cancer since conventional therapy has limitations resulting in unfavorable outcomes including side effects (Gavas et al., 2021).

4.1 How Nanoparticles Deliver Drugs to Cancer

Nano particles are beneficial in treatment, as it ensures that it gets to the cancer cells so therapy can be constitutional. They exploit features of tumors, for example, they penetrate the disordered vascular structure of tumors, they utilise the EPR effect that means that it accumulates in tumors due to the incompetent blood vessels in the tumor. Cancer cells are more often surrounded by vessels with larger size of gaps, thus making it possible for nanoparticles to penetrate inside the tumor sites than in the healthy tissues. This targeted delivery reduces the lethal impact to normal cells and improves therapeutic efficiency.This treatment can be endangered with many types of Amphiophilic nanoparticles containing numerous therapeutic loads Chemo paediatric, genetic, and immunologic. These particles are designed to deliver their payload in response to triggers associated with the tumor micro environment such as changes in pH or the presence of specific enzymes in the tumor. The treatment is delivered on a smart infrastructure to where it is required most; thus, the side effect is gently controlled (Sugahara *et al.,* 2009).

Liposomes, dendrimers and polymeric nanoparticles are deemed important nanocarriers in pancreatic cancer treatment. Liposomes, lipid vesicles, are used to convey both aqueous and lipid-soluble pharmaceuticals hence exhibiting an elongated shelf-life. Dendrimers which are branched macromolecules are primarily applied in terms of drug delivery either on the outer rim of dendrimers or within the body of dendrimers. Polymeric nanoparticles which are synthesized from biodegradable polymers make it possible to control the rate of release of the drug. These nanocarriers improve the solubility, stability, and hence the bioavailability for metabolism of the drugs. As it is revealed that nanoparticles do not harm the healthy tissues but instead it focuses on the tumors, cancer treatment is made precise, flexible and beneficial to the patients. These two characteristics make them a formidable weapon in cancer treatment.

4.2 Removing Barriers to Treatment: Safer and More Effective Options for Patients

This chapter focuses on ways by which nanotechnology enhances the management of pancreatic cancer by overcoming resistance and side effects of the treatment. Non-target therapies affect healthy cells adversely, while nano particles shield drug molecules and target them efficiently on the cancerous tissues minimizing side effects. This makes them capable of effectively delivering the administered drug to the target site which is surrounded by a tightly packed stroma. Nanoparticles are also imaging agents which facilitate monitoring of the treatment in the course of its implementation. Also, they allow the administration of a combinatorial treatment such as chemotherapy as well as immunotherapy. Nanotechnology increases the effectiveness of treatment by delivering accurate, safer and individualized treatments, and increases the patients' well-being during the cancer therapy.

5. GENE EDITING AND PERSONALIZED TREATMENT MODELS

Genetic deficiencies are the focus on individualizing treatment and gene editing in the management of pancreatic cancer. These create better and personalised therapy, hence a better way of handling a disease, which has always been challenging to treat while at the same time providing variety in the treatment of every patient.

5.1 CRISPR-Cas9: Repairing Damage to DNA That Leads to Cancer

CRISPR-Cas9 is relatively new technology that can modify the DNA sequences at certain position in the genome assignation. This tool known as molecular scissors may be used to remove, mend or replace unhealthy DNA strands is a tool that can trim the DNA at preferred locations. Research in pancreatic cancer is to make use of CRISPR-Cas9 to get rid of having the bad genes that lead to cancer development. For example, KRAS that is often mutated in pancreatic cancer may be targeted to decrease malignant growth promoting ability of it. Similarly, molecules like tumor suppressor genes including TP53 genes which are commonly mutated to develop cancer can be repaired to fight against cancer.

Nevertheless, in addition to editing the genes in cancer cells, CRISPR-Cas9 utilises the intensification of the immune response to pancreatic cancer. In details, they said that various methods in science can modify the immune cells to have better detection on the tumors and then attack them. In a therapeutic context, CRISPR-Cas9 is highly toxic to cancer cells and capable of modulating the immune system; in an analytical context, the same genes are lethal to cancer cells. Additionally, this technology is helping in describing the function of DNA alternations in the process of pancreatic cancer and also in writing experimental treatment plans employing model systems.

Table 4. Advancements in Pancreatic Cancer Therapies

Therapy Type	Mechanism	Benefits	Current Challenges
Immunotherapy	Enhances the immune system to attack tumors.	Durable responses in some patients.	Limited efficacy in dense stromal environments.
Nanotechnology	Sends medications straight to cancer cells.	The combination establishes both reduced side effects and enhanced drug effectiveness.	High production costs; scaling for clinical use.
CRISPR-Cas9 Gene Editing	The process both detects and removes faulty DNA patterns.	Targets cancer at the genetic level.	Ethical concerns; requires further testing.

5.2 Mini-Tumors in the Lab: Outlining the Right Treatment for Every Single Person

Organoids which many refer to as mini-tumors are laboratory generated models developed from a patient's malignant cells. These three-dimensional structures are very similar to the original tumor in terms of their architecture, genetics and molecular characteristic. By enabling the in vitro identification of optimal treatments and the assessment of a company's success in identifying drugs that are effective for a certain patient and a specific product, organoids are a very valuable tool in drug development.

It will briefly explain what organoid is to create an organoid tissue biopsy from the patient's tumor is collected and grown under controlled conditions in culture media that replicates the physiologic conditions within the human body. When the organoid is developed then it may be treated with any drug or can be put on different treatments. In this manner, the researchers are able to control the behavior of the mini-tumor and determine which treatment plan is good for this specific patient. Such an approach also avoids a trial and error when choosing the treatment and it reduces unnecessary side effects as well as enhances the possibility of success. In the case of pancreatic cancer, where patients have few treatment options, organoids give hope for better treatment results (Corrò *et al.*, 2020).

5.3 How Research is applied to Practical Use

In the current healthcare environment, for advances in promising research such as gene editing and organoid models to become applied in clinical practice, the respective scientists must incorporate clinicians into collaborations, as well as involve leaders in the private sector.The role of clinical trials proves essential to treatment development because they test experimental treatments on patients beyond the target patient category while therapeutic methods remain restricted. Clinical trials establish required evidence which regulatory bodies need for approval of new therapies to reach patients.Applications of CRISPR-Cas9 and organoids are a few reagent to face issues on manufacturability, training and costs. However, there is an indication that there is growth in bridging the gap between research and practice. Interactions between research centers and hospitals should be fostered for the improvement of personalized medicine. Organs on chip or organoids are changing the diagnosis and guaranteeing personalized treatment. These improved gene or tailored therapies for pancreatic cancer illustrates the role of science in bringing about positive change as well as offering hope and better survival to patients nor only in Northeast Ohio but across the globe.

6. BETTER SUPPORT FOR PATIENTS

The treatment of pancreatic cancer combines medical approaches with comprehensive patient care because pancreatic cancer requires personalized healthcare that addresses their physical and mental situations. In this way, the sick person and his or her family improve quality of support in health care services, which is achieved by the implementation of new strategies by health care providers.

6.1 Telehealth: Linking Patients with Doctors Anywhere

From the virtual care perspective, the patient gets to easily consult and there has also been enhanced patient involvement in communicating with the clinicians. Most pancreatic cancer patients would find this technology beneficial because they cannot travel because of their health limitations or because treatment facilities lie in remote areas. Telehealth offers a way to receive consultation from medical professionals, attend follow-up appointments and control symptoms without physical travel. This helps to reduce patient and caregiver burden, it also helps to ensure that quality of care that is being delivered is consistent. Besides that, with the help of telehealth platforms, the actual record of symptoms can be taken in real time, as well as the changes in the treatment strategies can be made considering the symptoms that are most common at the particular time, thus, early intervention to enhance outcomes for patients can be made (Lin *et al.*, 2018).

6.2 Full Understanding of New Approaches to Pain Relief and Comfort

The continued relevance of addressing the issue of pain relief for patients with pancreatic cancer is partly due to the fact that several patients that completed the survey expressed severe pain from the disease or its treatment. The management of this particular difficulty is getting much better solutions from other improvements of analgesia technologies. For instance, nerve blocks exclude specific pain tracts for an extended duration, while specific drug delivery systems ensure medicines work where pain is present without having undesirable side effects. For example, changes to the invasive treatments such as acupuncture, therapeutic massage, and the application of complementary modalities to decreased stress and improved patient relaxation in addition to conventional care is also under review (Nichols, 2018). With these knowledge and understandings of these methods, health care providers are in a meaningful position to develop client specific pain management interventions that does not only aim toward pain reduction but also toward the suffering and emocional quality of life of patients.

6.3 Caring for Both Body and Mind

The holistic care means that instead of attending only such things that have to do with sickness or diseases, the patient is seen as a whole entity or complete person. It gets worse that the pancreatic cancer is also toxic to the mental health of the patent, causing anxiety, depression, and loneliness. In order to resolve these problems, the Key service areas comprise Psychological support service including counseling and support/therapy groups. By providing these services the patients experience decreased loneliness and receive valuable coping mechanisms with their symptoms while maintaining a safe space for mutual sharing. Moreover, harmonizing practices such as, yoga, meditation or other mindfulness practices build the psychological robustness of the personal suffering from such diseases. Even more important is the relationship of nutrition to an integral concept, as pancreatic cancer can have an effect on digestion and appetite. We go on ensuring that patient obtain individual counselling so that they take the appropriate diet required to gain their nutritional health back.

Addressing the physical and mental health of the patient, the patient-centered, complementary, and integrative therapy only makes patients better and enables them to fight the diseases of pancreatic cancer. Altogether these supportive interventions are changing perceptions on the experience of cancer care for patients and their families as they embrace yet another ray of hope in combating this unpleasant disease (Nichols, 2018).

7. PREVENTION STRATEGIES INFORMING PRACTICE

Pancreatic cancer is a major global health issue, and prevention in addition to early diagnosis remains of paramount important in managing the disease. There are ongoing multidisciplinary approaches by different specialists and evolution in research to develop best practices in managing the disease.

7.1 How Specialists across Disciplines Collaborate

This means that, in the prevention regime, there must be collaboration between oncologists, geneticists, dietitians, and the primary care physicians. In this way, these specialists make sure that a patient is given uniform recommendations on how to change their lifestyle, genetic profiling, and the screening protocols. For instance, in case of risk factors such as smoking, obesity and family history, different discipline involvement is mandatory. Oncologists give information on how cancer progresses, geneticists tell patients when they are at risk for hereditary cancers, dietitians suggest modifications in diet to reduce the risk and primary care physicians include all of these into their recommendations to patients. Such coordination will help patients to have adequate information as well as recommendable tips that they may require in order reducing their risks of being diagnosed with pancreatic cancer (Minor, 2020).

7.2 Practical New Research and Favorable Trials

Current research and clinical trials are identifying new technologies and ways of avoiding pancreatic cancer. Some of the most useful piece of information has been obtained from research that focused on anti-inflammatory agents, diet specifics, and the discovery of early biomarkers. For instance, scientists are studying how some pieces of the diet plan have an effect on inflammation; this is a factor in the occurrence of cancer. Clinical biomarkers, and more specifically in the stage of early detection, are giving the tools to know who has a higher risk in order to avoid the corresponding risks before cancer is created.

These discoveries are also being disseminated in form of practical measures to be taken by health workers to encourage proper preventive measures amongst the community. Studies that involve patient education work concerning disease prevention and bringing forth change in risky behaviors such as smoking cessation and better dieting are already paying off. Other potential prevention strategies stem from clinical trials considering new therapeutic methodologies including anti-inflammatory medications or vaccines developments that can focus on precancerous diseases of the pancreas potentially holding other potential for decreasing the rates of pancreatic cancer. Implementing the presented data in actual clinical practice allows lowering the likelihood of pancreatic cancer onset and improving the quality of living among high-risk population (Sohal *et al.*, 2016).

Essential Measures for Risk Reduction and Prevention Comprise Risk

Figure 2.

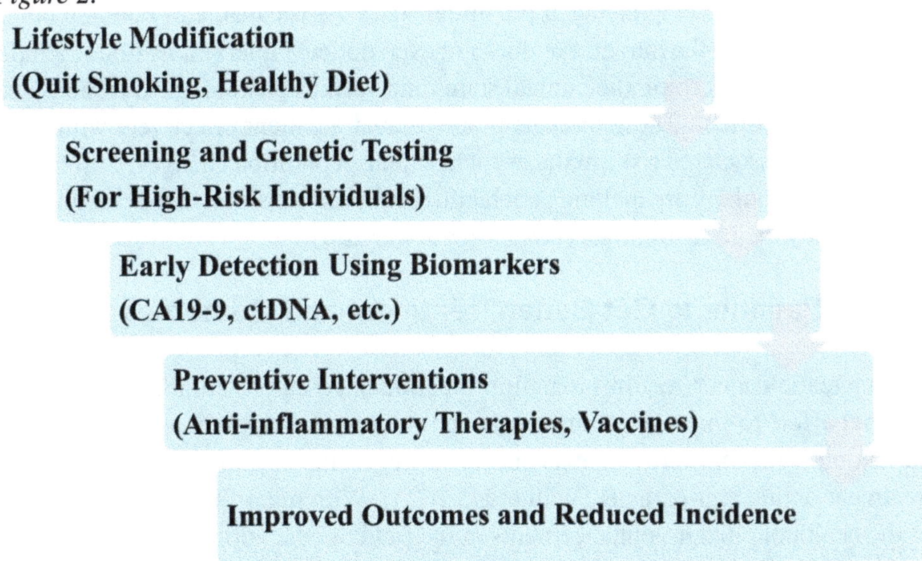

8. LOOKING AHEAD

Recent technological and research development and the model of care that is patient-focused are all creating better approaches to pancreatic cancer treatment.

8.1 Total Quality Management (TQM) Stand alongside New Key Innovations

Healthcare delivery through TQM research proposes an effective management concept which focuses on constant gradual enhancement of the quality and performance within the healthcare organizations. By introducing TQM principles in to the operations system within the hospitals and clinics, it becomes possible to enhance the performance and reduce the number of mistakes made. For the patients who have pancreatic cancer, this means more early diagnose precise therapeutic management, as well as efficient further treatment.

In the same manner, innovations in treatment process of pancreatic cancer cannot be ignored. Machine learning (ML) is redefining diagnostics where large data sets are used for predicting Individuals risk levels and chances of cancer at an early stage. First, let me share an example of how some biological activities might be improved Ag: To the extent of diagnosing at the initial stage, AI is capable of noticing other details in scans that the human eye does not even notice. Other innovations include wearables and concerning the clinical status and various physiological response of the particular patient. These tools help one to treat a patient effectively with least likelihood of associated risks in the event a patient's condition changes. Combined, TQM and technology are making pancreatic cancer a system that helps patients and delivers only the best solutions (Langabeer *et al.,* 2009).

8.2 For Patients to Get Better Treatment and Outcomes

Pancreatic cancer requires a multiprofessional, research, clinical, policy, and national effort to improve its diagnosis and treatment. It identifies how that collaboration helps in improving existence of novel therapies and availability of new treatment options for patients (Wall et al., 2023). With regard to the improvement of the health of citizens, enhancements in the field of education of health facilities and diagnostic instruments facilitate the minimization of inequalities and offer high-quality treatments for cancer.

Patient activation is as important as patient education, where the patient is informed about his disease, his experience in the hospital. Families choose the right kind of treatment for their kids when informed. The NM advocacy activities such as psychological support, counseling, meeting the patients, and providing them with necessary resources help to enhance the quality of life and hope among the patients. Thus, pancreatic cancer management today largely depends on available technologies, team work, and patient education. The gradual and sustained continued research and practice efforts contribute promising approaches to the disease and for the improvement of the patient condition.

Table 5. Challenges and Future Directions in Pancreatic Cancer Research

Challenge	Description	Future Directions
Late Diagnosis	Most cases are diagnosed at advanced stages.	Develop more reliable early detection methods like AI and biomarkers.
Drug Resistance	Tumors adapt to chemotherapy over time.	The exploration of new combination treatment strategies and the use of nanotechnology products should be pursued.
Dense Stromal Barrier	Prevents drugs from reaching the tumor.	Research stromal-disrupting therapies.
Patient Awareness	Lack of awareness leads to delayed diagnosis.	Public education campaigns must receive increased focus.

CONCLUSION

Pancreatic cancer is a very deadly cancer because of its invasiveness and the challenge to identify it at its earlier stages and minimal reaction to conventional medicine. But this situation is altering due to scientific and technological innovations. Combined with traditional treatments, namely, chemotherapy, radiation and surgery, precision medicine, targeting precise genetic alteration including BRCA1/2 mutation with drugs like PARP inhibitors, can enhance the efficiency of treatment and decrease side effects. Immunotherapy is also an upcoming hope as it beats the immune resistant condition of the tumor through the procedure of immune checkpoint blockers, cancer vaccines and combinations and chemotherapy or radiations. Nanotechnology enhances the drug delivery process in that the drug is used to attack specific cancerous cells by causing the least damage possible to the rest of the body, and it also offers the chance to diagnose the disease earlier due to skills of the advanced laboratory photographed method. The innovations are reinforced with prolonged patient care (relieving pain, feeding, and psychological support). The treatment of pancreatic cancer has become the topic of multidisciplinary cooperation of doctors, geneticists, immunologists, engineers, and other professionals to come up with new treatment options and test them in clinical trials. Needs based and preferences oriented care, or simply patient-centered care is also vital as it improves the quality of life. With scientific knowledge and the help of the so-called five Rs, which include Right patient, Right drug, Right dose, Right route, and Right time, the treatment difficulties may be minimized, survival rates may be increased, and the hope of the patients may be restored.

REFERENCES

Agarwal, R., & Epstein, A. S. (2017). Palliative care and advance care planning for pancreas and other cancers. *Linchuang Zhongliuxue Zazhi*, *6*(3), 32. PMID: 28705009

Bahrami, B., Hojjat-Farsangi, M., Mohammadi, H., Anvari, E., Ghalamfarsa, G., Yousefi, M., & Jadidi-Niaragh, F. (2017). Nanoparticles and targeted drug delivery in cancer therapy. *Immunology Letters*, *190*, 64–83. DOI: 10.1016/j.imlet.2017.07.015 PMID: 28760499

Borst, P. (2012). Cancer drug pan-resistance: Pumps, cancer stem cells, quiescence, epithelial to mesenchymal transition, blocked cell death pathways, persisters or what? *Open Biology*, *2*(5), 120066. DOI: 10.1098/rsob.120066 PMID: 22724067

Chen, Y., Gao, S. G., Chen, J. M., Wang, G. P., Wang, Z. F., Zhou, B., & Feng, X. S. (2015). Serum CA242, CA199, CA125, CEA, and TSGF are biomarkers for the efficacy and prognosis of cryoablation in pancreatic cancer patients. *Cell Biochemistry and Biophysics*, *71*(3), 1287–1291. DOI: 10.1007/s12013-014-0345-2 PMID: 25486903

Cives, M., & Strosberg, J. R. (2018). Gastroenteropancreatic neuroendocrine tumors. *CA: a Cancer Journal for Clinicians*, *68*(6), 471–487. DOI: 10.3322/caac.21493 PMID: 30295930

Corrò, C., Novellasdemunt, L., & Li, V. S. (2020). A brief history of organoids. *American Journal of Physiology. Cell Physiology*, *319*(1), C151–C165. DOI: 10.1152/ajpcell.00120.2020 PMID: 32459504

Cortesi, L., Rugo, H. S., & Jackisch, C. (2021). An overview of PARP inhibitors for the treatment of breast cancer. *Targeted Oncology*, *16*(3), 255–282. DOI: 10.1007/s11523-021-00796-4 PMID: 33710534

Duffy, D. J. (2016). Problems, challenges and promises: Perspectives on precision medicine. *Briefings in Bioinformatics*, *17*(3), 494–504. DOI: 10.1093/bib/bbv060 PMID: 26249224

Gavas, S., Quazi, S., & Karpiński, T. M. (2021). Nanoparticles for cancer therapy: Current progress and challenges. *Nanoscale Research Letters*, *16*(1), 173. DOI: 10.1186/s11671-021-03628-6 PMID: 34866166

Ginghina, O., Hudita, A., Zamfir, M., Spanu, A., Mardare, M., Bondoc, I., & Galateanu, B. (2022). Liquid biopsy and artificial intelligence as tools to detect signatures of colorectal malignancies: A modern approach in patient's stratification. *Frontiers in Oncology*, *12*, 856575. DOI: 10.3389/fonc.2022.856575 PMID: 35356214

Griffin, J. F., Poruk, K. E., & Wolfgang, C. L. (2015). Pancreatic cancer surgery: Past, present, and future. *Chinese Journal of Cancer Research = Chung-Kuo Yen Cheng Yen Chiu, 27*(4), 332. PMID: 26361403

Hameed, B. S., & Krishnan, U. M. (2022). Artificial intelligence-driven diagnosis of pancreatic cancer. *Cancers (Basel), 14*(21), 5382. DOI: 10.3390/cancers14215382 PMID: 36358800

Hunter, B., Hindocha, S., & Lee, R. W. (2022). The role of artificial intelligence in early cancer diagnosis. *Cancers (Basel), 14*(6), 1524. DOI: 10.3390/cancers14061524 PMID: 35326674

Kasban, H., El-Bendary, M. A. M., & Salama, D. H. (2015). A comparative study of medical imaging techniques. *International Journal of Information Science and Intelligent System, 4*(2), 37–58.

Kenner, B., Chari, S. T., Kelsen, D., Klimstra, D. S., Pandol, S. J., Rosenthal, M., & Wolpin, B. (2021). Artificial intelligence and early detection of pancreatic cancer: 2020 summative review. *Pancreas, 50*(3), 251–279. DOI: 10.1097/MPA.0000000000001762 PMID: 33835956

Kolbeinsson, H. M., Chandana, S., Wright, G. P., & Chung, M. (2023). Pancreatic cancer: A review of current treatment and novel therapies. *Journal of Investigative Surgery, 36*(1), 2129884. DOI: 10.1080/08941939.2022.2129884 PMID: 36191926

Koury, J., Lucero, M., Cato, C., Chang, L., Geiger, J., Henry, D., & Tran, A. (2018). Immunotherapies: Exploiting the immune system for cancer treatment. *Journal of Immunology Research, 2018*(1), 9585614. DOI: 10.1155/2018/9585614 PMID: 29725606

Langabeer, J. R., DelliFraine, J. L., Heineke, J., & Abbass, I. (2009). Implementation of Lean and Six Sigma quality initiatives in hospitals: A goal theoretic perspective. *Operations Management Research : Advancing Practice Through Research, 2*(1-4), 13–27. DOI: 10.1007/s12063-009-0021-7

Lin, C. C., Han, C. Y., & Pan, I. J. (2015). A qualitative approach of psychosocial adaptation process in patients undergoing long-term hemodialysis. *Asian Nursing Research, 9*(1), 35–41. DOI: 10.1016/j.anr.2014.10.007 PMID: 25829208

Lin, C. C. C., Dievler, A., Robbins, C., Sripipatana, A., Quinn, M., & Nair, S. (2018). Telehealth in health centers: Key adoption factors, barriers, and opportunities. *Health Affairs, 37*(12), 1967–1974. DOI: 10.1377/hlthaff.2018.05125 PMID: 30633683

Liu, W., Liu, Q., Wang, W., Wang, P., Chen, J., Hong, T., & He, X. (2018). Differential diagnostic roles of the serum CA19-9, total bilirubin (TBIL) and the ratio of CA19-9 to TBIL for benign and malignant. *Journal of Cancer*, *9*(10), 1804–1812. DOI: 10.7150/jca.25093 PMID: 29805707

Luchini, C., Grillo, F., Fassan, M., Vanoli, A., Capelli, P., Paolino, G., & Scarpa, A. (2020). Malignant epithelial/exocrine tumors of the pancreas. *Pathologica*, *112*(3), 210–226. DOI: 10.32074/1591-951X-167 PMID: 33179623

Madorsky Rowdo, F. P., Baron, A., Urrutia, M., & Mordoh, J. (2015). Immunotherapy in cancer: A combat between tumors and the immune system; you win some, you lose some. *Frontiers in Immunology*, *6*, 127. DOI: 10.3389/fimmu.2015.00127 PMID: 25859247

Malik, S., Muhammad, K., & Waheed, Y. (2023). Emerging applications of nanotechnology in healthcare and medicine. *Molecules (Basel, Switzerland)*, *28*(18), 6624. DOI: 10.3390/molecules28186624 PMID: 37764400

Minor, L. (2020). *Discovering precision health: predict, prevent, and cure to advance health and well-being*. John Wiley & Sons. DOI: 10.1002/9781119672715

Nersesyan, H., & Slavin, K. V. (2007). Current aproach to cancer pain management: Availability and implications of different treatment options. *Therapeutics and Clinical Risk Management*, *3*(3), 381–400. PMID: 18488078

Nichols, T. (2018). Comfort as a multidimensional construct for pain management. *Creative Nursing*, *24*(2), 88–98. DOI: 10.1891/1078-4535.24.2.88 PMID: 29871725

Olajubutu, O., Ogundipe, O. D., Adebayo, A., & Adesina, S. K. (2023). Drug delivery strategies for the treatment of pancreatic cancer. *Pharmaceutics*, *15*(5), 1318. DOI: 10.3390/pharmaceutics15051318 PMID: 37242560

Perkhofer, L., Gout, J., Roger, E., de Almeida, F. K., Simões, C. B., Wiesmüller, L., & Kleger, A. (2021). DNA damage repair as a target in pancreatic cancer: State-of-the-art and future perspectives. *Gut*, *70*(3), 606–617. DOI: 10.1136/gutjnl-2019-319984 PMID: 32855305

Qaid, M. M., & Abdelrahman, M. M. (2016). Role of insulin and other related hormones in energy metabolism—A review. *Cogent Food & Agriculture*, *2*(1), 1267691. DOI: 10.1080/23311932.2016.1267691

Rossi, G., Russo, A., Tagliamento, M., Tuzi, A., Nigro, O., Vallome, G., & Genova, C. (2020). Precision medicine for NSCLC in the era of immunotherapy: New biomarkers to select the most suitable treatment or the most suitable patient. *Cancers (Basel)*, *12*(5), 1125. DOI: 10.3390/cancers12051125 PMID: 32365882

Santarpia, M., Liguori, A., D'Aveni, A., Karachaliou, N., Gonzalez-Cao, M., Daffinà, M. G., & Rosell, R. (2018). Liquid biopsy for lung cancer early detection. *Journal of Thoracic Disease*, *10*(S7, Suppl 7), S882–S897. DOI: 10.21037/jtd.2018.03.81 PMID: 29780635

Sisodiya, S. M. (2021). Precision medicine and therapies of the future. *Epilepsia*, *62*(S2), S90–S105. DOI: 10.1111/epi.16539 PMID: 32776321

Sohal, D. P., Mangu, P. B., Khorana, A. A., Shah, M. A., Philip, P. A., O'Reilly, E. M., & Laheru, D. (2016). Metastatic pancreatic cancer: American Society of Clinical Oncology clinical practice guideline. *Journal of Clinical Oncology*, *34*(23), 2784–2796. DOI: 10.1200/JCO.2016.67.1412 PMID: 27247222

Stathis, A., & Moore, M. J. (2010). Advanced pancreatic carcinoma: Current treatment and future challenges. *Nature Reviews. Clinical Oncology*, *7*(3), 163–172. DOI: 10.1038/nrclinonc.2009.236 PMID: 20101258

Sugahara, K. N., Teesalu, T., Karmali, P. P., Kotamraju, V. R., Agemy, L., Girard, O. M., & Ruoslahti, E. (2009). Tissue-penetrating delivery of compounds and nanoparticles into tumors. *Cancer Cell*, *16*(6), 510–520. DOI: 10.1016/j.ccr.2009.10.013 PMID: 19962669

Talley, N. J., & O'connor, S. (2010). *Clinical examination: a systematic guide to physical diagnosis*. Elsevier Australia.

Tang, C. C., Von Ah, D., & Fulton, J. S. (2018). The symptom experience of patients with advanced pancreatic cancer: An integrative review. *Cancer Nursing*, *41*(1), 33–44. DOI: 10.1097/NCC.0000000000000463 PMID: 28059839

Tang, H., Yu, D., Zhang, J., Wang, M., Fu, M., Qian, Y., Zhang, X., Ji, R., Gu, J., & Zhang, X. (2024). The new advance of exosome-based liquid biopsy for cancer diagnosis. *Journal of Nanobiotechnology*, *22*(1), 610. DOI: 10.1186/s12951-024-02863-0 PMID: 39380060

Wall, N. R., Fuller, R. N., Morcos, A., & De Leon, M. (2023). Pancreatic Cancer Health Disparity: Pharmacologic Anthropology. *Cancers (Basel)*, *15*(20), 5070. DOI: 10.3390/cancers15205070 PMID: 37894437

Compilation of References

Abdelmohsin, O., Russell, T. B., Labib, P. L., & Aroori, S. (2024). SP4.3 - Pancreatoduodenectomy for malignancy with concomitant arterial resection: Results from the Recurrence After Whipple's (RAW) study. *British Journal of Surgery, 111*(Supplement_8), znae197.043. Advance online publication. DOI: 10.1093/bjs/znae197.043

Abraham, S. C., Wu, T. T., Klimstra, D. S., Finn, L. S., Lee, J.-H., Yeo, C. J., Cameron, J. L., & Hruban, R. H. (2002). Distinctive Molecular Genetic Alterations in Sporadic and Familial Adenomatous Polyposis-Associated Pancreatoblastomas. *American Journal of Pathology, 160*(5), 1619–1627. DOI: 10.1016/S0002-9440(10)63008-8 PMID: 11696422

Adem, B., Bastos, N., Ruivo, C. F., Sousa-Alves, S., Dias, C., Vieira, P. F., Batista, I. A., Cavadas, B., Saur, D., Machado, J. C., Cai, D., & Melo, S. A. (2024). Exosomes define a local and systemic communication network in healthy pancreas and pancreatic ductal adenocarcinoma. *Nature Communications, 15*(1), 1496–1502. DOI: 10.1038/s41467-024-45753-7

Adiseshaiah, P. P., Crist, R. M., Hook, S. S., & McNeil, S. E. (2016). Nanomedicine strategies to overcome the pathophysiological barriers of pancreatic cancer. *Nature Reviews. Clinical Oncology, 13*(12), 750–765. DOI: 10.1038/nrclinonc.2016.119

Adsay, N. V., Pierson, C., Sarkar, F., Abrams, J., Weaver, D., Conlon, K. C., Brennan, M. F., & Klimstra, D. S. (2001). Colloid (Mucinous Noncystic) Carcinoma of the Pancreas. *The American Journal of Surgical Pathology, 25*(1), 26–42. DOI: 10.1097/00000478-200101000-00003 PMID: 11145249

Afghani, E., & Klein, A. P. (2022). Pancreatic Adenocarcinoma. *Hematology/Oncology Clinics of North America, 36*(5), 879–895. DOI: 10.1016/j.hoc.2022.07.002 PMID: 36154788

Afshar-Kharghan, V. (2017). The role of the complement system in cancer. *The Journal of Clinical Investigation, 127*(3), 780–789. DOI: 10.1172/JCI90962

Aftab Alam, M., & Dhoundiyal, S. (2023). Overcoming the Limitations of Therapeutic Strategies to Combat Pancreatic Cancer Using Nanotechnology. *Current Cancer Drug Targets, 23*(9), 697–717. Advance online publication. DOI: 10.2174/1568009623666230329085618 PMID: 36999420

Agarwal, R., & Epstein, A. S. (2017). Palliative care and advance care planning for pancreas and other cancers. *Linchuang Zhongliuxue Zazhi, 6*(3), 32. PMID: 28705009

Aglietta, M., Barone, C., Sawyer, M. B., Moore, M. J., Miller, W. H.Jr, Bagalà, C., Colombi, F., Cagnazzo, C., Gioeni, L., Wang, E., Huang, B., Fly, K. D., & Leone, F. (2014). A phase I dose escalation trial of tremelimumab (CP-675,206) in combination with gemcitabine in chemotherapy-naive patients with metastatic pancreatic cancer. *Annals of Oncology : Official Journal of the European Society for Medical Oncology, 25*(9), 1750–1755. DOI: 10.1093/annonc/mdu205 PMID: 24907635

Agnihotri, S., Kumar, N., & Coudière, P. (2021). Acinar Cell Carcinoma of the Pancreas: A Comprehensive Review. *The Oncologist, 26*(7), e1122–e1132.

Ahmad, A., Imran, M., & Ahsan, H. (2023). Biomarkers as biomedical bioindicators: Approaches and techniques for the detection, analysis, and validation of novel biomarkers of diseases. *Pharmaceutics, 15*(6), 1630. DOI: 10.3390/pharmaceutics15061630 PMID: 37376078

Ahmad, N., Ahmad, R., Naqvi, A. A., Alam, M. A., Ashafaq, M., Samim, M., & Ahmad, F. J. (2020). Thymoquinone lipid nanocarrier for the treatment of *Nigella sativa*-induced neurotoxicity in experimental epilepsy: Behavioral and biochemical evidences. *Journal of Drug Delivery Science and Technology, 57*, 101696. DOI: 10.1016/j.jddst.2020.101696

Ahmed, S., Hasan, M. N., Altass, H. M., Bera, A., Alsantali, R., Pan, N., Alzahrani, A. Y. A., Bagchi, D., Al-Fahemi, J. H., Khder, A. S., & Pal, S. K. (2022). Tetracycline encapsulated in Au nanoparticle-decorated ZnO nanohybrids for enhanced antibacterial activity. *ACS Applied Nano Materials, 5*(3), 4484–4492. DOI: 10.1021/acsanm.2c00655

Ahn, J., Segers, S., & Hayes, R. B. (2012). Periodontal disease, *Porphyromonas gingivalis* serum antibody levels and orodigestive cancer mortality. *Carcinogenesis, 33*(5), 1055–1058. DOI: 10.1093/carcin/bgs112

Ahn, J., Sinha, R., Pei, Z., Dominianni, C., Wu, J., Shi, J., Goedert, J. J., Hayes, R. B., & Yang, L. (2013). Human gut microbiome and risk for colorectal cancer. *Journal of the National Cancer Institute*, *105*(24), 1907–1911. DOI: 10.1093/jnci/djt300

Ahuja, M., Schwartz, D. M., Tandon, M., Son, A., Zeng, M., Swaim, W., Eckhaus, M., Hoffman, V., Cui, Y., Xiao, B., Worley, P. F., & Muallem, S. (2017). Orai1-mediated antimicrobial secretion from pancreatic acini shapes the gut microbiome and regulates gut innate immunity. *Cell Metabolism*, *25*(3), 635–646. DOI: 10.1016/j.cmet.2017.02.007

Aier, I., Semwal, R., Sharma, A., & Varadwaj, P. K. (2019). A systematic assessment of statistics, risk factors, and underlying features involved in pancreatic cancer. *Cancer Epidemiology*, *58*, 104–110. DOI: 10.1016/j.canep.2018.12.001 PMID: 30537645

Al Balushi, H., Chowdhury, P., Babu, H. M., Rehman, A., Bokhari, S. F. H., Al-Tarawneh, L. M., Al-Adwan, A. J., Cheran, M., Chilla, S. P., Addula, A. R., & Amir, M. (2024). The Potential of Salivary Biomarkers in Early Detection of Pancreatic Ductal Adenocarcinoma: A Systematic Review. *Cureus*, *16*(2). Advance online publication. DOI: 10.7759/cureus.55003 PMID: 38550499

Alavi, M., & Nokhodchi, A. (2021). Micro and nano liposomal carriers for lung cancer therapy: An updated review. *Advanced Drug Delivery Reviews*, *174*, 73–102. DOI: 10.1016/j.addr.2021.04.006

Ali, A., & DiPersio, J. F. (2024). ReCARving the future: Bridging CAR T-cell therapy gaps with synthetic biology, engineering, and economic insights. *Frontiers in Immunology*, *15*, 1432799. DOI: 10.3389/fimmu.2024.1432799 PMID: 39301026

Ali, E. S., Sharker, S. M., Islam, M. T., Khan, I. N., Shaw, S., Rahman, A., Uddin, S. J., Shill, M. C., Rehman, S., Das, N., Ahmad, S., Shilpi, J. A., Tripathi, S., Mishra, S. K., & Mubarak, M. S. (2020). Targeting cancer cells with nanotherapeutics and nanodiagnostics: Current status and future perspectives. *Seminars in Cancer Biology*, *69*, 52–68. DOI: 10.1016/j.semcancer.2020.01.011 PMID: 32014609

Alkassis, S., Yazdanpanah, O., & Philip, P. A. (2021). BRCA mutations in pancreatic cancer and progress in their targeting. *Expert Opinion on Therapeutic Targets*, *25*(7), 547–557. DOI: 10.1080/14728222.2021.1957462

Allen, P. J., D'Angelica, M., Gonen, M., Jaques, D. P., Coit, D. G., Jarnagin, W. R., DeMatteo, R., Fong, Y., Blumgart, L. H., & Brennan, M. F. (2006). A selective approach to the resection of cystic lesions of the pancreas: Results from 539 consecutive patients. *Annals of Surgery*, *244*(4), 572–582. DOI: 10.1097/01.sla.0000237652.84466.54 PMID: 16998366

Allen, T. M., & Cullis, P. R. (2013). Liposomal drug delivery systems: From concept to clinical applications. *Advanced Drug Delivery Reviews, 65*(1), 36–48. DOI: 10.1016/j.addr.2012.09.037 PMID: 23036225

Alonso, I. J., Quinto, A. M., Maestro, O. C., Murillo, L. A., Conde, P. R., Fernández, C. F., & Romero, C. J. (2024). Duodenopancreatectomía cefálica tipo Whipple versus duodenopancreatectomía con preservación pilórica. Estudio retrospectivo. *Cirugía Española, 102*(5), 265–274. DOI: 10.1016/j.ciresp.2024.02.005 PMID: 38493929

Alturki, M. S., Tawfeeq, N., Alissa, A., Ahbail, Z., Gomaa, M. S., Al Khzem, A. H., & Alshehri, A. A. (2025). Targeting KRAS G12C and G12S mutations in lung cancer: In silico drug repurposing and antiproliferative assessment on A549 cells. *Informatics in Medicine Unlocked, 52*, 101612. DOI: 10.1016/j.imu.2024.101612

Amakye, D., Jagani, Z., & Dorsch, M. (2013). Unraveling the therapeutic potential of the Hedgehog pathway in cancer. *Nature Medicine, 19*(11), 1410–1422. DOI: 10.1038/nm.3389 PMID: 24202394

Amjad, M. W., Amin, M., Katas, H., Butt, A., Kesharwani, P., & Iyer, A. (2015). In vivo antitumor activity of folate-conjugated cholic acid-polyethylenimine micelles for the codelivery of doxorubicin and siRNA to colorectal adenocarcinomas. *Molecular Pharmaceutics, 12*(11), 4247–4258. DOI: 10.1021/acs.molpharmaceut.5b00827 PMID: 26567518

Ammer-Herrmenau, C., Pfisterer, N., Weingarten, M. F. J., & Neesse, A. (2020). The microbiome in pancreatic diseases: Recent advances and future perspectives. *United European Gastroenterology Journal, 8*(8), 878–885. DOI: 10.1177/2050640620944720

Annese, T., Tamma, R., Ruggieri, S., & Ribatti, D. (2019). Angiogenesis in pancreatic cancer: Pre-clinical and clinical studies. *Cancers (Basel), 11*(3), 381. DOI: 10.3390/cancers11030381

Arensman, M. D., Kovochich, A. N., Kulikauskas, R. M., Lay, A. R., Yang, P. T., Li, X., Donahue, T., Major, M. B., Moon, R. T., Chien, A. J., & Dawson, D. W. (2014). WNT7B mediates autocrine Wnt/β-catenin signaling and anchorage-independent growth in pancreatic adenocarcinoma. *Oncogene, 33*(7), 899–908. DOI: 10.1038/onc.2013.23

Artinyan, A., Anaya, D. A., McKenzie, S., Ellenhorn, J. D., & Kim, J. (2011). Neoadjuvant therapy is associated with improved survival in resectable pancreatic adenocarcinoma. *Cancer, 117*(10), 2044–2049. DOI: 10.1002/cncr.25763 PMID: 21523715

Aslan, M., Shahbazi, R., Ulubayram, K., & Ozpolat, B. (2018). Targeted therapies for pancreatic cancer and hurdles ahead. *Anticancer Research, 38*(12), 6591–6606. DOI: 10.21873/anticanres.13026

AstraZeneca. (2015). *Study of tremelimumab in patients with advanced solid tumors* (ClinicalTrials.gov Identifier No. NCT02527434). ClinicalTrials.gov. https://clinicaltrials.gov/show/NCT02527434

Au, M., Emeto, T. I., Power, J., Vangaveti, V. N., & Lai, H. (2016). Emerging therapeutic potential of nanoparticles in pancreatic cancer: A systematic review of clinical trials. *Biomedicines, 4*(3), 20. DOI: 10.3390/biomedicines4030020 PMID: 28536387

Awad, M. M., Liu, S., Rybkin, I. I., Arbour, K. C., Dilly, J., Zhu, V. W., & Riely, G. J. (2021). Acquired resistance to KRAS G12C inhibition in cancer. *The New England Journal of Medicine, 384*(25), 2382–2393. DOI: 10.1056/NEJMoa2105281 PMID: 34161704

Aykut, B., Pushalkar, S., Chen, R., Li, Q., Abengozar, R., Kim, J. I., Shadaloey, S. A., Wu, D., Preiss, P., Verma, N., Guo, Y., Saxena, A., Vardhan, M., Diskin, B., Wang, W., Leinwand, J., Kurz, E., Kochen Rossi, J. A., Hundeyin, M., & Miller, G. (2019). The fungal mycobiome promotes pancreatic oncogenesis via activation of MBL. *Nature, 574*(7777), 264–267. DOI: 10.1038/s41586-019-1608-2

Bahadar, H., Maqbool, F., Niaz, K., & Abdollahi, M. (2016). Toxicity of nanoparticles and an overview of current experimental models. *Iranian Biomedical Journal, 20*(1), 1–11. DOI: 10.22045/ibj.2016.01 PMID: 26286636

Bahar, M. E., Kim, H. J., & Kim, D. R. (2023). Targeting the RAS/RAF/MAPK pathway for cancer therapy: From mechanism to clinical studies. *Signal Transduction and Targeted Therapy, 455*(1), 455. DOI: 10.1038/s41392-023-01705-z PMID: 38105263

Bahrami, B., Hojjat-Farsangi, M., Mohammadi, H., Anvari, E., Ghalamfarsa, G., Yousefi, M., & Jadidi-Niaragh, F. (2017). Nanoparticles and targeted drug delivery in cancer therapy. *Immunology Letters, 190*, 64–83. DOI: 10.1016/j.imlet.2017.07.015 PMID: 28760499

Bakkevold, K. E., Arnesjo, B., Dahl, O., & Kambestad, B. (1993). Adjuvant combination chemotherapy (AMF) following radical resection of carcinoma of the pancreas and papilla of Vater: Results of a controlled, prospective, randomised multicentre study. *European Journal of Cancer, 29*(5), 698–703. DOI: 10.1016/S0959-8049(05)80349-1 PMID: 8471327

Balázs, K., Kis, E., Badie, C., Bogdándi, E. N., Candéias, S., Cruz Garcia, L., & Sáfrány, G. (2019). Radiotherapy-induced changes in the systemic immune and inflammation parameters of head and neck cancer patients. *Cancers (Basel), 11*(9), 1324. DOI: 10.3390/cancers11091324

Banerjee, K., Gautam, S. K., Kshirsagar, P., Ross, K. A., Spagnol, G., Sorgen, P., Wannemuehler, M. J., Narasimhan, B., Solheim, J. C., Kumar, S., Batra, S. K., & Jain, M. (2019). Amphiphilic polyanhydride-based recombinant MUC4β-nanovaccine activates dendritic cells. *Genes & Cancer, 10*(1-2), 52–62. DOI: 10.18632/genesandcancer.189 PMID: 31258832

Banigallapati, S. (2024). *Current Treatment Methods in Pancreatic Cancer and the Need for Improvement.* https://doi.org/DOI: 10.20944/preprints202410.1569.v1

Bannone, E., Romandini, E., Kleive, D., Marchegiani, G., Gilg, S., Sahakyan, M. A., Ghorbani, P., Perri, G., Sparrelid, E., Labori, K. J., & Salvia, R. (2023). Postpancreatectomy Acute Pancreatitis (PPAP) after Distal Pancreatectomy: A Tri-institutional International Cohort Study. *HPB : The Official Journal of the International Hepato Pancreato Biliary Association, 25*, S230–S231. DOI: 10.1016/j.hpb.2023.07.079

Banstola, A., Pham, T. T., Jeong, J. H., & Yook, S. (2019). Polydopamine-tailored paclitaxel-loaded polymeric microspheres with adhered NIR-controllable gold nanoparticles for chemo-phototherapy of pancreatic cancer. *Drug Delivery, 26*(1), 629–640. DOI: 10.1080/10717544.2019.1628118 PMID: 31237149

Barbour, A., Samra, J., Haghighi, K. S., Donoghoe, M. W., Burge, M., Harris, M. T., Chua, Y. J., Mitchell, J., O'Rourke, N., Chan, H., Gebski, V. J., Gananadha, S., Croagh, D. G., Kench, J. G., & Goldstein, D. (2020). The AGITG GAP study: A phase II study of perioperative gemcitabine and nab-paclitaxel for resectable pancreas cancer. *Annals of Surgical Oncology, 27*(7), 2506–2515. DOI: 10.1245/s10434-020-08205-2 PMID: 31997125

Barenholz, Y. (2012). Doxil® - The first FDA-approved nanodrug: Lessons learned. *Journal of Controlled Release, 160*(2), 117–134. DOI: 10.1016/j.jconrel.2012.03.020 PMID: 22484195

Barton, M. K. (2017). Symptoms, cancer-related distress, and overall distress may contribute to racial disparities in the outcomes of patients with early-stage breast cancer. *CA: a Cancer Journal for Clinicians, 67*(4), 257–258. DOI: 10.3322/caac.21371

Basturk, O., Hong, S. M., Wood, L. D., Adsay, N. V., Albores-Saavedra, J., Biankin, A. V., Brosens, L. A. A., Fukushima, N., Goggins, M., Hruban, R. H., Kato, Y., Klimstra, D. S., Klöppel, G., Krasinskas, A., Longnecker, D. S., Matthaei, H., Offerhaus, G. J. A., Shimizu, M., Takaori, K., & Furukawa, T. (2015). A Revised Classification System and Recommendations from the Baltimore Consensus Meeting for Neoplastic Precursor Lesions in the Pancreas. *The American Journal of Surgical Pathology*, *39*(12), 1730–1741. DOI: 10.1097/PAS.0000000000000533 PMID: 26559377

Basturk, O., Tang, L., & Hruban, R. H. (2015). Poorly Differentiated Neuroendocrine Carcinomas of the Pancreas: A Clinicopathologic Analysis of 44 Cases. *The American Journal of Surgical Pathology*, *39*(5), 683–690. DOI: 10.1097/PAS.0000000000000408 PMID: 25723112

Baumel, H., Huguier, M., Manderscheid, J. C., Fabre, J. M., Houry, S., & Fagot, H. (1994). Results of resection for cancer of the exocrine pancreas: A study from the French Association of Surgery. *British Journal of Surgery*, *81*(1), 102–107. DOI: 10.1002/bjs.1800810138 PMID: 7906180

Baunwall, S. M. D., Lee, M. M., Eriksen, M. K., Mullish, B. H., Marchesi, J. R., Dahlerup, J. F., & Hvas, C. L. (2020). Faecal microbiota transplantation for recurrent *Clostridioides difficile* infection: An updated systematic review and meta-analysis. *EClinicalMedicine*, *29*, 100642. DOI: 10.1016/j.eclinm.2020.100642

Bazeed, A. Y., Day, C. M., & Garg, S. (2022). Pancreatic Cancer: Challenges and Opportunities in Locoregional Therapies. *Cancers (Basel)*, *14*(17), 4257. DOI: 10.3390/cancers14174257 PMID: 36077794

Beatty, G. L. Safety and antitumor activity of chimeric antigen receptor modified T cells in patients with chemotherapy refractory metastatic pancreatic cancer. ASCO Annu. Meet. Proc. 33, 3007 (2015). DOI: 10.1200/jco.2015.33.15_suppl.3007

Beatty, G., Torigian, D., Chiorean, E., Saboury, B., Brothers, A., Alavi, A., Troxel, A. B., Sun, W., Teitelbaum, U. R., Vonderheide, R. H., & O'Dwyer, P. J. (2013). A phase I study of an agonist CD40 monoclonal antibody (CP-870,893) in combination with gemcitabine in patients with advanced pancreatic ductal adenocarcinoma. *Clinical Cancer Research*, *19*(22), 6286–6295. DOI: 10.1158/1078-0432.CCR-13-1320 PMID: 23983255

Bejarano, L., Jordão, M. J., & Joyce, J. A. (2021). Therapeutic targeting of the tumour microenvironment. *Cancer Discovery*, *11*(4), 933–959. DOI: 10.1158/2159-8290.CD-20-1808 PMID: 33811125

Bekaii-Saab, T. S., Yaeger, R., Spira, A. I., Pelster, M. S., Sabari, J. K., Hafez, N., Barve, M., Velastegui, K., Yan, X., Shetty, A., Der-Torossian, H., & Pant, S. (2023). Adagrasib in advanced solid tumors harboring a KRASG12C mutation. *Journal of Clinical Oncology*, *41*(20), 4097–4106. DOI: 10.1200/JCO.23.00434 PMID: 37099736

Benguigui, M., Weitz, I. S., Timaner, M., Kan, T., Shechter, D., Perlman, O., Sivan, S., Raviv, Z., Azhari, H., & Shaked, Y. (2019). Copper oxide nanoparticles inhibit pancreatic tumour growth primarily by targeting tumour-initiating cells. *Scientific Reports*, *9*(1), 12613. DOI: 10.1038/s41598-019-48959-8 PMID: 31471546

Ben, Q., Li, Z., Liu, C., Cai, Q., Yuan, Y., & Wang, K. (2011). Hepatitis B virus status and risk of pancreatic ductal adenocarcinoma: A case-control study from China. *Pancreas*, (5), 675–680. DOI: 10.1097/MPA.0b013e318214f834

Bhat, G. R., Sethi, I., Sadida, H. Q., Rah, B., Mir, R., Algehainy, N., Albalawi, I. A., Masoodi, T., Subbaraj, G. K., Jamal, F., Singh, M., Kumar, R., Macha, M. A., Uddin, S., Akil, A. S. A., Haris, M., & Bhat, A. A. (2024). Cancer cell plasticity: From cellular, molecular, and genetic mechanisms to tumor heterogeneity and drug resistance. *Cancer and Metastasis Reviews*, *43*(1), 197–228. DOI: 10.1007/s10555-024-10172-z PMID: 38329598

Bhinder, B., Gilvary, C., Madhukar, N. S., & Elemento, O. (2021). Artificial intelligence in cancer research and precision medicine. *Cancer Discovery*, *11*(4), 900–915. DOI: 10.1158/2159-8290.CD-21-0090 PMID: 33811123

Biagi, J. J., Cosby, R., Bahl, M., Elfiki, T., Goodwin, R., Hallet, J., Hirmiz, K., & Mahmud, A. (2023). Adjuvant Chemotherapy and Radiotherapy in Resected Pancreatic Ductal Adenocarcinoma: A Systematic Review and Clinical Practice Guideline. *Current Oncology (Toronto, Ont.)*, *30*(7), 6575–6586. DOI: 10.3390/curroncol30070482 PMID: 37504342

Biesel, E. A., Sundheimer, J., Badr, M. T., Posadas-Cantera, S., Chikhladze, S., Fichtner-Feigl, S., & Wittel, U. A. (2025). Microbiological colonization of the pancreatic tumor affects postoperative complications and outcome after pancreatic surgery. *Frontiers in Cellular and Infection Microbiology*, *15*, 1521952. DOI: 10.3389/fcimb.2025.1521952

Binenbaum, Y., Na'ara, S., & Gil, Z. (2015). Gemcitabine resistance in pancreatic ductal adenocarcinoma. *Drug Resistance Updates*, *23*, 55–68. DOI: 10.1016/j.drup.2015.10.002 PMID: 26690340

Biray Avci, C., Goker Bagca, B., Nikanfar, M., Takanlou, L. S., Takanlou, M. S., & Nourazarian, A. (2024). Tumor microenvironment and cancer metastasis: Molecular mechanisms and therapeutic implications. *Frontiers in Pharmacology*, *15*, 1442888. DOI: 10.3389/fphar.2024.1442888 PMID: 39600368

Blanco, E., Hsiao, A., Mann, A. P., Landry, M. G., Meric-Bernstam, F., & Ferrari, M. (2011). Nanomedicine in cancer therapy: Innovative trends and prospects. *Cancer Science*, *102*(7), 1247–1252. DOI: 10.1111/j.1349-7006.2011.01941.x PMID: 21447010

Blanquicett, J, C., & E. Aguirre, L. (. (2021). Therapeutic Advances for Pancreatic Cancer: A Slow and Challenging Feat that Continues to Evolve. *Acta Scientific Gastrointestinal Disorders*, *4*(7), 50–52. DOI: 10.31080/ASGIS.2021.04.0268 PMID: 34414366

Blaser, M. J. (1992). Hypotheses on the pathogenesis and natural history of *Helicobacter pylori* - induced inflammation. *Gastroenterology*, *102*(2), 720–727. DOI: 10.1016/0016-5085(92)90126-J

Bloomston, M., Zervos, E. E., & Rosemurgy, A. S.II. (2002). Matrix metalloproteinases and their role in pancreatic cancer: A review of preclinical studies and clinical trials. *Annals of Surgical Oncology*, *9*(7), 668–674. DOI: 10.1007/BF02574483

Blyuss, O., Zaikin, A., Cherepanova, V., Munblit, D., Kiseleva, E. M., Prytomanova, O. M., Duffy, S. W., & Crnogorac-Jurcevic, T. (2020). Development of PancRISK, a urine biomarker-based risk score for stratified screening of pancreatic cancer patients. *British Journal of Cancer*, *122*(5), 692–696. DOI: 10.1038/s41416-019-0694-0 PMID: 31857725

Boeck, S., Ankerst, D. P., & Heinemann, V. (2007). The role of adjuvant chemotherapy for patients with resected pancreatic cancer: Systematic review of randomized controlled trials and meta-analysis. *Oncology*, *72*(6), 314–321. DOI: 10.1159/000113054 PMID: 18187951

Boone, B. A. (2024). Employing Advanced Technology to Reduce Postoperative Pancreatic Fistula. *Annals of Surgery Open : Perspectives of Surgical History, Education, and Clinical Approaches*, *5*(1), e373–e373. DOI: 10.1097/AS9.0000000000000373 PMID: 38883937

Boone, B. A., Steve, J., Krasinskas, A. M., Zureikat, A. H., Lembersky, B. C., Gibson, M. K., Stoller, R. G., Zeh, H. J., & Bahary, N. (2013). Outcomes with FOLFIRINOX for borderline resectable and locally unresectable pancreatic cancer. *Journal of Surgical Oncology*, *108*(4), 236–241. DOI: 10.1002/jso.23392 PMID: 23955427

Borsig, L. (2018). Selectins in cancer immunity. *Glycobiology, 28*(9), 648–655. DOI: 10.1093/glycob/cwx105 PMID: 29272415

Borst, P. (2012). Cancer drug pan-resistance: Pumps, cancer stem cells, quiescence, epithelial to mesenchymal transition, blocked cell death pathways, persisters or what? *Open Biology, 2*(5), 120066. DOI: 10.1098/rsob.120066 PMID: 22724067

Bozzuto, G., & Molinari, A. (2015). Liposomes as nanomedical devices. *International Journal of Nanomedicine, 10*, 975–999. DOI: 10.2147/IJN.S68861 PMID: 25678787

Bracci, P. M. (2017). Oral health and the oral microbiome in pancreatic cancer: An overview of epidemiological studies. *Cancer Journal (Sudbury, Mass.), 23*(6), 310–314. DOI: 10.1097/PPO.0000000000000287

Bray, F., Ferlay, J., Soerjomataram, I., Siegel, R. L., Torre, L. A., & Jemal, A. (2018). Global cancer statistics 2018: GLOBOCAN estimates of incidence and mortality worldwide for 36 cancers in 185 countries. *CA: a Cancer Journal for Clinicians, 68*(6), 394–424. DOI: 10.3322/caac.21492 PMID: 30207593

Breslin, T. M., Hess, K. R., Harbison, D. B., Jean, M. E., Cleary, K. R., Dackiw, A. P., Wolff, R. A., Abbruzzese, J. L., Janjan, N. A., Crane, C. H., Vauthey, J. N., Lee, J. E., Pisters, P. W. T., & Evans, D. B. (2001). Neoadjuvant chemoradiotherapy for adenocarcinoma of the pancreas: Treatment variables and survival duration. *Annals of Surgical Oncology, 8*(2), 123–132. DOI: 10.1007/s10434-001-0123-4 PMID: 11258776

Brigger, I., Dubernet, C., & Couvreur, P. (2012). Nanoparticles in cancer therapy and diagnosis. *Advanced Drug Delivery Reviews, 64*, 24–36. DOI: 10.1016/j.addr.2012.09.006 PMID: 12204596

Bristol-Myers Squibb. (2013). *A study of nivolumab by itself or nivolumab combined with ipilimumab in patients with advanced or metastatic solid tumors* (ClinicalTrials.gov Identifier: NCT01928394). ClinicalTrials.gov. https://clinicaltrials.gov/show/NCT01928394

Brusselaers, N., Sadr-Azodi, O., & Engstrand, L. (2020). Long-term proton pump inhibitor usage and the association with pancreatic cancer in Sweden. *Journal of Gastroenterology, 55*(4), 453–461. DOI: 10.1007/s00535-019-01652-z

Bryant, J. M., Nakashima, J., Khatri, V. M., Sinnamon, A. J., Denbo, J. W., Hodul, P., Malafa, M., Hoffe, S., & Frakes, J. M. (2024). The Evolving Role of Neoadjuvant Radiation Therapy in Pancreatic Adenocarcinoma. *Journal of Clinical Medicine, 13*(22), 6800–6800. DOI: 10.3390/jcm13226800 PMID: 39597944

Büchler, P., Gazdhar, A., Schubert, M., Giese, N., Reber, H. A., Hines, O. J., & Friess, H. (2005). The Notch signaling pathway is related to neurovascular progression of pancreatic cancer. *Annals of Surgery, 242*(6), 791–801. DOI: 10.1097/01.sla.0000189115.94847.f1

Buchta, R. C., Feng, T. Y., Azar, F. N., & Rutkowski, M. R. (2019). Impact of the microbiome on cancer progression and response to anti-cancer therapies. *Advances in Cancer Research, 143*, 255–294. DOI: 10.1016/bs.acr.2019.03.005

Bunduc, S., Gede, N., Vancsa, S., Lillik, V., Kiss, S., Juhász, M. F., Erőss, B., Szakács, Z., Gheorghe, C., Mikó, A., & Hegyi, P. (2022). Exosomes as prognostic biomarkers in pancreatic ductal adenocarcinoma—A systematic review and meta-analysis. *Translational Research; the Journal of Laboratory and Clinical Medicine, 244*, 126–136. DOI: 10.1016/j.trsl.2022.01.001 PMID: 35066189

Buscail, L., Bournet, B., & Cordelier, P. (2020). Role of oncogenic KRAS in the diagnosis, prognosis, and treatment of pancreatic cancer. *Nature Reviews. Gastroenterology & Hepatology, 17*(3), 153–168. DOI: 10.1038/s41575-019-0245-4

Butt, A. M., Amin, M., Katas, H., Abdul Murad, N. A., Jamal, R., & Kesharwani, P. (2016). Doxorubicin and siRNA codelivery via chitosan-coated pH-responsive mixed micellar polyplexes for enhanced cancer therapy in multidrug-resistant tumors. *Molecular Pharmaceutics, 13*(2), 4179–4190. DOI: 10.1021/acs.molpharmaceut.6b00776 PMID: 27934479

Butturini, G., Stocken, D. D., Wente, M. N., Jeekel, H., Klinkenbijl, J. H. G., Bakkevold, K. E., Takada, T., Amano, H., Dervenis, C., Bassi, C., Büchler, M. W., & Neoptolemos, J. P.Pancreatic Cancer Meta-Analysis Group. (2008). Influence of resection margins and treatment on survival in patients with pancreatic cancer: Meta-analysis of randomized controlled trials. *Archives of Surgery, 143*(1), 75–83. DOI: 10.1001/archsurg.2007.17 PMID: 18209156

Caccialanza, R., Lobascio, F., Brugnatelli, S., & Pedrazzoli, P. (2020). Nutritional support in pancreatic cancer. *Cancer, 126*(8), 1810–1811. DOI: 10.1002/cncr.32713

Caccialanza, R., Pedrazzoli, P., Cereda, E., Gavazzi, C., Pinto, C., Paccagnella, A., Beretta, G. D., Nardi, M., Laviano, A., & Zagonel, V. (2016). Nutritional support in cancer patients: A position paper from the Italian Society of Medical Oncology (AIOM) and the Italian Society of Artificial Nutrition and Metabolism (SINPE). *Journal of Cancer, 7*(2), 131–135. DOI: 10.7150/jca.13818

Caldas, C., & Kern, S. E. (1995). K-ras mutation and pancreatic adenocarcinoma. *International Journal of Pancreatology, 18*(1), 1–6. DOI: 10.1007/BF02825415

Campbell, A. S., Albo, D., Kimsey, T. F., White, S. L., & Wang, T. N. (2005). Macrophage inflammatory protein-3alpha promotes pancreatic cancer cell invasion. *The Journal of Surgical Research, 123*(1), 96–101. DOI: 10.1016/j.jss.2004.07.013

Cao, D., Song, Q., Li, J., Jiang, Y., Wang, Z., & Lu, S. (2021). Opportunities and challenges in targeted therapy and immunotherapy for pancreatic cancer. *Expert Reviews in Molecular Medicine, 23*, e21. DOI: 10.1017/erm.2021.26

Cao, J., Yang, P., Wang, P., Xu, S., Cheng, Y., Qian, K., Xu, M., Sheng, D., Li, Y., Wei, Y., & Zhang, Q. (2021). 'Adhesion and release' nanoparticle-mediated efficient inhibition of platelet activation disrupts endothelial barriers for enhanced drug delivery in tumours. *Biomaterials, 269*, 120620. DOI: 10.1016/j.biomaterials.2020.120620 PMID: 33421709

Cao, L., Huang, X., Yu, J., Liao, Z., & Zhang, J. (2023). Cell-free DNA methylation markers in plasma for early detection of pancreatic cancer. *Biomarker Research, 11*(1), 88. DOI: 10.1186/s40364-023-00528-y

Cao, X., Hu, Y., Luo, S., Wang, Y., Gong, T., Sun, X., Fu, Y., & Zhang, Z. (2019). Neutrophil-mimicking therapeutic nanoparticles for targeted chemotherapy of pancreatic carcinoma. *Acta Pharmaceutica Sinica. B, 9*(3), 575–589. DOI: 10.1016/j.apsb.2018.12.009 PMID: 31193785

Capasso, M., Franceschi, M., Rodriguez-Castro, K. I., Crafa, P., Cambiè, G., Miraglia, C., Barchi, A., Nouvenne, A., Leandro, G., & Meschi, T., De' Angelis, G. L., & Di Mario, F. (2018). Epidemiology and risk factors of pancreatic cancer. *Acta Biomedica, 89*(9-S), 141–146. DOI: 10.23750/abm.v89i9-S.7923 PMID: 30561407

Casà, C., Portik, D., Abbasi, A. N., & Micciché, F. (2025). Radiomics in early detection of bilio-pancreatic lesions: A narrative review. *Best Practice & Research. Clinical Gastroenterology, 65*, 101997. DOI: 10.1016/j.bpg.2025.101997 PMID: 40210337

Casucci, M., Nicolis di Robilant, B., Falcone, L., Camisa, B., Norelli, M., Genovese, P., Gentner, B., Gullotta, F., Ponzoni, M., Bernardi, M., Marcatti, M., Saudemont, A., Bordignon, C., Savoldo, B., Ciceri, F., Naldini, L., Dotti, G., Bonini, C., & Bondanza, A. (2013). CD44v6-targeted T cells mediate potent antitumor effects against acute myeloid leukemia and multiple myeloma. *Blood, 122*(20), 3461–3472. DOI: 10.1182/blood-2013-04-493361 PMID: 24016461

Catenacci, D. V.. (2015). Randomized phase IB/II study of gemcitabine plus placebo or vismodegib in patients with metastatic pancreatic cancer. *PLoS One, 10*(4), e0127770. DOI: 10.1371/journal.pone.0127770

Cecchini, M., Salem, R. R., Robert, M., Czerniak, S., Blaha, O., Zelterman, D., Rajaei, M., Townsend, J. P., Cai, G., Chowdhury, S., Yugawa, D., Tseng, R., Mejia Arbelaez, C., Jiao, J., Shroyer, K., Thumar, J., Kortmansky, J., Zaheer, W., Fischbach, N., & Lacy, J. (2024). Perioperative Modified FOLFIRINOX for Resectable Pancreatic Cancer: A Nonrandomized Controlled Trial. *JAMA Oncology*, *10*(8), 1027. Advance online publication. DOI: 10.1001/jamaoncol.2024.1575 PMID: 38900452

Chakrabarti, S., Kamgar, M., & Mahipal, A. (2022). Systemic Therapy of Metastatic Pancreatic Adenocarcinoma: Current Status, Challenges, and Opportunities. *Cancers (Basel)*, *14*(11), 2588. DOI: 10.3390/cancers14112588 PMID: 35681565

Chandana, S. R., Woods, L. M., Maxwell, F., Gandolfo, R., & Bekaii-Saab, T. (2023). Risk factors for early-onset pancreatic ductal adenocarcinoma: A systematic literature review. *European Journal of Cancer*, *198*, 113471. DOI: 10.1016/j.ejca.2023.113471 PMID: 38154392

Chang, C. (2010). The immune effects of naturally occurring and synthetic nanoparticles. *Journal of Autoimmunity*, *34*(3), J234–J246. DOI: 10.1016/j.jaut.2009.11.009 PMID: 19995678

Chang, M. C., Chen, C. H., Liang, J. D., Tien, Y. W., Hsu, C., & Wong, J. M. (2014). Hepatitis B and C viruses are not risks for pancreatic adenocarcinoma. *World Journal of Gastroenterology*, *20*(17), 5060–5065. DOI: 10.3748/wjg.v20.i17.5060

Cheerla, A., & Gevaert, O. (2019). Deep learning with multimodal representation for pancancer prognosis prediction. *Bioinformatics (Oxford, England)*, *35*(14), 446–454. DOI: 10.1093/bioinformatics/btz342 PMID: 31510656

Chen, D., Wu, J., Jin, D., Wang, B., & Cao, H. (2019). Fecal microbiota transplantation in cancer management: Current status and perspectives. *International Journal of Cancer*, *145*(8), 2021–2031. DOI: 10.1002/ijc.32003

Cheng, F., Su, L., & Qian, C. (2016). Circulating tumor DNA: A promising biomarker in the liquid biopsy of cancer. *Oncotarget*, *7*(30), 48832–48841. DOI: 10.18632/oncotarget.9453 PMID: 27223063

Cheng, W. Y., Wu, C. Y., & Yu, J. (2020). The role of gut microbiota in cancer treatment: Friend or foe? *Gut*, *69*(10), 1867–1876. DOI: 10.1136/gutjnl-2020-321153

Chen, L., Xu, Z., Li, Q., Feng, Q., Zheng, C., Du, Y., Yuan, R., & Peng, X. (2021). USP28 facilitates pancreatic cancer progression through activation of the Wnt/β-catenin pathway via stabilising FOXM1. *Cell Death & Disease*, *12*(10), 887. DOI: 10.1038/s41419-021-04163-z

Chen, M., Liu, H., Xiao, Y., Liang, R., Xu, H., Hong, B., & Qian, Y. (2025). Predictive biomarkers of pancreatic cancer metastasis: A comprehensive review. *Clinica Chimica Acta, 550*, 120176. DOI: 10.1016/j.cca.2025.120176 PMID: 39914505

Chen, S. M., Chieng, W. W., Huang, S. W., Hsu, L. J., & Jan, M. S. (2020). The synergistic tumor growth-inhibitory effect of probiotic *Lactobacillus* on transgenic mouse model of pancreatic cancer treated with gemcitabine. *Scientific Reports, 10*(1), 20319–20326. DOI: 10.1038/s41598-020-77322-5

Chen, T., Carter, J., Mahmud, M., & Khuman, A. S. (2022). *Artificial intelligence in healthcare: Recent applications and developments*. Springer Nature., DOI: 10.1007/978-981-19-5272-2

Chen, W., Butler, R. K., Zhou, Y., Parker, R. A., Jeon, C. Y., & Wu, B. U. (2020). Prediction of pancreatic cancer based on imaging features in patients with duct abnormalities. *Pancreas, 49*(4), 413–419. DOI: 10.1097/MPA.0000000000001499 PMID: 32132511

Chen, X., Zeh, H. J., Kang, R., Kroemer, G., & Tang, D. (2021). Cell death in pancreatic cancer: From pathogenesis to therapy. *Nature Reviews. Gastroenterology & Hepatology, 18*(11), 804–823. DOI: 10.1038/s41575-021-00486-6

Chen, Y., Gao, S. G., Chen, J. M., Wang, G. P., Wang, Z. F., Zhou, B., & Feng, X. S. (2015). Serum CA242, CA199, CA125, CEA, and TSGF are biomarkers for the efficacy and prognosis of cryoablation in pancreatic cancer patients. *Cell Biochemistry and Biophysics, 71*(3), 1287–1291. DOI: 10.1007/s12013-014-0345-2 PMID: 25486903

Chen, Z., & Lin, Y. (2023). A commentary on "Minimally invasive versus open total pancreatectomy: A systematic review and meta-analysis.". *International Journal of Surgery, 110*(1), 600–601. DOI: 10.1097/JS9.0000000000000770 PMID: 37738018

Chen, Z., Zhang, S., Dong, S., Xu, H., & Zhou, W. (2022). Association of the microbiota and pancreatic cancer: Opportunities and limitations. *Frontiers in Immunology, 13*, 844401. DOI: 10.3389/fimmu.2022.844401

Chi, J., Chung, S. Y., Parakrama, R., Fayyaz, F., Jose, J., & Saif, M. W. (2021). The role of PARP inhibitors in BRCA mutated pancreatic cancer. *Therapeutic Advances in Gastroenterology, 14*, 175628482110148. DOI: 10.1177/17562848211014818 PMID: 34025781

Chikkaveeraiah, B. V., Bhirde, A. A., Morgan, N. Y., Eden, H. S., & Chen, X. (2012). Electrochemical immune sensors for the detection of cancer protein biomarkers. *ACS Nano, 6*(8), 6546–6561. DOI: 10.1021/nn3023969 PMID: 22835068

Chinnadurai, R. K., Khan, N., Meghwanshi, G. K., Ponne, S., Althobiti, M., & Kumar, R. (2023). Current research status of anti-cancer peptides: Mechanism of action, production, and clinical applications. *Biomedicine and Pharmacotherapy*, *164*, 114996. DOI: 10.1016/j.biopha.2023.114996 PMID: 37311281

Chmielewski, M., Kopecky, C., Hombach, A. A., & Abken, H. (2011). IL-12 release by engineered T cells expressing chimeric antigen receptors can effectively Muster an antigen-independent macrophage response on tumor cells that have shut down tumor antigen expression. *Cancer Research*, *71*(17), 5697–5706. DOI: 10.1158/0008-5472.CAN-11-0103 PMID: 21742772

Choi, D., Gonzalez-Suarez, A. M., Dumbrava, M. G., Medlyn, M., de Hoyos-Vega, J. M., Cichocki, F., Miller, J. S., Ding, L., Zhu, M., Stybayeva, G., Gaspar-Maia, A., Billadeau, D. D., Ma, W. W., & Revzin, A. (2024). Microfluidic organoid cultures derived from pancreatic cancer biopsies for personalized testing of chemotherapy and immunotherapy. *Advancement of Science*, *11*(5), 2303088. Advance online publication. DOI: 10.1002/advs.202303088 PMID: 38018486

Choi, I. J., Kook, M.-C., Kim, Y.-I., Cho, S.-J., Lee, J. Y., Kim, C. G., Park, B., & Nam, B. H. (2018). *Helicobacter pylori* therapy for the prevention of metachronous gastric cancer. *The New England Journal of Medicine*, *378*(12), 1085–1095. DOI: 10.1056/NEJMoa1708423

Choteau, L., Parny, M., Francois, N., Bertin, B., Fumery, M., Dubuquoy, L., Takahashi, K., Colombel, J.-F., Jouault, T., Poulain, D., Sendid, B., & Jawhara, S. (2016). Role of mannose-binding lectin in intestinal homeostasis and fungal elimination. *Mucosal Immunology*, *9*(3), 767–776. DOI: 10.1038/mi.2015.100

Choudhury, A., & Asan, O. (2020). Role of artificial intelligence in patient safety outcomes: Systematic literature review. *JMIR Medical Informatics*, *8*(7), 18599. DOI: 10.2196/18599 PMID: 32706688

Chour, A., Toffart, A. C., Berton, E., & Duruisseaux, M. (2024). Mechanisms of resistance to KRASG12C inhibitors in KRASG12C-mutated non-small cell lung cancer. *Frontiers in Oncology*, *14*, 1328728. DOI: 10.3389/fonc.2024.1328728 PMID: 39301544

Christenson, E. S., Jaffee, E., & Azad, N. S. (2020). Current and emerging therapies for patients with advanced pancreatic ductal adenocarcinoma: A bright future. *The Lancet. Oncology*, *21*(5), e135–e145. DOI: 10.1016/S1470-2045(19)30795-8 PMID: 32135117

Chua, T. C., & Saxena, A. (2010). Extended pancreaticoduodenectomy with vascular resection for pancreatic cancer: A systematic review. *Journal of Gastrointestinal Surgery, 14*(9), 1442–1452. DOI: 10.1007/s11605-009-1129-7 PMID: 20379794

Chung, L. M., Liang, J.-A., Lin, C.-L., Sun, L.-M., & Kao, C.-H. (2017). Cancer risk in patients with candidiasis: A nationwide population-based cohort study. *Oncotarget, 8*(38), 63562–63573. DOI: 10.18632/oncotarget.18855

Cives, M., & Strosberg, J. R. (2018). Gastroenteropancreatic neuroendocrine tumors. *CA: a Cancer Journal for Clinicians, 68*(6), 471–487. DOI: 10.3322/caac.21493 PMID: 30295930

Clarke, J. M., & Hurwitz, H. I. (2013). Targeted inhibition of VEGF receptor 2: An update on ramucirumab. *Expert Opinion on Biological Therapy, 13*(8), 1187–1196. DOI: 10.1517/14712598.2013.810717 PMID: 23803182

ClinicalTrials.gov. [Internet]. Bethesda (MD): National Library of Medicine (US). Identifier NCT06241352, A Study of Modified FOLFIRINOX With Simvastatin in Metastatic Pancreatic Adenocarcinoma; 2024 [cited 2025 Apr 29]. Available from: https://clinicaltrials.gov/ct2/show/NCT06241352

Collins, I., & Workman, P. (2006). New approaches to molecular cancer therapeutics. *Nature Chemical Biology, 2*(12), 689–700. DOI: 10.1038/nchembio840 PMID: 17108987

Conroy, T., Bachet, J.-B., Ayav, A., Huguet, F., Lambert, A., Caramella, C., Maréchal, R., Van Laethem, J.-L., & Ducreux, M. (2016). Current standards and new innovative approaches for treatment of pancreatic cancer. *European Journal of Cancer, 57*, 10–22. DOI: 10.1016/j.ejca.2015.12.026 PMID: 26851397

Conroy, T., Hammel, P., Hebbar, M., Abdelghani, M. B., Wei, A. C., & Raoul, J. L. (2018). FOLFIRINOX or gemcitabine as adjuvant therapy for pancreatic cancer. *The New England Journal of Medicine, 379*(25), 2395–2406. DOI: 10.1056/NEJMoa1809775 PMID: 30575490

Conroy, T., Pfeiffer, P., Vilgrain, V., Lamarca, A., Seufferlein, T., O'Reilly, E. M., Hackert, T., Golan, T., Prager, G., Haustermans, K., Vogel, A., & Ducreux, M. (2023). Pancreatic cancer: ESMO Clinical Practice Guideline for diagnosis, treatment and follow-up†. *Annals of Oncology : Official Journal of the European Society for Medical Oncology, 34*(11), 987–1002. Advance online publication. DOI: 10.1016/j.annonc.2023.08.009 PMID: 37678671

Conte, M., & Cauda, V. (2022). Multimodal therapies against pancreatic ductal adenocarcinoma: A review on synergistic approaches toward ultimate nanomedicine treatments. *Advanced Therapeutics*, *5*(11), 2200079. DOI: 10.1002/adtp.202200079

Coquard, R., Ayzac, L., Gilly, F. N., Romestaing, P., Ardiet, J. M., Sondaz, C., Sotton, M. P., Sentenac, I., Braillon, G., & Gerard, J. P. (1997). Intraoperative radiotherapy in resected pancreatic cancer: Feasibility and results. *Radiotherapy and Oncology : Journal of the European Society for Therapeutic Radiology and Oncology*, *44*(3), 271–275. DOI: 10.1016/S0167-8140(97)00107-2 PMID: 9380827

Corrò, C., Novellasdemunt, L., & Li, V. S. (2020). A brief history of organoids. *American Journal of Physiology. Cell Physiology*, *319*(1), C151–C165. DOI: 10.1152/ajpcell.00120.2020 PMID: 32459504

Cortesi, L., Rugo, H. S., & Jackisch, C. (2021). An overview of PARP inhibitors for the treatment of breast cancer. *Targeted Oncology*, *16*(3), 255–282. DOI: 10.1007/s11523-021-00796-4 PMID: 33710534

Cortiana, V., Abbas, R. H., Chorya, H., Gambill, J., Mahendru, D., Park, C. H., & Leyfman, Y. (2024). Personalized medicine in pancreatic cancer: The promise of biomarkers and molecular targeting with dr. *Michael J. Pishvaian. Cancers*, *16*(13), 2329. PMID: 39001391

Craven, K. E., Gore, J., & Korc, M. (2016). Overview of pre-clinical and clinical studies targeting angiogenesis in pancreatic ductal adenocarcinoma. *Cancer Letters*, *381*(1), 201–210. DOI: 10.1016/j.canlet.2015.11.047

Cress, R. D., Yin, D., Clarke, L., Bold, R., & Holly, E. A. (2006). Survival among patients with adenocarcinoma of the pancreas: A population-based study (United States). *Cancer Causes & Control*, *17*(4), 403–409. DOI: 10.1007/s10552-005-0539-4 PMID: 16596292

Crippa, S., Piccioli, A., Guarneri, G., Longo, E., & Falconi, M. (2017). Pancreatic ductal adenocarcinoma in 2017: Time to change the therapeutic algorithm? *Endoscopic Ultrasound*, *6*(9), S62–S65. DOI: 10.4103/eus.eus_61_17 PMID: 29387691

Cruz, M. S., Tintelnot, J., & Gagliani, N. (2024). Roles of microbiota in pancreatic cancer development and treatment. *Gut Microbes*, *16*(1), 2320280. DOI: 10.1080/19490976.2024.2320280

Cui, J., Jiang, W., Wang, S., Wang, L., & Xie, K. (2012). Role of Wnt/β-catenin signaling in drug resistance of pancreatic cancer. *Current Pharmaceutical Design*, *18*(17), 2464–2471. DOI: 10.2174/13816128112092464

Cullinan, S., Moertel, C. G., Wieand, H. S., Schutt, A. J., Krook, J. E., Foley, J. F., Norris, B. D., Kardinal, C. G., Tschetter, L. K., & Barlow, J. F. (1990). A phase III trial on the therapy of advanced pancreatic carcinoma: Evaluations of the Mallinson regimen and combined 5-fluorouracil, doxorubicin, and cisplatin. *Cancer*, *65*(10), 2207–2212. DOI: 10.1002/1097-0142(19900515)65:10<2207::AID-CNCR2820651007>3.0.CO;2-Y PMID: 2189551

Cunningham, D., Allum, W., Stenning, S. P., Thompson, J. N., Van de Velde, C. J. H., Nicolson, M., Scarffe, J. H., Lofts, F. J., Falk, S. J., Iveson, T. J., Smith, D. B., Langley, R. E., Verma, M., Weeden, S., & Chua, Y. J. (2006). Perioperative chemotherapy versus surgery alone for resectable gastroesophageal cancer. *The New England Journal of Medicine*, *355*(1), 11–20. DOI: 10.1056/NEJMoa055531 PMID: 16822992

Cunningham, D., Chau, I., Stocken, D. D., Valle, J. W., Smith, D., Steward, W., Harper, P. G., Dunn, J., Tudur-Smith, C., West, J., Falk, S., Crellin, A., Adab, F., Thompson, J., Leonard, P., Ostrowski, J., Eatock, M., Scheithauer, W., Herrmann, R., & Neoptolemos, J. P. (2009). Phase III randomized comparison of gemcitabine versus gemcitabine plus capecitabine in patients with advanced pancreatic cancer. *Journal of Clinical Oncology*, *27*(33), 5513–5518. DOI: 10.1200/JCO.2009.24.2446 PMID: 19858379

Cun, X., Chen, J., Li, M., He, X., Tang, X., Guo, R., Deng, M., Li, M., Zhang, Z., & He, Q. (2019). Tumour-associated fibroblast-targeted regulation and deep tumour delivery of chemotherapeutic drugs with a multifunctional size-switchable nanoparticle. *ACS Applied Materials & Interfaces*, *11*(44), 39545–39559. DOI: 10.1021/acsami.9b13957 PMID: 31617997

Czaplicka, A., Lachota, M., Pączek, L., Zagożdżon, R., & Kaleta, B. (2024). Chimeric Antigen Receptor T Cell Therapy for Pancreatic Cancer: A Review of Current Evidence. *Cells*, *13*(1), 101. DOI: 10.3390/cells13010101 PMID: 38201305

Daamen, L. A., Molenaar, I. Q., & Groot, V. P. (2023). Recent Advances and Future Challenges in Pancreatic Cancer Care: Early Detection, Liquid Biopsies, Precision Medicine and Artificial Intelligence. *Journal of Clinical Medicine*, *12*(23), 7485. Advance online publication. DOI: 10.3390/jcm12237485 PMID: 38068536

Dai, W., Qiao, X., Fang, Y., Guo, R., Bai, P., Liu, S., Li, T., Jiang, Y., Wei, S., Na, Z., Xiao, X., & Li, D. (2024). Epigenetics-targeted drugs: Current paradigms and future challenges. *Signal Transduction and Targeted Therapy*, *9*(1), 332. DOI: 10.1038/s41392-024-02039-0 PMID: 39592582

Dalmasso, B., Puccini, A., Catalano, F., Borea, R., Iaia, M. L., Bruno, W., Fornarini, G., Sciallero, S., Rebuzzi, S. E., & Ghiorzo, P. (2022). Beyond BRCA: The emerging significance of DNA damage response and personalized treatment in pancreatic and prostate cancer patients. *International Journal of Molecular Sciences*, *23*(9), 4709–4710. DOI: 10.3390/ijms23094709 PMID: 35563100

Dambuza, I. M., & Brown, G. D. (2019). Fungi accelerate pancreatic cancer. *Nature*, *574*(7777), 184–185. https://Doi.org/10.1038/d41586-019-02892-y. DOI: 10.1038/d41586-019-02892-y

Davis, M. E., Zuckerman, J. E., Choi, C. H. J., Seligson, D., Tolcher, A., Alabi, C. A., Yen, Y., Heidel, J. D., & Ribas, A. (2010). Evidence of RNAi in humans from systemically administered siRNA via targeted nanoparticles. *Nature*, *464*(7291), 1067–1070. DOI: 10.1038/nature08956 PMID: 20305636

De Dosso, S., Siebenhüner, A. R., Winder, T., Meisel, A., Fritsch, R., Astaras, C., Szturz, P., & Borner, M. (2021). Treatment landscape of metastatic pancreatic cancer. *Cancer Treatment Reviews*, *96*, 102180. DOI: 10.1016/j.ctrv.2021.102180 PMID: 33812339

de Jesus, V. H. F., Camandaroba, M. P. G., Donadio, M. D. S., Cabral, A., Muniz, T. P., de Moura Leite, L., & Sant'Ana, L. F. (2018). Retrospective analysis of efficacy and safety of gemcitabine-based chemotherapy in patients with metastatic pancreatic adenocarcinoma experiencing disease progression on FOLFIRINOX. *Journal of Gastrointestinal Oncology*, *9*(5), 806–819. DOI: 10.21037/jgo.2018.06.08 PMID: 30505579

de Jesus, V. H. F., Mathias-Machado, M. C., de Farias, J. P. F., Aruquipa, M. P. S., Jácome, A. A., & Peixoto, R. D. (2023). Targeting KRAS in Pancreatic Ductal Adenocarcinoma: The Long Road to Cure. *Cancers (Basel)*, *15*(20), 5015. DOI: 10.3390/cancers15205015 PMID: 37894382

del Rivero, J., & Kohn, E. C. (2017). PARP Inhibitors: The Cornerstone of DNA Repair-Targeted Therapies. *Oncology (Williston Park, N.Y.)*, *31*(4), 265–273. PMID: 28412778

Desai, M. P., Labhasetwar, V., Amidon, G. L., & Levy, R. J. (1996). Gastrointestinal uptake of biodegradable microparticles: Effect of particle size. *Pharmaceutical Research*, *13*(12), 1838–1845. DOI: 10.1023/A:1016085108889 PMID: 8987081

Desgrosellier, J. S., & Cheresh, D. A. (2010). Integrins in cancer: Biological implications and therapeutic opportunities. *Nature Reviews. Cancer*, *10*(1), 9–22. DOI: 10.1038/nrc2748 PMID: 20029421

Dhamija, K., Awuah, K.-F. B., Marwaha, A., Kharoud, H., & Monga, D. K. (2025). Neoadjuvant therapy in borderline resectable and resectable pancreatic cancer. *Journal of Clinical Oncology*, *43*(4, suppl), 735–735. DOI: 10.1200/JCO.2025.43.4_suppl.735

Dhudum, R., Ganeshpurkar, A., & Pawar, A. (2024). Revolutionizing Drug Discovery: A Comprehensive Review of AI Applications. *Drugs and Drug Candidates*, *3*(1), 148–171. DOI: 10.3390/ddc3010009

Dibitetto, D., Widmer, C. A., & Rottenberg, S. (2024). PARPi, BRCA, and gaps: Controversies and future research. *Trends in Cancer*, *10*(9), 857–869. DOI: 10.1016/j.trecan.2024.06.008 PMID: 39004561

Diken, M., Kreiter, S., Selmi, A., Britten, C. M., Huber, C., Türeci, Ö., & Sahin, U. (2011). Selective uptake of naked vaccine RNA by dendritic cells is driven by macropinocytosis and abrogated upon DC maturation. *Gene Therapy*, *18*(7), 702–708. DOI: 10.1038/gt.2011.17 PMID: 21368901

Ding, S. Z., Goldberg, J. B., & Hatakeyama, M. (2010). Helicobacter pylori infection, oncogenic pathways and epigenetic mechanisms in gastric carcinogenesis. *Future Oncology (London, England)*, *6*(5), 851–862. DOI: 10.2217/fon.10.37

Ding, Y., Xu, H., Xu, C., Tong, Z., Zhang, S., Bai, Y., Chen, Y., Xu, Q., Zhou, L., Ding, H., Sun, Z., Yan, S., Mao, Z., & Wang, W. (2020). A nanomedicine fabricated from gold nanoparticles-decorated metal–organic framework for cascade chemo/chemodynamic cancer therapy. *Advancement of Science*, *7*(17), 2001060. DOI: 10.1002/advs.202001060 PMID: 32995124

Disis, M. L. (2010). Immune regulation of cancer. *Journal of Clinical Oncology*, *28*(29), 4531–4538. DOI: 10.1200/JCO.2009.27.2146 PMID: 20516428

Doe, J., & Smith, A. (2023). Exploring new methodologies in data science. *Journal of Data Science : JDS*, *15*(2), 123–134. DOI: 10.1016/j.jds.2023.01.001

Dosch, J. S., Pasca di Magliano, M., & Simeone, D. M. (2010). Pancreatic cancer and hedgehog pathway signaling: new insights. *Pancreatology: official journal of the International Association of Pancreatology (IAP) ... [et al.]*, *10*(2-3), 151–157. DOI: 10.1159/000225923

Dreaden, E. C., Alkilany, A. M., Huang, X., Murphy, C. J., & El-Sayed, M. A. (2012). The golden age: Gold nanoparticles for biomedicine. *Chemical Society Reviews*, *41*(7), 2740–2779. DOI: 10.1039/C1CS15237H PMID: 22109657

Duan, H., Li, L., & He, S. (2023). Advances and prospects in the treatment of pancreatic cancer. *International Journal of Nanomedicine*, *18*, 3973–3988. DOI: 10.2147/IJN.S413496 PMID: 37489138

Du, C., Qi, Y., Zhang, Y., Wang, Y., Zhao, X., Min, H., Han, X., Lang, J., Qin, H., Shi, Q., Zhang, Z., Tian, X., Anderson, G. J., Zhao, Y., Nie, G., & Yang, Y. (2018). Epidermal growth factor receptor-targeting peptide nanoparticles simultaneously deliver gemcitabine and olaparib to treat pancreatic cancer with breast cancer 2 (BRCA2) mutation. *ACS Nano, 12*(11), 10785–10796. DOI: 10.1021/acsnano.8b01573 PMID: 30407790

Ducreux, M., Cuhna, A. S., Caramella, C., Hollebecque, A., Burtin, P., Goere, D., Seufferlein, T., Haustermans, K., Van Laethem, J. L., Conroy, T., & Arnold, D. (2015). Cancer of the pancreas: ESMO Clinical Practice Guidelines for diagnosis, treatment and follow-up. *Annals of Oncology : Official Journal of the European Society for Medical Oncology, 26*, 56–68. DOI: 10.1093/annonc/mdv295

Duffy, D. J. (2016). Problems, challenges and promises: Perspectives on precision medicine. *Briefings in Bioinformatics, 17*(3), 494–504. DOI: 10.1093/bib/bbv060 PMID: 26249224

Du, J., An, Z. J., Huang, Z. F., Yang, Y. C., Zhang, M. H., Fu, X. H., Shi, W.-Y., & Hou, J. (2023). Novel insights from spatial transcriptome analysis in solid tumors. *International Journal of Biological Sciences, 19*(15), 4778–4792. DOI: 10.7150/ijbs.83098 PMID: 37781515

Durack, J., & Lynch, S. V. (2019). The gut microbiome: Relationships with disease and opportunities for therapy. *The Journal of Experimental Medicine, 216*(1), 20–40. DOI: 10.1084/jem.20180448

Eash, K. J., Greenbaum, A. M., Gopalan, P. K., & Link, D. C. (2010). CXCR2 and CXCR4 antagonistically regulate neutrophil trafficking from murine bone marrow. *The Journal of Clinical Investigation, 120*(7), 2423–2431. DOI: 10.1172/JCI41649

Elgogary, A., Xu, Q., Poore, B., Alt, J., Zimmermann, S. C., Zhao, L., Fu, J., Chen, B., Xia, S., Liu, Y., Neisser, M., Nguyen, C., Lee, R., Park, J. K., Reyes, J., Hartung, T., Rojas, C., & Alexander, R. K. Yuan, & Hanes, J. (2016). Combination therapy with BPTES nanoparticles and metformin targets the metabolic heterogeneity of pancreatic cancer. *Proceedings of the National Academy of Sciences, 113*(36), E5328–E5336. https://doi.org/DOI: 10.1073/pnas.1611406113

El-Zahaby, S. A., Elnaggar, Y. S. R., & Abdallah, O. Y. (2018). Reviewing two decades of nanomedicine implementations in targeted treatment and diagnosis of pancreatic cancer: An emphasis on state-of-the-art. *Journal of Controlled Release, 293*, 21–35. DOI: 10.1016/j.jconrel.2018.11.013 PMID: 30445002

Elzoghby, A. O., Samy, W. M., & Elgindy, N. A. (2012). Albumin-based nanoparticles as potential controlled release drug delivery systems. *Journal of Controlled Release*, *157*(2), 168–182. DOI: 10.1016/j.jconrel.2011.07.031 PMID: 21839127

Eribe, E. R., & Olsen, I. (2008). *Leptotrichia* species in human infections. *Anaerobe*, *14*(3), 131–137. DOI: 10.1016/j.anaerobe.2008.04.004

Erkan, M., Hausmann, S., Michalski, C. W., Fingerle, A. A., Dobritz, M., Kleeff, J., & Friess, H. (2012). The role of stroma in pancreatic cancer: Diagnostic and therapeutic implications. *Nature Reviews. Gastroenterology & Hepatology*, *9*(8), 454–467. DOI: 10.1038/nrgastro.2012.115 PMID: 22710569

Ertz-Archambault, N., Keim, P., & Von Hoff, D. (2017). Microbiome and pancreatic cancer: A comprehensive topic review of literature. *World Journal of Gastroenterology*, *23*(10), 1899–1908. DOI: 10.3748/wjg.v23.i10.1899

Ettrich, T. J., & Seufferlein, T. (2021). Systemic Therapy for Metastatic Pancreatic Cancer. *Current Treatment Options in Oncology*, *22*(11), 106. Advance online publication. DOI: 10.1007/s11864-021-00895-4 PMID: 34665339

Evans, D. B., Rich, T. A., Byrd, D. R., Ames, F. C., & Cleary, K. R. (1992). Preoperative chemoradiation and pancreaticoduodenectomy for adenocarcinoma of the pancreas. *Archives of Surgery*, *127*(11), 1335–1339. DOI: 10.1001/archsurg.1992.01420110083017 PMID: 1359851

Evans, D. B., Varadhachary, G. R., Crane, C. H., Sun, C. C., Lee, J. E., Pisters, P. W. T., Vauthey, J.-N., Wang, H., Cleary, K. R., Staerkel, G. A., Charnsangavej, C., Lano, E. A., Ho, L., Lenzi, R., Abbruzzese, J. L., & Wolff, R. A. (2008). Preoperative gemcitabine-based chemoradiation for patients with resectable adenocarcinoma of the pancreatic head. *Journal of Clinical Oncology*, *26*(21), 3496–3502. DOI: 10.1200/JCO.2007.15.8634 PMID: 18640930

Fagman, J. B., Ljungman, D., Falk, P., Iresjö, B. M., Engström, C., Naredi, P., & Lundholm, K. (2019, June). EGFR, but not COX-2, protein in resected pancreatic ductal adenocarcinoma is associated with poor survival. *Oncology Letters*, *17*(6), 5361–5368. DOI: 10.3892/ol.2019.10224 PMID: 31186753

Falconi, M., Eriksson, B., Kaltsas, G., Bartsch, D. K., Capdevila, J., Caplin, M., Kos-Kudla, B., Kwekkeboom, D., Rindi, G., Klöppel, G., Reed, N., Kianmanesh, R., & Jensen, R. T. (2016). ENETS Consensus Guidelines Update for the Management of Patients with Functional Pancreatic Neuroendocrine Tumors and Non-Functional Pancreatic Neuroendocrine Tumors. *Neuroendocrinology*, *103*(2), 153–171. DOI: 10.1159/000443171 PMID: 26742109

Fan, X., Alekseyenko, A. V., Wu, J., Peters, B. A., Jacobs, E. J., Gapstur, S. M., Purdue, M. P., Abnet, C. C., Stolzenberg-Solomon, R., Miller, G., Ravel, J., Hayes, R. B., & Ahn, J. (2018). Human oral microbiome and prospective risk for pancreatic cancer: A population-based nested case-control study. *Gut*, *67*(1), 120–127. DOI: 10.1136/gutjnl-2016-312580

Fan, Z., Xiao, Y., Du, Y., Zhang, Y., & Zhou, W. (2025). Pancreatic cancer subtyping - the keystone of precision treatment. *Frontiers in Immunology*, *16*, 1563725. DOI: 10.3389/fimmu.2025.1563725 PMID: 40264765

Farnell, M. B., Pearson, R. K., Sarr, M. G., DiMagno, E. P., Burgart, L. J., Dahl, T. R., Foster, N., & Sargent, D. J.the Pancreas Cancer Working Group. (2005). A prospective randomized trial comparing standard pancreatoduodenectomy with pancreatoduodenectomy with extended lymphadenectomy in resectable pancreatic head adenocarcinoma. *Surgery*, *138*(4), 618–628. DOI: 10.1016/j.surg.2005.06.044 PMID: 16269290

Farrell, J. J., Elsaleh, H., Garcia, M., Lai, R., Ammar, A., Regine, W. F., Abrams, R., Benson, A. B., Macdonald, J., Cass, C. E., Dicker, A. P., & Mackey, J. R. (2009). Human equilibrative nucleoside transporter 1 levels predict response to gemcitabine in patients with pancreatic cancer. *Gastroenterology*, *136*(1), 187–195. DOI: 10.1053/j.gastro.2008.09.067 PMID: 18992248

Fatima, M., Abourehab, M. A. S., Aggarwal, G., Jain, G. K., Sahebkar, A., & Kesharwani, P. (2022). Advancement of cell-penetrating peptides in combating triple-negative breast cancer. *Drug Discovery Today*, *27*(11), 103353. DOI: 10.1016/j.drudis.2022.103353 PMID: 36099963

Feig, C., Gopinathan, A., Neesse, A., Chan, D., Cook, N., & Tuveson, D. (2012). The pancreas cancer microenvironment. *Clinical Cancer Research*, *18*(16), 4266–4276. DOI: 10.1158/1078-0432.CCR-11-3114 PMID: 22896693

Feng, Z., Prentice, R., & Srivastava, S. (2004). Research issues and strategies for genomic and proteomic biomarker discovery and validation: A statistical perspective. *Pharmacogenomics*, *5*(6), 709–719. DOI: 10.1517/14622416.5.6.709 PMID: 15335291

Ferrone, C. R., Marchegiani, G., Hong, T. S., Ryan, D. P., Deshpande, V., McDonnell, E. I., Sabbatino, F., Santos, D. D., Allen, J. N., Blaszkowsky, L. S., Clark, J. W., Faris, J. E., Goyal, L., Kwak, E. L., Murphy, J. E., Ting, D. T., Wo, J. Y., Zhu, A. X., Warshaw, A. L., & Castillo, C. F. (2015). Radiological and surgical implications of neoadjuvant treatment with FOLFIRINOX for locally advanced and borderline resectable pancreatic cancer. *Annals of Surgery*, *261*(1), 12–17. DOI: 10.1097/SLA.0000000000000867 PMID: 25599322

Ferry, D. R., Deakin, M., Babb, J., & Kerr, D. J. (2000). A Phase II study of the 5-lipoxygenase inhibitor, CV6504, in advanced pancreatic cancer: Correlation of clinical data with pharmacokinetic and pharmacodynamic endpoints. *Annals of Oncology : Official Journal of the European Society for Medical Oncology*, *11*(10), 1165–1170. DOI: 10.1023/A:1008303715515 PMID: 11061613

Fiorino, S., Bacchi-Reggiani, L., Pontoriero, M., Gallo, C., Chili, E., Masetti, M., Zanini, N., Grondona, A. G., Silvestri, T., Cuppini, A., Jovine, E., & de Biase, D. (2018). Association between Hepatitis B or Hepatitis C Virus Infection and Risk of Pancreatic Adenocarcinoma Development: A Systematic Review and Meta-Analysis. *Pancreatology*, (6), 647–655. DOI: 10.1016/j.pan.2018.05.006

Fiorino, S., Chili, E., Bacchi-Reggiani, L., Masetti, M., Deleonardi, G., Grondona, A. G., Silvestri, T., Magrini, E., Zanini, N., Cuppini, A., Nardi, R., & Jovine, E. (2013). Association between Hepatitis B or Hepatitis C virus infection and risk of pancreatic adenocarcinoma development: A systematic review and meta-analysis. *Pancreatology*, *13*(2), 147–160. DOI: 10.1016/j.pan.2013.01.005

Foley, K., Kim, V., Jaffee, E., & Zheng, L. (2016). Current progress in immunotherapy for pancreatic cancer. *Cancer Letters*, *381*(1), 244–251. DOI: 10.1016/j.canlet.2015.12.020 PMID: 26723878

Fossati, V., Cattaneo, G. M., & Clarke, L. (1995). The role of intraoperative therapy by electron beam and combination of Adjuvant Chemotherapy and External Radiotherapy in carcinoma of the Pancreas. *Tumori*, *81*(1), 23–31. DOI: 10.1177/030089169508100106 PMID: 7754537

Fraher, M. H., O'Toole, P. W., & Quigley, E. M. (2012). Techniques used to characterize the gut microbiota: A guide for the clinician. *Nature Reviews. Gastroenterology & Hepatology*, *9*(6), 312–322. https:// Doi.org/10.1038/nrgastro.2012.44. DOI: 10.1038/nrgastro.2012.44

Furnari, F. B., Cloughesy, T. F., Cavenee, W. K., & Mischel, P. S. (2015). Heterogeneity of epidermal growth factor receptor signalling networks in glioblastoma. *Nature Reviews. Cancer*, *15*(5), 302–310. DOI: 10.1038/nrc3918 PMID: 25855404

Furukawa, T., Hatori, T., Fujita, I., Yamamoto, M., Kobayashi, M., Ohike, N., Morohoshi, T., Egawa, S., Unno, M., Takao, S., Osako, M., Yonezawa, S., Mino-Kenudson, M., Lauwers, G. Y., Yamaguchi, H., Ban, S., & Shimizu, M. (2011). Prognostic relevance of morphological types of intraductal papillary mucinous neoplasms of the pancreas. *Gut*, *60*(4), 509–516. DOI: 10.1136/gut.2010.210567 PMID: 21193453

Gao, J., Long, B., & Wang, Z. (2017). Role of Notch signaling pathway in pancreatic cancer. *American Journal of Cancer Research*, *7*(2), 173.

Garcia-Sampedro, A., Gaggia, G., Ney, A., Mahamed, I., & Acedo, P. (2021). The State-of-the-Art of Phase II/III Clinical Trials for Targeted Pancreatic Cancer Therapies. *Journal of Clinical Medicine*, *10*(4), 566–566. DOI: 10.3390/jcm10040566 PMID: 33546207

Garg, P., Pareek, S., Kulkarni, P., Horne, D., Salgia, R., & Singhal, S. S. (2024). Next-Generation Immunotherapy: Advancing Clinical Applications in Cancer Treatment. *Journal of Clinical Medicine*, *13*(21), 6537. DOI: 10.3390/jcm13216537 PMID: 39518676

Garrido-Laguna, I., & Hidalgo, M. (2015). Pancreatic cancer: From state-of-the-art treatments to promising novel therapies. *Nature Reviews. Clinical Oncology*, *12*(6), 319–334. DOI: 10.1038/nrclinonc.2015.53 PMID: 25824606

Gavas, S., Quazi, S., & Karpiński, T. M. (2021). Nanoparticles for cancer therapy: Current progress and challenges. *Nanoscale Research Letters*, *16*(1), 173. DOI: 10.1186/s11671-021-03628-6 PMID: 34866166

Geier, B., Sogin, E. M., Michellod, D., Janda, M., Kompauer, M., Spengler, B., Dubilier, N., & Liebeke, M. (2020). Spatial metabolomics of in situ host–microbe interactions at the micrometre scale. *Nature Microbiology*, *5*(3), 498–510. DOI: 10.1038/s41564-019-0664-6 PMID: 32015496

Geller, L. T., Barzily-Rokni, M., Danino, T., Jonas, O. H., Shental, N., Nejman, D., Gavert, N., Zwang, Y., Cooper, Z. A., Shee, K., Thaiss, C. A., Reuben, A., Livny, J., Avraham, R., Frederick, D. T., Ligorio, M., Chatman, K., Johnston, S. E., Mosher, C. M., & Straussman, R. (2017). Potential role of intratumor bacteria in mediating tumor resistance to the chemotherapeutic drug gemcitabine. *Science*, *357*(6356), 1156–1160. DOI: 10.1126/science.aah5043

Genton, L., Lazarevic, V., Stojanovic, O., Spiljar, M., Djaafar, S., Koessler, T., Dutoit, V., Gaïa, N., Mareschal, J., Macpherson, A. J., Herrmann, F., Trajkovski, M., & Schrenzel, J. (2021). Metataxonomic and metabolic impact of fecal microbiota transplantation from patients with pancreatic cancer into germ-free mice: A pilot study. *Frontiers in Cellular and Infection Microbiology*, *11*, 752889. DOI: 10.3389/fcimb.2021.752889

Gerriets, V., & Kasi, A. (2025 Jan). Bevacizumab. [Updated 2023 Aug 28] In *StatPearls* [Internet]. StatPearls Publishing., Available from https://www.ncbi.nlm.nih.gov/books/NBK482126/

Ge, Y., Wang, X., Guo, Y., Yan, J., Abuduwaili, A., Aximujiang, K., Yan, J., & Wu, M. (2021). Gut microbiota influence tumor development and Alter interactions with the human immune system. *Journal of Experimental & Clinical Cancer Research : CR*, *40*(1), 42. DOI: 10.1186/s13046-021-01845-6

Ghaneh, P., Palmer, D. H., Cicconi, S., Halloran, C., Psarelli, E. E., Rawcliffe, C. L., Sripadam, R., Mukherjee, S., Wadsley, J., Al-Mukhtar, A., Jiao, L. R., Wasan, H. S., Carter, R., Graham, J. S., Ammad, F., Evans, J., Tjaden, C., Hackert, T., Buchler, M. W., & Neoptolemos, J. P. (2020). ESPAC-5F: Four-arm, prospective, multicenter, international randomized phase II trial of immediate surgery compared with neoadjuvant gemcitabine plus capecitabine (GEMCAP) or FOLFIRINOX or chemoradiotherapy (CRT) in patients with borderline resectable pancreatic cancer. *Journal of Clinical Oncology*, *38*(15, suppl), 4505. DOI: 10.1200/JCO.2020.38.15_suppl.4505

Gheorghe, G., Bungau, S., Ilie, M., Behl, T., Vesa, C. M., Brisc, C., Bacalbasa, N., Turi, V., Costache, R. S., & Diaconu, C. C. (2020). Early diagnosis of pancreatic cancer: The key to survival. *Diagnostics (Basel)*, *10*(11), 869. DOI: 10.3390/diagnostics10110869 PMID: 33114412

Gianella, A., Jarzyna, P. A., Mani, V., Ramachandran, S., Calcagno, C., Tang, J., Kann, B., Dijk, W. J. R., Thijssen, V. L., Griffioen, A. W., Storm, G., Fayad, Z. A., & Mulder, W. J. M. (2011). Multifunctional nanoemulsion platform for imaging-guided therapy evaluated in experimental cancer. *ACS Nano*, *5*(6), 4422–4433. DOI: 10.1021/nn103336a PMID: 21557611

Gibson, G. R., Scott, K. P., Rastall, R. A., Tuohy, K. M., Hotchkiss, A., Dubert-Ferrandon, A., Gareau, M., Murphy, E. F., Saulnier, D., Loh, G., Macfarlane, S., Delzenne, N., Ringel, Y., Kozianowski, G., Dickmann, R., Lenoir-Wijnkoop, I., Walker, C., & Buddington, R. (2010). Dietary prebiotics: Current status and new definition. *Food Science and Technology Bulletin*, *7*(1), 1–19. DOI: 10.1616/1476-2137.15880

Gill, S., Tasian, S. K., Ruella, M., Shestova, O., Li, Y., Porter, D. L., Carroll, M., Danet-Desnoyers, G., Scholler, J., Grupp, S. A., June, C. H., & Kalos, M. (2014). Preclinical targeting of human acute myeloid leukemia and myeloablation using chimeric antigen receptor–modified T cells. *Blood*, *123*(15), 2343–2354. DOI: 10.1182/blood-2013-09-529537 PMID: 24596416

Ginghina, O., Hudita, A., Zamfir, M., Spanu, A., Mardare, M., Bondoc, I., & Galateanu, B. (2022). Liquid biopsy and artificial intelligence as tools to detect signatures of colorectal malignancies: A modern approach in patient's stratification. *Frontiers in Oncology*, *12*, 856575. DOI: 10.3389/fonc.2022.856575 PMID: 35356214

Gjertsen, M. K., Buanes, T., & Rosseland, A. R. (2001). Intradermal ras peptide vaccination with granulocyte-macrophage colony-stimulating factor as adjuvant: Clinical and immunological responses in patients with pancreatic adenocarcinoma. *International Journal of Cancer*, *92*(3), 441–450. DOI: 10.1002/ijc.1205 PMID: 11291084

Glimelius, B., Hoffman, K., Sjoden, P. O., Jacobsson, G., Sellstrom, H., Enander, L. K., Linne, T., & Svensson, C. (1996). Chemotherapy improves survival and quality of life in advanced pancreatic and biliary cancer. *Annals of Oncology : Official Journal of the European Society for Medical Oncology*, *7*(6), 593–600. DOI: 10.1093/oxfordjournals.annonc.a010676 PMID: 8879373

Goicoechea, S. M., Garcia-Mata, R., Staub, J., Valdivia, A., Sharek, L., McCulloch, C. G., Hwang, R. F., Urrutia, R., Yeh, J. J., Kim, H. J., & Otey, C. A. (2014). Palladin promotes invasion of pancreatic cancer cells by enhancing invadopodia formation in cancer-associated fibroblasts. *Oncogene*, *33*(10), 1265–1273. DOI: 10.1038/onc.2013.68

Golan, T., Hammel, P., Reni, M., Van Cutsem, E., Macarulla, T., Hall, M. J., Park, J. O., Hochhauser, D., Arnold, D., Oh, D. Y., Reinacher-Schick, A., Tortora, G., Algül, H., O'Reilly, E. M., McGuinness, D., Cui, K. Y., Schlienger, K., Locker, G. Y., & Kindler, H. L. (2019). Maintenance olaparib for germline BRCA-mutated metastatic pancreatic cancer. *The New England Journal of Medicine*, *381*(4), 317–327. DOI: 10.1056/NEJMoa1903387 PMID: 31157963

Gong, M., Meng, H., Tan, D., Li, P., Qin, J., An, Q., Shi, C., & An, J. (2023). Establishment of organoid models for pancreatic ductal adenocarcinoma and screening of individualized therapy strategy. *Animal Models and Experimental Medicine*, *6*(5), 409–418. DOI: 10.1002/ame2.12352 PMID: 37890865

Gopalakrishnan, V., Spencer, C. N., Nezi, L., Reuben, A., Andrews, M. C., Karpinets, T. V., & Wargo, J. A. (2018). Gut microbiome modulates response to anti–PD-1 immunotherapy in melanoma patients. *Science, 359*(6371), 97–103. DOI: 10.1126/science.aan4236

Gopinathan, A., Morton, J. P., Jodrell, D. I., & Sansom, O. J. (2015). GEMMs as preclinical models for testing pancreatic cancer therapies. *Disease Models & Mechanisms, 8*(10), 1185–1200. DOI: 10.1242/dmm.021055

Gresham, G. K., Wells, G. A., Gill, S., Cameron, C., & Jonker, D. J. (2014). Chemotherapy regimens for advanced pancreatic cancer: A systematic review and network meta-analysis. *BMC Cancer, 14*(1), 471. Advance online publication. DOI: 10.1186/1471-2407-14-471 PMID: 24972449

Griffin, J. F., Poruk, K. E., & Wolfgang, C. L. (2015). Pancreatic cancer surgery: Past, present, and future. *Chinese Journal of Cancer Research = Chung-Kuo Yen Cheng Yen Chiu, 27*(4), 332. PMID: 26361403

Groot Koerkamp, B., Sadot, E., Kemeny, N., Gönen, M., Leal, J. N., Allen, P. J., Cercek, A., DeMatteo, R. P., Kingham, T. P., Jarnagin, W. R., & D'Angelica, M. I. (2017). Perioperative hepatic arterial infusion pump chemotherapy is associated with longer survival after resection of colorectal liver metastases: A propensity score analysis. *Journal of Clinical Oncology, 35*(17), 1938–1944. DOI: 10.1200/JCO.2016.71.8346 PMID: 28426374

Grosser, R., Cherkassky, L., Chintala, N., & Adusumilli, P. S. (2019). Combination Immunotherapy with CAR T Cells and Checkpoint Blockade for the Treatment of Solid Tumors. *Cancer Cell, 36*(5), 471–482. DOI: 10.1016/j.ccell.2019.09.006 PMID: 31715131

Guan, S., Deng, G., Sun, J., Han, Q., Lv, Y., Xue, T., Ding, L., Yang, T., Qian, N., & Dai, G. (2022). Evaluation of circulating tumor DNA as a prognostic biomarker for metastatic pancreatic adenocarcinoma. *Frontiers in Oncology, 12*, 926260. DOI: 10.3389/fonc.2022.926260 PMID: 36081557

Gunderson, L. L., Martin, J. K., Kvols, L. K., Nagorney, D. M., Fieck, J. M., Wieand, H. S., Martinez, A., O'Connell, M. J., Earle, J. D., & McIlrath, D. C. (1987). Intraoperative and external beam irradiation ± 5-FU for locally advanced Pancreatic Cancer. *International Journal of Radiation Oncology, Biology, Physics, 13*(3), 319–329. DOI: 10.1016/0360-3016(87)90005-8 PMID: 3104244

Gunderson, L. L., Nagorney, D. M., Martenson, J. A., Donohue, J. H., Garton, G. R., Nelson, H., & Fieck, J. (1995). External beam plus intraoperative irradiation for gastrointestinal cancers. *World Journal of Surgery, 19*(2), 191–197. DOI: 10.1007/BF00308625 PMID: 7754622

Guo, Y. J., Pan, W. W., Liu, S. B., Shen, Z. F., Xu, Y., & Hu, L. L. (2020). ERK/MAPK signalling pathway and tumorigenesis. *Experimental and Therapeutic Medicine, 19*(3), 1997–2007. PMID: 32104259

Gupta, A. K., & Gupta, M. (2005). Synthesis and surface engineering of iron oxide nanoparticles for biomedical applications. *Biomaterials, 26*(18), 3995–4021. DOI: 10.1016/j.biomaterials.2004.10.012 PMID: 15626447

Hackeng, W. M., Hruban, R. H., Offerhaus, G. J. A., & Brosens, L. A. A. (2016). Surgical and molecular pathology of pancreatic neoplasms. *Diagnostic Pathology, 11*(1), 47. DOI: 10.1186/s13000-016-0497-z PMID: 27267993

Halder, S., Basu, S., Lall, S. P., Ganti, A. K., Batra, S. K., & Seshacharyulu, P. (2023). Targeting the EGFR signaling pathway in cancer therapy: What's new in 2023? *Expert Opinion on Therapeutic Targets, 27*(4-5), 305–324. DOI: 10.1080/14728222.2023.2218613 PMID: 37243489

Halfdanarson, T. R., Rabe, K. G., Rubin, J., & Petersen, G. M. (2008). Pancreatic Neuroendocrine Tumors (PNETs): Incidence, Prognosis, and Recent Trend Toward Improved Survival. *Annals of Oncology : Official Journal of the European Society for Medical Oncology, 19*(10), 1727–1733. DOI: 10.1093/annonc/mdn351 PMID: 18515795

Halimi, A., Gabarrini, G., Sobkowiak, M. J., Ateeb, Z., Davanian, H., Gaiser, R. A., Arnelo, U., Valente, R., Wong, A. Y. W., Moro, C. F., Del Chiaro, M., Özenci, V., & Sällberg Chen, M. (2021). Isolation of pancreatic microbiota from cystic precursors of pancreatic cancer with intracellular growth and DNA-damaging properties. *Gut Microbes, 13*(1), 1983101. DOI: 10.1080/19490976.2021.1983101

Haller, D. G. (2002, December). Future directions in the treatment of pancreatic cancer. [). WB Saunders.]. *Seminars in Oncology, 29*(6), 31–39. DOI: 10.1016/S0093-7754(02)70024-9

Hallin, J., Engstrom, L. D., Hargis, L., Calinisan, A., Aranda, R., Briere, D. M., Sudhakar, N., Bowcut, V., Baer, B. R., Ballard, J. A., Burkard, M. R., Fell, J. B., Fischer, J. P., Vigers, G. P., Xue, Y., Gatto, S., Fernandez-Banet, J., Pavlicek, A., Velastagui, K., & Christensen, J. G. (2020). The KRASG12C inhibitor MRTX849 provides insight toward therapeutic susceptibility of KRAS-mutant cancers in mouse models and patients. *Cancer Discovery*, *10*(1), 54–71. DOI: 10.1158/2159-8290.CD-19-1167 PMID: 31658955

Hamada, T., Nowak, J. A., Milner, D. J.Jr, Song, M. Y., & Ogino, S. J. (2019). Integration of microbiology, molecular pathology, and epidemiology: A new paradigm to explore the pathogenesis of microbiome-driven neoplasms. *The Journal of Pathology*, *247*(5), 615–628. DOI: 10.1002/path.5236

Hameed, B. S., & Krishnan, U. M. (2022). Artificial intelligence-driven diagnosis of pancreatic cancer. *Cancers (Basel)*, *14*(21), 5382. DOI: 10.3390/cancers14215382 PMID: 36358800

Hammel, P., Huguet, F., Van Laethem, J. L., Goldstein, D., Glimelius, B., Artru, P., Borbath, I., Bouché, O., Shannon, J., André, T., Mineur, L., Chibaudel, B., Bonnetain, F., & Louvet, C. (2016). Effect of chemoradiotherapy vs chemotherapy on survival in patients with locally advanced pancreatic cancer controlled after 4 months of gemcitabine with or without erlotinib: The LAP07 randomized clinical trial. *Journal of the American Medical Association*, *315*(17), 1844–1853. DOI: 10.1001/jama.2016.4324

Hanaf-Bojd, M. Y., Ansari, L., & Malaekeh-Nikouei, B. (2016). Codelivery of anticancer drugs and siRNA by mesoporous silica nanoparticles. *Therapeutic Delivery*, *7*(9), 649–655. DOI: 10.4155/tde-2016-0045 PMID: 27582236

Hanahan, D., & Weinberg, R. A. (2011). Hallmarks of cancer: The next generation. *Cell*, *144*(5), 646–674. DOI: 10.1016/j.cell.2011.02.013

Han, X., Li, Y., Xu, Y., Zhao, X., Zhang, Y., Yang, X., Wang, Y., Zhao, R., Anderson, G. J., Zhao, Y., & Nie, G. (2018). Reversal of pancreatic desmoplasia by re-educating stellate cells with a tumour microenvironment-activated nanosystem. *Nature Communications*, *9*(1), 3390. DOI: 10.1038/s41467-018-05906-x PMID: 30139933

Harrison, P. T., Vyse, S., & Huang, P. H. (2020). Rare epidermal growth factor receptor (EGFR) mutations in non-small cell lung cancer. *Seminars in Cancer Biology*, *61*, 167–179. DOI: 10.1016/j.semcancer.2019.09.015 PMID: 31562956

Hayat, U., Croce, P. S., Saadeh, A., Desai, K., Appiah, J., Khan, S., Khan, Y. I., Kumar, K., & Hanif, A. (2025). Current and emerging treatment options for pancreatic cancer: A comprehensive review. *Journal of Clinical Medicine*, *14*(4), 1129. DOI: 10.3390/jcm14041129 PMID: 40004658

Haycox, A., Lombard, M., Neoptolemos, J. P., & Walley, T. (1998). Review article: Current treatment and optimal patient management in pancreatic cancer. *Alimentary Pharmacology & Therapeutics*, *12*(10), 949–964. DOI: 10.1046/j.1365-2036.1998.00390.x PMID: 9798799

Hegde, S., Krisnawan, V. E., Herzog, B. H., Zuo, C., Breden, M. A., Knolhoff, B. L., Hogg, G. D., Tang, J. P., Baer, J. M., Mpoy, C., Lee, K. B., Alexander, K. A., Rogers, B. E., Murphy, K. M., Hawkins, W. G., Fields, R. C., DeSelm, C. J., Schwarz, J. K., & DeNardo, D. G. (2020). Dendritic cell paucity leads to dysfunctional immune surveillance in pancreatic cancer. *Cancer Cell*, *37*(3), 289–307. DOI: 10.1016/j.ccell.2020.02.008

Heinemann, V., Haas, M., & Boeck, S. (2013). Neoadjuvant treatment of borderline resectable and non-resectable pancreatic cancer. *Annals of Oncology : Official Journal of the European Society for Medical Oncology*, *24*(10), 2484–2492. DOI: 10.1093/annonc/mdt239 PMID: 23852311

Heinz, H., Pramanik, C., Heinz, O., Ding, Y., Mishra, R. K., Marchon, D., Flatt, R. J., Estrela-Lopis, I., Llop, J., Moya, S., & Ziolo, R. F. (2017). Nanoparticle decoration with surfactants: Molecular interactions, assembly, and applications. *Surface Science Reports*, *72*(1), 1–58. DOI: 10.1016/j.surfrep.2017.02.001

He, J., Mo, Z., Mai, Q., & Chen, X. (2021). Serum neutrophil/lymphocyte ratio as a potential predictor of treatment response for immune checkpoint inhibitors in patients with advanced hepatocellular carcinoma. *Journal of Clinical Oncology*, *39*(15, suppl), e16156. Advance online publication. DOI: 10.1200/JCO.2021.39.15_suppl.e16156

Hentic, O., Hammel, P., & Couvelard, A. (2012). FOLFIRI Regimen in Metastatic Pancreatic Adenocarcinoma Resistant to Gemcitabine and Platinum-Salts. *World Journal of Gastroenterology*, *18*(33), 4533–4541. DOI: 10.3748/wjg.v18.i33.4533 PMID: 22969226

Herbst, B., & Zheng, L. (2019). Precision medicine in pancreatic cancer: treating every patient as an exception. *The lancet. Gastroenterology & hepatology*, *4*(10), 805–810. doi:.1016/S2468-1253(19)30175-X

Heredia-Soto, V., Rodríguez-Salas, N., & Feliu, J. (2021). Liquid biopsy in pancreatic cancer: Are we ready to apply it in the clinical practice? *Cancers (Basel)*, *13*(8), 1986. DOI: 10.3390/cancers13081986 PMID: 33924143

Hester, C. A., Augustine, M. M., & Choti, M. A. (2020). Comparative Outcomes of Acinar Cell Carcinoma and Pancreatic Adenocarcinoma: A Population-Based Analysis. *Journal of Surgical Oncology*, *121*(5), 821–829.

He, Y., Sun, M. M., Zhang, G. G., Yang, J., Chen, K. S., Xu, W. W., & Li, B. (2021). Targeting PI3K/Akt signal transduction for cancer therapy. *Signal Transduction and Targeted Therapy*, *6*(1), 425. DOI: 10.1038/s41392-021-00828-5 PMID: 34916492

Hill, C., Guarner, F., Reid, G., Gibson, G. R., Merenstein, D. J., Pot, B., Morelli, L., Canani, R. B., Flint, H. J., Salminen, S., Calder, P. C., & Sanders, M. E. (2014). Expert consensus document: The International Scientific Association for Probiotics and Prebiotics consensus statement on the scope and appropriate use of the term probiotic. *Nature Reviews. Gastroenterology & Hepatology*, *11*(8), 506–514. DOI: 10.1038/nrgastro.2014.66

Hiraoka, T. (1990). Extended radical resection of cancer of the pancreas with intra-operative radiotherapy. *Bailliere's Clinical Gastroenterology*, *4*(4), 985–993. DOI: 10.1016/0950-3528(90)90031-B PMID: 2078795

Hiraoka, T., Uchino, R., Kanemitsu, K., Toyonaga, M., Saitoh, N., Nakamura, I., Tashiro, S., & Miyauchi, Y. (1990). Combination of intraoperative radiation with resection of cancer of the pancreas. *International Journal of Pancreatology*, *7*(3), 201–207. DOI: 10.1007/BF02924238 PMID: 1964472

Hirooka, Y., Kasuya, H., Ishikawa, T., Kawashima, H., Ohno, E., Villalobos, I. B., Naoe, Y., Ichinose, T., Koyama, N., Tanaka, M., Kodera, Y., & Goto, H. (2022). A Phase I clinical trial of EUS-guided intratumoral injection of the oncolytic virus, HF10 for unresectable locally advanced pancreatic cancer. *BMC Cancer*, *18*(1), 596. DOI: 10.1186/s12885-018-4453-z

Hoffman, J. P., Lipsitz, S., Pisansky, T., Weese, J. L., Solin, L., & Benson, A. B.III. (1998). Phase II trial of preoperative radiation therapy and chemotherapy for patients with localized, resectable adenocarcinoma of the pancreas: An Eastern Cooperative Oncology Group Study. *Journal of Clinical Oncology*, *16*(1), 317–323. DOI: 10.1200/JCO.1998.16.1.317 PMID: 9440759

Hosein, A. N., Brekken, R. A., & Maitra, A. (2020). Pancreatic cancer stroma: An update on therapeutic targeting strategies. *Nature Reviews. Gastroenterology & Hepatology*, *17*(8), 487–505. DOI: 10.1038/s41575-020-0300-1

Hosein, P. J., de Lima Lopes, G., Pastorini, V. H., Gomez, C., Macintyre, J., Zayas, G., Reis, I., Montero, A. J., Merchan, J. R., & Rocha Lima, C. M. (2013). A phase II trial of nab-Paclitaxel as second-line therapy in patients with advanced pancreatic cancer. *American Journal of Clinical Oncology*, *36*(2), 151–156. DOI: 10.1097/COC.0b013e3182436e8c PMID: 22307213

Hossen, N., Rao, G., Dey, A., Robertson, J. D., Bhattacharya, R., & Mukherjee, P. (2019). Gold nanoparticle transforms activated cancer-associated fibroblasts to quiescence. *ACS Applied Materials & Interfaces*, *11*(30), 26060–26068. DOI: 10.1021/acsami.9b03313 PMID: 31117437

Hou, X., Zaks, T., Langer, R., & Dong, Y. (2021). Lipid nanoparticles for mRNA delivery. *Nature Reviews. Materials*, *6*(12), 1078–1094. DOI: 10.1038/s41578-021-00358-0 PMID: 34394960

Ho, W. J., Jaffee, E. M., & Zheng, L. (2020). The tumour microenvironment in pancreatic cancer clinical challenges and opportunities. *Nature Reviews. Clinical Oncology*, *17*(9), 527–540. DOI: 10.1038/s41571-020-0363-5

Huang, J., Liu, J., Chen-Xiao, K., Zhang, X., Lee, W. P., Go, V. L. W., & Xiao, G. G. (2016). Advance in microRNA as a potential biomarker for early detection of pancreatic cancer. *Biomarker Research*, *4*(1), 1–5. DOI: 10.1186/s40364-016-0074-3 PMID: 27795830

Huang, J., Zhan, J., Ye, B., Hu, W., Zhang, J., Wang, S., & Wang, L. (2018). Autophagy induced by curcumin and caffeine ameliorates oxidative stress-induced aging. *Cellular Physiology and Biochemistry*, *47*(3), 1241–1252. DOI: 10.1159/000490189

Huber, M., Brehm, C. U., Gress, T. M., Buchholz, M., Alhamwe, B. A., von Strandmann, E. P., Slater, E. P., Bartsch, J. W., Bauer, C., & Lauth, M. (2020). The immune microenvironment in pancreatic cancer. *International Journal of Molecular Sciences*, *21*(19), 7307. DOI: 10.3390/ijms21197307 PMID: 33022971

Hu, J.-X., Zhao, C.-F., Chen, W.-B., Liu, Q.-C., Li, Q.-W., Lin, Y.-Y., & Gao, F. (2021). Pancreatic cancer: A review of epidemiology, trend, and risk factors. *World Journal of Gastroenterology*, *27*(27), 4298–4321. DOI: 10.3748/wjg.v27.i27.4298 PMID: 34366606

Hujoel, P. P., Drangsholt, M., Spiekerman, C., & Weiss, N. S. (2003). An exploration of the periodontitis–cancer association. *Annals of Epidemiology*, *13*(5), 312–316. DOI: 10.1016/S1047-2797(02)00425-8

Hu, M., Wang, Y., Xu, L., An, S., Tang, Y., Zhou, X., Li, J., Liu, R., Dan, H., & Huang, L. (2019). Relaxin gene delivery mitigates liver metastasis and synergises with checkpoint therapy. *Nature Communications*, *10*(1), 2993. DOI: 10.1038/s41467-019-10893-8 PMID: 31278269

Hunter, B., Hindocha, S., & Lee, R. W. (2022). The role of artificial intelligence in early cancer diagnosis. *Cancers (Basel)*, *14*(6), 1524. DOI: 10.3390/cancers14061524 PMID: 35326674

Hussain, M. S., Prajapati, B. G., Gandhi, S. M., Sharma, M., Kapoor, D. U., Elossaily, G. M., & Garg, S. (2025). Overcoming obstacles: The role of lipid nanocarriers in therapeutic approaches for pancreatic cancer. *BioNanoScience*, *15*(2), 262. DOI: 10.1007/s12668-025-01873-y

Hu, Z. I., Shia, J., & Stadler, Z. K. (2020). Evaluating Mismatch Repair Deficiency in Pancreatic Adenocarcinoma: Challenges and Recommendations. *Clinical Cancer Research*, *26*(6), 1346–1354. DOI: 10.1158/1078-0432.CCR-17-3099 PMID: 29367431

Iida, N., Dzutsev, A., Stewart, C. A., Smith, L., Bouladoux, N., Weingarten, R. A., Molina, D. A., Salcedo, R., Back, T., Cramer, S., Dai, R.-M., Kiu, H., Cardone, M., Naik, S., Patri, A. K., Wang, E., Marincola, F. M., Frank, K. M., Belkaid, Y., & Goldszmid, R. S. (2013). Commensal bacteria control cancer response to therapy by modulating the tumor microenvironment. *Science*, *342*(6161), 967–970. DOI: 10.1126/science.1240527

Ilic, I., & Ilic, M. (2022). International patterns in incidence and mortality trends of pancreatic cancer in the last three decades: A joinpoint regression analysis. *World Journal of Gastroenterology*, *28*(32), 4698–4715. DOI: 10.3748/wjg.v28.i32.4698 PMID: 36157927

Imtiaz, S., Ferdous, U. T., Nizela, A., Hasan, A., Shakoor, A., Zia, A. W., & Uddin, S. (2025). Mechanistic study of cancer drug delivery: Current techniques, limitations, and future prospects. *European Journal of Medicinal Chemistry*, *290*, 117535. DOI: 10.1016/j.ejmech.2025.117535 PMID: 40132495

Ino, Y., Yamazaki-Itoh, R., Shimada, K., Iwasaki, M., Kosuge, T., Kanai, Y., & Hiraoka, N. (2013). Immune cell infiltration as an indicator of the immune microenvironment of pancreatic cancer. *British Journal of Cancer*, *108*(4), 914–923. DOI: 10.1038/bjc.2013.32 PMID: 23385730

Iravani, S. (2011). Green synthesis of metal nanoparticles using plants. *Green Chemistry*, *13*(10), 2638–2650. DOI: 10.1039/c1gc15386b

Ishikawa, O., Ohhigashi, H., Teshima, T., Chatani, M., Inoue, T., Tanaka, S., Kitamura, T., Wada, A., Sasaki, Y., Imaoka, S., & Iwanaga, T. (1989). Clinical and histopathological appraisal of preoperative irradiation for adenocarcinoma of the pancreatoduodenal region. *Journal of Surgical Oncology*, *40*(3), 143–151. DOI: 10.1002/jso.2930400303 PMID: 2918720

Ishikawa, T., Okayama, T., Oka, K., Mizushima, K., Yasuda, T., Sakamoto, N., & Itoh, Y. (2017). The JAK/STAT pathway is involved in the upregulation of PD-L1 expression in pancreatic cancer cell lines. *Oncology Reports*, *37*(3), 1545–1554. DOI: 10.3892/or.2017.5399

Iwai, T. (2009). Periodontal bacteremia and various vascular diseases. *Journal of Periodontal Research*, *44*(6), 689–694. DOI: 10.1111/j.1600-0765.2008.01165.x

Jaaks, P., Coker, E. A., Vis, D. J., Edwards, O., Carpenter, E. F., Leto, S. M., Dwane, L., Sassi, F., Lightfoot, H., Barthorpe, S., van der Meer, D., Yang, W., Beck, A., Mironenko, T., Hall, C., Hall, J., Mali, I., Richardson, L., Tolley, C., & Garnett, M. J. (2022). Effective drug combinations in breast, colon and pancreatic cancer cells. *Nature*, *603*(7899), 166–173. DOI: 10.1038/s41586-022-04437-2 PMID: 35197630

Jabłońska, B., Pawlicki, K., & Mrowiec, S. (2021). Associations between Nutritional and Immune Status and Clinicopathologic Factors in Patients with Pancreatic Cancer: A Comprehensive Analysis. *Cancers (Basel)*, *13*(20), 5041. DOI: 10.3390/cancers13205041 PMID: 34680194

Jackson, H. J., Rafiq, S., & Brentjens, R. J. (2016). Driving CAR T-cells forward. *Nature Reviews. Clinical Oncology*, *13*(6), 370–383. DOI: 10.1038/nrclinonc.2016.36 PMID: 27000958

Jain, A., Jain, A., Parajuli, P., Mishra, V., Ghoshal, G., Singh, B., Shivhare, U. S., Katare, O. P., & Kesharwani, P. (2017). Recent advances in galactose-engineered nanocarriers for the site-specific delivery of siRNA and anticancer drugs. *Drug Discovery Today*, *23*(5), 960–973. DOI: 10.1016/j.drudis.2017.11.003 PMID: 29129804

Jamal, M. H., & Khan, M. N. (2025). Developments in pancreatic cancer emerging therapies, diagnostic methods, and epidemiology. *Pathology, Research and Practice*, *156012*, 156012. Advance online publication. DOI: 10.1016/j.prp.2025.156012

Jang, J.-E., Hajdu, C. H., Liot, C., Miller, G., Dustin, M. L., & Bar-Sagi, D. (2017). Crosstalk between regulatory T cells and tumour-associated dendritic cells negates anti-tumour immunity in pancreatic cancer. *Cell Reports*, *20*(3), 558–571. DOI: 10.1016/j.celrep.2017.06.062 PMID: 28723561

Jarboe, J. S., Johnson, K. R., Choi, Y., Lonser, R. R., & Park, J. K. (2007). Expression of interleukin-13 receptor α2 in glioblastoma multiforme: Implications for targeted therapies. *Cancer Research, 67*(17), 7983–7986. DOI: 10.1158/0008-5472.CAN-07-1493 PMID: 17804706

Javadinia, S. A., Shahidsales, S., Fanipakdel, A., Joudi-Mashhad, M., Mehramiz, M., Talebian, S., Maftouh, M., Mardani, R., Hassanian, S. M., Khazaei, M., Ferns, G. A., & Avan, A. (2019). Therapeutic potential of targeting the Wnt/β-catenin pathway in the treatment of pancreatic cancer. *Journal of Cellular Biochemistry, 120*(5), 6833–6840. DOI: 10.1002/jcb.27835

Javle, M., Li, Y., Tan, D., Dong, X., Chang, P., Kar, S., & Li, D. (2014). Biomarkers of TGF-β signaling pathway and prognosis of pancreatic cancer. *PLoS One, 9*(1), e85942. DOI: 10.1371/journal.pone.0085942

Jeekel, J., Garofalo, M. C., Regine, W. F., & Tan, M. T. (2006). Upon statistical reanalysis, the EORTC trial was found to bepositive for Adjuvant Chemoradiation in Pancreatic Cancer. *Annals of Surgery, 244*, 332–333. DOI: 10.1097/00000658-200608000-00036 PMID: 16858208

Jemal, A., Bray, F., Center, M. M., Ferlay, J., Ward, E., & Forman, D. (2011). Global cancer statistics. *CA: a Cancer Journal for Clinicians, 61*(2), 69–90. DOI: 10.3322/caac.20107

Jessup, J. M., Steele, G. J., & Mayer, R. J. (1993). Neoadjuvant therapy for unresectable Pancreatic Adenocarcinoma. *Archives of Surgery, 128*(5), 559–564. DOI: 10.1001/archsurg.1993.01420170093014 PMID: 8098206

Jiang, H., Liu, X., Knolhoff, B. L., Hegde, S., Lee, K. B., Jiang, H., Fields, R. C., Pachter, J. A., Lim, K.-H., & DeNardo, D. G. (2019). Development of resistance to FAK inhibition in pancreatic cancer is linked to stromal depletion. *Gut, 69*(1), 122–132. DOI: 10.1136/gutjnl-2018-317424 PMID: 31076405

Jiang, W., Zhao, X., Wang, L., & Li, W. (2014). Hormone receptor-targeted nanoparticles for cancer imaging and therapy. *Journal of Controlled Release, 193*, 139–153. DOI: 10.1016/j.jconrel.2014.05.032

Jiao, Y., Yonescu, R., & Offerhaus, G. J. (2018). Whole-Exome Sequencing of Pancreatic Neoplasms with Acinar Differentiation. *The Journal of Pathology, 234*(4), 545–555. DOI: 10.1002/path.4310 PMID: 24293293

Jindal, A., Sarkar, S., & Alam, A. (2021). Nanomaterials-mediated immunomodulation for cancer therapeutics. *Frontiers in Chemistry, 9*, 629635. DOI: 10.3389/fchem.2021.629635 PMID: 33708759

Jing, J., Wu, Z., Wang, J., Luo, G., Lin, H., Fan, Y., & Zhou, C. (2023). Hedgehog signaling in tissue homeostasis, cancers and targeted therapies. *Signal Transduction and Targeted Therapy*, *8*(1), 315. DOI: 10.1038/s41392-023-01559-5 PMID: 37596267

Jin, Y., Gao, H., Chen, H., Wang, J., Chen, M., Li, G., Wang, L., Gu, J., & Tu, H. (2013). Identification and impact of hepatitis B virus DNA and antigens in pancreatic cancer tissues and adjacent non-cancerous tissues. *Cancer Letters*, *335*(2), 447–454. DOI: 10.1016/j.canlet.2013.03.001

Johansson, H., Andersson, R., Bauden, M., Hammes, S., Holdenrieder, S., & Ansari, D. (2016). Immune checkpoint therapy for pancreatic cancer. *World Journal of Gastroenterology*, *22*(43), 9457. DOI: 10.3748/wjg.v22.i43.9457 PMID: 27920468

John, K. M., Tenner, J., Franco, Y., Croocks, R., Perez, M., McEvoy, T., Zavadsky, T., Beyer, K., Mercieca, R., Nadella, S., Carvino, A., Barish, M., & King, D. A. (2024). Abstract PR01: Implementation of a real-time AI-guided navigation service for pancreas cancer. *Cancer Research*, *84*(2, Supplement), PR01–PR01. DOI: 10.1158/1538-7445.PANCA2023-PR01

Judge, A. D., Robbins, M., Tavakoli, I., Levi, J., Hu, L., Fronda, A., Ambegia, E., McClintock, K., & MacLachlan, I. (2009). Confirming the RNAi-mediated mechanism of action of siRNA-based cancer therapeutics in mice. *The Journal of Clinical Investigation*, *119*(3), 661–673. DOI: 10.1172/JCI37515 PMID: 19229107

Juiz, N. A., Iovanna, J., & Dusetti, N. (2019). Pancreatic cancer heterogeneity can be explained beyond the genome. *Frontiers in Oncology*, *9*, 246. DOI: 10.3389/fonc.2019.00246 PMID: 31024848

Kalser, M. H., & Ellenberg, S. S. (1985). Pancreatic cancer: Adjuvant combined radiation and chemotherapy following curative resection. *Archives of Surgery*, *120*(8), 899–903. DOI: 10.1001/archsurg.1985.01390320023003 PMID: 4015380

Kamarajah, S. K., Gopalan, V., Khan, Z., Baker, D. M., Lucas, A., Hawkins, D., Munnelly, S., Hollyman, M., Magill, L., & Lee, M. J. (2025). Gaps and uncertainties in the management of acute pancreatitis: A scoping review and quality assessment of clinical practice guidelines. *EClinicalMedicine*, *84*, 103216. Advance online publication. DOI: 10.1016/j.eclinm.2025.103216

Kamisawa, T., Wood, L. D., Itoi, T., & Takaori, K. (2016). Pancreatic cancer. *Lancet*, *388*(10039), 73–85. DOI: 10.1016/S0140-6736(16)00141-0

Karamitopoulou, E. (2020). Pancreatic ductal adenocarcinoma: Almost a century of attempting to solve the mystery of its early dissemination. *Cancers (Basel), 12*(4), 1021. DOI: 10.3390/cancers12041021 PMID: 32326377

Karpiński, T. M. (2019). Role of oral microbiota in cancer development. *Microorganisms, 7*(1), 20. DOI: 10.3390/microorganisms7010020

Karthika, C., Sureshkumar, R., Zehravi, M., Akter, R., Ali, F., Ramproshad, S., Mondal, B., Tagde, P., Ahmed, Z., Khan, F. S., Rahman, M. H., & Cavalu, S. (2022). Multidrug Resistance of Cancer Cells and the Vital Role of P-Glycoprotein. *Life (Basel, Switzerland), 12*(6), 897. doi:3390/life12060897

Kasban, H., El-Bendary, M. A. M., & Salama, D. H. (2015). A comparative study of medical imaging techniques. *International Journal of Information Science and Intelligent System, 4*(2), 37–58.

Kashida, Y., Sasaki, Y. F., Ohsawa, K. I., Yokohama, N., Takahashi, A., & Watanabe, T. (2002). Mechanistic study on flumequine hepatocarcinogenicity focusing on DNA damage in mice. *Toxicological Sciences, 69*(2), 317–321. DOI: 10.1093/toxsci/69.2.317

Katayama, E. S., Hue, J. J., Bajor, D. L., Ocuin, L. M., Ammori, J. B., Hardacre, J. M., & Winter, J. M. (2020). A comprehensive analysis of clinical trials in pancreatic cancer: What is coming down the pike? *Oncotarget, 11*(38), 3489–3501. DOI: 10.18632/oncotarget.27727 PMID: 33014285

Katz, M. H. G., Shi, Q., Meyers, J. P., Herman, J. M., Choung, M., Wolpin, B. M., Ahmad, S., Marsh, R. W., Schwartz, L. H., Behr, S., Frankel, W. L., Collisson, E. A., Leenstra, J. L., Williams, T. M., Vaccaro, G. M., Venook, A. P., Meyerhardt, J. A., & O'Reilly, E. M. (2021). Alliance A021501: Preoperative mFOLFIRINOX or mFOLFIRINOX plus hypofractionated radiation therapy (RT) for borderline resectable (BR) adenocarcinoma of the pancreas. *Journal of Clinical Oncology, 39*(3, suppl), 377. DOI: 10.1200/JCO.2021.39.3_suppl.377

Kaufman, H. L., Kim-Schulze, S., Manson, K., DeRaffele, G., Mitcham, J., Seo, K. S., Kim, D. W., & Marshall, J. (2007). Poxvirus-based vaccine therapy for patients with advanced pancreatic cancer. *Journal of Translational Medicine, 5*(1), 1–10. DOI: 10.1186/1479-5876-5-60 PMID: 18039393

Kaur, S., Kumar, S., Momi, N., Sasson, A. R., & Batra, S. K. (2013). Mucins in Pancreatic Cancer and Its Microenvironment. *Nature Reviews. Gastroenterology & Hepatology, 10*(10), 607–620. DOI: 10.1038/nrgastro.2013.120 PMID: 23856888

Kaźmierczak-Siedlecka, K., Dvořák, A., Folwarski, M., Daca, A., Przewłócka, K., & Makarewicz, W. (2020). Fungal gut microbiota dysbiosis and its role in colorectal, oral, and pancreatic carcinogenesis. *Cancers (Basel)*, *12*(5), 1326. DOI: 10.3390/cancers12051326

Kelleher, F. C. (2011). Hedgehog signaling and therapeutics in pancreatic cancer. *Carcinogenesis*, *32*(4), 445–451. DOI: 10.1093/carcin/bgq280

Kelley, R. K., & Ko, A. H. (2008). Erlotinib in the treatment of advanced pancreatic cancer. *Biologics*, *2*(1), 83–95. DOI: 10.2147/BTT.S1832 PMID: 19707431

Kenner, B., Chari, S. T., Kelsen, D., Klimstra, D. S., Pandol, S. J., Rosenthal, M., Rustgi, A. K., Taylor, J. A., Yala, A., Abul-Husn, N., Andersen, D. K., Bernstein, D., Brunak, S., Canto, M. I., Eldar, Y. C., Fishman, E. K., Fleshman, J., Go, V. L. W., Holt, J. M., & Wolpin, B. (2021). Artificial intelligence and early detection of pancreatic cancer: 2020 summative review. *Pancreas*, *50*(3), 251–279. DOI: 10.1097/MPA.0000000000001762

Kerr, K. M., Bibeau, F., Thunnissen, E., Botling, J., Ryska, A., Wolf, J., Öhrling, K., Burdon, P., Malapelle, U., & Büttner, R. (2021). The evolving landscape of biomarker testing for non-small cell lung cancer in Europe. *Lung Cancer (Amsterdam, Netherlands)*, *154*, 161–175. DOI: 10.1016/j.lungcan.2021.02.026 PMID: 33690091

Khder, A., Ashour, S., Altass, H., & Khairou, K. S. (2016). Pd nanoparticles supported on iron oxide nanorods for CO oxidation: Effect of preparation method. *Journal of Environmental Chemical Engineering*, *4*(1), 4794–4800. DOI: 10.1016/j.jece.2016.10.019

Khomiak, A., Brunner, M., Kordes, M., Lindblad, S., Miksch, R. C., Öhlund, D., & Regel, I. (2020). Recent discoveries of diagnostic, prognostic and predictive biomarkers for pancreatic cancer. *Cancers (Basel)*, *12*(11), 3234. DOI: 10.3390/cancers12113234 PMID: 33147766

Kim, H. J., Lee, H. N., Jeong, M. S., & Jang, S. B. (2021). Oncogenic KRAS: Signaling and Drug Resistance. *Cancers (Basel)*, *13*(22), 5599. DOI: 10.3390/cancers13225599 PMID: 34830757

Kim, J. Y., Lim, Y., Cho, S., & Kim, J. (2024). Multiomics analysis identifies AQP1 as a prognostic marker and potential therapeutic target in pancreatic cancer. *Experimental & Molecular Medicine*, *56*, 13. https://www.nature.com/articles/s12276-024-01378-w

Kim, J., Bamlet, W. R., Oberg, A. L., Chaffee, K. G., & Petersen, G. M. (2023). CA 19-9 and emerging biomarkers for the early detection of pancreatic cancer. *World Journal of Gastroenterology*, *29*(10), 1387–1400.

Kim, S. H., Lee, S. M., Jeung, H. C., Lee, I. J., Park, J. S., Song, M., Lee, D. K., & Lee, S.-M. (2019). The effect of nutrition intervention with oral nutritional supplements on pancreatic and bile duct cancer patients undergoing chemotherapy. *Nutrients*, *11*(6), 1145. DOI: 10.3390/nu11051145

Kimura, I., Ichimura, A., Ohue-Kitano, R., & Igarashi, M. (2020). Free fatty acid receptors in health and disease. *Physiological Reviews*, *100*(1), 171–210. DOI: 10.1152/physrev.00041.2018

Kipanyula, M. J., Seke, E. P., Vecchio, L., Farahna, M., Nukenine, E. N., & Nwabo Kamdje, A. H. (2013). Signaling pathways bridging microbial-triggered inflammation and cancer. *Cellular Signalling*, *25*(2), 403–416. DOI: 10.1016/j.cellsig.2012.10.014

Kita, A., Fujiya, M., Konishi, H., Tanaka, H., Kashima, S., Iwama, T., Ijiri, M., Murakami, Y., Takauji, S., Goto, T., Sakatani, A., Ando, K., Ueno, N., Ogawa, N., & Okumura, T. (2020). Probiotic-derived ferrichrome inhibits the growth of refractory pancreatic cancer cells. *International Journal of Oncology*, *57*(3), 721–732. DOI: 10.3892/ijo.2020.5096

Kitago, M., Endo, Y., Aiura, K., Takigawa, Y., Tani, N., Matsui, J., Suzuki, K., Nishiyama, R., Nakano, Y., Abe, Y., Yagi, H., Shinoda, M., Itano, O., Tanabe, M., & Kitagawa, Y. (2024). Adjuvant 5-fluorouracil and portal vein infusion chemotherapy followed by gemcitabine for pancreatic cancer. *Cancer Medicine*, *13*(14), e7459. Advance online publication. DOI: 10.1002/cam4.7459 PMID: 39030993

Klaiber, U., Leonhardt, C. S., Strobel, O., Tjaden, C., Hackert, T., & Neoptolemos, J. P. (2018). Neoadjuvant and adjuvant chemotherapy in pancreatic cancer. *Langenbeck's Archives of Surgery*, *403*(8), 917–932. DOI: 10.1007/s00423-018-1724-8 PMID: 30397779

Kleeff, J., Korc, M., Apte, M., La Vecchia, C., Johnson, C. D., Biankin, A. V., Neale, R. E., Tempero, M., Tuveson, D. A., Hruban, R. H., & Neoptolemos, J. P. (2016). Pancreatic cancer. *Nature Reviews. Disease Primers*, *2*(1), 16022. DOI: 10.1038/nrdp.2016.22

Klein, A. P. (2021). Pancreatic cancer epidemiology: Understanding the role of lifestyle and inherited risk factors. *Nature Reviews. Gastroenterology & Hepatology*, *18*(7), 493–502. DOI: 10.1038/s41575-021-00457-x PMID: 34002083

Klieser, E., Swierczynski, S., Mayr, C., Jäger, T., Schmidt, J., Neureiter, D., Kiesslich, T., & Illig, R. (2016). Differential role of Hedgehog signaling in human pancreatic (patho-) physiology: An up-to-date review. *World Journal of Gastrointestinal Pathophysiology*, *7*(2), 199–210. DOI: 10.4291/wjgp.v7.i2.199 PMID: 27190692

Klimstra, D. S., Heffess, C. S., Oertel, J. E., & Rosai, J. (1992). Acinar Cell Carcinoma of the Pancreas: A Clinicopathologic Study of 28 Cases. *The American Journal of Surgical Pathology*, *16*(9), 815–837. DOI: 10.1097/00000478-199209000-00001 PMID: 1384374

Klimstra, D. S., Modlin, I. R., Coppola, D., Lloyd, R. V., & Suster, S. (2010). The Pathologic Classification of Neuroendocrine Tumors: A Review of Nomenclature, Grading, and Staging Systems. *Pancreas*, *39*(6), 707–712. DOI: 10.1097/MPA.0b013e3181ec124e PMID: 20664470

Klinkenbijl, J. H., Jeekel, J., Sahmoud, T., van Pel, R., Couvreur, M. L., Veenhof, C. H., Arnaud, J. P., Gonzalez Gonzalez, D., de Wit, L. T., Hennipman, A., & Wils, J. (1999). Adjuvant radiotherapy and 5-fluorouracil after curative resection of cancer of the pancreas and periampullary region: Phase III trial of the EORTC gastrointestinal tract cancer cooperative group. *Annals of Surgery*, *230*(6), 776–782. DOI: 10.1097/00000658-199912000-00006 PMID: 10615932

Klomp, J. E., Klomp, J. A., & Der, C. J. (2021). The ERK mitogen-activated protein kinase signaling network: The final frontier in RAS signal transduction. *Biochemical Society Transactions*, *49*(1), 253–267. DOI: 10.1042/BST20200507 PMID: 33544118

Kolbeinsson, H. M., Chandana, S., Wright, G. P., & Chung, M. (2023). Pancreatic cancer: A review of current treatment and novel therapies. *Journal of Investigative Surgery*, *36*(1), 2129884. DOI: 10.1080/08941939.2022.2129884

Kolemen, S., Ozdemir, T., Lee, D., Kim, G. M., Karatas, T., Yoon, J., & Akkaya, E. U. (2016). Remote-controlled release of singlet oxygen by the plasmonic heating of endoperoxide-modified gold nanorods: Towards a paradigm change in photodynamic therapy. *Angewandte Chemie International Edition*, *55*(11), 3606–3610. DOI: 10.1002/anie.201510064 PMID: 26845734

Kopelson, G. (1983). Curative surgery for adenocarcinoma of the pancreas/ampulla of Vater: The role of adjuvant pre- or postoperative radiation therapy. *International Journal of Radiation Oncology, Biology, Physics*, *9*(6), 911–915. DOI: 10.1016/0360-3016(83)90018-4 PMID: 6408038

Kosuge, T., Kiuchi, T., Mukai, K., & Kakizoe, T. (2006). A multicenter randomized controlled trial to evaluate the effect of adjuvant cisplatin and 5-fluorouracil therapy after curative resection in cases of pancreatic cancer. *Japanese Journal of Clinical Oncology*, *36*(3), 159–165. DOI: 10.1093/jjco/hyi234 PMID: 16490736

Koumarianou, A., Kaltsas, G., Kulke, M. H., Oberg, K., Strosberg, J. R., Spada, F., Galdy, S., Barberis, M., Fumagalli, C., Berruti, A., & Fazio, N. (2017). Temozolomide in Advanced Neuroendocrine Neoplasms: Pharmacological and Clinical Aspects. *Neuroendocrinology*, *105*(3), 274–288. DOI: 10.1159/000430816 PMID: 25924937

Koury, J., Lucero, M., Cato, C., Chang, L., Geiger, J., Henry, D., & Tran, A. (2018). Immunotherapies: Exploiting the immune system for cancer treatment. *Journal of Immunology Research*, *2018*(1), 9585614. DOI: 10.1155/2018/9585614 PMID: 29725606

Kumar, Y., Gupta, S., Singla, R., & Hu, Y.-C. (2022). A systematic review of artificial intelligence techniques in cancer prediction and diagnosis. *Archives of Computational Methods in Engineering*, *29*(4), 2043–2070. DOI: 10.1007/s11831-021-09648-w PMID: 34602811

Kurilshikov, A., Wijmenga, C., Fu, J., & Zhernakova, A. (2017). Host genetics and gut microbiome: Challenges and perspectives. *Trends in Immunology*, *38*(9), 633–647. DOI: 10.1016/j.it.2017.06.003

Kuwahara, T., Hara, K., Mizuno, N., Okuno, N., Matsumoto, S., Obata, M., Kurita, Y., Koda, H., Toriyama, K., Onishi, S., Ishihara, M., Tanaka, T., Tajika, M., & Niwa, Y. (2019). Usefulness of deep learning analysis for the diagnosis of malignancy in intraductal papillary mucinous neoplasms of the pancreas. *Clinical and Translational Gastroenterology*, *10*(5), 1–8. DOI: 10.14309/ctg.0000000000000045 PMID: 31117111

La Rosa, S., Adsay, V., & Albarello, L. (2016). Clinicopathologic Study of 62 Acinar Cell Carcinomas of the Pancreas: Insights into the Morphology and Immunophenotype and Search for Prognostic Markers. *Modern Pathology*, *25*(7), 1038–1052. DOI: 10.1097/PAS.0b013e318263209d PMID: 23026929

Lambert, A., Schwarz, L., Borbath, I., Henry, A., Van Laethem, J.-L., Malka, D., Ducreux, M., & Conroy, T. (2019). An update on treatment options for pancreatic adenocarcinoma. *Therapeutic Advances in Medical Oncology*, *11*, 1758835919875568. DOI: 10.1177/1758835919875568 PMID: 31598142

Langabeer, J. R., DelliFraine, J. L., Heineke, J., & Abbass, I. (2009). Implementation of Lean and Six Sigma quality initiatives in hospitals: A goal theoretic perspective. *Operations Management Research : Advancing Practice Through Research, 2*(1-4), 13–27. DOI: 10.1007/s12063-009-0021-7

Lanitis, E., Poussin, M., Hagemann, I. S., Coukos, G., Sandaltzopoulos, R., Scholler, N., & Powell, D. J.Jr. (2012). Redirected antitumor activity of primary human lymphocytes transduced with a fully human anti-mesothelin chimeric receptor. *Molecular Therapy : the Journal of the American Society of Gene Therapy, 20*(3), 633–643. DOI: 10.1038/mt.2011.256 PMID: 22127019

Laranjo, L., Dunn, A. G., Tong, H. L., Kocaballi, A. B., Chen, J., Bashir, R., Surian, D., Gallego, B., Magrabi, F., Lau, A. Y. S., & Coiera, E. (2018). Conversational agents in healthcare: A systematic review. *Journal of the American Medical Informatics Association : JAMIA, 25*(9), 1248–1258. DOI: 10.1093/jamia/ocy072 PMID: 30010941

Leamon, C. P., Lovejoy, C. D., & Nguyen, B. (2013). Patient selection and targeted treatment in the management of platinum-resistant ovarian cancer. *Pharmacogenomics and Personalized Medicine, 6*, 113–125. DOI: 10.2147/PGPM.S24943 PMID: 24109193

Lebre, F., de Lima, M. P., Lavelle, E., & Borges, O. (2018). Mechanistic study of the adjuvant effect of chitosan-aluminium nanoparticles. *International Journal of Pharmaceutics, 552*(1-2), 7–15. DOI: 10.1016/j.ijpharm.2018.09.044 PMID: 30244149

Lee, D. U., Han, B. S., Jung, K. H., & Hong, S.-S. (2024). Tumor Stroma as a Therapeutic Target for Pancreatic Ductal Adenocarcinoma. *Biomolecules & Therapeutics, 32*(3), 281–290. Advance online publication. DOI: 10.4062/biomolther.2024.029 PMID: 38590092

Lee, J. J., Perera, R. M., Wang, H., Wu, D. C., Liu, X. S., Han, S., Fitamant, J., Jones, P. D., Ghanta, K. S., Kawano, S., Nagle, J. M., Deshpande, V., Boucher, Y., Kato, T., Chen, J. K., Willmann, J. K., Bardeesy, N., & Beachy, P. A. (2014). Stromal response to Hedgehog signaling restrains pancreatic cancer progression. *Proceedings of the National Academy of Sciences of the United States of America, 111*(30), E3091–E3100. DOI: 10.1073/pnas.1411679111

Lee, K. S., Jang, J. Y., Yu, Y. D., Heo, J. S., Han, H. S., Yoon, Y. S., Kang, C. M., Hwang, H. K., & Kang, S. (2021). Usefulness of artificial intelligence for predicting recurrence following surgery for pancreatic cancer: Retrospective cohort study. *International Journal of Surgery, 93*, 106050. DOI: 10.1016/j.ijsu.2021.106050 PMID: 34388677

Lee, T., Teng, T. Z. J., & Shelat, V. G. (2020). Carbohydrate antigen 19-9 - tumor marker: Past, present, and future. *World Journal of Gastrointestinal Surgery*, *12*(12), 468–490. DOI: 10.4240/wjgs.v12.i12.468 PMID: 33437400

Lekan, A. A., & Weiner, L. M. (2024). The role of chemokines in orchestrating the immune response to pancreatic ductal adenocarcinoma. *Cancers (Basel)*, *16*(3), 559. DOI: 10.3390/cancers16030559

Leroux, C., & Konstantinidou, G. (2021). Targeted Therapies for Pancreatic Cancer: Overview of Current Treatments and New Opportunities for Personalized Oncology. *Cancers (Basel)*, *13*(4), 799. DOI: 10.3390/cancers13040799 PMID: 33672917

Lewis, B., Guta, A., Shin, J., Ji, Z., Kim, J. S., & Kim, T. (2023). Evaluating motion of pancreatic tumors and anatomical surrogates using cine MRI in 0.35T MRgRT under free breathing conditions. *Journal of Applied Clinical Medical Physics*, *24*(6), e13930. Advance online publication. DOI: 10.1002/acm2.13930 PMID: 37073428

Liang, S. C., Tan, X. Y., Luxenberg, D. P., Karim, R., Dunussi-Joannopoulos, K., Collins, M., & Fouser, L. A. (2006). Interleukin (IL)-22 and IL-17 are co-expressed by Th17 cells and cooperatively enhance expression of antimicrobial peptides. *The Journal of Experimental Medicine*, *203*(10), 2271–2279. DOI: 10.1084/jem.20061308

Li, B., Zhang, Q., Castaneda, C., & Cook, S. (2024). Targeted Therapies in Pancreatic Cancer: A New Era of Precision Medicine. *Biomedicines*, *12*(10), 2175. DOI: 10.3390/biomedicines12102175 PMID: 39457488

Lideståhl, A., Permert, J., Linder, S., Bylund, H., Edsborg, N., & Lind, P. (2006). Efficacy of systemic therapy in advanced pancreatic carcinoma. *Acta Oncologica*, *45*(2), 136–143. DOI: 10.1080/02841860500537861 PMID: 16546858

Li, H., He, J., & Jia, W. (2016). The influence of gut microbiota on drug metabolism and toxicity. *Expert Opinion on Drug Metabolism & Toxicology*, *12*(1), 31–40. DOI: 10.1517/17425255.2016.1121234

Li, J. W. H., & Vederas, J. C. (2009). Drug discovery and natural products: End of an era or an endless frontier? *Science*, *325*(5937), 161–165. DOI: 10.1126/science.1168243 PMID: 19589993

Li, J., Liu, J., Zhou, Z., Wu, R., Chen, X., Yu, C., Stockwell, B., Kroemer, G., Kang, R., & Tang, D. (2023). Tumor-specific GPX4 degradation enhances ferroptosis-initiated antitumor immune response in mouse models of pancreatic cancer. *Science Translational Medicine*, *15*(720), eadg3049. DOI: 10.1126/scitranslmed.adg3049

Li, K., Shi, H., Zhang, B., Ou, X., Ma, Q., Chen, Y., Shu, P., Li, D., & Wang, Y. (2021). Myeloid-derived suppressor cells as immunosuppressive regulators and therapeutic targets in cancer. *Signal Transduction and Targeted Therapy*, *6*(1), 362. DOI: 10.1038/s41392-021-00670-9 PMID: 34620838

Lin, C. C. C., Dievler, A., Robbins, C., Sripipatana, A., Quinn, M., & Nair, S. (2018). Telehealth in health centers: Key adoption factors, barriers, and opportunities. *Health Affairs*, *37*(12), 1967–1974. DOI: 10.1377/hlthaff.2018.05125 PMID: 30633683

Lin, C. C., Han, C. Y., & Pan, I. J. (2015). A qualitative approach of psychosocial adaptation process in patients undergoing long-term hemodialysis. *Asian Nursing Research*, *9*(1), 35–41. DOI: 10.1016/j.anr.2014.10.007 PMID: 25829208

Linehan, A., O'Reilly, M., McDermott, R., & O'Kane, G. M. (2024). Targeting KRAS mutations in pancreatic cancer: Opportunities for future strategies. *Frontiers in Medicine*, *11*, 1369136. DOI: 10.3389/fmed.2024.1369136

Lin, G., Hu, R., Law, W. C., Chen, C.-K., Wang, Y., Li Chin, H., Nguyen, Q. T., Lai, C. K., Yoon, H. S., Wang, X., Xu, G., Ye, L., Cheng, C., & Yong, K.-T. (2013). Biodegradable nanocapsules as siRNA carriers for mutant K-Ras gene silencing of human pancreatic carcinoma cells. *Small*, *9*(16), 2757–2763. DOI: 10.1002/smll.201201716 PMID: 23427041

Lin, H. J., Liang, T. L., Chang, Y. Y., Liu, D. Z., Fan, J. Y., Roffler, S. R., & Lin, S. Y. (2022). Development of irinotecan liposome armed with dual-target anti-epidermal growth factor receptor and anti-fibroblast activation protein-specific antibody for pancreatic cancer treatment. *Pharmaceutics*, *14*(6), 1202. DOI: 10.3390/pharmaceutics14061202 PMID: 35745775

Lin, L., Fan, Y., Gao, F., Jin, L., Li, D., Sun, W., Li, F., Qin, P., Shi, Q., Shi, X., & Du, L. (2018). UTMD promoted the delivery of dendrimer-entrapped gold nanoparticles for pancreatic cancer therapy. *Theranostics*, *8*(7), 1923–1939. DOI: 10.7150/thno.22834 PMID: 29556365

Li, Q., Geng, S., Luo, H., Wang, W., Mo, Y. Q., Luo, Q., Wang, L., Song, G.-B., Sheng, J.-P., & Xu, B. (2024). Signaling pathways involved in colorectal cancer: Pathogenesis and targeted therapy. *Signal Transduction and Targeted Therapy*, *9*(1), 266. DOI: 10.1038/s41392-024-01953-7 PMID: 39370455

Liu, J., Liu, C., & Yue, J. (2021). Radiotherapy and the gut microbiome: Facts and fiction. *Radiation Oncology (London, England)*, *16*(1), 9–17. DOI: 10.1186/s13014-020-01735-9

Liu, L., Huang, X., Shi, F., Song, J., Guo, C., Yang, J., Liang, T., & Bai, X. (2022). Combination therapy for pancreatic cancer: anti-PD-(L) 1-based strategy. *Journal of Experimental & Clinical Cancer Research : CR, 41*(1), 56. DOI: 10.1186/s13046-022-02273-w

Liu, L., Wang, K., Zhu, Z. M., & Shao, J. H. (2011). Associations between P53 Arg72Pro and development of digestive tract cancers: A meta-analysis. *Archives of Medical Research, 42*(1), 60–69. DOI: 10.1016/j.arcmed.2011.01.008

Liu, L., Wang, W. Q., & Lou, W. H. (2022). [Ten directions for improving clinical therapeutic effect of pancreatic cancer in the future]. *PubMed, 60*(1), 10–16. DOI: 10.3760/cma.j.cn112139-20211109-00525 PMID: 34954940

Liu, W., Liu, Q., Wang, W., Wang, P., Chen, J., Hong, T., & He, X. (2018). Differential diagnostic roles of the serum CA19-9, total bilirubin (TBIL) and the ratio of CA19-9 to TBIL for benign and malignant. *Journal of Cancer, 9*(10), 1804–1812. DOI: 10.7150/jca.25093 PMID: 29805707

Liu, X., Jiang, J., Liao, Y. P., Tang, I., Zheng, E., Qiu, W., Lin, M., Wang, X., Ji, Y., Mei, K. C., & Nel, A. E. (2021). Combination chemo-immunotherapy for pancreatic cancer using the immunogenic effects of an irinotecan silicasome nanocarrier plus anti-PD-1. *Advancement of Science, 8*(6), 2002147. DOI: 10.1002/advs.202002147 PMID: 33747719

Liu, X., Sun, L., & Zhang, W. (2020). The role of nanotechnology in pancreatic cancer treatment: A review of nanoparticle-based drug delivery systems. *Journal of Cancer Research and Clinical Oncology, 146*(9), 2165–2177. DOI: 10.1007/s00432-020-03288-x

Liu, Z. L., Chen, H. H., Zheng, L. L., Sun, L. P., & Shi, L. (2023). Angiogenic signaling pathways and anti-angiogenic therapy for cancer. *Signal Transduction and Targeted Therapy, 8*(1), 198. DOI: 10.1038/s41392-023-01460-1 PMID: 37169756

Li, X., Zhou, E., Dong, X., Zhao, C., Han, Y., Cui, B., & Lin, X. (2023). Adjuvant chemotherapy in pancreatic cancer at different AJCC stages: A propensity score matching analysis. *European Journal of Medical Research, 28*(1), 606. Advance online publication. DOI: 10.1186/s40001-023-01572-y PMID: 38115156

Li, Y. J., Wu, J. Y., Wang, J. M., Xiang, D. X., & Jia, Y. B. (2020). Emerging nanomedicine-based strategies for preventing metastasis of pancreatic cancer. *Journal of Controlled Release, 320*, 105–111. DOI: 10.1016/j.jconrel.2020.01.041 PMID: 31978441

Long, J., Zhang, Y., Yu, X., Yang, J., LeBrun, D. G., Chen, C., Yao, Q., & Li, M. (2011). Overcoming drug resistance in pancreatic cancer. *Expert Opinion on Therapeutic Targets*, *15*(7), 817–828. DOI: 10.1517/14728222.2011.566216 PMID: 21391891

Lorentzen, C. L., Haanen, J. B., Met, Ö., & Svane, I. M. (2022). Clinical advances and ongoing trials of mRNA vaccines for cancer treatment. *The Lancet. Oncology*, *23*(10), e450–e458. DOI: 10.1016/S1470-2045(22)00372-2 PMID: 36174631

Lorkowski, M. E., Atukorale, P. U., Bielecki, P. A., Tong, K. H., Covarrubias, G., Zhang, Y., Loutrianakis, G., Moon, T. J., Santulli, A. R., Becicka, W. M., & Karathanasis, E. (2021). Immunostimulatory nanoparticle incorporating two immune agonists for the treatment of pancreatic tumours. *Journal of Controlled Release*, *330*, 1095–1105. DOI: 10.1016/j.jconrel.2020.11.014 PMID: 33188827

Lowenfels, A. B., Maisonneuve, P., Cavallini, G., Ammann, R. W., Lankisch, P. G., Andersen, J. R., Dimagno, E. P., Andrén-Sandberg, A., & Domellöf, L. (1993). Pancreatitis and the risk of pancreatic cancer. *The New England Journal of Medicine*, *328*(20), 1433–1437. DOI: 10.1056/NEJM199305203282001

Lowenfels, A. B., Maisonneuve, P., DiMagno, E. P., Elitsur, Y., Gates, L. K., Perrault, J., & Whitcomb, D. C. (1997). Hereditary pancreatitis and the risk of pancreatic cancer. *Journal of the National Cancer Institute*, *89*(6), 442–446. DOI: 10.1093/jnci/89.6.442 PMID: 9091646

Lowenfels, A. B., Maisonneuve, P., Whitcomb, D. C., Lerch, M. M., & DiMagno, E. P. (2001). Cigarette smoking as a risk factor for Pancreatic cancer in patients with hereditary pancreatitis. *Journal of the American Medical Association*, *286*(2), 169–170. DOI: 10.1001/jama.286.2.169 PMID: 11448279

Lowery, M. A., Klimstra, D. S., Shia, J., Yu, K. H., Allen, P. J., Brennan, M. F., & O'Reilly, E. M. (2011). Acinar Cell Carcinoma of the Pancreas: New Genetic and Treatment Insights into a Rare Malignancy. *The Oncologist*, *16*(12), 1714–1720. DOI: 10.1634/theoncologist.2011-0231 PMID: 22042785

Lowery, M. A., & O'Reilly, E. M. (2011). Pancreatic cancer: The role of molecular markers in diagnosis and management. *Clinical Advances in Hematology & Oncology*, *9*(12), 900–908. PMID: 22252658

Luchini, C., Grillo, F., Fassan, M., Vanoli, A., Capelli, P., Paolino, G., & Scarpa, A. (2020). Malignant epithelial/exocrine tumors of the pancreas. *Pathologica*, *112*(3), 210–226. DOI: 10.32074/1591-951X-167 PMID: 33179623

Lu, J., Liu, X., Liao, Y. P., Salazar, F., Sun, B., Jiang, W., Chang, C. H., Jiang, J., Wang, X., Wu, A. M., & Nel, A. E. (2017). Nano-enabled pancreas cancer immunotherapy using immunogenic cell death and reversing immunosuppression. *Nature Communications*, *8*(1), 1811. DOI: 10.1038/s41467-017-01651-9 PMID: 29180759

Luo, J. (2021). KRAS mutation in pancreatic cancer. *Seminars in Oncology*, *48*(1), 10–18. DOI: 10.1053/j.seminoncol.2021.02.003 PMID: 33676749

Luo, Q., Hu, Z., Zhao, H., Fan, Y., Tu, X., Wang, Y., & Liu, X. (2023). The role of TGF-β in the tumor microenvironment of pancreatic cancer. *Genes & Diseases*, *10*(4), 1513–1524. DOI: 10.1016/j.gendis.2022.10.019

Luo, W., Wen, T., & Qu, X. (2024). Tumor immune microenvironment-based therapies in pancreatic ductal adenocarcinoma: Time to update the concept. *Journal of Experimental & Clinical Cancer Research : CR*, *43*(1), 1–32. DOI: 10.1186/s13046-024-02835-x

Lu, S. Y., Hua, J., Xu, J., Wei, M. Y., Liang, C., Meng, Q. C., Liu, J., Zhang, B., Wang, W., Yu, X.-J., & Shi, S. (2021). Microorganisms in chemotherapy for pancreatic cancer: An overview of current research and future directions. *International Journal of Biological Sciences*, *17*(10), 2666–2682. DOI: 10.7150/ijbs.59117

Lu, Y., Yuan, X., Wang, M., He, Z., Li, H., Wang, J., & Li, Q. (2022). Gut microbiota influence immunotherapy responses: Mechanisms and therapeutic strategies. *Journal of Hematology & Oncology*, *15*(1), 47–56. DOI: 10.1186/s13045-022-01273-9

Lv, H., Zhang, S., Wang, B., Cui, S., & Yan, J. (2006). Toxicity of cationic lipids and cationic polymers in gene delivery. *Journal of Controlled Release*, *114*(1), 100–109. DOI: 10.1016/j.jconrel.2006.04.014 PMID: 16831482

Lyman, G. H., & Moses, H. L. (2016). Biomarker tests for molecularly targeted therapies-the key to unlocking precision medicine. *The New England Journal of Medicine*, *375*(1), 4–6. DOI: 10.1056/NEJMp1604033 PMID: 27353537

Madorsky Rowdo, F. P., Baron, A., Urrutia, M., & Mordoh, J. (2015). Immunotherapy in cancer: A combat between tumors and the immune system; you win some, you lose some. *Frontiers in Immunology*, *6*, 127. DOI: 10.3389/fimmu.2015.00127 PMID: 25859247

Maekawa, T., Fukaya, R., Takamatsu, S., Itoyama, S., Fukuoka, T., Yamada, M., Hata, T., Nagaoka, S., Kawamoto, K., Eguchi, H., Murata, K., Kumada, T., Ito, T., Tanemura, M., Fujimoto, K., Tomita, Y., Tobe, T., Kamada, Y., & Miyoshi, E. (2018). Possible involvement of *Enterococcus* infection in the pathogenesis of chronic pancreatitis and cancer. *Biochemical and Biophysical Research Communications, 506*(4), 962–969. DOI: 10.1016/j.bbrc.2018.10.169

Ma, H., Liu, Z. X., Zhang, J., Wu, F. T., Xu, C. F., Shen, Z., Yu, C.-H., & Li, Y.-M. (2020). Construction of a convolutional neural network classifier developed by computed tomography images for pancreatic cancer diagnosis. *World Journal of Gastroenterology, 26*(34), 5156–5168. DOI: 10.3748/wjg.v26.i34.5156 PMID: 32982116

Ma, J., Xia, J., Miele, L., Sarkar, F. H., & Wang, Z. (2013). Notch signaling pathway in pancreatic cancer progression. *Pancreatic Disorders & Therapy, 3*(114), 1000114. DOI: 10.4172/2165-7092.1000114

Ma, L., Guo, H., Zhao, Y., Liu, Z., Wang, C., Bu, J., Sun, T., & Wei, J. (2024). Liquid biopsy in cancer current: Status, challenges and future prospects. *Signal Transduction and Targeted Therapy, 9*(1), 336. DOI: 10.1038/s41392-024-02021-w PMID: 39617822

Malhotra, R., Patel, V., Chikkaveeraiah, B. V., Munge, B. S., Cheong, S. C., Zain, R. B., Abraham, M. T., Dey, D. K., Gutkind, J. S., & Rusling, J. F. (2012). Ultrasensitive detection of cancer biomarkers in the clinic by use of a nanostructured microfluidic array. *Analytical Chemistry, 84*(14), 6249–6255. DOI: 10.1021/ac301392g PMID: 22697359

Malik, S., Muhammad, K., & Waheed, Y. (2023). Emerging applications of nanotechnology in healthcare and medicine. *Molecules (Basel, Switzerland), 28*(18), 6624. DOI: 10.3390/molecules28186624 PMID: 37764400

Malla, M., Fekrmandi, F., Malik, N., Hatoum, H., George, S., Goldberg, R. M., & Mukherjee, S. (2023). The evolving role of radiation in pancreatic cancer. *Frontiers in Oncology, 12*, 1060885. DOI: 10.3389/fonc.2022.1060885 PMID: 36713520

Mallinson, C. N., Rake, M. D., Cocking, J. B., Fox, C. A., Cwynarski, M. T., Diffey, B. L., Jackson, G. A., & Wass, V. J. (1980). Chemotherapy in pancreatic cancer: Results of a controlled, prospective, randomised, multicentre trial. *British Medical Journal, 281*(6255), 1589–1591. DOI: 10.1136/bmj.281.6255.1589 PMID: 7004559

Mann, K., Jones, R. P., Ghaneh, P., & Neoptolemos, J. P. (2023). Adjuvant Chemotherapy in Pancreatic Cancer. In *Pancreas* (pp. 1143–1152). Lippincott Williams & Wilkins., DOI: 10.1002/9781119876007.ch148

Mantovani, A., Allavena, P., Sica, A., & Balkwill, F. (2008). Cancer-related inflammation. *Nature, 454*(7203), 436–444. DOI: 10.1038/nature07205

Marabelle, A., Le, D. T., Ascierto, P. A., Di Giacomo, A. M., De Jesus-Acosta, A., Delord, J. P., Geva, R., Gottfried, M., Penel, N., Hansen, A. R., Piha-Paul, S. A., Doi, T., Gao, B., Chung, H. C., Lopez-Martin, J., Bang, Y.-J., Frommer, R. S., Shah, M., Ghori, R., & Diaz, L. A.Jr. (2020). Efficacy of pembrolizumab in patients with noncolorectal high microsatellite instability/mismatch repair–deficient cancer: Results from the phase II KEYNOTE-158 study. *Journal of Clinical Oncology, 38*(1), 1–0. DOI: 10.1200/JCO.19.02105 PMID: 31682550

Marchese, A., Orhan, I. E., Daglia, M., Barbieri, R., Di Lorenzo, A., Nabavi, S. F., Gortzi, O., Izadi, M., & Nabavi, S. M. (2017). Antibacterial and antifungal activities of thymol: A brief review of the literature. *Food Chemistry, 210*, 402–414. DOI: 10.1016/j.foodchem.2016.04.111 PMID: 27211664

Mardhian, D. F., Vrynas, A., Storm, G., Bansal, R., & Prakash, J. (2020). FGF2-engineered SPIONs attenuate tumour stroma and potentiate the effect of chemotherapy in a 3D heterospheroidal model of pancreatic tumour. *Nanotheranostics, 4*(1), 26–39. DOI: 10.7150/ntno.38092 PMID: 31911892

Marquart, J., Chen, E. Y., & Prasad, V. (2018). Estimation of the percentage of US patients with cancer who benefit from genome-driven oncology. *JAMA Oncology, 4*(8), 1093–1098. DOI: 10.1001/jamaoncol.2018.1660 PMID: 29710180

Marroncini, G., Naldi, L., Martinelli, S., & Amedei, A. (2024). Gut-liver-pancreas axis crosstalk in health and disease: From the role of microbial metabolites to innovative microbiota manipulating strategies. *Biomedicines, 12*(7), 189–198. DOI: 10.3390/biomedicines12071398

Marya, N. B., Powers, P. D., Chari, S. T., Gleeson, F. C., Leggett, C. L., Abu Dayyeh, B. K., Chandrasekhara, V., Iyer, P. G., Majumder, S., Pearson, R. K., Petersen, B. T., Rajan, E., Sawas, T., Storm, A. C., Vege, S. S., Chen, S., Long, Z., Hough, D. M., Mara, K., & Levy, M. J. (2021). Utilisation of artificial intelligence for the development of an EUS-convolutional neural network model trained to enhance the diagnosis of autoimmune pancreatitis. *Gut, 70*(7), 1335–1344. DOI: 10.1136/gutjnl-2020-322821 PMID: 33028668

Matson, V., Fessler, J., Bao, R., Chongsuwat, T., Zha, Y., Alegre, M.-L., Luke, J. J., & Gajewski, T. F. (2018). The commensal microbiome is associated with anti-PD-1 efficacy in metastatic melanoma patients. *Science, 359*(6371), 104–108. DOI: 10.1126/science.aao3290

Matthaei, H., Norris, A. L., Tsiatis, A. C., Olino, K., Hong, S.-M., dal Molin, M., Goggins, M. G., Canto, M., Horton, K. M., Jackson, K. D., Capelli, P., Zamboni, G., Bortesi, L., Furukawa, T., Egawa, S., Ishida, M., Ottomo, S., Unno, M., Motoi, F., & Hruban, R. H. (2012). Clinicopathological Characteristics and Molecular Analyses of Multifocal Intraductal Papillary Mucinous Neoplasms of the Pancreas. *Annals of Surgery, 255*(2), 326–333. DOI: 10.1097/SLA.0b013e3182378a18 PMID: 22167000

Matuszewska, K., Pereira, M., Petrik, D., Lawler, J., & Petrik, J. (2021). Normalizing Tumor Vasculature to Reduce Hypoxia, Enhance Perfusion, and Optimize Therapy Uptake. *Cancers (Basel), 13*(17), 4444. DOI: 10.3390/cancers13174444 PMID: 34503254

Ma, W. W., & Hidalgo, M. (2013). The winning formulation: The development of paclitaxel in pancreatic cancer. *Clinical Cancer Research, 19*(22), 5572–5579. DOI: 10.1158/1078-0432.CCR-13-1356 PMID: 23918602

Ma, Y., Zhang, F., & Yang, Y. (2024). Recent advances in the treatment of pancreatic cancer. *Holistic Integrative Oncology., 3*(1), 34. DOI: 10.1007/s44178-024-00089-6

McCarthy, E. F. (2006). The toxins of William B. Coley and the treatment of bone and soft-tissue sarcomas. *The Iowa Orthopaedic Journal, 26*, 154. PMID: 16789469

McGuigan, A., Kelly, P., Turkington, R. C., Jones, C., Coleman, H. G., & McCain, R. S. (2018). Pancreatic cancer: A review of clinical diagnosis, epidemiology, treatment, and outcomes. *World Journal of Gastroenterology, 24*(43), 4846–4861. DOI: 10.3748/wjg.v24.i43.4846

Mehta, K. Y., Wu, H. J., Menon, S. S., Fallah, Y., Zhong, X., Rizk, N., Unger, K., Mapstone, M., Fiandaca, M. S., Federoff, H. J., & Cheema, A. K. (2017). Metabolomic biomarkers of pancreatic cancer: A meta-analysis study. *Oncotarget, 8*(40), 68899–68915. DOI: 10.18632/oncotarget.20324 PMID: 28978166

Mehta, V. K., Fisher, G., Ford, J. A., Poen, J., Koong, A., & Bastidas, J. A. (2001). Preoperative chemoradiation for marginally resectable adenocarcinoma of the pancreas. *Journal of Gastrointestinal Surgery, 5*(1), 27–35. DOI: 10.1016/S1091-255X(01)80010-X PMID: 11309645

Melisi, D.. (2018). Galunisertib plus gemcitabine vs. gemcitabine for first-line treatment of unresectable pancreatic cancer: A randomized phase II study. *British Journal of Cancer, 119*(10), 1208–1214. DOI: 10.1038/s41416-018-0246-z

Memorial Sloan Kettering Cancer Center. (n.d.). *Pancreatic cancer clinical trials & research*. https://www.mskcc.org/cancer-care/types/pancreatic/clinical-trials

Mendez, R., Kesh, K., Arora, N., Di Martino, L., McAllister, F., Merchant, N., Banerjee, S., & Banerjee, S. (2020). Microbial dysbiosis and polyamine metabolism as predictive markers for early detection of pancreatic cancer. *Carcinogenesis*, *41*(5), 561–570. DOI: 10.1093/carcin/bgz116

Meng, H., Zhao, Y., Dong, J., Xue, M., Lin, Y. S., Ji, Z., Mai, W. X., Zhang, H., Chang, C. H., Brinker, C. J., Zink, J. I., & Nel, A. E. (2013). Two-wave nanotherapy to target the stroma and optimise gemcitabine delivery to a human pancreatic cancer model in mice. *ACS Nano*, *7*(12), 10048–10065. DOI: 10.1021/nn404083m PMID: 24295225

Mengistu, B. A., Tsegaw, T., Demessie, Y., Getnet, K., Bitew, A. B., Kinde, M. Z., Beirhun, A. M., Mebratu, A. S., Mekasha, Y. T., Feleke, M. G., & Fenta, M. D. (2024). Comprehensive review of drug resistance in mammalian cancer stem cells: Implications for cancer therapy. *Cancer Cell International*, *24*(1), 406. DOI: 10.1186/s12935-024-03558-0 PMID: 39695669

Menis, J., Hasan, B., & Besse, B. (2014). New clinical research strategies in thoracic oncology: Clinical trial design, adaptive, basket and umbrella trials, new end-points and new evaluations of response. *European Respiratory Review : an Official Journal of the European Respiratory Society*, *23*(133), 367–378. DOI: 10.1183/09059180.00004214 PMID: 25176973

Michaud, D. S., Izard, J., Wilhelm-Benartzi, C. S., You, D. H., Grote, V. A., Tjonneland, A., Dahm, C. C., Overvad, K., Jenab, M., Fedirko, V., Boutron-Ruault, M. C., Clavel-Chapelon, F., Racine, A., Kaaks, R., Boeing, H., Foerster, J., Trichopoulou, A., Lagiou, P., Trichopoulos, D., & Riboli, E. (2013). Plasma antibodies to oral bacteria and risk of pancreatic cancer in a large European prospective cohort study. *Gut*, *62*(12), 1764–1770. DOI: 10.1136/gutjnl-2012-303006

Michaud, D. S., Joshipura, K., Giovannucci, E., & Fuchs, C. S. (2007). A prospective study of periodontal disease and pancreatic cancer in US male health professionals. *Journal of the National Cancer Institute*, *99*(2), 171–175. DOI: 10.1093/jnci/djk021

Mikdadi, D., O'Connell, K. A., Meacham, P. J., Dugan, M. A., Ojiere, M. O., Carlson, T. B., & Klenk, J. A. (2022). Applications of artificial intelligence (AI) in ovarian cancer, pancreatic cancer, and image biomarker discovery. *Cancer Biomarkers*, *33*(2), 173–184. DOI: 10.3233/CBM-210301 PMID: 35213360

Mima, K., Nishihara, R., Qian, Z. R., Cao, Y., Sukawa, Y., Nowak, J. A., Yang, J., Dou, R., Masugi, Y., Song, M., Kostic, A. D., Giannakis, M., Bullman, S., Milner, D. A., Baba, H., Giovannucci, E. L., Garraway, L. A., Freeman, G. J., Dranoff, G., & Ogino, S. (2016). *Fusobacterium nucleatum* in colorectal carcinoma tissue and patient prognosis. *Gut, 65*(12), 1973–1980. DOI: 10.1136/gutjnl-2015-310101

Mino-Kenudson, M., Fernández-del Castillo, C., & Baba, Y. (2010). Prognosis of Invasive Intraductal Papillary Mucinous Neoplasm Depends on Histologic Subtype. *Human Pathology, 41*(6), 810–819. DOI: 10.1136/gut.2010.232272 PMID: 21508421

Minor, L. (2020). *Discovering precision health: predict, prevent, and cure to advance health and well-being*. John Wiley & Sons. DOI: 10.1002/9781119672715

Mishra, V., Kesharwani, P., & Jain, N. K. (2014). siRNA nanotherapeutics: A Trojan horse approach against HIV. *Drug Discovery Today, 19*(12), 1913–1920. DOI: 10.1016/j.drudis.2014.09.019 PMID: 25281591

Mitsuhashi, K., Nosho, K., Sukawa, Y., Matsunaga, Y., Ito, M., Kurihara, H., Kanno, S., Igarashi, H., Naito, T., Adachi, Y., Tachibana, M., Tanuma, T., Maguchi, H., Shinohara, T., Hasegawa, T., Imamura, M., Kimura, Y., Hirata, K., Maruyama, R., & Ogino, S. (2015). Association of Fusobacterium species in pancreatic cancer tissues with molecular features and prognosis. *Oncotarget, 6*(9), 7209–7220. DOI: 10.18632/oncotarget.3109

Miyashita, H., Kato, S., & Hong, D. S. (2024). KRAS G12C inhibitor combination therapies: Current evidence and challenge. *Frontiers in Oncology, 14*, 1380584. DOI: 10.3389/fonc.2024.1380584 PMID: 38756650

Mizugaki, H., Yamamoto, N., Murakami, H., Kenmotsu, H., Fujiwara, Y., Ishida, Y., Kawakami, T., & Takahashi, T. (2016). Phase I dose-finding study of monotherapy with atezolizumab, an engineered immunoglobulin monoclonal antibody targeting PD-L1, in Japanese patients with advanced solid tumors. *Investigational New Drugs, 34*(4), 596–603. DOI: 10.1007/s10637-016-0371-6 PMID: 27363843

Moertel, C. G., Childs, D. S., Reitemeier, R. J., Colby, M. Y., & Holbrook, M. A. (1969). Combined 5-fluorouracil and supervoltage radiation therapy of locally unresectable gastrointestinal cancer. *Lancet, 294*(7626), 865–867. DOI: 10.1016/S0140-6736(69)92326-5 PMID: 4186452

Mohindra, N. A., Kircher, S. M., Nimeiri, H. S., Benson, A. B., Rademaker, A., Alonso, E., Blatner, N., Khazaie, K., & Mulcahy, M. F. (2015). Results of the phase Ib study of ipilimumab and gemcitabine for advanced pancreas cancer. *Journal of Clinical Oncology, 33*(15, suppl), e15281. DOI: 10.1200/jco.2015.33.15_suppl.e15281

Mokdad, A. A., Minter, R. M., Zhu, H., Augustine, M. M., Porembka, M. R., Wang, S. C., Yopp, A. C., Mansour, J. C., Choti, M. A., & Polanco, P. M. (2017). Neoadjuvant therapy followed by resection versus upfront resection for resectable pancreatic cancer: A propensity score matched analysis. *Journal of Clinical Oncology*, *35*(5), 515–522. DOI: 10.1200/JCO.2016.68.5081 PMID: 27621388

Montoya Mira, J., Bayani, N., Kesavan, M., Zhu, Y., Chen, L., & Housman, G.. (2023, April 5). A multimodal blood test for early detection of pancreatic cancer. *Science Translational Medicine*, *15*(693), eabq5734. Advance online publication. DOI: 10.1126/scitranslmed.abq5734

Moore, M. J., Andersen, J. S., Burris, H. A., Tarassoff, P., Green, M. R., & Casper, E. S. (1997). A randomized trial of gemcitabine versus 5-FU as first-line therapy in advanced pancreatic cancer. *Journal of Clinical Oncology*, *15*(6), 2403–2410. DOI: 10.1200/JCO.1997.15.6.2403 PMID: 9196156

Morrison, A., Byrne, K., & Vonderheide, R. (2018). Immunotherapy and prevention of pancreatic cancer. *Trends in Cancer*, *4*(6), 418–428. DOI: 10.1016/j.trecan.2018.04.001 PMID: 29860986

Morrison, D. J., & Preston, T. (2016). Formation of short chain fatty acids by the gut microbiota and their impact on human metabolism. *Gut Microbes*, *7*(3), 189–200. DOI: 10.1080/19490976.2015.1134082

Moss, R. A., & Lee, C. (2010). Current and emerging therapies for the treatment of pancreatic cancer. *OncoTargets and Therapy*, •••, 111–127. DOI: 10.2147/OTT.S7203 PMID: 20856847

Motoori, M., Yano, M., Miyata, H., Sugimura, K., Saito, T., Omori, T., Fujiwara, Y., Miyoshi, N., Akita, H., Gotoh, K., Takahashi, H., Kobayashi, S., Noura, S., Ohue, M., Asahara, T., Nomoto, K., Ishikawa, O., & Sakon, M. (2017). Randomized study of the effect of synbiotics during neoadjuvant chemotherapy on adverse events in esophageal cancer patients. *Clinical Nutrition (Edinburgh, Lothian)*, *36*(1), 93–99. DOI: 10.1016/j.clnu.2015.11.008

Motzer, R. J., Porta, C., Eto, M., Powles, T., Grünwald, V., Hutson, T. E., Alekseev, B., Rha, S. Y., Merchan, J. R., Goh, J. C., Kapoor, A., De Giorgi, U., Melichar, B., Hong, S.-H., Gurney, H., Rodriguez-Lopez, K., He, C. S., Okpara, C., McKenzie, J., & Choueiri, T. K. (2023). Final prespecified overall survival (OS) analysis of CLEAR: 4-year follow-up of lenvatinib plus pembrolizumab (L+ P) vs sunitinib (S) in patients (pts) with advanced renal cell carcinoma (aRCC). *Journal of Clinical Oncology*, *41*(16, suppl), 4502. Advance online publication. DOI: 10.1200/JCO.2023.41.16_suppl.4502

Moussa, A. S. A., Hafez, A. H. A., Aziz, A. A. R. A., & Rayan, M. T. (2024). Open distal pancreatectomy stump closure by linear stapling versus continuous suturing: A retrospective–prospective comparative study. *The Egyptian Journal of Surgery*, *43*(2), 413–420. DOI: 10.4103/ejs.ejs_298_23

Moutardier, V., Magnin, V., Turrini, O., Viret, F., Hennekinne-Mucci, S., Gonçalves, A., Pesenti, C., Guiramand, J., Lelong, B., Giovannini, M., Monges, G., Houvenaeghel, G., & Delpero, J.-R. (2004). Assessment of pathologic response after Preoperative Chemoradiotherapy and Surgery in Pancreatic Adenocarcinoma. *International Journal of Radiation Oncology, Biology, Physics*, *60*(2), 437–443. DOI: 10.1016/j.ijrobp.2004.04.004 PMID: 15380577

Mukherjee, S., Patra, A., Khasawneh, H., Korfiatis, P., Rajamohan, N., Suman, G., Majumder, S., Panda, A., Johnson, M. P., Larson, N. B., Wright, D. E., Kline, T. L., Fletcher, J. G., Chari, S. T., & Goenka, A. H. (2022). Radiomics-based machine-learning models can detect pancreatic cancer on prediagnostic computed tomography scans at a substantial lead time before clinical diagnosis. *Gastroenterology*, *163*(5), 1435–1446.e3. DOI: 10.1053/j.gastro.2022.06.066 PMID: 35788343

Muratović, B., & Nikolić, A. (2023). Epidemiology of pancreatic cancer. *Zdravstvena Zastita*, *52*(4), 36–49. DOI: 10.5937/zdravzast52-47366

Murphy, J., Wo, J., Ryan, D., Jiang, W., Yeap, B. Y., Drapek, L. C., Blaszkowsky, L. S., Kwak, E. L., Allen, J. N., Clark, J. W., Faris, J. E., Zhu, A. X., Goyal, L., Lillemoe, K. D., DeLaney, T. F., Fernández-del Castillo, C., Ferrone, C. R., & Hong, T. S. (2018). Total neoadjuvant therapy with FOLFIRINOX followed by individualized chemoradiotherapy for borderline resectable pancreatic adenocarcinoma: A phase 2 clinical trial. *JAMA Oncology*, *4*(7), 963–969. DOI: 10.1001/jamaoncol.2018.0329 PMID: 29800971

Murray, C. J., & López, A. D. (1994). Global and regional cause-of-death patterns in 1990. *Bulletin of the World Health Organization*, *72*(3), 447. PMID: 8062402

Murtaugh, L. C. (2008). The what, where, when, and how of Wnt/β-catenin signaling in pancreas development. *Organogenesis*, *4*(2), 81–86. DOI: 10.4161/org.4.2.5853

Mustafa, M., Abbas, K., Alam, M., Habib, S., Zulfareen, , Hasan, G. M., Islam, S., Shamsi, A., & Hassan, I. (2024). Investigating underlying molecular mechanisms, signaling pathways, emerging therapeutic approaches in pancreatic cancer. *Frontiers in Oncology*, *14*, 1427802. DOI: 10.3389/fonc.2024.1427802 PMID: 39087024

Myo Min, K. K., Ffrench, C. B., Jessup, C. F., Shepherdson, M., Barreto, S. G., & Bonder, C. S. (2023). Overcoming the Fibrotic Fortress in Pancreatic Ductal Adenocarcinoma: Challenges and Opportunities. *Cancers (Basel), 15*(8), 2354. DOI: 10.3390/cancers15082354 PMID: 37190281

Narayanan, G., Ucar, A., Gandhi, R. T., Nasiri, A., Inampudi, P., Wilson, N. M., & Asbun, H. J. (2020). Emerging Ablative and Transarterial Therapies for Pancreatic Cancer. *Digestive Disease Interventions, 04*(04), 389–394. DOI: 10.1055/s-0040-1721415

National Institutes of Health. (n.d.). *A study of nivolumab by itself or nivolumab combined with ipilimumab in patients with advanced or metastatic solid tumors* (ClinicalTrials.gov Identifier: NCT01928394). ClinicalTrials.gov. https://clinicaltrials.gov/show/NCT01928394

Neesse, A., Algül, H., Tuveson, D. A., & Gress, T. M. (2015). Stromal biology and therapy in pancreatic cancer: A changing paradigm. *Gut, 64*(9), 1476–1484. DOI: 10.1136/gutjnl-2015-309304 PMID: 25994217

Nejman, D., Livyatan, I., Fuks, G., Gavert, N., Zwang, Y., Geller, L. T., Rotter-Maskowitz, A., Weiser, R., Mallel, G., Gigi, E., Meltser, A., Douglas, G. M., Kamer, I., Gopalakrishnan, V., Dadosh, T., Levin-Zaidman, S., Avnet, S., Atlan, T., Cooper, Z. A., & Straussman, R. (2020). The human tumor microbiome is composed of tumor type-specific intracellular bacteria. *Science, 368*(6494), 973–980. DOI: 10.1126/science.aay9189

Němeček, R., & Eid, M. (2024). The role of neoadjuvant treatment in localized pancreatic cancer. *Rozhledy v Chirurgii, 103*(11), 429–436. DOI: 10.48095/ccrvch2024429 PMID: 39645401

Neoptolemos, J. P., Cunningham, D., & Friess, H. (2001). Adjuvant 5-fluorouracil plus folinic acid vs observation in resected pancreatic cancer: ESPAC-1 results. *Lancet, 357*(9268), 1559–1565. DOI: 10.1016/S0140-6736(00)04639-6

Neoptolemos, J. P., Kleeff, J., Michl, P., Costello, E., Greenhalf, W., & Palmer, D. H. (2018). Therapeutic developments in pancreatic cancer: Current and future perspectives. *Nature Reviews. Gastroenterology & Hepatology, 15*(6), 333–348. DOI: 10.1038/s41575-018-0005-x

Neoptolemos, J. P., Palmer, D. H., Ghaneh, P., Psarelli, E. E., Valle, J. W., Halloran, C. M., Faluyi, O., O'Reilly, D. A., Cunningham, D., Wadsley, J., Darby, S., Meyer, T., Gillmore, R., Anthoney, A., Lind, P., Glimelius, B., Falk, S., Izbicki, J. R., Middleton, G. W., & Büchler, M. W. (2017). Comparison of adjuvant gemcitabine and capecitabine with gemcitabine monotherapy in patients with resected pancreatic cancer (ESPAC-4): A multicentre, open-label, randomised, phase 3 trial. *Lancet*, *389*(10073), 1011–1024. DOI: 10.1016/S0140-6736(16)32409-6 PMID: 28129987

Neoptolemos, J. P., Stocken, D. D., Bassi, C., Ghaneh, P., Cunningham, D., Goldstein, D., Padbury, R., Moore, M. J., Gallinger, S., Mariette, C., Wente, M. N., Izbicki, J. R., Friess, H., Lerch, M. M., Dervenis, C., Oláh, A., Butturini, G., Doi, R., Lind, P. A., & European Study Group for Pancreatic Cancer, . (2010). Adjuvant chemotherapy with fluorouracil plus folinic acid vs gemcitabine following pancreatic cancer resection: A randomized controlled trial. *Journal of the American Medical Association*, *304*(10), 1073–1081. DOI: 10.1001/jama.2010.1275 PMID: 20823433

Neoptolemos, J. P., Stocken, D. D., Dunn, J., Almond, J., Beger, H. G., Pederzoli, P., Bassi, C., Dervenis, C., Fernandez-Cruz, L., Lacaine, F., Buckels, J., Deakin, M., Adab, F. A., Sutton, R., Imrie, C., Ihse, I., Tihanyi, T., Olah, A., Pedrazzoli, S., & Büchler, M. W. (2001). Influence of resection margins on survival for patients with pancreatic cancer treated by adjuvant chemoradiation and chemotherapy in the ESPAC-1 randomized controlled trial. *Annals of Surgery*, *234*(6), 758–768. DOI: 10.1097/00000658-200112000-00007 PMID: 11729382

Neoptolemos, J., Stocken, D., Friess, H., Bassi, C., Dunn, J. A., Hickey, H., Beger, H., Fernandez-Cruz, L., Dervenis, C., Lacaine, F., Falconi, M., Pederzoli, P., Pap, A., Spooner, D., Kerr, D. J., & Büchler, M. W. (2004). A randomized trial of chemoradiotherapy and chemotherapy after resection of pancreatic cancer. *The New England Journal of Medicine*, *350*(12), 1200–1210. DOI: 10.1056/NEJMoa032295 PMID: 15028824

Nersesyan, H., & Slavin, K. V. (2007). Current aproach to cancer pain management: Availability and implications of different treatment options. *Therapeutics and Clinical Risk Management*, *3*(3), 381–400. PMID: 18488078

Ngiam, K. Y., & Khor, I. W. (2019). Big data and machine learning algorithms for health-care delivery. *The Lancet. Oncology*, *20*(5), e262–e273. DOI: 10.1016/S1470-2045(19)30149-4 PMID: 31044724

Nichetti, F., Rota, S., Ambrosini, P., Pircher, C., Gusmaroli, E., Droz Dit Busset, M., Pusceddu, S., Sposito, C., Coppa, J., Morano, F., Pietrantonio, F., Di Bartolomeo, M., Mariani, L., Mazzaferro, V., de Braud, F., & Niger, M. (2024). NALIRIFOX, FOLFIRINOX, and Gemcitabine With Nab-Paclitaxel as First-Line Chemotherapy for Metastatic Pancreatic Cancer: A Systematic Review and Meta-Analysis. *JAMA Network Open*, *7*(1), e2350756. DOI: 10.1001/jamanetworkopen.2023.50756 PMID: 38190183

Nichols, T. (2018). Comfort as a multidimensional construct for pain management. *Creative Nursing*, *24*(2), 88–98. DOI: 10.1891/1078-4535.24.2.88 PMID: 29871725

Nigam Joshi, P., Agawane, S., Athalye, M. C., Jadhav, V., Sarkar, D., & Prakash, R. (2017). Multifunctional inulin-tethered silver-graphene quantum dots nanotheranostic module for pancreatic cancer therapy. *Materials Science and Engineering C*, *78*, 1203–1211. DOI: 10.1016/j.msec.2017.03.176 PMID: 28575959

Nisar, M., Paracha, R. Z., Adil, S., Qureshi, S. N., & Janjua, H. A. (2022). An extensive review of preclinical and clinical trials of oncolytic virus therapy for pancreatic cancer. *Frontiers in Oncology*, *12*, 875188. DOI: 10.3389/fonc.2022.875188

Nishimoto, A. (2022). Effective combinations of anti-cancer and targeted drugs for pancreatic cancer treatment. *World Journal of Gastroenterology*, *28*(28), 3637–3643. DOI: 10.3748/wjg.v28.i28.3637

Nomi, T., Sho, M., Akahori, T., Hamada, K., Kubo, A., Kanehiro, H., Nakamura, S., Enomoto, K., Yagita, H., Azuma, M., & Nakajima, Y. (2007). Clinical significance and therapeutic potential of the programmed death-1 ligand/programmed death-1 pathway in human pancreatic cancer. *Clinical Cancer Research*, *13*(7), 2151–2157. DOI: 10.1158/1078-0432.CCR-06-2746 PMID: 17404099

Nsairat, H., Khater, D., Sayed, U., Odeh, F., Al Bawab, A., & Alshaer, W. (2022). Liposomes: Structure, Composition, Types, and Clinical Applications. *Heliyon*, *8*(9), e09394. DOI: 10.1016/j.heliyon.2022.e09394 PMID: 35600452

Nunes-Xavier, C. E., & Pulido, R. (2020). Targeting EMT in pancreatic cancer. *Cancers (Basel)*, *12*(6), 1374. DOI: 10.3390/cancers12061374 PMID: 32471123

Nussbaum, D. P., Adam, M. A., Youngwirth, L. M., Ganapathi, A. M., Roman, S. A., Tyler, D. S., Sosa, J. A., & Blazer, D. G.III. (2016). Minimally invasive pancreaticoduodenectomy does not improve use or time to initiation of adjuvant chemotherapy for patients with pancreatic adenocarcinoma. *Annals of Surgical Oncology*, *23*(3), 1026–1033. DOI: 10.1245/s10434-015-4937-x PMID: 26542590

O'connor, J. P., Aboagye, E. O., Adams, J. E., Aerts, H. J., Barrington, S. F., Beer, A. J., Boellaard, R., Bohndiek, S. E., Brady, M., Brown, G., Buckley, D. L., Chenevert, T. L., Clarke, L. P., Collette, S., Cook, G. J., deSouza, N. M., Dickson, J. C., Dive, C., Evelhoch, J. L., & Waterton, J. C. (2017). Imaging biomarker roadmap for cancer studies. *Nature Reviews. Clinical Oncology*, *14*(3), 169–186. DOI: 10.1038/nrclinonc.2016.162 PMID: 27725679

O'Neill, R. S., & Stoita, A. (2021). Biomarkers in the diagnosis of pancreatic cancer: Are we closer to finding the golden ticket? *World Journal of Gastroenterology*, *27*(26), 4045–4087. DOI: 10.3748/wjg.v27.i26.4045 PMID: 34326612

O'Reilly, E. M., & Buckley, C. W. (2024). Next-generation therapies for pancreatic cancer. *Expert Review of Gastroenterology & Hepatology*, *18*(1–3), 55–72.

O'Reilly, E. M., Oh, D. Y., Dhani, N., Renouf, D. J., Lee, M. A., Sun, W., Fisher, G., Hezel, A., Chang, S.-C., Vlahovic, G., Takahashi, O., Yang, Y., Fitts, D., & Philip, P. A. (2019). Durvalumab with or without tremelimumab for patients with metastatic pancreatic ductal adenocarcinoma: A phase 2 randomized clinical trial. *JAMA Oncology*, *5*(10), 1431–1438. DOI: 10.1001/jamaoncol.2019.1588 PMID: 31318392

Ochi, A., Nguyen, A. H., Bedrosian, A. S., Mushlin, H. M., Zarbakhsh, S., Barilla, R., Zambirinis, C. P., Fallon, N. C., Rehman, A., Pylayeva-Gupta, Y., Badar, S., Hajdu, C. H., Frey, A. B., Bar-Sagi, D., & Miller, G. (2012). MyD88 inhibition amplifies dendritic cell capacity to promote pancreatic carcinogenesis *via* Th2 cells. *The Journal of Experimental Medicine*, *209*(9), 1671–1687. DOI: 10.1084/jem.20111706

Oettle, H., Neuhaus, P., Hochhaus, A., Hartmann, J. T., Gellert, K., Ridwelski, K., Niedergethmann, M., Zülke, C., Fahlke, J., Arning, M. B., Sinn, M., Hinke, A., & Riess, H. (2013). Adjuvant chemotherapy with gemcitabine and long-term outcomes among patients with resected pancreatic cancer: The CONKO-001 randomized trial. *Journal of the American Medical Association*, *310*(14), 1473–1481. DOI: 10.1001/jama.2013.279201 PMID: 24104372

Oettle, H., Post, S., Neuhaus, P., Gellert, K., Langrehr, J., Ridwelski, K., Schramm, H., Fahlke, J., Zuelke, C., Burkart, C., Gutberlet, K., Kettner, E., Schmalenberg, H., Weigang-Koehler, K., Bechstein, W.-O., Niedergethmann, M., Schmidt-Wolf, I., Roll, L., Doerken, B., & Riess, H. (2007). Adjuvant chemotherapy with gemcitabine vs observation in patients undergoing curative-intent resection of pancreatic cancer: A randomized controlled trial. *Journal of the American Medical Association*, *297*(3), 267–277. DOI: 10.1001/jama.297.3.267 PMID: 17227978

Okuda, S., Hirose, Y., Takihara, H., Okuda, A., Ling, Y., Tajima, Y., Shimada, Y., Ichikawa, H., Takizawa, K., Sakata, J., & Wakai, T. (2022). Unveiling microbiome profiles in human inner body fluids and tumor tissues with pancreatic or biliary tract cancer. *Scientific Reports, 12*(1), 8766–8775. DOI: 10.1038/s41598-022-12658-8

Oláh, A., Belágyi, T., Issekutz, Á., Gamal, M. E., & Bengmark, S. (2002). Randomized clinical trial of specific *Lactobacillus* and fibre supplement to early enteral nutrition in patients with acute pancreatitis. *British Journal of Surgery, 89*(9), 1103–1107. DOI: 10.1046/j.1365-2168.2002.02189.x

Olajubutu, O., Ogundipe, O. D., Adebayo, A., & Adesina, S. K. (2023). Drug delivery strategies for the treatment of pancreatic cancer. *Pharmaceutics, 15*(5), 1318. DOI: 10.3390/pharmaceutics15051318 PMID: 37242560

Olsen, I., Taubman, M. A., & Singhrao, S. K. (2016). *Porphyromonas gingivalis* suppresses adaptive immunity in periodontitis, atherosclerosis, and Alzheimer's disease. *Journal of Oral Microbiology, 8*(1), 33029–33036. DOI: 10.3402/jom.v8.33029

Onishi, H., & Katano, M. (2014). Hedgehog signaling pathway as a new therapeutic target in pancreatic cancer. World journal of gastroenterology. *World Journal of Gastroenterology, 20*(9), 2335. DOI: 10.3748/wjg.v20.i9.2335

Paisey, S. A., & Bateman, A. R. (2024). Neoadjuvant chemoradiotherapy for pancreatic cancer. *CRC Press EBooks*, 71–82. DOI: 10.1201/9781003579755-9

Palagani, V., Bozko, P., El Khatib, M., Belahmer, H., Giese, N., Sipos, B., Malek, N. P., & Plentz, R. R. (2014). Combined inhibition of Notch and JAK/STAT is superior to monotherapies and impairs pancreatic cancer progression. *Carcinogenesis, 35*(4), 859–866. DOI: 10.1093/carcin/bgt394

Palumbo, M. O., Kavan, P., Miller, W. H., Panasci, L., Assouline, S., Johnson, N., Cohen, V., Patenaude, F., Pollak, M., Jagoe, R. T., & Batist, G. (2013). Systemic cancer therapy: Achievements and challenges that lie ahead. *Frontiers in Pharmacology, 4*. Advance online publication. DOI: 10.3389/fphar.2013.00057 PMID: 23675348

Pancreatic Cancer Action Network. (2025, January 16). *What is pancreatic cancer? – Pancreatic Cancer Action Network*. https://pancan.org/facing-pancreatic-cancer/about-pancreatic-cancer/what-is-pancreatic-cancer/

Pancreatic cancer treatment. (2024, August 28). Cancer.gov. https://www.cancer.gov/types/pancreatic/patient/pancreatic-treatment-pdq

Panebianco, C., Villani, A., & Pazienza, V. (2019). High levels of prebiotic resistant starch in diet modulate gene expression and metabolomic profile in pancreatic cancer xenograft mice. *Nutrients, 11*(4), 709–717. DOI: 10.3390/nu11040709

Panni, R. Z., Sanford, D. E., Belt, B. A., Mitchem, J. B., Worley, L. A., Goetz, B. D., Mukherjee, P., Wang-Gillam, A., Link, D. C., DeNardo, D. G., Goedegebuure, S. P., & Linehan, D. C. (2014). Tumor-induced STAT3 activation in monocytic myeloid-derived suppressor cells enhances stemness and mesenchymal properties in human pancreatic cancer. *Cancer Immunology, Immunotherapy : CII, 63*(5), 513–528. DOI: 10.1007/s00262-014-1527-x PMID: 24652403

Paparo, L., Tripodi, L., Bruno, C., D'Agostino, L., Di Costanzo, M., Cosenza, L., & Nocerino, R. (2020). Protective action of *Bacillus clausii* probiotic strains in an in vitro model of rotavirus infection. *Scientific Reports, 10*(1), 12636. DOI: 10.1038/s41598-020-69533-7

Park, W., Chawla, A., & O'Reilly, E. M. (2021). Pancreatic cancer: A review. *Journal of the American Medical Association, 326*(9), 851–862. DOI: 10.1001/jama.2021.13027

Pavel, M., Öberg, K., & Falconi, M. (2020). ENETS Consensus Guidelines Update for the Management of Distant Metastatic Disease of Intestinal, Pancreatic, and Bronchial Neuroendocrine Neoplasms. *Neuroendocrinology, 110*(9–10), 988–1008. DOI: 10.1159/000443167 PMID: 26731013

Pearce, T. R., Shroff, K., & Kokkoli, E. (2012). Peptide-targeted lipid nanoparticles for anticancer drug delivery. *Advanced Materials, 24*(28), 3803–3822. DOI: 10.1002/adma.201200832 PMID: 22674563

Pei, X., Song, F., & Wang, Z. (2019). Emerging incidence trends and application of curative treatments of pancreatic cancer in the USA. *Medicine, 98*(51), e17175. DOI: 10.1097/MD.0000000000017175

Pelzer, U., Hempel, C., Stieler, J., & Oettle, H. (2002). Oxaliplatin (OXA) in combination with high-dose 5-FU (24 h)/folinic acid (FA) as salvage therapy in patients with gemzar-refractory advanced pancreatic cancer. *Proceedings of the American Society of Clinical Oncology, 21*, 172–180.

Perazzoli, G., García-Valdeavero, O. M., Pena, M., Prados, J., Melguizo, C., & Jimenez-Luna, C. (2023). Evaluating metabolite-based biomarkers for early diagnosis of pancreatic cancer: A systematic review. *Metabolites, 13*(7), 872. DOI: 10.3390/metabo13070872 PMID: 37512579

Pereira, N. P., & Corrêa, J. R. (2018). Pancreatic cancer: Treatment approaches and trends. [N-A.]. *Journal of Cancer Metastasis and Treatment*, •••, 4.

Perello-Reus, C. M., Rubio-Tomás, T., Cisneros-Barroso, E., Ibargüen-González, L., Segura-Sampedro, J. J., Morales-Soriano, R., & Barceló, C. (2022). Challenges in precision medicine in pancreatic cancer: A focus in cancer stem cells and microbiota. *Frontiers in oncology, 12*, 995357. doi:.3389/fonc.2022.995357

Perkhofer, L., Gout, J., Roger, E., de Almeida, F. K., Simões, C. B., Wiesmüller, L., & Kleger, A. (2021). DNA damage repair as a target in pancreatic cancer: State-of-the-art and future perspectives. *Gut, 70*(3), 606–617. DOI: 10.1136/gutjnl-2019-319984 PMID: 32855305

Petros, R. A., & DeSimone, J. M. (2010). Strategies in the design of nanoparticles for therapeutic applications. *Nature Reviews. Drug Discovery, 9*(8), 615–627. DOI: 10.1038/nrd2591 PMID: 20616808

Pflüger, M. J., Jamouss, K. T., Afghani, E., Lim, S. J., Franco, S. R., Mayo, H., & Wood, L. D. (2023). Predictive ability of pancreatic cyst fluid biomarkers: A systematic review and meta-analysis. *Pancreatology, 23*(7), 868–877. DOI: 10.1016/j.pan.2023.05.005 PMID: 37230894

Philipp, L. M., Yesilyurt, U. U., Surrow, A., Künstner, A., Mehdorn, A. S., Hauser, C., Gundlach, J. P., Will, O., Hoffmann, P., Stahmer, L., Franzenburg, S., Knaack, H., Schumacher, U., Busch, H., & Sebens, S. (2024). Epithelial and Mesenchymal-like Pancreatic Cancer Cells Exhibit Different Stem Cell Phenotypes Associated with Different Metastatic Propensities. *Cancers (Basel), 16*(4), 686. DOI: 10.3390/cancers16040686 PMID: 38398077

Pilepich, M. V., & Miller, H. H. (1980). Preoperative irradiation in carcinoma of the pancreas. *Cancer, 46*(9), 1945–1949. DOI: 10.1002/1097-0142(19801101)46:9<1945::AID-CNCR2820460908>3.0.CO;2-X PMID: 7427900

Pino, M. S., Milella, M., Gelibter, A., Sperduti, I., De Marco, S., Nuzzo, C., Bria, E., Carpanese, L., Ruggeri, E. M., Carlini, P., & Cognetti, F. (2009). Capecitabine and celecoxib as second-line treatment of advanced pancreatic and biliary tract cancers. *Oncology, 76*(4), 254–261. DOI: 10.1159/000205388 PMID: 19246950

Pishvaian, M. J., Blais, E. M., Brody, J. R., Lyons, E., DeArbeloa, P., Hendifar, A., Mikhail, S., Chung, V., Sahai, V., Sohal, D. P. S., Bellakbira, S., Thach, D., Rahib, L., Madhavan, S., Matrisian, L. M., & Petricoin, E. F.III. (2020). Overall survival in patients with pancreatic cancer receiving matched therapies following molecular profiling: A retrospective analysis of the Know Your Tumor registry trial. *The Lancet. Oncology, 21*(4), 508–518. DOI: 10.1016/S1470-2045(20)30074-7 PMID: 32135080

Pisters, P. W., Abbruzzese, J. L., Janjan, N. A., Cleary, K. R., Charnsangavej, C., Goswitz, M. S., Rich, T. A., Raijman, I., Wolff, R. A., Lenzi, R., Lee, J. E., & Evans, D. B. (1998). Rapid-fractionation preoperative chemoradiation, pancreaticoduodenectomy, and intraoperative radiation therapy for resectable Pancreatic adenocarcinoma. *Journal of Clinical Oncology*, *16*(12), 3843–3850. DOI: 10.1200/JCO.1998.16.12.3843 PMID: 9850029

Plana, D., Palmer, A. C., & Sorger, P. K. (2022). Independent drug action in combination therapy: Implications for precision oncology. *Cancer Discovery*, *12*(3), 606–624. DOI: 10.1158/2159-8290.CD-21-0212 PMID: 34983746

Pourmousa, M., Jain, S., Barnaeva, E., Jin, W., Hochuli, J., Itkin, Z., Maxfield, T., Melo-Filho, C., Thieme, A., Wilson, K., Klumpp-Thomas, C., Michael, S., Southall, N., Jaakkola, T., Muratov, E. N., Barzilay, R., Tropsha, A., Ferrer, M., & Zakharov, A. V. (2025). AI-driven discovery of synergistic drug combinations against pancreatic cancer. *Nature Communications*, *16*(1), 4020. DOI: 10.1038/s41467-025-56818-6

Principe, D. R., Underwood, P. W., Korc, M., Trevino, J. G., Munshi, H. G., & Rana, A. (2021). The current treatment paradigm for pancreatic ductal adenocarcinoma and barriers to therapeutic efficacy. *Frontiers in Oncology*, *11*, 688377. DOI: 10.3389/fonc.2021.688377 PMID: 34336673

Priyadarshini, M., Villa, S. R., Fuller, M., Wicksteed, B., Mackay, C. R., Alquier, T., Poitout, V., Mancebo, H., Mirmira, R. G., Gilchrist, A., & Layden, B. T. (2015). An acetate-specific GPCR, FFAR2, regulates insulin secretion. *Molecular Endocrinology (Baltimore, Md.)*, *29*(7), 1055–1066. DOI: 10.1210/me.2015-1007

Provenzano, P. P., Cuevas, C., Chang, A. E., Goel, V. K., Von Hoff, D. D., & Hingorani, S. R. (2012). Enzymatic Targeting of the Stroma Ablates Physical Barriers to Treatment of Pancreatic Ductal Adenocarcinoma. *Cancer Cell*, *21*(3), 418–429. DOI: 10.1016/j.ccr.2012.01.007 PMID: 22439937

Provenzano, P. P., & Hingorani, S. R. (2013). Hyaluronan, fluid pressure, and stromal resistance in pancreatic cancer. *British Journal of Cancer*, *108*(1), 1–8. DOI: 10.1038/bjc.2012.569 PMID: 23299539

Pushalkar, S., Hundeyin, M., Daley, D., Zambirinis, C. P., Kurz, E., Mishra, A., Mohan, N., Aykut, B., Usyk, M., Torres, L. E., Werba, G., Zhang, K., Guo, Y., Li, Q., Akkad, N., Lall, S., Wadowski, B., Gutierrez, J., Kochen Rossi, J. A., & Miller, G. (2018). The Pancreatic Cancer Microbiome Promotes Oncogenesis by Induction of Innate and Adaptive Immune Suppression. *Cancer Discovery*, *8*(4), 403–416. DOI: 10.1158/2159-8290.CD-17-1134

Qaid, M. M., & Abdelrahman, M. M. (2016). Role of insulin and other related hormones in energy metabolism—A review. *Cogent Food & Agriculture, 2*(1), 1267691. DOI: 10.1080/23311932.2016.1267691

Qian, Z. M., Li, H., Sun, H., & Ho, K. (2002). Targeted drug delivery via the transferrin receptor-mediated endocytosis pathway. *Pharmacological Reviews, 54*(4), 561–587. DOI: 10.1124/pr.54.4.561 PMID: 12429868

Rad, A. H., Maleki, L. A., Kafil, H. S., Zavoshti, H. F., & Abbasi, A. (2021). Postbiotics as promising tools for cancer adjuvant therapy. *Advanced Pharmaceutical Bulletin, 11*(1), 1–5. DOI: 10.34172/apb.2021.001

Raderer, M., Wrba, F., Kornek, G., Maca, T., Koller, D. Y., Weinlaender, G., Hejna, M., & Scheithauer, W. (1998). Association between helicobacter pylori infection and pancreatic cancer. *Oncology, 55*(1), 16–19. DOI: 10.1159/000011830

Radon, T. P., Massat, N. J., Jones, R., Alrawashdeh, W., Dumartin, L., & Ennis, D. (2015). Identification of a three-biomarker panel in urine for early detection of pancreatic adenocarcinoma. *Clinical Cancer Research, 21*(15), 3512–3521. DOI: 10.1158/1078-0432.CCR-14-2467 PMID: 26240291

Rahib, L., Smith, B. D., Aizenberg, R., Rosenzweig, A. B., Fleshman, J. M., & Matrisian, L. M. (2014). Projecting cancer incidence and deaths to 2030: The unexpected burden of thyroid, liver, and pancreas cancers in the United States. *Cancer Research, 74*(11), 2913–2921. DOI: 10.1158/0008-5472.CAN-14-0155

Rahmani, N., Pourali, G., Hosseini, N., Fiuji, H., Maftooh, M., Hassanian, S. M., Ferns, G. A., Khazaei, M., & Avan, A. (2023). Probiotics as a therapeutic approach in colorectal cancer. *Current Cancer Drug Targets, 23*(10), 764–777. DOI: 10.2174/1568009623666230413081513

Rajpoot, M., Sharma, A. K., Sharma, A., & Gupta, G. K. (2018). Understanding the microbiome: Emerging biomarkers for exploiting the microbiota for personalized medicine against cancer. *Seminars in Cancer Biology, 52*, 1–8. DOI: 10.1016/j.semcancer.2018.02.003

Ram Makena, M., Gatla, H., Verlekar, D., Sukhavasi, S., & Pandey, K., M., & C. Pramanik, K. (. (2019). Wnt/β-catenin signaling: The culprit in pancreatic carcinogenesis and therapeutic resistance. *International Journal of Molecular Sciences, 20*(17), 4242. DOI: 10.3390/ijms20174242

Ramirez-Garcia, A., Rementeria, A., Aguirre-Urizar, J. M., Moragues, M. D., Antoran, A., Pellon, A., Abad-Diaz-de-Cerio, A., & Hernando, F. L. (2016). *Candida albicans* and cancer: Can this yeast induce cancer development or progression? *Critical Reviews in Microbiology, 42*, 182–193. DOI: 10.3109/1040841X.2014.913004

Rana, T. M. (2007). Illuminating the silence: Understanding the structure and function of small RNAs. *Nature Reviews. Molecular Cell Biology, 8*(1), 23–36. DOI: 10.1038/nrm2085 PMID: 17183358

Ravikumar, R., Sabin, C., Hilal, M. A., Bramhall, S., White, S., Wigmore, S., Imber, C. J., & Fusai, G. (2014). Portal Vein Resection in Borderline Resectable Pancreatic Cancer: A United Kingdom Multicenter Study. *Journal of the American College of Surgeons, 218*(3), 401–411. DOI: 10.1016/j.jamcollsurg.2013.11.017 PMID: 24484730

Rawla, P., Sunkara, T., & Gaduputi, V. (2019). Epidemiology of pancreatic cancer: Global trends, etiology and risk factors. *World Journal of Oncology, 10*(1), 10–27. DOI: 10.14740/wjon1166 PMID: 30834048

Regine, W. F. (2001). Postoperative adjuvant therapy: past, present, and future trial development. In Evans, D. B., Pisters, P. W. T., Abbruzzese, J. L., & Pollock, R. E. (Eds.), *MD Anderson Solid Tumor Oncology Series: Pancreatic Cancer* (pp. 235–242). Springer-Verlag., DOI: 10.1007/978-1-4613-0089-0_20

Reni, M., Panucci, M. G., Ferreri, A. J. M., Balzano, G., Passoni, P., Cattaneo, G. M., Cordio, S., Scaglietti, U., Zerbi, A., Ceresoli, G. L., Fiorino, C., Calandrino, R., Staudacher, C., Villa, E., & Di Carlo, V. (2001). Effect on local control and survival of electron beam intraoperative irradiation for resectable pancreatic adenocarcinoma. *International Journal of Radiation Oncology, Biology, Physics, 50*(3), 651–658. DOI: 10.1016/S0360-3016(01)01470-5 PMID: 11395232

Rennick, J. J., Johnston, A. P. R., & Parton, R. G. (2021). Key principles and methods for studying the endocytosis of biological and nanoparticle therapeutics. *Nature Nanotechnology, 16*(3), 266–276. DOI: 10.1038/s41565-021-00858-8 PMID: 33712737

Richter, J., & Saif, M. W. (2010). Updates in adjuvant therapy in pancreatic cancer: Gemcitabine and beyond. Highlights from the "2010 ASCO Gastrointestinal Cancers Symposium". Orlando, FL, USA. January 22–24, 2010. *Journal of the Pancreas, 11(2),* 144–147. doi:pubmed.ncbi.nlm.nih.gov/20208323/

Riquelme, E., Maitra, A., & McAllister, F. (2018). Immunotherapy for pancreatic cancer: More than just a gut feeling. *Cancer Discovery, 8*(4), 386–388. DOI: 10.1158/2159-8290.CD-18-0123

Riquelme, E., Zhang, Y., Zhang, L., Montiel, M., Zoltan, M., Dong, W., Quesada, P., Sahin, I., Chandra, V., San Lucas, A., Scheet, P., Xu, H., Hanash, S. M., Feng, L., Burks, J. K., Do, K. A., Peterson, C. B., Nejman, D., Tzeng, C. D., & McAllister, F. (2019). Tumor Microbiome Diversity and Composition Influence Pancreatic Cancer Outcomes. *Cell, 178*(4), 795–806.e12. DOI: 10.1016/j.cell.2019.07.008

Risch, H. A., Yu, H., Lu, L., & Kidd, M. S. (2014). Detectable Serum Antibodies to Helicobacter pylori and the CagA Protein Do Not Correlate with Long-Term Risk of Pancreatic Cancer in a Prospective Cohort. *Cancer Epidemiology, Biomarkers & Prevention*, (11), 2461–2464. DOI: 10.1158/1055-9965.EPI-14-0559

Ristorcelli, E., & Lombardo, D. (2010). Targeting Notch signaling in pancreatic cancer. *Expert Opinion on Therapeutic Targets*, *14*(5), 541–552. DOI: 10.1517/14728221003769895

Robatel, S., & Schenk, M. (2022). Current limitations and novel perspectives in pancreatic cancer treatment. *Cancers (Basel)*, *14*(4), 985. DOI: 10.3390/cancers14040985

Robey, R. W., Pluchino, K. M., Hall, M. D., Fojo, A. T., Bates, S. E., & Gottesman, M. M. (2018). Revisiting the role of ABC transporters in multidrug-resistant cancer. *Nature Reviews. Cancer*, *18*(7), 452–464. DOI: 10.1038/s41568-018-0005-8 PMID: 29643473

Robinson, K., Lambiase, L., Li, J., Monteiro, C., & Schiff, M. (2003). Fatal cholestatic liver failure associated with gemcitabine therapy. *Digestive Diseases and Sciences*, *48*(9), 1804–1808. DOI: 10.1023/A:1025415616592 PMID: 14561005

Ro, C., Chai, W., Yu, V. E., & Yu, R. (2013). Pancreatic neuroendocrine tumors: Biology, diagnosis, and treatment. *Chinese Journal of Cancer*, *32*(6), 312–324. DOI: 10.5732/cjc.012.10295

Roh, Y. J., Kim, J. H., Kim, I. W., Na, K., Park, J. M., & Choi, M. G. (2017). Photodynamic therapy using photosensitizer-encapsulated polymeric nanoparticles to overcome ATP-binding cassette transporter subfamily G2 function in pancreatic cancer. *Molecular Cancer Therapeutics*, *16*(7), 1487–1496. DOI: 10.1158/1535-7163.MCT-16-0642 PMID: 28416605

Rojas, L. A., Sethna, Z., Soares, K. C., Olcese, C., Pang, N., Patterson, E., Lihm, J., Ceglia, N., Guasp, P., Chu, A., Yu, R., Chandra, A. K., Waters, T., Ruan, J., Amisaki, M., Zebboudj, A., Odgerel, Z., Payne, G., Derhovanessian, E., & Balachandran, V. P. (2023). Personalized RNA neoantigen vaccines stimulate T cells in pancreatic cancer. *Nature*, *618*(7963), 144–150. DOI: 10.1038/s41586-023-06063-y PMID: 37165196

Rose, M., Burgess, J. T., O'Byrne, K., Richard, D. J., & Bolderson, E. (2020). PARP Inhibitors: Clinical Relevance, Mechanisms of Action and Tumor Resistance. *Frontiers in Cell and Developmental Biology, 8*, 564601. DOI: 10.3389/fcell.2020.564601 PMID: 33015058

Rossi, G., Russo, A., Tagliamento, M., Tuzi, A., Nigro, O., Vallome, G., & Genova, C. (2020). Precision medicine for NSCLC in the era of immunotherapy: New biomarkers to select the most suitable treatment or the most suitable patient. *Cancers (Basel), 12*(5), 1125. DOI: 10.3390/cancers12051125 PMID: 32365882

Round, J. L., & Mazmanian, S. K. (2009). The gut microbiota shapes intestinal immune responses during health and disease. *Nature Reviews. Immunology, 9*(5), 313–323. DOI: 10.1038/nri2515

Royal, R. E., Levy, C., Turner, K., Mathur, A., Hughes, M., Kammula, U. S., Sherry, R. M., Topalian, S. L., Yang, J. C., Lowy, I., & Rosenberg, S. A. (2010). Phase 2 trial of single agent ipilimumab (anti-CTLA-4) for locally advanced or metastatic pancreatic adenocarcinoma. *Journal of Immunotherapy, 33*(8), 828–833. DOI: 10.1097/CJI.0b013e3181eec14c PMID: 20842054

Rubinsky, B., Onik, G., & Mikus, P. (2007). Irreversible electroporation: A new ablation modality - clinical implications. *Technology in Cancer Research & Treatment, 6*(1), 37–48. DOI: 10.1177/153303460700600106 PMID: 17241099

Rump, A., Morikawa, Y., Tanaka, M., Minami, S., Umesaki, N., Takeuchi, M., & Miyajima, A. (2004). Binding of ovarian cancer antigen CA125/MUC16 to mesothelin mediates cell adhesion. *The Journal of Biological Chemistry, 279*(10), 9190–9198. DOI: 10.1074/jbc.M312372200 PMID: 14676194

Ryan, D. P., Eder, J. P., Winkelmann, J., & Clark, J. W. (2002). Pharmacokinetic and pharmacodynamic Phase I study of PS-341 and gemcitabine in patients with advanced solid tumors. *Proceedings of the American Society of Clinical Oncology, 21*, 95–102.

Ryan, D. P., Hong, T. S., & Bardeesy, N. (2014). Pancreatic adenocarcinoma. *The New England Journal of Medicine, 371*(11), 1039–1049. DOI: 10.1056/NEJMra1404198 PMID: 25207767

Ryan, M. B., Fece de la Cruz, F., Phat, S., Myers, D. T., Wong, E., Shahzade, H. A., Hong, C. B., & Corcoran, R. B. (2020). Vertical pathway inhibition overcomes adaptive feedback resistance to KRASG12C inhibition. *Clinical Cancer Research, 26*(7), 1633–1643. DOI: 10.1158/1078-0432.CCR-19-3523

Ryu, J. H., Lee, S., Son, S., Kim, S. H., Leary, J. F., Choi, K., & Kwon, I. C. (2014). Theranostic nanoparticles for future personalised medicine. *Journal of Controlled Release, 190*, 477–484. DOI: 10.1016/j.jconrel.2014.04.027 PMID: 24780269

Saha, S., Xiong, X., Chakraborty, P. K., Shameer, K., Arvizo, R. R., Kudgus, R. A., Dwivedi, S. K. D., Hossen, M. N., Gillies, E. M., Robertson, J. D., & Mukherjee, P. (2016). Gold nanoparticle reprograms pancreatic tumour microenvironment and inhibits tumour growth. *ACS Nano, 10*(12), 10636–10651. DOI: 10.1021/acsnano.6b02231 PMID: 27758098

Salman, B., Zhou, D., Jaffee, E. M., Edil, B. H., & Zheng, L. (2013). Vaccine therapy for pancreatic cancer. *OncoImmunology, 2*(12), e26662. DOI: 10.4161/onci.26662 PMID: 24498551

Sano, M., Driscoll, D. R., DeJesus-Monge, W. E., Quattrochi, B., Appleman, V. A., Ou, J., Zhu, L. J., Yoshida, N., Yamazaki, S., Takayama, T., Sugitani, M., Nemoto, N., Klimstra, D. S., & Lewis, B. C. (2016). Activation of WNT/β-catenin signaling enhances pancreatic cancer development and the malignant potential via up-regulation of Cyr61. *Neoplasia : an International Journal for Oncology Research, 18*(12), 785–794. DOI: 10.1016/j.neo.2016.11.004

Santarpia, M., Liguori, A., D'Aveni, A., Karachaliou, N., Gonzalez-Cao, M., Daffinà, M. G., & Rosell, R. (2018). Liquid biopsy for lung cancer early detection. *Journal of Thoracic Disease, 10*(S7, Suppl 7), S882–S897. DOI: 10.21037/jtd.2018.03.81 PMID: 29780635

Santos-Rebelo, A., Garcia, C., Eleutério, C., Bastos, A., Coelho, S. C., Coelho, M. A. N., Molpeceres, J., Viana, A. S., Ascensão, L., & Pinto, J. F. (2018). Development of Parvifloron D-loaded smart nanoparticles to target pancreatic cancer. *Pharmaceutics, 10*(4), 216. DOI: 10.3390/pharmaceutics10040216 PMID: 30400382

Sauer-Heilborn, A., Kath, R., Schneider, C. P., & Höffken, K. (1999). Severe non-haematological toxicity after treatment with gemcitabine. *Journal of Cancer Research and Clinical Oncology, 125*(11), 637–640. DOI: 10.1007/s004320050327 PMID: 10541971

Saung, M. T., Muth, S., Ding, D., & Armstrong, T. D. (2020). Targeting the tumour microenvironment in pancreatic ductal adenocarcinoma: Rationale and current status. *Cancers (Basel), 12*(5), 1156. DOI: 10.3390/cancers12051156

Scarpa, A., Chang, D. K., Nones, K., Corbo, V., Patch, A.-M., Bailey, P., Lawlor, R. T., Johns, A. L., Miller, D. K., Mafficini, A., Rusev, B., Scardoni, M., Antonello, D., Barbi, S., Sikora, K. O., Cingarlini, S., Vicentini, C., McKay, S., Quinn, M. C. J., & Grimmond, S. M. (2017). Whole-Genome Landscape of Pancreatic Neuroendocrine Tumors. *Nature*, *543*(7643), 65–71. DOI: 10.1038/nature21063 PMID: 28199314

Schawkat, K., Manning, M. A., Glickman, J. N., & Mortele, K. J. (2020). Pancreatic ductal adenocarcinoma and its variants: Pearls and perils. *Radiographics*, *40*(1), 121–140. DOI: 10.1148/rg.2020190184

Schmidt, C. M., Matos, J. M., & Bentrem, D. J. (2007). Acinar Cell Carcinoma of the Pancreas in the United States: Prognostic Factors and Comparison to Ductal Adenocarcinoma. *Journal of Gastrointestinal Surgery*, *11*(7), 829–836. DOI: 10.1007/s11605-008-0705-6 PMID: 18836784

Schober, M., Jesenofsky, R., Faissner, R., Weidenauer, C., Hagmann, W., Michl, P., Heuchel, R. L., Haas, S. L., & Löhr, J. M. (2014). Desmoplasia and chemoresistance in pancreatic cancer. *Cancers (Basel)*, *6*(4), 2137–2154. DOI: 10.3390/cancers6042137 PMID: 25337831

Schroeder, A., Levins, C. G., Cortez, C., Langer, R., & Anderson, D. G. (2010). Lipid-based nanotherapeutics for siRNA delivery. *Journal of Internal Medicine*, *267*(1), 9–21. DOI: 10.1111/j.1365-2796.2009.02189.x PMID: 20059641

Schuurmans, M., Alves, N., Vendittelli, P., Huisman, H., & Hermans, J. (2022). Setting the research agenda for clinical artificial intelligence in pancreatic adenocarcinoma imaging. *Cancers (Basel)*, *14*(14), 3498. DOI: 10.3390/cancers14143498 PMID: 35884559

Seicean, A. (2015). New targeted therapies in pancreatic cancer. *World Journal of Gastroenterology*, *21*(20), 6127. DOI: 10.3748/wjg.v21.i20.6127 PMID: 26034349

Seidel, G., Zahurak, M., Iacobuzio-Donahue, C., Sohn, T. A., Adsay, N. V., Yeo, C. J., Lillemoe, K. D., Cameron, J. L., Hruban, R. H., & Wilentz, R. E. (2002). Almost All Infiltrating Colloid Carcinomas of the Pancreas and Periampullary Region Arise from In Situ Papillary Neoplasms: A Study of 39 Cases. *The American Journal of Surgical Pathology*, *26*(1), 56–63. DOI: 10.1097/00000478-200201000-00006 PMID: 11756769

Shah, M. H., Goldner, W. S., Benson, A. B., Bergsland, E., Blaszkowsky, L. S., Brock, P., Chan, J., Das, S., Dickson, P. V., Fanta, P., Giordano, T., Halfdanarson, T. R., Halperin, D., He, J., Heaney, A., Heslin, M. J., Kandeel, F., Kardan, A., Khan, S. A., & Hochstetler, C. (2021). Neuroendocrine and Adrenal Tumors, Version 2.2021, NCCN Clinical Practice Guidelines in Oncology. *Journal of the National Comprehensive Cancer Network : JNCCN*, *19*(7), 839–868. DOI: 10.6004/jnccn.2021.0032 PMID: 34340212

Sharma, A., Kandlakunta, H., Nagpal, S., Feng, Z., Hoos, W., Petersen, G. M., & Chari, S. T. (2018). Model to determine risk of pancreatic cancer in patients with new-onset diabetes. *Gastroenterology*, *155*(3), 730–739. DOI: 10.1053/j.gastro.2018.05.023 PMID: 29775599

Sharma, R., Ghosh, R., Kumar, S., Komal, K., & Kumar, M. (2025). Decoding pancreatic cancer: Key risk factors across genetics and lifestyle. *Expert Review of Molecular Diagnostics*, *25*(4), 95–99. Advance online publication. DOI: 10.1080/14737159.2025.2464563 PMID: 39918844

Shen, W., Tao, G. Q., Zhang, Y., Cai, B., Sun, J., & Tian, Z. Q. (2017). TGF-β in pancreatic cancer initiation and progression: Two sides of the same coin. *Cell & Bioscience*, *7*(1), 1–7. DOI: 10.1186/s13578-017-0168-0

Sherman, M. H., & Beatty, G. L. (2023). Tumor microenvironment in pancreatic cancer pathogenesis and therapeutic resistance. *Annual Review of Pathology*, *18*(1), 123–148. DOI: 10.1146/annurev-pathmechdis-031621-024600

Shi, M., Yu, D. H., Chen, Y., Zhao, C. Y., Zhang, J., Liu, Q. H., & Zhu, M. H. (2012). Expression of fibroblast activation protein in human pancreatic adenocarcinoma and its clinicopathological significance. *World Journal of Gastroenterology*, *18*(8), 840–846. DOI: 10.3748/wjg.v18.i8.840

Shoaf, K., Mulvey, G. L., Armstrong, G. D., & Hutkins, R. W. (2006). Prebiotic galacto-oligosaccharides reduce adherence of entero-pathogenic *Escherichia coli* to tissue culture cells. *Infection and Immunity*, *74*(12), 6920–6928. DOI: 10.1128/IAI.01030-06

Siddiqui, Z. R., Rahman, S., Verma, N., Srivastava, A., Jahan, N., Mohanty, S., & Suman, S. (2025). Gut–Oral microbial Dysbiosis: A correlated ecosystem. *Advanced Gut & Microbiome Research*, *2025*(1), 7351229. DOI: 10.1155/agm3/7351229

Siegel, R. L., Miller, K. D., Fuchs, H. E., & Jemal, A. (2021). Cancer statistics, 2021. *CA: a Cancer Journal for Clinicians*, *71*(1), 7–33. DOI: 10.3322/caac.21654

Siegel, R. L., Miller, K. D., & Jemal, A. (2019). Cancer statistics. *CA: a Cancer Journal for Clinicians*, *69*(1), 7–34. DOI: 10.3322/caac.21551 PMID: 30620402

Si, K., Xue, Y., Yu, X., Zhu, X., Li, Q., Gong, W., Liang, T., & Duan, S. (2021). Fully end-to-end deep learning-based diagnosis of pancreatic tumors. *Theranostics*, *11*(4), 1982–1990. DOI: 10.7150/thno.52508 PMID: 33408793

Sindelar, W. F., & Kinsella, T. J. (1999). Studies of intraoperative radiotherapy in carcinoma of the pancreas. *Annals of Oncology : Official Journal of the European Society for Medical Oncology*, *10*(4), 226–230. DOI: 10.1093/annonc/10.suppl_4.S226 PMID: 10436828

Singhi, A. D., Liu, T. C., Roncaioli, J. L., Cao, D., Zeh, H. J., Zureikat, A. H., Tsung, A., Marsh, J. W., Lee, K. K., Hogg, M. E., Bahary, N., Brand, R. E., McGrath, K. M., Slivka, A., Cressman, K. L., Fuhrer, K., & O'Sullivan, R. J. (2017). Alternative Lengthening of Telomeres and Loss of DAXX/ATRX Expression Predicts Metastatic Disease and Poor Survival in Patients with Pancreatic Neuroendocrine Tumors. *Clinical Cancer Research*, *23*(2), 600–609. DOI: 10.1158/1078-0432.CCR-16-1113 PMID: 27407094

Singhi, A. D., & Wood, L. D. (2021). Early detection of pancreatic cancer using DNA-based molecular approaches. *Nature Reviews. Gastroenterology & Hepatology*, *18*(7), 457–468. DOI: 10.1038/s41575-021-00470-0 PMID: 34099908

Singh, V., Sheikh, A., Abourehab, M. A. S., & Kesharwani, P. (2022). Dostarlimab as a miracle drug: Rising hope against cancer treatment. *Biosensors (Basel)*, *12*(8), 617. DOI: 10.3390/bios12080617 PMID: 36005013

Sisodiya, S. M. (2021). Precision medicine and therapies of the future. *Epilepsia*, *62*(S2), S90–S105. DOI: 10.1111/epi.16539 PMID: 32776321

Sivakumar, S., Jainarayanan, A., Arbe-Barnes, E., Sharma, P. K., Leathlobhair, M. N., Amin, S., Reiss, D. J., Heij, L., Hegde, S., Magen, A., Tucci, F., Sun, B., Wu, S., Anand, N. M., Slawinski, H., Revale, S., Nassiri, I., Webber, J., Hoeltzel, G. D., & Bashford-Rogers, R. (2025). Distinct immune cell infiltration patterns in pancreatic ductal adenocarcinoma (PDAC) exhibit divergent immune cell selection and immunosuppressive mechanisms. *Nature Communications*, *16*(1), 1397. DOI: 10.1038/s41467-024-55424-2

Sivan, A., Corrales, L., Hubert, N., Williams, J. B., Aquino-Michaels, K., Earley, Z. M., Benyamin, F. W., Man Lei, Y., Jabri, B., Alegre, M.-L., Chang, E. B., & Gajewski, T. F. (2015). Commensal *Bifidobacterium* promotes antitumor immunity and facilitates anti–PD-L1 efficacy. *Science*, *350*(6264), 1084–1089. DOI: 10.1126/science.aac4255

Siveen, K. S., & Kuttan, G. (2009). Role of macrophages in tumour progression. *Immunology Letters*, *123*(2), 97–102. DOI: 10.1016/j.imlet.2009.02.011

Smeenk, H. G., van Eijck, C. H. J., Hop, W., Erdmann, J., Tran, K. C. K., Debois, M., van Cutsem, E., van Dekken, H., Klinkenbijl, J. H., & Jeekel, J. (2007). Long-term survival and metastatic pattern of pancreatic and periampullary cancer after adjuvant chemoradiation or observation: Long-term results of EORTC trial 40891. *Annals of Surgery*, *246*(5), 734–740. DOI: 10.1097/SLA.0b013e318156eef3 PMID: 17968163

Sofuni, A., Iijima, H., Moriyasu, F., Nakayama, D., Shimizu, M., Nakamura, K., Itokawa, F., & Itoi, T. (2005). Differential diagnosis of pancreatic tumours using ultrasound contrast imaging. *Journal of Gastroenterology*, *40*(5), 518–525. DOI: 10.1007/s00535-005-1578-z PMID: 15942718

Sohal, D. P. S., Duong, M., Ahmad, S. A., Gandhi, N. S., Beg, M. S., Wang-Gillam, A., Wade, J. L.III, Chiorean, E. G., Guthrie, K. A., Lowy, A. M., Philip, P. A., & Hochster, H. S. (2021). Efficacy of perioperative chemotherapy for resectable pancreatic adenocarcinoma: A phase 2 randomized clinical trial. *JAMA Oncology*, *7*(3), 421–427. DOI: 10.1001/jamaoncol.2020.7328 PMID: 33475684

Sohal, D. P., Mangu, P. B., Khorana, A. A., Shah, M. A., Philip, P. A., O'Reilly, E. M., & Laheru, D. (2016). Metastatic pancreatic cancer: American Society of Clinical Oncology clinical practice guideline. *Journal of Clinical Oncology*, *34*(23), 2784–2796. DOI: 10.1200/JCO.2016.67.1412 PMID: 27247222

Song, K. B., Kim, S. C., Hwang, D. W., Lee, J. H., Lee, D. J., Lee, J. W., Park, K.-M., & Lee, Y.-J. (2015). Matched case-control analysis comparing laparoscopic and open pylorus-preserving pancreaticoduodenectomy in patients with periampullary tumors. *Annals of Surgery*, *262*(1), 146–155. DOI: 10.1097/SLA.0000000000001079 PMID: 25563866

Song, X., Sun, X., Oh, S. F., Wu, M., Zhang, Y., Zheng, W., Geva-Zatorsky, N., Jupp, R., Mathis, D., Benoist, C., & Kasper, D. L. (2020). Microbial bile acid metabolites modulate gut RORγ+ regulatory T cell homeostasis. *Nature*, *577*(7790), 410–415. DOI: 10.1038/s41586-019-1865-0

Soo, R. A., Yong, W. P., & Innocenti, F. (2012). Systemic therapies for pancreatic cancer—The role of pharmacogenetics. *Current Drug Targets*, *13*(6), 811–828. DOI: 10.2174/138945012800564068 PMID: 22458528

Splinter, T. A. W., Obertop, H., Kok, T. C., & Jeekel, J. (1989). Adjuvant Chemotherapy after resection of Adenocarcinoma of the periampullary region and the head of the pancreas: A non-randomised pilot study. *Journal of Cancer Research and Clinical Oncology, 115*(2), 200–202. DOI: 10.1007/BF00397924 PMID: 2715169

Spring, B. Q., Bryan Sears, R., Zheng, L. Z., Mai, Z., Watanabe, R., Sherwood, M. E., Schoenfeld, D. A., Pogue, B. W., Pereira, S. P., Villa, E., & Hasan, T. (2016). A photoactivatable multi-inhibitor nanoliposome for tumour control and simultaneous inhibition of treatment escape pathways. *Nature Nanotechnology, 11*(4), 378–387. DOI: 10.1038/nnano.2015.311 PMID: 26780659

Springfeld, C., Jäger, D., Büchler, M. W., Strobel, O., Hackert, T., Palmer, D. H., & Neoptolemos, J. P. (2019). Chemotherapy for pancreatic cancer. *La Presse Medicale, 48*(3), e159–e174. DOI: 10.1016/j.lpm.2019.02.025 PMID: 30879894

Stasiewicz, M., Kwaśniewski, M., & Karpiński, T. M. (2021). Microbial associations with pancreatic cancer: A new frontier in biomarkers. *Cancers (Basel), 13*(15), 3784. DOI: 10.3390/cancers13153784

Stathis, A., & Moore, M. J. (2010). Advanced pancreatic carcinoma: Current treatment and future challenges. *Nature Reviews. Clinical Oncology, 7*(3), 163–172. DOI: 10.1038/nrclinonc.2009.236 PMID: 20101258

Stec, W. M., Kudas, Z., Górka, M., Wojtkiewicz, A., Piekarska, M., & Szerej, K. (2024). Advancements in Pancreatic Cancer Treatment: A Comprehensive Review of Current Therapies and Future Directions. *Quality in Sport, 27*, 54941. DOI: 10.12775/QS.2024.27.54941

Stefanoudakis, D., Frountzas, M., Schizas, D., Michalopoulos, N. V., Drakaki, A., & Toutouzas, K. G. (2024). Significance of TP53, CDKN2A, SMAD4 and KRAS in Pancreatic Cancer. *Current Issues in Molecular Biology, 46*(4), 2827–2844. DOI: 10.3390/cimb46040177 PMID: 38666907

Stocken, D. D., Büchler, M. W., Dervenis, C., Bassi, C., Jeekel, H., Klinkenbijl, J. H., Bakkevold, K. E., Takada, T., Amano, H., & Neoptolemos, J. P. (2005). Meta-analysis of Randomised Adjuvant Therapy trials for Pancreatic Cancer. *British Journal of Cancer, 92*(8), 1372–1381. DOI: 10.1038/sj.bjc.6602513 PMID: 15812554

Stone, M. L., & Beatty, G. L. (2019). Cellular determinants and therapeutic implications of inflammation in pancreatic cancer. *Pharmacology & Therapeutics, 201*, 202–213. DOI: 10.1016/j.pharmthera.2019.05.012

Strimpakos, A., Saif, M. W., & Syrigos, K. N. (2008). Pancreatic cancer: From molecular pathogenesis to targeted therapy. *Cancer and Metastasis Reviews*, *27*(3), 495–522. DOI: 10.1007/s10555-008-9134-y

Strobel, O., Neoptolemos, J., Jager, D., & Buchler, M. W. (2019). Optimizing the outcomes of Pancreatic Cancer Surgery. *Nature Reviews. Clinical Oncology*, *16*(1), 11–26. DOI: 10.1038/s41571-018-0112-1 PMID: 30341417

Stromnes, I., Brockenbrough, J., Izeradjene, K., Carlson, M. A., Cuevas, C., Simmons, R. M., Greenberg, P. D., & Hingorani, S. R. (2014). Targeted depletion of an MDSC subset unmasks pancreatic ductal adenocarcinoma to adaptive immunity. *Gut*, *63*(11), 1769–1781. DOI: 10.1136/gutjnl-2013-306271 PMID: 24555999

Strosberg, J. R., Halfdanarson, T. R., & Bellizzi, A. M. (2017). NANETS Consensus Guidelines for the Diagnosis and Management of Poorly Differentiated (High-Grade) Extrapulmonary Neuroendocrine Carcinomas. *Pancreas*, *46*(1), 1–12. DOI: 10.1097/MPA.0b013e3181ebb56f PMID: 27977625

Sudimack, J., & Lee, R. J. (2000). Targeted drug delivery via the folate receptor. *Advanced Drug Delivery Reviews*, *41*(2), 147–162. DOI: 10.1016/S0169-409X(99)00062-9 PMID: 10699311

Sugahara, K. N., Teesalu, T., Karmali, P. P., Kotamraju, V. R., Agemy, L., Girard, O. M., & Ruoslahti, E. (2009). Tissue-penetrating delivery of compounds and nanoparticles into tumors. *Cancer Cell*, *16*(6), 510–520. DOI: 10.1016/j.ccr.2009.10.013 PMID: 19962669

Sugimoto, M., Wong, D. T., Hirayama, A., Soga, T., & Tomita, M. (2010). Capillary electrophoresis mass spectrometry-based saliva metabolomics identified oral, breast and pancreatic cancer-specific profiles. *Metabolomics*, *6*(1), 78–95. DOI: 10.1007/s11306-009-0178-y PMID: 20300169

Suker, M., Beumer, B. R., Sadot, E., Marthey, L., Faris, J. E., Mellon, E. A., El-Rayes, B. F., Wang-Gillam, A., Lacy, J., Hosein, P. J., Moorcraft, S. Y., Conroy, T., Hohla, F., Allen, P., Taieb, J., Hong, T. S., Shridhar, R., Chau, I., van Eijck, C. H., & Koerkamp, B. G. (2016). FOLFIRINOX for locally advanced pancreatic cancer: A systematic review and patient-level meta-analysis. *The Lancet. Oncology*, *17*(6), 801–810. DOI: 10.1016/S1470-2045(16)00172-8 PMID: 27160474

Sun, C.. (2020). Targeting Wnt signaling in cancer stem cells for cancer therapy. *Pharmaceuticals*, *13*(6), 137. DOI: 10.3390/ph13060137

Sun, Q., Zhou, S., Zhao, J., Deng, C., Teng, R., Zhao, Y., Chen, J., Dong, J., Yin, M., Bai, Y., Deng, H., & Wen, J. (2018). Engineered T lymphocytes eliminate lung metastases in models of pancreatic cancer. *Oncotarget, 9*(17), 13694–13705. DOI: 10.18632/oncotarget.24122 PMID: 29568387

Symeonidis, D., Zacharoulis, D., Kissa, L., Samara, A. A., Petsa, E., & Tepetes, K. (2023). From Classic Whipple to Pylorus Preserving Pancreaticoduodenectomy and Ultimately to Pylorus Resecting - Stomach Preserving Pancreaticoduodenectomy. *Revue de Chirurgie, 118*(4), 335. DOI: 10.21614/chirurgia.2023.v.118.i.4.p.335 PMID: 37697996

Tabernero, J., Shapiro, G. I., Lorusso, P. M., Cervantes, A., Schwartz, G. K., Weiss, G. J., Paz-Ares, L., Cho, D. C., Infante, J. R., Alsina, M., Gounder, M. M., Falzone, R., Harrop, J., White, A. C. S., Toudjarska, I., Bumcrot, D., Meyers, R. E., Hinkle, G., Svrzikapa, N., & de Sauvage, F. J. (2013). First-in-human trial of an RNA interference therapeutic targeting VEGF and KSP in cancer patients with liver involvement. *Cancer Discovery, 3*(4), 406–417. DOI: 10.1158/2159-8290.CD-12-0429 PMID: 23358650

Taieb, J., Prager, G. W., Melisi, D., Westphalen, C. B., D'Esquermes, N., Ferreras, A., Carrato, A., & Macarulla, T. (2020). First-line and second-line treatment of patients with metastatic pancreatic adenocarcinoma in routine clinical practice across Europe: A retrospective, observational chart review study. *ESMO Open, 5*(1), e000698. DOI: 10.1136/esmoopen-2019-000587 PMID: 31958291

Takada, T., Amano, H., Yasuda, H., Nimura, Y., Matsushiro, T., Kato, H., Nagakawa, T., & Nakayama, T. (2002). Is postoperative adjuvant chemotherapy useful for gallbladder carcinoma? A Phase III multicenter prospective randomized controlled trial in patients with resected Pancreaticobiliary Carcinoma. *Cancer, 95*(8), 1685–1695. DOI: 10.1002/cncr.10831 PMID: 12365016

Takeichi, M. (1991). Cadherin cell adhesion receptors as a morphogenetic regulator. *Science, 251*(5000), 1451–1455. DOI: 10.1126/science.2006419 PMID: 2006419

Talley, N. J., & O'connor, S. (2010). *Clinical examination: a systematic guide to physical diagnosis*. Elsevier Australia.

Tang, C. C., Von Ah, D., & Fulton, J. S. (2018). The symptom experience of patients with advanced pancreatic cancer: An integrative review. *Cancer Nursing, 41*(1), 33–44. DOI: 10.1097/NCC.0000000000000463 PMID: 28059839

Tang, H., Yu, D., Zhang, J., Wang, M., Fu, M., Qian, Y., Zhang, X., Ji, R., Gu, J., & Zhang, X. (2024). The new advance of exosome-based liquid biopsy for cancer diagnosis. *Journal of Nanobiotechnology*, *22*(1), 610. DOI: 10.1186/s12951-024-02863-0 PMID: 39380060

Tangutoori, S., Spring, B. Q., Mai, Z., Palanisami, A., Mensah, L. B., & Hasan, T. (2016). Simultaneous delivery of cytotoxic and biologic therapeutics using nanophotoactivatable liposomes enhances treatment efficacy in a mouse model of pancreatic cancer. *Nanomedicine (London)*, *12*(1), 223–234. DOI: 10.1016/j.nano.2015.08.007 PMID: 26390832

Tarannum, M., Holtzman, K., Dréau, D., Mukherjee, P., & Vivero-Escoto, J. L. (2022). Nanoparticle combination for precise stroma modulation and improved delivery for pancreatic cancer. *Journal of Controlled Release*, *347*(1), 425–434. DOI: 10.1016/j.jconrel.2022.05.019 PMID: 35569588

Tarasiuk, A., Mackiewicz, T., Małecka-Panas, E., & Fichna, J. (2021). Biomarkers for early detection of pancreatic cancer–miRNAs as a potential diagnostic and therapeutic tool? *Cancer Biology & Therapy*, *22*(5-6), 347–356. DOI: 10.1080/15384047.2021.1941584 PMID: 34224317

Tariq, S., & Badar, A. (2019). Immune evasion strategies of pancreatic cancer and the emerging role of immunotherapy. *Journal of Experimental & Clinical Cancer Research : CR*, *38*, 162. DOI: 10.1186/s13046-019-1153-8

Temel, H. Y., Kaymak, Ö., Kaplan, S., Bahcivanci, B., Gkoutos, G. V., & Acharjee, A. (2023). Role of microbiota and microbiota derived short-chain fatty acids in PDAC. *Cancer Medicine*, *12*(5), 5661–5675. DOI: 10.1002/cam4.5323

Tempero, M. A., Malafa, M. P., Al-Hawary, M., Behrman, S. W., Benson, A. B., Cardin, D. B., Chiorean, E. G., Chung, V., Czito, B., Del Chiaro, M., Dillhoff, M., Donahue, T. R., Dotan, E., Ferrone, C. R., Fountzilas, C., Hardacre, J., Hawkins, W. G., Klute, K., Ko, A. H., & George, G. V. (2021). Pancreatic Adenocarcinoma, Version 2.2021, NCCN Clinical Practice Guidelines in Oncology. *Journal of the National Comprehensive Cancer Network : JNCCN*, *19*(4), 439–457. DOI: 10.6004/jnccn.2021.0017 PMID: 33845462

Tempero, M. A., Malafa, M. P., Chiorean, E. G., Czito, B., Scaife, C., Narang, A. K., Bartholomew, M. J., & Bekaii-Saab, T. (2019). Pancreatic Adenocarcinoma, Version 1.2019. *Journal of the National Comprehensive Cancer Network : JNCCN*, *17*(3), 202–210. DOI: 10.6004/jnccn.2019.0014 PMID: 30865919

Teng, T., Lin, R., Lin, Z., Ke, K., Lin, X., Pan, M., Zhang, D., & Huang, H. (2020). Photothermal augment stromal disrupting effects for enhanced Abraxane synergy chemotherapy in pancreatic cancer PDX model. *Biomaterials Science*, *8*(12), 3278–3285. DOI: 10.1039/D0BM00549E PMID: 32355947

Thapa, R. K., Nguyen, H. T., Gautam, M., Shrestha, A., Lee, E. S., Ku, S. K., Choi, H.-G., Yong, C. S., & Kim, J. O. (2017). Hydrophobic binding peptide-conjugated hybrid lipid-mesoporous silica nanoparticles for effective chemo-photothermal therapy of pancreatic cancer. *Drug Delivery*, *24*(1), 1690–1702. DOI: 10.1080/10717544.2017.1396382 PMID: 29098877

Thomas, R. M., & Jobin, C. (2020). Microbiota in pancreatic health and disease: The next frontier in microbiome research. *Nature Reviews. Gastroenterology & Hepatology*, *17*(1), 53–64. DOI: 10.1038/s41575-019-0242-7

Tilg, H., Adolph, T. E., & Trauner, M. (2022). Gut-liver axis: Pathophysiological concepts and clinical implications. *Cell Metabolism*, *34*(11), 1700–1718. DOI: 10.1016/j.cmet.2022.09.017

Timmer, F. E., Geboers, B., Nieuwenhuizen, S., Dijkstra, M., Schouten, E. A., Puijk, R. S., de Vries, J. J. J., van den Tol, M. P., Bruynzeel, A. M. E., Streppel, M. M., Wilmink, J. W., van der Vliet, H. J., Meijerink, M. R., Scheffer, H. J., & de Gruijl, T. D. (2021). Pancreatic cancer and immunotherapy: A clinical overview. *Cancers (Basel)*, *13*(16), 4138. DOI: 10.3390/cancers13164138

Tiriac, H., Belleau, P., Engle, D. D., Plenker, D., Deschênes, A., Somerville, T. D. D., Froeling, F. E. M., Burkhart, R. A., Denroche, R. E., Jang, G.-H., Miyabayashi, K., Young, C. M., Patel, H., Ma, M., LaComb, J. F., Palmaira, R. L. D., Javed, A. A., Huynh, J. C., Johnson, M., & Tuveson, D. A. (2018). Organoid profiling identifies common responders to Chemotherapy in Pancreatic Cancer. *Cancer Discovery*, *8*(9), 1112–1129. DOI: 10.1158/2159-8290.CD-18-0349 PMID: 29853643

Tolstonog, G. V., & Krupitza, G. (2019). HGF/c-MET as a therapeutic target in pancreatic cancer: Past achievements and future perspectives. *Frontiers in Oncology*, *9*, 1227. DOI: 10.3389/fonc.2019.01227

Tong, Z., Liu, Y., Ma, H., Zhang, J., Lin, B., Bao, X., Xu, X., Gu, C., Zheng, Y., Liu, L., Fang, W., Deng, S., & Zhao, P. (2020). Development, validation and comparison of artificial neural network models and logistic regression models predicting survival of unresectable pancreatic cancer. *Frontiers in Bioengineering and Biotechnology*, *8*, 196. DOI: 10.3389/fbioe.2020.00196 PMID: 32232040

Topol, E. J. (2019). High-performance medicine: The convergence of human and artificial intelligence. *Nature Medicine*, *25*(1), 44–56. DOI: 10.1038/s41591-018-0300-7 PMID: 30617339

Torphy, R. J., Zhu, Y., & Schulick, R. D. (2018). Immunotherapy for pancreatic cancer: Barriers and breakthroughs. *Annals of Gastroenterological Surgery*, *2*(4), 274–281. DOI: 10.1002/ags3.12176 PMID: 30003190

Torres, P. J., Fletcher, E. M., Gibbons, S. M., Bouvet, M., Doran, K. S., & Kelley, S. T. (2015). Characterization of the salivary microbiome in patients with pancreatic cancer. *PeerJ*, *1373*, e1373. Advance online publication. DOI: 10.7717/peerj.1373

Tripathi, S. (2021). Artificial intelligence: A brief review. In *Analyzing future applications of AI, sensors, and robotics in society* (pp. 1–22). IGI Global., DOI: 10.4018/978-1-7998-3499-1.ch001

Trivieri, N., Panebianco, C., Villani, A., Pracella, R., Latiano, T. P., Perri, F., Binda, E., & Pazienza, V. (2020). High levels of prebiotic resistant starch in diet modulate a specific pattern of miRNAs expression profile associated with a better overall survival in pancreatic cancer. *Biomolecules*, *11*(1), 26–38. DOI: 10.3390/biom11010026

Tyagi, A. K., Prasad, S., Majeed, M., & Aggarwal, B. B. (2015). Curcumin, a component of turmeric: From farm to pharmacy. *BioFactors (Oxford, England)*, *41*(1), 1–9. DOI: 10.1002/biof.1214 PMID: 25545372

Uehata, T., & Takeuchi, O. (2020). RNA recognition and immunity—Innate immune sensing and its posttranscriptional regulation mechanisms. *Cells*, *9*(7), 1701. DOI: 10.3390/cells9071701 PMID: 32708595

Ueno, H., Kosuge, T., Matsuyama, Y., Yamamoto, J., Nakao, A., Egawa, S., Doi, R., Monden, M., Hatori, T., Tanaka, M., Shimada, M., & Kanemitsu, K. (2009). A randomised Phase III trial comparing gemcitabine with surgery-only in patients with resected Pancreatic Cancer: Japanese Study Group of Adjuvant Therapy for Pancreatic Cancer. *British Journal of Cancer*, *101*(6), 908–915. DOI: 10.1038/sj.bjc.6605256 PMID: 19690548

Uesato, Y., Sasahira, N., Ozaka, M., Sasaki, T., Takatsuki, M., & Zembutsu, H. (2020). Evaluation of circulating tumor DNA as a biomarker in pancreatic cancer with liver metastasis. *PLoS One*, *15*(7), e0235623. DOI: 10.1371/journal.pone.0235623 PMID: 32614932

Valle, J. W., Palmer, D., Jackson, R., Cox, T., Neoptolemos, J. P., Ghaneh, P., Rawcliffe, C. L., Bassi, C., Stocken, D. D., Cunningham, D., O'Reilly, D., Goldstein, D., Robinson, B. A., Karapetis, C., Scarfe, A., Lacaine, F., Sand, J., Izbicki, J. R., Mayerle, J., & Büchler, M. W. (2014). Optimal duration and timing of Adjuvant Chemotherapy after definitive surgery for ductal adenocarcinoma of the pancreas: Ongoing lessons from the ESPAC-3 study. *Journal of Clinical Oncology*, *32*(6), 504–512. DOI: 10.1200/JCO.2013.50.7657 PMID: 24419109

van der Sijde, F., Mustafa, D. A., Vietsch, E. E., Katsikis, P. D., & van Eijck, C. H. (2021). Circulating immunological biomarkers: Prognosis of pancreatic cancer patients reflected by the immune system. *Pancreas*, *50*(7), 933–941. DOI: 10.1097/MPA.0000000000001862 PMID: 34643608

van Heek, N. T., Kuhlmann, K. F. D., Scholten, R. J. P. M., de Castro, S. M. M., Busch, O. R. C., van Gulik, T. M., Obertop, H., & Gouma, D. J. (2005). Hospital volume and mortality after pancreatic resection: A systematic review and an evaluation of intervention in the Netherlands. *Annals of Surgery*, *242*(6), 781–788. DOI: 10.1097/01.sla.0000188462.00249.36 PMID: 16327488

Vennin, C., Murphy, K. J., Morton, J. P., Cox, T. R., Pajic, M., & Timpson, P. (2018). Reshaping the tumour stroma for treatment of pancreatic cancer. *Gastroenterology*, *154*(4), 820–838. DOI: 10.1053/j.gastro.2017.11.280 PMID: 29287624

Verma, R. K., Yu, W., Shrivastava, A., Shankar, S., & Srivastava, R. K. (2016). α-Mangostin-encapsulated PLGA nanoparticles inhibit pancreatic carcinogenesis by targeting cancer stem cells in human, and transgenic (KrasG12D, and KrasG12D/tp53R270H) mice. *Scientific Reports*, *6*(1), 32743. DOI: 10.1038/srep32743 PMID: 27624879

Vétil, R.. (2023). Non-redundant combination of hand-crafted and deep learning radiomics: Application to early detection of pancreatic cancer. *Scientific Reports*, *13*(1), 2175.

Viaud, S., Saccheri, F., Mignot, G., Yamazaki, T., Daillère, R., Hannani, D., Enot, D. P., Pfirschke, C., Engblom, C., Pittet, M. J., Schlitzer, A., Ginhoux, F., Apetoh, L., Chachaty, E., Woerther, P.-L., Eberl, G., Bérard, M., Ecobichon, C., Clermont, D., & Zitvogel, L. (2013). The intestinal microbiota modulates the anticancer immune effects of cyclophosphamide. *Science*, *342*(6161), 971–976. DOI: 10.1126/science.1240537

Villanueva, A., García, C., Paules, A. B., Vicente, M., Megías, M., Reyes, G., de Villalonga, P., Agell, N., Lluís, F., Bachs, O., & Capellá, G. (1998). Disruption of the antiproliferative TGF-β signaling pathways in human pancreatic cancer cells. *Oncogene*, *17*(15), 1969–1978. DOI: 10.1038/sj.onc.1202118

Vitale, F., Dal Verme, L. Z., Paratore, M., Negri, M., Nista, E. C., Ainora, M. E., & Nicoletti, A. (2024). The Past, Present, and Future of Biomarkers for the Early Diagnosis of Pancreatic Cancer. *Biomedicines*, *12*(12), 2840. DOI: 10.3390/biomedicines12122840 PMID: 39767746

Vogtmann, E., Han, Y., Caporaso, J. G., Bokulich, N., Mohamadkhani, A., Moayyedkazemi, A., & Pourshams, A. (2020). Oral microbial community composition is associated with pancreatic cancer: A case-control study in Iran. *Cancer Medicine*, *9*(2), 797–806. DOI: 10.1002/cam4.2660

Von Hoff, D. D., Ramanathan, R. K., Borad, M. J., Laheru, D. A., Smith, L. S., Wood, T. E., Korn, R. L., Desai, N., Trieu, V., Iglesias, J. L., Zhang, H., Soon-Shiong, P., Shi, T., Rajeshkumar, N. V., Maitra, A., & Hidalgo, M. (2011). Gemcitabine plus nab-paclitaxel is an active regimen in patients with advanced pancreatic cancer: A phase I/II trial. *Journal of Clinical Oncology*, *29*(34), 4548–4554. DOI: 10.1200/JCO.2011.36.5742 PMID: 21969517

Waddell, N., Pajic, M., Patch, A. M., Chang, D. K., Kassahn, K. S., Bailey, P., Johns, A. L., Miller, D., Nones, K., Quek, K., Quinn, M. C. J., Robertson, A. J., Fadlullah, M. Z. H., Bruxner, T. J. C., Christ, A. N., Harliwong, I., Idrisoglu, S., Manning, S., Nourse, C., & Grimmond, S. M. (2015). Whole genomes redefine the mutational landscape of pancreatic cancer. *Nature*, *518*(7540), 495–501. DOI: 10.1038/nature14169

Wadhwa, A., Aljabbari, A., Lokras, A., Foged, C., & Thakur, A. (2020). Opportunities and challenges in the delivery of mRNA-based vaccines. *Pharmaceutics*, *12*(2), 102. DOI: 10.3390/pharmaceutics12020102 PMID: 32013049

Wainberg, Z. A., Hochster, H. S., Kim, E. J., George, B., Kaylan, A., Chiorean, E. G., Waterhouse, D. M., Guiterrez, M., Parikh, A., Jain, R., Carrizosa, D. R., Soliman, H. H., Lila, T., Reiss, D. J., Pierce, D. W., Bhore, R., Banerjee, S., Lyons, L., Louis, C. U., & O'Dwyer, P. J. (2020). Open-label, Phase I Study of Nivolumab Combined with *nab*-Paclitaxel Plus Gemcitabine in Advanced Pancreatic Cancer. *Clinical Cancer Research*, *26*(18), 4814–4822. DOI: 10.1158/1078-0432.CCR-20-0099 PMID: 32554514

Wall, N. R., Fuller, R. N., Morcos, A., & De Leon, M. (2023). Pancreatic Cancer Health Disparity: Pharmacologic Anthropology. *Cancers (Basel), 15*(20), 5070. DOI: 10.3390/cancers15205070 PMID: 37894437

Walsh, N., Kennedy, S., Larkin, A., Corkery, B., O'Driscoll, L., Clynes, M., Crown, J., & O'Donovan, N. (2012). EGFR and HER2 inhibition in pancreatic cancer. *Investigational New Drugs, 31*(3), 558–566. DOI: 10.1007/s10637-012-9891-x PMID: 23076814

Wandmacher, A. M., Letsch, A., & Sebens, S. (2021). Challenges and future perspectives of immunotherapy in pancreatic cancer. *Cancers (Basel), 13*(16), 4235. DOI: 10.3390/cancers13164235 PMID: 34439389

Wang, F., Li, L., Liu, B., Xin, H., & Cheng, L. (2015). Advances with liposomal carriers for paclitaxel: A review. *Journal of Nanoscience and Nanotechnology, 15*(1), 1–12. DOI: 10.1166/jnn.2015.10289 PMID: 26328301

Wang-Gillam, A., Li, C. P., Bodoky, G., Dean, A., Shan, Y. S., Jameson, G., Macarulla, T., Lee, K. H., Cunningham, D., Blanc, J. F., Hubner, R. A., Chiu, C.-F., Schwartsmann, G., Siveke, J. T., Braiteh, F., Moyo, V., Belanger, B., Dhindsa, N., Bayever, E., & Wong, M. (2016). Nanoliposomal irinotecan with fluorouracil and folinic acid in metastatic pancreatic cancer after previous gemcitabine-based therapy (NAPOLI-1): A global, randomised, open-label, phase 3 trial. *Lancet, 387*(10018), 545–557. DOI: 10.1016/S0140-6736(15)00986-1 PMID: 26615328

Wang, H., Liang, Y., Yin, Y., Zhang, J., Su, W., White, A. M., Jiang, B., Xu, J., Zhang, Y., Stewart, S., & Li, Y. (2021). Carbon nano-onion-mediated dual targeting of P-selectin and P-glycoprotein to overcome cancer drug resistance. *Nature Communications, 12*(1), 312. DOI: 10.1038/s41467-020-20588-0 PMID: 33436622

Wang, J., Mao, W., Lock, L. L., & Tang, J. (2021). Targeted delivery strategies for precision medicines. *Nature Reviews. Materials, 6*(11), 924–939. DOI: 10.1038/s41578-021-00317-6 PMID: 34950512

Wang, L., Wang, H., Zhang, Q., & Zhang, H. (2021). Recent advances in nanomedicine for cancer therapy. *Biomaterials Science, 9*(4), 1137–1152. DOI: 10.1039/D0BM01928K

Wang, S., Zheng, Y., Yang, F., Zhu, L., Zhu, X., Wang, Z., Wu, X.-L., Zhou, C.-H., Yan, J.-Y., Hu, B.-Y., Kong, B., Fu, D.-L., Bruns, C., Zhao, Y., Qin, L.-X., & Dong, Q.-Z. (2021). The molecular biology of pancreatic adenocarcinoma: Translational challenges and clinical perspectives. *Signal Transduction and Targeted Therapy, 6*(1), 1–23. DOI: 10.1038/s41392-021-00659-4 PMID: 34219130

Wang, X., Zhang, Y., & Luo, Y. (2021). Toxicity concerns and stability of nanoparticles in pancreatic cancer therapy. *Cancer Nanotechnology*, *8*(6), 289–296. DOI: 10.1002/cncr.33698

Wang, Z., Li, Y., Kong, D., Banerjee, S., Ahmad, A., Azmi, A. S., Ali, S., Abbruzzese, J. L., Gallick, G. E., & Sarkar, F. H. (2009). Acquisition of epithelial-mesenchymal transition phenotype of gemcitabine-resistant pancreatic cancer cells is linked with activation of the notch signaling pathway. *Cancer Research*, *69*(6), 2400–2407. DOI: 10.1158/0008-5472.CAN-08-4312

Waterhouse, D. M., Richards, D., & Wagener, D. J. (2002). CA 19-9 levels in patients with Advanced Pancreatic Cancer (APC) treated in a randomized, Phase II trial with the histone deacetylase inhibitor CI-994 + gemcitabine (CI-994 + G) versus placebo + gemcitabine (P + G). *Proceedings of the American Society of Clinical Oncology*, *21*, 148–156.

Waters, A. M., & Der, C. J. (2018). KRAS: The critical driver and therapeutic target for pancreatic cancer. *Cold Spring Harbor Perspectives in Medicine*, *8*(9), a031435. DOI: 10.1101/cshperspect.a031435

Weber, J. S. (2014). Current perspectives on immunotherapy. *Seminars in Oncology*, *41*(5), S14–S29. DOI: 10.1053/j.seminoncol.2014.09.003

Wei, M. Y., Shi, S., Liang, C., Meng, Q. C., Hua, J., Zhang, Y. Y., Liu, J., Zhang, B., Xu, J., & Yu, X.-J. (2019). The microbiota and microbiome in pancreatic cancer: More influential than expected. *Molecular Cancer*, *18*(1), 97–106. DOI: 10.1186/s12943-019-1008-0

Weiss, G. J., Blaydorn, L., Beck, J., Bornemann-Kolatzki, K., Urnovitz, H., Schütz, E., & Khemka, V. (2019). Correction to: Phase Ib/II study of gemcitabine, nab-paclitaxel, and pembrolizumab in metastatic pancreatic adenocarcinoma. *Investigational New Drugs*, *37*(4), 761. DOI: 10.1007/s10637-019-00763-x PMID: 31020607

Wenzel, P., Mogler, C., Görgülü, K., & Algül, H. (2024). Pancreatic Cancer: Current Concepts, Trends, and Future Directions. *The Turkish Journal of Gastroenterology : the Official Journal of Turkish Society of Gastroenterology*, *36*(2), 69–81. DOI: 10.5152/tjg.2024.24544

Whipple, A. O., Parsons, W. B., & Mullins, C. R. (1935). Treatment of carcinoma of the ampulla of Vater. *Annals of Surgery*, *102*(4), 763–777. DOI: 10.1097/00000658-193510000-00023 PMID: 17856666

Willett, C. G., & Warshaw, A. L. (1998). Intraoperative radiation therapy of pancreatic cancer. In Beger, H. G., Warshaw, A. L., Büchler, M. W., Carr-Locke, D. L., Neoptolemos, J. P., Russell, C., & Sarr, M. G. (Eds.), *The Pancreas: A Clinical.*, Textbook.

Winter, J. M., Jiang, W., & Basturk, O. (2013). Recurrence and Survival After Resection of Small Intraductal Papillary Mucinous Neoplasm-associated Carcinomas (≤20 mm Invasive Component). *Annals of Surgery, 258*(2), 313–320. DOI: 10.1097/SLA.0000000000001319 PMID: 23360922

Wisnoski, N. C., Townsend, C. M.Jr, Nealon, W. H., Freeman, J. L., & Riall, T. S. (2008). 672 Patients with Acinar Cell Carcinoma of the Pancreas: A Population-Based Comparison to Pancreatic Adenocarcinoma. *Surgery, 144*(2), 141–148. DOI: 10.1016/j.surg.2008.03.006 PMID: 18656619

Wolfgang, C. L., Herman, J. M., Laheru, D. A., Klein, A. P., Erdek, M. A., Fishman, E. K., & Hruban, R. H. (2013). Recent progress in pancreatic cancer. *CA: a Cancer Journal for Clinicians, 63*(5), 318–348. DOI: 10.3322/caac.21190 PMID: 23856911

Wong, T., Howes, N., Threadgold, J., Smart, H. L., Lombard, M. G., Gilmore, I., Sutton, R., Greenhalf, W., Ellis, I., & Neoptolemos, J. P. (2001). Molecular diagnosis of early pancreatic ductal adenocarcinoma in high-risk patients. *Pancreatology, 1*(5), 486–509. DOI: 10.1159/000055852 PMID: 12120229

Wood, L. D., Canto, M. I., Jaffee, E. M., & Simeone, D. M. (2022). Pancreatic Cancer: Pathogenesis, Screening, Diagnosis, and Treatment. *Gastroenterology, 163*(2), 386–402.e1. DOI: 10.1053/j.gastro.2022.03.056 PMID: 35398344

Wu, J., Matthaei, H., Maitra, A., Dal Molin, M., Wood, L. D., Eshleman, J. R., Goggins, M., Canto, M. I., Schulick, R. D., Edil, B. H., Wolfgang, C. L., Klein, A. P., Diaz, L. A.Jr, Allen, P. J., Schmidt, C. M., Kinzler, K. W., Papadopoulos, N., Hruban, R. H., & Vogelstein, B. (2011). Recurrent GNAS mutations define an unexpected pathway for pancreatic cyst development. *Science Translational Medicine, 3*(92), 92ra66. Advance online publication. DOI: 10.1126/scitranslmed.3002543 PMID: 21775669

Wu, L., Zhou, W. B., Zhou, J., Wei, Y., Wang, H. M., Liu, X. D., Chen, X.-C., Wang, W., Ye, L., Yao, L., Chen, Q.-H., & Tang, Z. G. (2020). Circulating exosomal microRNAs as novel potential detection biomarkers in pancreatic cancer. *Oncology Letters, 20*(2), 1432–1440. DOI: 10.3892/ol.2020.11691 PMID: 32724386

Wu, M., Liu, J., Wu, S., Xie, H., Wang, Y., Zhang, J., & Zhang, Y. (2021). Systemic immune activation and responses of irradiation to different metastatic sites combined with immunotherapy in advanced non-small cell lung cancer. *Frontiers in Immunology*, *12*, 803247. DOI: 10.3389/fimmu.2021.803247

Wu, Y. S., Chung, I., Wong, W. F., Masamune, A., Sim, M. S., & Looi, C. Y. (2017). Paracrine IL-6 signaling mediates the effects of pancreatic stellate cells on epithelial-mesenchymal transition via Stat3/Nrf2 pathway in pancreatic cancer cells. *Biochimica et Biophysica Acta (BBA) -. Biochimica et Biophysica Acta. G, General Subjects*, *1861*(2), 296–306. DOI: 10.1016/j.bbagen.2016.10.006

Wu, Y., Han, W., Dong, H., Liu, X., & Su, X. (2024). The rising roles of exosomes in the tumor microenvironment reprogramming and cancer immunotherapy. *MedComm*, *5*(4), e541–e550. DOI: 10.1002/mco2.541

Xiang, X., Chen, X., He, Y., Wang, Y., Xia, W., Ye, S., Wang, S., Xiao, Y., Li, Q., Wang, X., Luo, W., & Li, J. (2023). Pancreatic cancer challenge in 52 Asian countries: Age-centric insights and the role of modifiable risk factors (1990-2019). *Frontiers in Oncology*, *13*, 1271370. Advance online publication. DOI: 10.3389/fonc.2023.1271370 PMID: 37849795

Xiao, Q., Zhang, F., Xu, L., Yue, L., Kon, O. L., Zhu, Y., & Guo, T. (2021). High-throughput proteomics and AI for cancer biomarker discovery. *Advanced Drug Delivery Reviews*, *176*, 113844. DOI: 10.1016/j.addr.2021.113844 PMID: 34182017

Xie, Y., Hang, Y., Wang, Y., Sleightholm, R., Prajapati, D. R., Bader, J., Yu, A., Tang, W., Jaramillo, L., Li, J., Singh, R. K., & Oupický, D. (2020). Stromal modulation and treatment of metastatic pancreatic cancer with local intraperitoneal triple miRNA/siRNA nanotherapy. *ACS Nano*, *14*(1), 255–271. DOI: 10.1021/acsnano.9b03978 PMID: 31927946

Xiong, H. Q., Du, M., Wolff, R. A., & Abbruzzese, J. L. (2002). Pharmacology study of celecoxib in combination with gemcitabine for advanced pancreatic cancer. *Proceedings of the American Society of Clinical Oncology*, *21*, 113–118.

Xue, Y., Xiao, H., Guo, S., Xu, B., Liao, Y., Wu, Y., & Zhang, G. (2018). The association between Helicobacter pylori infection and pancreatic cancer: A meta-analysis. *Journal of Cancer Research and Therapeutics*, *14*, S428–S432. DOI: 10.4103/0973-1482.202888

Xu, H., Banerjee, P., Khan, S. A., Ahsan, F., Yadav, D., & Das, S. (2025). Unveiling circulating targets in pancreatic cancer: Insights from proteogenomic evidence and clinical cohorts. *iScience*, *102304*. Advance online publication. DOI: 10.1016/j.isci.2025.102304

Xu, K., Jin, L., Xu, L., Zhu, Y., Hong, L., Pan, C., Li, Y., Yao, J., Zou, R., Tang, W., Wang, J., Wu, A., & Ren, W. (2022). IGF1 receptor-targeted black TiO2 nanoprobes for MRI-guided synergetic photothermal-chemotherapy in drug resistant pancreatic tumor. *Journal of Nanobiotechnology*, *20*(1), 315–316. DOI: 10.1186/s12951-022-01525-3 PMID: 35794573

Xu, Q., Zhou, Y., Zhang, H., Li, H., Qin, H., & Wang, H. (2023). Bibliometric analysis of hotspots and frontiers of immunotherapy in pancreatic cancer. *Health Care*, *11*(3), 304. DOI: 10.3390/healthcare11030304 PMID: 36766879

Xu, Z. H., Wang, W. Q., Lou, W. H., & Liu, L. (2022). Insight of pancreatic cancer: Recommendations for improving its therapeutic efficacy in the next decade. *Journal of Pancreatology*, *5*(02), 58–68. DOI: 10.1097/JP9.0000000000000093

Yabuuchi, S., Pai, S. G., Campbell, N. R., De Wilde, R. F., De Oliveira, E., Korangath, P., Streppel, M. M., Rasheed, Z. A., Hidalgo, M., Maitra, A., & Rajeshkumar, N. V. (2013). Notch signaling pathway targeted therapy suppresses tumor progression and metastatic spread in pancreatic cancer. *Cancer Letters*, *335*(1), 41–51. DOI: 10.1016/j.canlet.2013.01.054

Yamamoto, J., Saiura, A., Koga, R., Seki, M., Katori, M., Kato, Y., Sakamoto, Y., Kokudo, N., & Yamaguchi, T. (2010). Improved survival of left-sided pancreatic cancer after surgery. *Japanese Journal of Clinical Oncology*, *40*(6), 530–536. DOI: 10.1093/jjco/hyq015 PMID: 20363769

Yamamura, R., & Sonoshita, M. (2025). Fecal microbiota transplantation as a novel therapeutic strategy for pancreatic cancer. *Translational and Regulatory Sciences*, *7*(1), 37–45. DOI: 10.33611/trs.2025-003

Yang, C., Chan, K., Xu, G., Yin, M., Lin, G., Wang, X., Lin, W.-J., Birowosuto, M. D., Zeng, S., Ogi, T., Okuyama, K., Permatasari, F. A., Iskandar, F., Chen, C.-K., & Yong, K.-T. (2019). Biodegradable polymer-coated multifunctional graphene quantum dots for light-triggered synergetic therapy of pancreatic cancer. *ACS Applied Materials & Interfaces*, *11*(3), 2768–2781. DOI: 10.1021/acsami.8b16168 PMID: 30589254

Yang, F., Liu, D. Y., Guo, J. T., Ge, N., Zhu, P., Liu, X., Wang, S., Wang, G.-X., & Sun, S. Y. (2017). Circular RNA circ-LDLRAD3 as a biomarker in diagnosis of pancreatic cancer. *World Journal of Gastroenterology*, *23*(47), 8345–8354. DOI: 10.3748/wjg.v23.i47.8345 PMID: 29307994

Yang, J., Li, S., Li, J., Wang, F., Chen, K., Zheng, Y., Wang, J., Lu, W., Zhou, Y., Yin, Q., Zhang, H., & Guo, C. (2016). A meta-analysis of the diagnostic value of detecting K-ras mutation in pancreatic juice as a molecular marker for pancreatic cancer. *Pancreatology*, *16*(4), 605–614. DOI: 10.1016/j.pan.2016.04.033 PMID: 27237100

Yang, J., Xu, R., Wang, C., Qiu, J., Ren, B., & You, L. (2021). Early screening and diagnosis strategies of pancreatic cancer: A comprehensive review. *Cancer Communications*, *41*(12), 1257–1274. DOI: 10.1002/cac2.12204 PMID: 34331845

Yang, X., & Wu, H. (2024, November 9). RAS signaling in carcinogenesis, cancer therapy and resistance mechanisms. *Journal of Hematology & Oncology*, *17*(1), 108. DOI: 10.1186/s13045-024-01631-9 PMID: 39522047

Yang, Y., Tian, X., Xie, X., Zhuang, Y., Wu, W., & Wang, W. (2010). Expression and regulation of the hedgehog signaling pathway in pancreatic cancer. *Langenbeck's Archives of Surgery*, *395*(5), 515–525. DOI: 10.1007/s00423-009-0493-9

Yao, J. C., Fazio, N., Singh, S., Buzzoni, R., Carnaghi, C., Wolin, E., Tomasek, J., Raderer, M., Lahner, H., Voi, M., Pacaud, L. B., Rouyrre, N., Sachs, C., Valle, J. W., Fave, G. D., Van Cutsem, E., Tesselaar, M., Shimada, Y., Oh, D.-Y., & Pavel, M. E. (2016). Everolimus for the Treatment of Advanced, Non-Functional Neuroendocrine Tumours of the Lung or Gastrointestinal Tract (RADIANT-4): A Randomised, Placebo-Controlled, Phase 3 Study. *Lancet*, *387*(10022), 968–977. DOI: 10.1016/S0140-6736(15)00817-X PMID: 26703889

Ychou, M., Conroy, T., Seitz, J. F., Gourgou, S., Hua, A., Mery-Mignard, D., & Kramar, A. (2003). An open phase I study assessing the feasibility of the triple combination: Oxaliplatin plus irinotecan plus leucovorin/5-fluorouracil every 2 weeks in patients with advanced solid tumors. *Annals of Oncology : Official Journal of the European Society for Medical Oncology*, *14*(3), 481–489. DOI: 10.1093/annonc/mdg119 PMID: 12598357

Yin, F., Hu, K., Chen, Y., Yu, M., Wang, D., Wang, Q., Yong, K.-T., Lu, F., Liang, Y., & Li, Z. (2017). siRNA delivery with PEGylated graphene oxide nanosheets for combined photothermal and gene therapy for pancreatic cancer. *Theranostics*, *7*(5), 1133–1148. DOI: 10.7150/thno.17841 PMID: 28435453

Yin, F., Yang, C., Wang, Q., Zeng, S., Hu, R., Lin, G., Tian, J., Hu, S., Lan, R. F., Yoon, H. S., Lu, F., Wang, K., & Yong, K.-T. (2015). A light-driven therapy of pancreatic adenocarcinoma using gold nanorods-based nanocarriers for co-delivery of doxorubicin and siRNA. *Theranostics*, *5*(8), 818–833. DOI: 10.7150/thno.11335 PMID: 26000055

Yin, J., Ngiam, K. Y., & Teo, H. H. (2021). Role of artificial intelligence applications in real-life clinical practice: Systematic review. *Journal of Medical Internet Research, 23*(4), e25759. DOI: 10.2196/25759 PMID: 33885365

Yopp, A. C., Katabi, N., Janakos, M., Klimstra, D. S., D'Angelica, M. I., DeMatteo, R. P., Fong, Y., Brennan, M. F., Jarnagin, W. R., & Allen, P. J. (2011). Invasive carcinoma arising in intraductal papillary mucinous neoplasms of the pancreas: A matched control study with conventional pancreatic ductal adenocarcinoma. *Annals of Surgery, 253*(5), 968–974. DOI: 10.1097/SLA.0b013e318214bcb4 PMID: 21422912

Young, M. R., Abrams, N., Ghosh, S., Rinaudo, J. A. S., Marquez, G., & Srivastava, S. (2020). Pre-diagnostic image data, artificial intelligence, and pancreatic cancer: A tell-tale sign to early detection. *Pancreas, 49*(7), 882–886. DOI: 10.1097/MPA.0000000000001603 PMID: 32675784

Yuan, X., Curtin, J., Xiong, Y., Liu, G., Waschsmann-Hogiu, S., Farkas, D. L., Black, K. L., & Yu, J. S. (2004). Isolation of cancer stem cells from adult glioblastoma multiforme. *Oncogene, 23*(58), 9392–9400. DOI: 10.1038/sj.onc.1208311 PMID: 15558011

Yu, B., Shao, S., & Ma, W. (2024). Frontiers in pancreatic cancer on biomarkers, microenvironment, and immunotherapy. *Cancer Letters*, •••, 217350. PMID: 39581219

Yu, Q., Qiu, Y., Li, J., Tang, X., Wang, X., Cun, X., Xu, S., Liu, Y., Li, M., Zhang, Z., & He, Q. (2020). Targeting cancer-associated fibroblast by dual-responsive lipid-albumin nanoparticles to enhance drug perfusion for pancreatic tumour therapy. *Journal of Controlled Release, 321*, 564–575. DOI: 10.1016/j.jconrel.2020.02.040 PMID: 32112854

Zeitouni, D., Pylayeva-Gupta, Y., Der, C., & Bryant, K. (2016). KRAS Mutant Pancreatic Cancer: No Lone Path to an Effective Treatment. *Cancers (Basel), 8*(4), 45. DOI: 10.3390/cancers8040045 PMID: 27096871

Zeng, G., Germinaro, M., Micsenyi, A., Monga, N. K., Bell, A., Sood, A., Malhotra, V., Sood, N., Midda, V., Monga, D. K., Kokkinakis, D. M., & Monga, S. P. (2006). Aberrant Wnt/β-catenin signaling in pancreatic adenocarcinoma. *Neoplasia : an International Journal for Oncology Research, 8*(4), 279–289. DOI: 10.1593/neo.05607

Zerbi, A., Fossati, V., Parolini, D., Carlucci, M., Balzano, G., Bordogna, G., Staudacher, C., & Di Carlo, V. (1994). Intraoperative radiation therapy adjuvant to resection in the treatment of Pancreatic Cancer. *Cancer, 73*(12), 2930–2935. DOI: 10.1002/1097-0142(19940615)73:12<2930::AID-CNCR2820731209>3.0.CO;2-M PMID: 8199990

Zhang, L., Sanagapalli, S., & Stoita, A. (2018). Challenges in diagnosis of pancreatic cancer. *World Journal of Gastroenterology, 24*(19), 2047–2060. DOI: 10.3748/wjg.v24.i19.2047

Zhang, Q., Lou, Y., Zhang, J., Fu, Q., Wei, T., Sun, X., Chen, Q., Yang, J., Bai, X., & Liang, T. (2017). Hypoxia-inducible factor-2α promotes tumor progression and has crosstalk with Wnt/β-catenin signaling in pancreatic cancer. *Molecular Cancer, 16*(1), 1–14. DOI: 10.1186/s12943-017-0689-5

Zhang, T., Gao, G., Sakandar, H. A., Kwok, L.-Y., & Sun, Z. (2022). Gut dysbiosis in pancreatic diseases: A causative factor and a novel therapeutic target. *Frontiers in Nutrition, 9*, 814269. DOI: 10.3389/fnut.2022.814269

Zhang, T., Liu, Q., & Zhou, S. (2020). Nanomedicine: An overview of nanotechnology in cancer treatment. *Journal of Nanoscience and Nanotechnology, 20*(5), 2691–2704. DOI: 10.1166/jnn.2020.18113

Zhang, X., Shi, S., Zhang, B., Ni, Q. X., & Xu, J. (2018). Circulating biomarkers for early diagnosis of pancreatic cancer: Facts and hopes. *American Journal of Cancer Research, 8*, 332–353.

Zhang, X., Zhang, T., Wang, S., Jiang, C., & Yu, X. (2022). Advances in polymeric nanoparticles for drug delivery: An updated review. *International Journal of Molecular Sciences, 23*(4), 1906. DOI: 10.3390/ijms23041906

Zhang, Y., Liu, X., Wang, L., & Chen, H. (2024). Advanced nanomaterials for targeted cancer therapy: A comprehensive review. *International Journal of Pharmaceutics, 635*, 122845. DOI: 10.1016/j.ijpharm.2024.122845

Zhang, Y., Zhou, M., Wei, H., Zhou, H., He, J., Lu, Y., Wang, D., Chen, B., Zeng, J., Peng, W., Du, F., Gong, A., & Xu, M. (2017). Furin promotes epithelial-mesenchymal transition in pancreatic cancer cells via Hippo-YAP pathway. *International Journal of Oncology, 50*(4), 1352–1362. DOI: 10.3892/ijo.2017.3896

Zhang, Z., Gao, S., Xu, Y., & Zhao, C. (2021). Regulation of ABCG2 expression by Wnt5a through FZD7 in human pancreatic cancer cells. *Molecular Medicine Reports, 23*(1), 1–11. DOI: 10.3892/mmr.2020.11690 PMID: 33200805

Zhan, X., Nie, X., Gao, F., Zhang, C., You, Y.-Z., & Yu, Y. (2020). An NIR-activated polymeric nanoplatform with ROS- and temperature-sensitivity for combined photothermal therapy and chemotherapy of pancreatic cancer. *Biomaterials Science, 8*(21), 5931–5940. DOI: 10.1039/D0BM01324B PMID: 32966381

Zhao, K., & Hu, Y. (2020). Microbiome harbored within tumors: A new chance to revisit our understanding of cancer pathogenesis and treatment. *Signal Transduction and Targeted Therapy*, *5*(1), 136–145. DOI: 10.1038/s41392-020-00244-1

Zhao, Q., Ahmed, M., Tassev, D. V., Hasan, A., Kuo, T. Y., Guo, H. F., O'Reilly, R. J., & Cheung, N. K. (2015). Affinity maturation of T-cell receptor-like antibodies for Wilms tumor 1 peptide greatly enhances therapeutic potential. *Leukemia*, *29*(11), 2238–2247. DOI: 10.1038/leu.2015.125 PMID: 25987253

Zhao, X., Li, F., Li, Y., Wang, H., Ren, H., Chen, J., Nie, G., & Hao, J. (2015). Co-delivery of HIF1α siRNA and gemcitabine via biocompatible lipid-polymer hybrid nanoparticles for effective treatment of pancreatic cancer. *Biomaterials*, *46*, 13–25. DOI: 10.1016/j.biomaterials.2014.12.028 PMID: 25678112

Zhao, X., Yang, K., Zhao, R., Ji, T., Wang, X., Yang, X., Zhang, Y., Cheng, K., Liu, S., Hao, J., Ren, H., & Nie, G. (2016). Inducing enhanced immunogenic cell death with nanocarrier-based drug delivery systems for pancreatic cancer therapy. *Biomaterials*, *102*, 187–197. DOI: 10.1016/j.biomaterials.2016.06.032 PMID: 27343466

Zhao, Z., Zheng, L., Chen, W., Weng, W., Song, J., & Ji, J. (2019). Delivery strategies of cancer immunotherapy: Recent advances and future perspectives. *Journal of Hematology & Oncology*, *12*(1), 126–127. DOI: 10.1186/s13045-019-0817-3 PMID: 31779642

Zheng, R., Liu, X., Zhang, Y., Liu, Y., Wang, Y., Guo, S., Jin, X., Zhang, J., Guan, Y., & Liu, Y. (2024). Frontiers and future of immunotherapy for pancreatic cancer: From molecular mechanisms to clinical application. *Frontiers in Immunology*, *15*, 1383978. Advance online publication. DOI: 10.3389/fimmu.2024.1383978 PMID: 38756774

Zheng, R., Zhang, S., Zeng, H., Wang, S., Sun, K., Chen, R., Li, L., Wei, W., & He, J. (2022). Cancer incidence and mortality in China, 2016. *Journal of the National Cancer Center*, *2*(1), 1–9. DOI: 10.1016/j.jncc.2022.02.002 PMID: 39035212

Zhong, G., Zhang, X., Zhao, R., Guo, Z., Wang, C., Yu, C., Liu, D., Hu, K., Gao, Y., Zhao, B., Liu, X., Shi, X., Chen, L., Li, Y., & Yu, L. (2025). The high efficacy of claudin18.2-targeted CAR-T cell therapy in advanced pancreatic cancer with an antibody-dependent safety strategy. *Molecular Therapy : the Journal of the American Society of Gene Therapy*, *33*(6), 2778–2788. Advance online publication. DOI: 10.1016/j.ymthe.2025.01.012 PMID: 39797399

Zhong, Y., Goltsche, K., Cheng, L., Xie, F., & Morsbach, S. (2022). Nanostructured lipid carriers in cancer therapy: Advances and challenges. *Journal of Controlled Release*, *351*, 370–389. DOI: 10.1016/j.jconrel.2022.09.019

Zhou, F., Yang, J., Zhang, Y., Liu, M., Lang, M. L., Li, M., & Chen, W. R. (2018). Local phototherapy synergizes with immunoadjuvant for treatment of pancreatic cancer through induced immunogenic tumor vaccine. *Clinical Cancer Research, 24*(21), 5335–5346. DOI: 10.1158/1078-0432.CCR-18-1126 PMID: 30068705

Zhou, P., Li, Y., Li, B., Zhang, M., Liu, Y., Yao, Y., & Li, D. (2019). NMIIA promotes tumor growth and metastasis by activating the Wnt/β-catenin signaling pathway and EMT in pancreatic cancer. *Oncogene, 38*(27), 5500–5515. DOI: 10.1038/s41388-019-0806-6

Zhou, W., Zhou, Y., Chen, X., Ning, T., Chen, H., Guo, Q., Zhang, Y., Liu, P., Zhang, Y., Li, C., & Zhang, Z. (2021). Pancreatic cancer-targeting exosomes for enhancing immunotherapy and reprogramming tumour microenvironment. *Biomaterials, 268*, 120546. DOI: 10.1016/j.biomaterials.2020.120546 PMID: 33253966

Zhou, X., Wang, X., Yang, S., & Huang, Z. (2025). Advances in immunotherapy and targeted therapy for pancreatic cancer. *Oncology and Translational Medicine, 11*(2), 81–91. DOI: 10.1097/ot9.0000000000000074

Zhou, Y., Kuang, Y., Wang, C., Yu, Y., Pan, L., & Hu, X. (2024). Impact of KRAS mutation on the tumor microenvironment in colorectal cancer. *International Journal of Biological Sciences, 20*(5), 1947–1964. DOI: 10.7150/ijbs.88779 PMID: 38481800

Zhou, Y., Ma, Y., Sheng, J., Ma, Y., Ding, J., & Zhou, W. (2024). Breaking Down Barriers in Drug Delivery by Stromal Remodeling Approaches in Pancreatic Cancer. *Molecular Pharmaceutics, 21*(8), 3764–3776. Advance online publication. DOI: 10.1021/acs.molpharmaceut.4c00329 PMID: 39049481

Zhou, Y., Shan, T., Ding, W., Hua, Z., Shen, Y., Lu, Z., Chen, B., & Dai, T. (2018). Study on mechanism about long noncoding RNA MALAT1 affecting pancreatic cancer by regulating Hippo-YAP signaling. *Journal of Cellular Physiology, 233*(8), 5805–5814. DOI: 10.1002/jcp.26357

Zhou, Y., Tao, L., Qiu, J., Xu, J., Yang, X., Zhang, Y., Tian, X., Guan, X., Cen, X., & Zhao, Y. (2024). Tumor biomarkers for diagnosis, prognosis and targeted therapy. *Signal Transduction and Targeted Therapy, 9*(1), 132. DOI: 10.1038/s41392-024-01823-2 PMID: 38763973

Zhu, C., Guan, X., Zhang, X., Luan, X., Song, Z., Cheng, X., Zhang, W., & Qin, J.-J. (2022). Targeting KRAS mutant cancers: From druggable therapy to drug resistance. *Molecular Cancer, 21*(1), 159. DOI: 10.1186/s12943-022-01629-2 PMID: 35922812

Zhu, H., Wei, M., Xu, J., Hua, J., Liang, C., Meng, Q., Zhang, Y., Liu, J., Zhang, B., Yu, X., & Shi, S. (2020). PARP inhibitors in pancreatic cancer: Molecular mechanisms and clinical applications. *Molecular Cancer*, *19*(1), 49. Advance online publication. DOI: 10.1186/s12943-020-01167-9 PMID: 32122376

Zhu, Y., Luo, T. M., Jobin, C., & Young, H. A. (2011). Gut microbiota and probiotics in colon tumorigenesis. *Cancer Letters*, *309*(2), 119–127. DOI: 10.1016/j.canlet.2011.06.004

Zonneville, J., Safina, A., Truskinovsky, A. M., Arteaga, C. L., & Bakin, A. V. (2018). TGF-β signalling promotes tumour vasculature by enhancing the pericyte-endothelium association. *BMC Cancer*, *18*(1), 670. DOI: 10.1186/s12885-018-4587-z PMID: 29921235

About the Contributors

Pallavi Singh has been a Seasoned academician and versatile Researcher with more than 17 years of experience in teaching, research, Innovation, and leadership experience in the domain of Biotechnology. She holds B.Tech, M.Tech and Ph.D degree in Biotechnology. She is currently serving as Professor and Program Coordinator (B.Tech. Biotechnology) in Department of Biotechnology at Graphic Era Deemed to be University, Uttarakhand, India. She has published over 57 research papers in reputed National and International journals which includes journals like International Journal of Surgery, Frontiers in Microbiology, Current Issues in Molecular Biology, Computational Toxicology, Journal of Nanomaterials Scientific Reports, Plant Science Today etc. She has further published 2 Books, 5 Book chapters along with many International and National conference presentations. Further, She has published 9 patents in the domain of computational biology, Cancer and Bioprocess Engineering. 4 of her patents have been granted in years 2023 and 2024. She has h index of 11 and i10 index of 11 and is in Editorial Board of many Scopus and SCI journals. She has guided 35 projects at B.Tech and M.Tech level and 5 students are currently pursuing their Ph.D under her guidance.

Shiva Prasad Kollur is working as Associate Professor in Chemistry at Amrita Vishwa Vidyapeetham, Mysuru Campus, India. His research interests included Anticancer therapeutics, Bioinorganic and Materials Chemistry. He has published over 250 scientific research articles in international peer-reviewed journals and several of his research findings are patented. He has mentored more than 40 scholars (Grads/Postgrads) for their degree fulfilment and 8 PhD scholars are presently working under his supervision.

Raghavendra G. Amachawadi is currently working as an Associate Professor in Department of Clinical Sciences, Kansas State University, Manhattan. He has published 116 research articles and has h index of 28 and i10 index of 65. He has handled National level projects in United states and has obtained total funding of dollars14,244,503 from prominent agencies in United states like USDA-NIFA, USAID-Global Food Systems, FDA, National Pork Board, Elanco Animal Health, National Cattlemen's Beef Association (Beef check-off), ICASA-FFAR, and Animal Health Commodity groups.He has expertise in microbiome, metagenomics, and metabolomics research, and investigates the complex interactions between host, microbial communities, and pathogens, aiming to develop innovative, antibiotic-free intervention strategies to control critical issues such as liver abscesses in feedlot cattle, bovine respiratory disease, and swine colibacillosis. He has thorough expertise in animal research and translational medicine.

***

Sayan Acharyya is a dedicated and workaholic individual with a deep passion for the field of biotechnology and bioinformatics. With a strong academic background, Sayan completed a Bachelor of Technology (B.Tech) in Biotechnology from Adamas University and is currently pursuing a Master of Technology (M.Tech) in Bioinformatics from Maulana Abul Kalam Azad University of Technology. Driven by a strong interest in scientific research and technological innovation, Sayan has focused on gaining expertise in areas such as Structural Biology and Next-Generation Sequencing (NGS). Their dedication to these fields is evident in their academic achievements, where they have excelled in integrating computational tools with biological data to understand complex biological systems. Through their educational journey, Sayan has developed a keen interest in structural biology, which involves understanding the three-dimensional structure of proteins, nucleic acids, and other macromolecules, as well as how these structures relate to their functions in living organisms. Additionally, they have developed a strong understanding of NGS technologies, which are revolutionizing the way we analyze and interpret genetic information. Sayan is passionate about contributing to the advancements in healthcare and biotechnology through research and technological development. With a work ethic driven by commitment and dedication, they are eager to apply their knowledge and skills in the field, aiming to make a significant impact in scientific research and industry. As a future professional in bioinformatics and biotechnology, Sayan is committed to furthering their understanding of the molecular mechanisms of diseases, applying innovative technologies to solve biological challenges, and contributing to the cutting-edge developments in bioinformatics and structural biology.

Hridoy Ranjan Bairagya is currently an Associate Professor in the Department of Bioinformatics at Maulana Abul Kalam Azad University of Technology, Government of West Bengal, formerly known as West Bengal University of

Technology. His research focuses on Cancer Bioinformatics, Computational Drug Discovery, Biomolecular Simulation, and Computational Structural Bioinformatics. He has participated in several high-profile research projects related to human CML (Chronic Myeloid Leukemia) cancerous proteins and has designed various inhibitors for these proteins using novel computational tools and techniques. Dr. Bairagya earned his Ph.D. in 2012 from the National Institute of Technology, Durgapur, in the Department of Biotechnology, specializing in Engineering Biotechnology with a focus on Bioinformatics. His research experience includes roles (i) as a Young Scientist at the Molecular Biophysics Unit of the Indian Institute of Science in Bangalore, (ii) as a Research Associate in the Department of Chemistry at the University of Cambridge (UK), and (iii) as a CSIR-Pool Scientist in the Department of Biophysics at the All India Institute of Medical Sciences in New Delhi. Dr. Bairagya has published over 50 research papers in various international journals and has authored two international books. Additionally, he serves as a reviewer for different scientific journals.

Tejal Bele is an accomplished academic and research scholar with a deep passion for pharmacology, currently pursuing her Ph.D. at Savitribai Phule University, Pune, with an M.Pharm in Pharmacology, where she was awarded a Gold Medal for her academic excellence. With over six years of experience in both research and teaching, she has contributed significantly to advancing the field of pharmacology. Her work is focused on preclinical evaluation of potential neuropharmacological agents and utilizing cutting-edge computational methods such as network pharmacology, molecular docking and simulation to predict the interaction between therapeutic molecules and biological targets. As a researcher, she had the privilege of presenting her work at an international & national conference and received the Best Oral Presentation Award. She has published several research papers in peer-reviewed journals and is actively involved in research activities. Also, she guides students on their research projects, encouraging them to pursue innovative research and contributing to their academic growth.

Shraddha Devarshi is a Doctor of Pharmacy graduate from BVDU's Poona College of Pharmacy in 2016. During this tenure, she has worked on a project titled quality of life of Beta-thalassemia patients. She has been awarded Gold medal for her academic excellence. She is currently working as Assistant Professor in SCES's Indira College of Pharmacy, Pune. She has 9 years of teaching experience. She has 5 research articles, 2 case reports, and 1 book chapter published in national and international journals with total citation of 10 and hi-index of 2. She has also presented her work in national and international conferences. She guides Pharm.D. students in their project work, demonstrating her keen interest in research. She had delivered guest lecture on Writing SOAP notes, how to teach Pharmacotherapeutics effectively?, Do's & Don't of Project & Clerkship. She was also a panelist at Clinical Pharmacy Summit 2024 focused on bridging gap between academia and clinical practice. Her areas of research include drug utilisation pattern studies, quality of life studies, and health services. Her areas of expertise in Cardiology, Pulmonology, infectious diseases, Pharmacotherapeutics, Clinical Research, Clinical Pharmacy, Patient Counselling.

Aarti Dwivedi, B.Sc., M.Sc., Ph.D. from Purvanchal University (Jaunpur, UP), is a dedicated chemistry educator with over 13 years of teaching experience. Currently serving as Assistant Professor (Grade III) in the Department of Chemistry at Amity University, Gwalior, MP, she brings a rich background in chemical sciences to her role .Her academic journey began with a B.Sc. and M.Sc. in Chemistry from Purvanchal University, culminating in a Ph.D. focused on organic chemistry. Over more than a decade of teaching, Dr. Dwivedi has developed and delivered undergraduate and postgraduate courses, mentoring students and fostering a dynamic classroom environment.An active researcher, she has authored six publications in peer-reviewed scientific journals and holds two patents, reflecting her commitment to expanding the frontiers of chemistry. Her research emphasis lies in organic synthesis and applications relevant to education and industry, guiding student research projects and contributing to Amity's growing scholarly output.At Amity University, Gwalior, Dr. Dwivedi balances her responsibilities as an educator and researcher. In the classroom, she inspires students with practical insights and real-world relevance, while in the lab, she pursues innovative projects with academic and societal impact. Her dual focus on teaching excellence and scientific inquiry makes her a valued member of academia in central India.

Vinay Dwivedi is a renowned academician and administrator with over 23 years of distinguished experience in higher education. He has served in various capacities, including Lecturer, Associate Professor, Professor, Dean, and Director at esteemed institutions. A university topper in both graduation and post-graduation, Dr. Dwivedi also excelled in the GATE examination, securing an impressive All India Rank of 52. Beyond academics, Dr. Dwivedi has demonstrated exemplary leadership, serving as an NSS Program Officer, Director of Placements, Chairman of the Board of Studies, Chairman of the Doctoral Research Committee (DRC), and a member of advisory boards for various committees. His research contributions are substantial, with more than 65 publications in SCOPUS and SCI-indexed journals. He has authored one book, contributed 15 book chapters, and holds 12 patents to his credit. Dr. Dwivedi's commitment to mentorship is evident, with 5 Ph.D. scholars successfully completing their research under his guidance and four more currently pursuing their doctorates. As a sought-after keynote speaker, he has addressed over 30 national and international conferences. His excellence in academia and research has been recognized with five prestigious national and international awards. Dr. Dwivedi's career reflects a harmonious blend of scholarly achievement, administrative acumen, and dedication to advancing education and research.

Rutuja Kamble is a dynamic and dedicated professional with 15 years of experience. Her contributions encompass teaching, with a deep passion for inspiring and mentoring young minds, as well as fostering the growth and development of the institution. She has published several papers in national and international journals, presented numerous posters at various national and international platforms, and received Special Appreciation, secured First Rank, and been awarded Best Presenter at both national and international levels. Actively engaged in continuous professional development, she regularly participates in Faculty Development Programmes to further enhance her expertise and teaching practices. Her research interests include the synthesis, purification, and characterization of organic compounds, as well as online in silico studies and docking studies

Gayatri Abhay Kerkar is a research scholar at Amity Institute of Biotechnology at amity University Madhya Pradesh

Deepak Kumar, an accomplished M. Pharm graduate in Pharmacology, is a dedicated researcher and academician with extensive experience in pharmaceutical sciences. Currently serving as an Assistant Professor at Shri Gopichand College of Pharmacy Baghpat, U.P., he is passionate about advancing pharmacological research, mentoring budding scientists, and exploring innovative medical approaches. He has contributed significantly to the field through his research on novel drug formulations and targeted therapies, including the development of emulates for anti-psoriatic activity and investigations into the role of AI in Healthcare. Deepak has co-authored several peer-reviewed publications and holds certifications in drug safety, pharmacovigilance, and quality assurance.

Puneet Kumar is an Associate Professor of Pharmaceutical Chemistry at Shri Gopichand College of Pharmacy, affiliated with Dr. APJ Abdul Kalam Technical University, Lucknow. He holds a Bachelor's degree in Pharmacy (2015) and a Master's degree in Pharmacy (2017) from IFTM University, Moradabad. With over 7 years of teaching experience, he has published 8 research articles and 19 review articles in peer-reviewed journals. His research interests focus on Synthetic Organic Chemistry, Synthetic Medicinal Chemistry, Medicinal and Pharmaceutical Chemistry, and Chromatography. He is also actively involved in studying diseases such as Middle East Respiratory Syndrome Coronavirus (MERS-CoV), COVID-19, and Epilepsy, particularly Absence Epilepsy and the development of Antiepileptic Drugs.

Yuvalakshmi Logesan, Assistant Professor, PG and Research Department of Microbiology (Autonomous), Sacred Heart College (Autonomous), Tirupattur, Tamil Nadu, India.

Arun Kumar Mishra, completed B.Pharm and M.Pharm from U P Technical University in years 2006 and 2009 respectively. He has completed Ph.D in Pharmacy. After qualifying GATE 2006 and 2009 Dr. Mishra received a fellowship of Rs 120000/ from AICTE. He is having 16 Years of teaching experience with an experience of supervising 26 M.Pharm students. Under his supervision, 8 students have been awarded Ph.D, 2 students have submitted the Ph.D thesis and 6 are working for Ph.D degree. His area of interest is Pharmacotherapeutics, Analytical Chemistry, Dermatology, Synthetic Medicinal Chemistry, Natural Product Chemistry and Nanotechnology based formulations. Dr. Mishra is recipient of workshop grant from DBT, authored thirteen books, two books chapter and got published 10 Indian patents. He has to his credit 84 research and 32 review articles in various journals of high repute with cumulative impact factor 60.07 in SCI indexed journals. Apart from this, Dr Mishra received Bentham Brand Ambassador Award, Shikshak Shree Award, Bharat Jyoti Award, Best Researcher Award, Acharya Siromani Award etc. In addition to academic responsibility as Professor and Head (Pharmacy), Dr. Mishra is also engaged in administrative work as Dean, Students Welfare etc.

Raghvendra Kumar Mishra, Ph.D., is a Professor at the Amity Institute of Biotechnology, Gwalior. He completed his Ph.D. at the National Institute of Plant Genome Research (NIPGR), JNU Campus, New Delhi, under the supervision of Prof. Sushil Kumar (former Director of CIMAP and NBRI, Lucknow). Before joining Amity University Gwalior, Dr. Mishra worked as an Assistant Professor in the Molecular Biotechnology Department at Konkuk University, Seoul, South Korea, and as a Research Associate in the School of Life Sciences (SLS), JNU, New Delhi, with Professor Neera Bhalla Sarin. He has over 21 years of teaching and research experience. His research interests include crop improvement and the study of secondary metabolites in medicinal plants and their role in cancer research. Dr. Mishra has co-supervised two Ph.D. scholars and supervised one Ph.D. student. He has published 59 research papers in reputed journals and has participated in national and international seminars and conferences. Four US patents credited in in his account and 07 more Indian patents he has filed or published. Additionally, he has published one book and two laboratory manuals. He has also authored in 03 book chapters. He is in the editorial board and reviewer of reputed journals and has life memberships of various International and National Scientific bodies.

P. Saranraj, Head, PG and Research Department of Microbiology, Sacred Heart College (Autonomous), Tirupattur – 635 601, Tamil Nadu, India E.

Bikram Sarkar is a graduate student pursuing a Master of Science in Bioinformatics. With a strong foundation in computational biology and data analysis, Bikram is passionate about applying bioinformatics tools to solve complex biological problems. This marks my first contribution to academic literature through a book chapter. My research interests include genomic data analysis, molecular biology, and exploring innovative solutions for personalized medicine. My aims to advance the understanding of disease mechanisms and improve therapeutic strategies through interdisciplinary research.

Diksha Shrivastava is a research scholar at Amity Institute of Biotechnology, Amity University Madhya Pradesh

Niharika Singh, Research Scholar, Junior Research Fellow (JRF), Amity Institute of Biotechnology, Amity University Madhya Pradesh, Gwalior.

Sangam Singh is a distinguished pharmacy professional and academician with a Master's degree in Pharmacy specializing in Pharmaceutical Chemistry. With over 10 years of experience in academia and research, she has made significant contributions to the advancement of pharmaceutical sciences. Currently serving as an Associate Professor at Oxford College of Pharmacy, Hapur. An accomplished researcher, she has authored five research papers and seven review articles published in reputed international Scopus-indexed journals, and one book chapter.

Ragini Singh is a research scholar of Amity Institute of Biotechnology at Amity University Madhya Pradesh

Pallavi Singh Chouhan is a highly skilled academician and researcher with 8 years 10 months of professional experience. For the past 8 years, she has been serving as an Assistant Professor in the Department of Pharmaceutical Chemistry at Indira College of Pharmacy. Additionally, she has gained valuable industry experience as a QA executive in the Packaging and Manufacturing department. She is a university approved guide and involved in mentoring M. Pharm Quality Assurance students through their research projects and dissertations. Her research interests lie in the application of Quality by Design (QBD), analytical method development, stability testing in pharmaceuticals, and Pharmaceutical Validation. She has filed a patent and has authored one research and 3 review publications

Amruta Walvekar is an academician and researcher with 9 years of professional experience, including 8 years at Indira College of Pharmacy, Pune. She is Passionate about mentoring students, fostering academic excellence, and accomplishing institutional goals. She has contributed extensively to teaching, delivering well-structured and engaging lectures in pharmaceutical chemistry related subjects. She has authored 2 research and 2 review papers in reputed journals with citation index of 7 and h-index of 2. She has contributed to 1 book chapter which is indexed in international publication in the field of pharmaceutical science. She has been actively involved and participated in poster and oral presentation at various conferences to forecast innovative ideas. She has keen interest to attend various seminars and FDPs organized by various organization at national and international levels. She has guided under graduate and post graduate students on academic projects, career planning, personal development, emphasizing practical knowledge and innovative thinking.

Index

A

B

C

D

E

F

I

K

M

N

P

R

www.ingramcontent.com/pod-product-compliance
Lightning Source LLC
LaVergne TN
LVHW062336300926
849161LV00007B/1712
* 9 7 9 8 3 3 7 3 1 4 6 9 3 *